Preneoplasia of the Breast
A New Conceptual Approach to Proliferative Breast Disease

Werner Boecker

Preneoplasia of the Breast

A New Conceptual Approach
to Proliferative Breast Disease

Werner Boecker, MD, PhD
Professor of Pathology
Director, Department of Pathology
University Hospital Muenster
Muenster, Germany

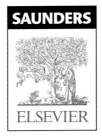

SAUNDERS

ELSEVIER

ELSEVIER
SAUNDERS

All business correspondence should be made with:
Elsevier GmbH, Urban & Fischer Verlag, Lektorat Medizin, Karlstr. 45, 80333 Munich, Germany
medizin@elsevier.de

Preneoplasia of the Breast
A New Conceptual Approach to Proliferative Breast Disease

Bibliographic information published by Die Deutsche Bibliothek
Die Deutsche Bibliothek lists this publication in the Deutsche Nationalbibliografie;
Detailed bibliographic data is available in the Internet at http://dnb.ddb.de.

Project managing editor: Dr. Barbara Heiden
Book production: Sibylle Hartl
Typesetting: Kösel
Printed and bound by: Appl GmbH
Graphics: Nieschlag + Wentrup, Susanne Adler (Credits *see* p XVII)
Cover design: Spiesz-Design
Cover photography: Prof. Werner Boecker

ISBN-13: 978-0-7020-2892-2
ISBN-10:   0-7020-2892-4

Printed in Germany

Current information by **www.elsevier.de** and **www.elsevier.com**

This book is dedicated to my wife Christiane, my daughter Almuth,
my sons Christian and Joerg, and my granddaughter Annanine:
for their love and never-ending support.

Contributors

Werner Boecker, MD, PhD
Professor of Pathology
Director, Department of Pathology
University Hospital Muenster
Muenster, Germany

Burkhard H. Brandt, PhD
Professor of Tumor Biology
Deputy Director, Institute of Tumor Biology
University Medical Center
Center of Experimental Medicine
Institute for Tumor Biology
Hamburg, Germany

Michael Buehner, MD
Consultant Gynecologist
Department of Obstetrics and Gynecology
Bayreuth University Hospital
Bayreuth, Germany

Horst Buerger, MD, PhD
Associate Professor
Department of Pathology
University Hospital Muenster
Muenster, Germany

Thomas Decker, MD
Consultant Pathologist
Department of Pathology
University Hospital Muenster
Muenster, Germany

Ian O. Ellis, BM, BS, FRCPath
Professor of Cancer Pathology, University of Nottingham
Honorary Consultant Pathologist
Nottingham City Hospital
Department of Histopathology
Nottingham, UK

Andrew Evans, MD, MRCP, FRCR
Consultant Radiologist
Nottingham Breast Institute
Nottingham, UK

Walter Heindel, MD
Professor of Radiology
Director, Institute of Radiology
Department of Clinical Radiology
University Hospital Muenster
Muenster, Germany

Hermann Herbst, FRCPath
Professor of Radiology
Director, Institute of Radiology
Vivantes-Klinikum Neukoelln
Institute of Pathology
Berlin, Germany

Sylvia Heywang-Koebrunner, MD
Professor of Radiology
Department of Breast Imaging and Intervention
Radiology
Klinikum Rechts der Isar
Technical University Munich
Munich, Germany

Thomas Huettner, MD
Consultant Radiologist
Department of Radiology
Department of Obstetrics and Gynecology
University Hospital Bayreuth
Bayreuth, Germany

Daniela Hungermann, MD
Resident
Department of Pathology
University Hospital Muenster
Muenster, Germany

Heike Jacob, MD
Consultant Radiologist
Diagnostic Center Halensee
Berlin, Germany

Elke Keil, MD
Consultant Gynecologist
Department of Obstetrics and Gynecology
HELIOS Klinikum Berlin-Buch
Berlin, Germany

Ute Kettritz, MD
Consultant Radiologist
Institute of Diagnostic Radiology
HELIOS Klinikum Berlin-Buch
Berlin, Germany

Arno Kuijper, MD, PhD
Associate Research Assistant
Department of Pathology
University Medical Center
Department of Pathology
Utrecht, The Netherlands

Douglas R. Macmillan, MD, FRCS
Consultant Breast Surgeon
Associate Clinical Director
Nottingham Breast Institute
Nottingham, UK

Guenter Morack, MD
Director, Department of Gynecology and Obstetrics
HELIOS Klinikum Berlin-Buch
Berlin, Germany

Contributors

Rainer Obenaus, MD
Consultant Gynecologist
Department of Obstetrics and Gynecology
HELIOS Klinikum Berlin-Buch
Berlin, Germany

Steve Parker, MD, FACR
Director, Institute of Radiology
The Sally Jobe Breast Centre
Greenwood Village, USA

Sarah E. Pinder, MD, FRCPath
Consultant Breast Pathologist
Department of Histopathology
Addenbrooke's NHS Trust
Cambridge, UK

Rajendra S. Rampaul, MD, MRCS
Specialist Registrar
Nottingham Breast Institute
Nottingham, UK

John F. R. Robertson, MD
Professor of Surgery
Head of the Academic Division of Breast Surgery
Nottingham Breast Institute
Nottingham, UK

Katy Roterberg, MD
Consultant Gynecologist
Interdisciplinary Breast Center Gifhorn
Department of Obstetrics and Gynecology
Gifhorn, Germany

Monika Ruhnke, MD
Consultant Breast Pathologist
Pathology Department
University College Hospital
Galway, Ireland

Stuart J. Schnitt, MD
Professor of Pathology
Harvard Medical School
Director, Division of Anatomic Pathology
Department of Pathology
Beth Israel Hospital
Boston, USA

Wolfgang Schulze, MD
Attending Radiation Therapist
Department of Radiation Therapy
University Hospital Bayreuth
Bayreuth, Germany

Ruediger Schulz-Wendtland, MD
Professor of Radiology
Director, Institute of Gynecological Radiology
Institute of Diagnostic Radiology
University Erlangen-Nuremberg
Erlangen, Germany

Melvin J. Silverstein, MD, FACS
Professor of Surgery
Henrietta C. Lee Chair
in Breast Cancer Research
Director, Lee Breast Center
USC-Norris Cancer Center
Los Angeles, USA

Petra Stute, MD
Consultant Gynecologist
Department of Obstetrics and Gynecology
University of Muenster
Muenster, Germany

Augustinus Harjanto Tulusan, MD
Professor of Gynecology
Director, Department of Gynecology
Bayreuth University Hospital
Bayreuth, Germany

Elsken van der Wall, MD, PhD
Professor of Medicine
Department of Internal Medicine and Dermatology
Utrecht, The Netherlands

Paul S. van Diest, MD, PhD
Professor of Pathology
University Medical Center
Utrecht, The Netherlands

Hildegard Volkholz, MD
Consultant Pathologist
Division of Gynecological Pathology
Department of Pathology
Bayreuth University Hospital
Bayreuth, Germany

Stefanie Weigel, MD
Consultant Radiologist
Department of Diagnostic Radiology
Muenster University Hospital
Muenster, Germany

Clive Wells, MD
Consultant Pathologist
Department of Histopathology
St Bartholomew's Hospital
Medical School
London, UK

Robin Wilson, MD, MB ChB, FRCR, FRCP
Consultant Radiologist and Clinical Director
Nottingham National Breast Screening Training Centre
City Hospital
Nottingham, UK

Krisztina Zels, Dipl. Med.
Consultant Pathologist
Koenigs Wusterhausen, Germany

Foreword

During my career, spanning more than 40 years, I have been fortunate to participate in the renaissance of all aspects of diagnostic histopathology. This is particularly true of breast pathology, which has evolved considerably in that time and has now emerged as a subspeciality in its own right. There are a number of different but interconnected factors for this change but the driving force, even in this molecular age, has been the need to obtain an accurate tissue diagnosis before definitive therapy is given.

Originally the management of patients with breast disease was the preserve of general surgeons who were only interested in establishing a diagnosis of cancer, usually by means of frozen section. Since most breast lumps are non-malignant this practice led to a large number of unnecessary breast excisions but gave pathologists insight into the morphology of benign breast lesions. The introduction of fine-needle aspiration cytology and then needle core biopsy led to radical improvements in pre- and non-operative diagnosis and reduced excisions for benign lesions. A further change occurred with the development of mammography as both a diagnostic and screening procedure which led to the need to sample smaller palpable and impalpable lesions. More precise targeting was provided by high-resolution ultrasound allied to sophisticated biopsy techniques such as automated needle core biopsy and vacuum-assisted mammotomy. Paradoxically these modern approaches have rekindled interest in the pathological processes occupying the 'borderland' between overtly benign and clearly malignant disease, such as columnar cell change and flat epithelial atypia. This, in turn, has highlighted the importance of appropriate multidisciplinary management for patients with these preneoplastic conditions.

The publication of textbooks relating to breast pathology has largely followed a similar pattern to that described above. Thirty or forty years ago breast lesions were covered in one chapter in a general systemic pathology book or at best as a section in a clinical volume on breast disease. The mould was broken by the publication of monographs such as John Azzopardi's 'Problems in Breast Pathology' in 1979. Since then a succession of breast pathology books has appeared, all covering both benign and malignant disease with the main emphasis on the latter. This volume breaks the mould again, devoted as it is to preneoplastic lesions of the breast and its publication serves to reinforce the importance that this area of breast disease has assumed.

I can think of no better person to mastermind such a volume than Werner Boecker. He has an impeccable background and experience in breast pathology in general but he has also made an enormous contribution to the literature with his original and elegant double immunostaining technique applied to breast epithelium. The progenitor cell concept has had a profound influence on our understanding of breast physiology and provides a cell biological explanation for almost all epithelial proliferative lesions. In addition such data, coupled with careful epidemiological studies and, more recently, exciting developments in molecular biology and gene expression techniques have clarified the neoplastic potential of these lesions.

Despite the obvious interest in epithelial proliferation as a precursor of malignancy, the book gives a comprehensive account of all aspects of benign breast disease, including fibroepithelial lesions and inflammatory conditions. Professor Boecker has assembled an impressive list of co-authors, largely but not exclusively European and the volume has a truly international flavour. Not surprisingly it is beautifully illustrated in colour with clear diagrams and an extensive reference list. It will make essential reading for a wide audience: histopathologists who are particularly concerned with diagnostic criteria and clinical management issues; cell and molecular biologists who need to understand the pathological basis for the diseases which they study; and, dare I say it, clinicians who also require a sound knowledge of pathological processes to enable them to give their patients appropriate treatment. I have every confidence that 'Boecker' will rightly take its place amongst the classics of breast pathology literature.

Christopher Elston, MD, FRCPath
Professor of Tumour Pathology,
Nottingham University Medical School
Consultant Histopathologist, City Hospital,
Nottingham, UK

Preface

The intention of this book is to provide a comprehensive introduction to pathology, cell biology, radiology and treatment of preneoplasia and related proliferative diseases of the breast, including all lesions that must be considered in differential diagnosis. An explosion of knowledge has dramatically altered breast medicine over the past 20 years. Whereas our conceptual knowledge of diagnosis and treatment of invasive breast cancer has reached a certain level of consensus and consistency, our knowledge of even normal breast physiology, let alone benign proliferative breast disease and precursor lesions of breast carcinoma, is still limited.

Key to the study and understanding of proliferative breast disease is the depth of knowledge of normal breast epithelium. Recent in situ studies and elegant cell culture studies on normal human breast epithelium have provided evidence that Ck5/14+ progenitor cells give rise to either the Ck8/18+ glandular or sm-actin+ myoepithelial cell lineages. In this book we explain this progenitor cell concept in detail, focusing on the way in which it helps us to better understand the different types of benign and malignant proliferative breast lesions. Using this model as a foundation, we attempt to explain the various types of proliferative breast disease in a completely novel way and, crucially, as an adjunct to traditional pattern recognition.

It is immediately obvious that this concept has novel features that are of considerable theoretical and practical interest: it provides us with explanations for a whole range of previously unaccounted phenomena in our daily hematoxylin-eosin histology, and, furthermore, using just a small panel of antibodies it represents a rationale for immunohistochemical analyses of a given lesion. In consequence, antibodies against basal Ck5/14 and glandular Ck8/18 cytokeratins as well as against myoepithelial lineage-specific differentiation markers (sm-actin and others) can be used as powerful immunohistochemical tools to define distinct disease entities by analyzing the differentiative state of cells of a given lesion. Most importantly, it allows us to distinguish between benign and malignant lesions in a given context. Based on our experience of more than 25 years with Ck5/14 immunohistochemistry, we strongly feel that the introduction of this concept into our differential diagnostic view and its practical application is a great advantage in daily routine pathology and will bring about more objectivity into the practice of breast pathology.

Breast carcinoma development follows different genetic pathways. As in all fields of medical science, molecular pathology is becoming increasingly dominant. This rapid change is not only the result of the method's novelty; it has engendered real progress in our knowledge and understanding of the molecular mechanisms leading to malignant transformation of cells. The method has helped us to come to a first approximation as to how genetic alterations are responsible for the multitude of genetic pathways leading to breast carcinoma. Furthermore, the molecular data has provided evidence that benign breast lesions, for example usual ductal hyperplasia, show striking differences compared to carcinomas. These observations have led us to modify the basic concept as to how breast carcinoma develops. The tremendous implications of this knowledge in both theory and practice are described in the corresponding chapters.

Breast medicine as an interdisciplinary task. The relevance of radiology for ideal management of patients with breast diseases is clearly obvious. Among the radiologic criteria that indicate suspicion of cancer are the presence of microcalcifications, architectural distortions and mass lesions. It must, however, be emphasized that 50–70% of radiologically suspect lesions prove benign, and some 20% of malignant breast lesions are currently found to be intraepithelial neoplasias.

With the improvement of interventional technologies in radiology – especially stereotactically obtained core and vacuum-assisted needle biopsies – the extent to which pathology plays a role in the management and care of patients has become increasingly evident. To provide clinically relevant diagnoses, therefore, the pathologist must be deeply versed not only in his own field and the new types of tissue available but also in both radiology and the therapeutic options at the clinician's disposal, the stratifications of which are constantly broadening. In this context, appropriate correlation of radiologic and pathologic findings, pre- and postoperatively, is a prerequisite of good medical practice.

The main emphasis and the foundation upon which this textbook is based are therefore the morphology and immunohistochemistry of lesions, set against a background of molecular and cell biological data, the respective radiologic data and finally the appropriate treatment options. We employ the traditional classification system of proliferative breast disease lesions as used in the most recent WHO Histological Classification of Tumors of the Breast, with only slight adaptations to give the reader a better understanding of the respective lesions. This book also includes chapters on the techniques and diagnosis of minimal invasive biopsy, work-up of operative specimens, therapy of ductal carcinoma in situ, and, in each chapter, a clinical paragraph with the main radiologic findings.

The target audiences are therefore practising breast pathologists, radiologists and breast surgeons who are intimately concerned with the management of breast patients on a daily basis. This book should also be useful to scientists and other health workers providing care for women in their practices.

Werner Boecker, MD, PhD
Professor of Pathology
Director, Department of Pathology
University Hospital Muenster

Acknowledgements

First and foremost the editor is grateful to all those who co-operated, from start to finish, in the creation of this book. I was fortunate that all the outstanding individuals listed in the contributors' page were prepared to take part in this project, and I am very grateful for their generous contributions to this book.

I was most fortunate when I was accepted for a residency at the Institute of Pathology at the University of Hamburg with the then current chairholder Professor Gerhard Seifert – one of the pioneers in salivary gland tumors. I am most grateful to him and his team of dedicated young pathologists who introduced me to pathology. They all had a great impact on my career. My first teacher in breast pathology was Professor Hans-Egon Stegner, Head of the Department of Gynecopathology at the University of Hamburg. My own interest in and understanding of breast medicine were greatly influenced by the interdisciplinary teamwork at this clinic.

The current list of great textbooks on breast pathology is extensive, and I do not pretend to replace any of them. The excellent monograph by John G. Azzopardi, *Problems in Breast Pathology*, and that by David L. Page and Thomas J. Anderson, *Diagnostic Histopathology of the Breast*, published in 1979 and 1987 respectively, were among the seminal works that helped shape my understanding of breast pathology. These works were immensely valuable, and I read them again and again. Christopher W. Elston's and Ian O. Ellis's book *The Breast* was a concise guide in my daily routine work. It subsequently introduced me to further aspects of breast pathology, for example the grading and pathology of screen-detected mammographic abnormalities.

I also studied the now classic textbooks by Fattaneh A. Tavassoli, *Breast Pathology*, and Paul P. Rosen, *Rosen's Breast Pathology*, with great interest – they were an inexhaustible wealth of knowledge. I am grateful to Noel Weidner for his inspiring chapter on the differential diagnosis of breast diseases in *The Difficult Diagnosis in Surgical Pathology* and to Rosemary Millis for the concepts underlying her *Atlas of Breast Pathology*. Last but not least, Ronald Baessler's German textbook, *Pathologie der Brustdrüse* (vol. 11 of the series *Spezielle Pathologische Anatomie* edited by Doerr, Seifert and Uehlinger), was always a reassuring work of reference.

I am deeply indebted to the members of the 'European Working Group on Breast Screening Pathology' (EWGBSP) of the European Commission who were ever willing to engage in lively debate and share their knowledge of breast pathology (Isabel Amendoeira, Nikiforos Apostolikas, Jean Pierre Bellocq, Simonetta Bianchi, Charles E. Connolly, Gabor Cserni, Thomas Decker, Conchita De Miguel, Peter Dervan, Maria Drijkoningen, Ian O. Ellis, Christopher W. Elston, Vincenzo Eusebi, Daniel Faverly, the late Adel Gad, Paivi Heikkila, Roland Holland, Jocelyne Jacquemier, Janina Kulka, Manuela Lacerda, José Martinez-Peñuela, Hans Nordgren, Hans Peterse, Fritz Rank, Peter Regitnig, Angelika Reiner, Anna Sapino, Brigitte Sigal-Zafrani, the late John P. Sloane, Anne-Marie Tanous, Sten Thorstenson, Clive Alan Wells, Vicki Kerner and Bettina Borisch). I have learned a great deal from them and have tried to incorporate many of their ideas into this book. I am deeply grateful, in particular, to the first chairman of this group, the late John P. Sloane who encouraged me from the beginning and who witnessed our first, as yet unpublished, ideas on the progenitor cell concept of human breast epithelium, as well as to his successor as chairman, Clive Wells. I also owe a great deal to the editorial board members for their valuable discussion of classification problems whenever we met in Lyon in the run-up to the most recent WHO classification of breast tumors. I am deeply indebted to the outstanding pathologists, scientists and clinicians who contributed to the ideas discussed in this book by way of their invaluable publications, and I apologize for any errors that remain my own. I hope to hear from readers concerning errors that may have inadvertently crept into the final text; their suggestions will be utilized in improving future written work.

Although this book follows a new conceptual approach to the understanding of proliferative breast pathology that is primarily based on the progenitor cell concept, the above-mentioned works remain the background against which we developed our theories.

The cases included in this book are those that I have seen in my own daily routine work, in second-opinion practice or discovered in second reading of the German mammography screening program. I am immensely grateful to the many pathologists whose cases and material I have been permitted to use.

I have received invaluable assistance from our technical and secretarial staff, especially from my secretary Michaela Kemper who kept the daily routine here at the Institute running smoothly whenever I was otherwise preoccupied. I would also like to thank

Susanne Koelsch, who had to cope with my less than perfect English, for her invaluable editorial work. I would like to thank Nicholas Hariades for his excellent work as a linguistic editor of the text – quite a challenge considering the various nationalities of those contributing. I thank Dr. Annette Staebler for her thorough revision of some of the pivotal chapters. Professor Igor Buchwalov assisted with the organization of the photo collection for some figures in Chapters 1 and 17 and helped to finalize a number of figures when time was running short.

A special mention is due the editorial staff at Elsevier/Saunders for their courtesy, co-operation and valuable assistance throughout the creation of this book. Our special thanks go to Dr. Barbara Heiden, who supervised the entire production process. I would also like to mention the Elsevier production team in Munich who skillfully edited and assembled the book. I also thank Lisa Nieschlag and Christian Wentrup (*Büro für Gestaltung*, Muenster, Germany) for their involvement in the production of the first design draft of this book.

My apologies go to many colleagues at the faculty, to the different societies I am member of and to the entire staff at the Institute of Pathology of the University of Muenster for the long periods of time during which I was unable to answer my e-mails, keep deadlines or, without their assistance, even do my daily routine work.

Introduction

This book is principally concerned with the conceptual and diagnostic problems of benign proliferative breast disease and precursor lesions of breast carcinoma. Thus the title invokes only one of the book's topics: precursor lesions of breast carcinomas. It must be understood that the existence of both benign and malignant proliferative breast lesions is predicated by their historical continuity with normal breast epithelial cells. Our intent is to provide and utilize the progenitor cell model as a starting point for explaining how these lesions are cellularly constructed and how they can be characterized and distinguished from one another.

With only a few exceptions, all of the chapters in this book have been constructed on the same paragraph structure.

The first paragraph of each chapter is devoted to problems associated with clearly defining the lesion in question. The second paragraph, on conceptual approach, details the cell biology of lesions based on the progenitor cell concept and is, therefore, novel. I believe this to be of special importance, as the nature of proliferative lesions, both at a theoretical and practical level, can only be understood by employing such a cellular model. Subsequently, we discuss the clinical findings, and in particular the radiologic data. The following main paragraphs detail and discuss morphologic features and differential diagnosis. Immunohistochemistry, which is addressed in a special paragraph, is the most valuable tool in clarifying problems in daily practice that remain unanswered at the light microscopic level. The principal molecular data are summarized in the paragraph on molecular genetics. The development of atypical ductal or lobular type proliferation in primarily benign lesions is addressed in a special paragraph. Finally the diagnostic difficulties in core biopsies and differential diagnosis are discussed in the final paragraphs.

Many of the chapters can be read in a single sitting. We suggest, however, that readers use Chapters 1, 7 and 17 as the starting point for explaining how the progenitor cell model is constructed and how it operates.

Breast epithelium is a prime example of tissue with a high capacity for self-renewal – turnover is a constant process. The progenitor (adult stem) cell model detailed in **Chapter 1** provides a new conceptual basis for normal regeneration, terminal differentiation during pregnancy and lactation as well as involution after weaning. In **Chapters 2 and 3** we discuss lesions such as fibrocystic change and aberrations of normal development and involution (ANDI). The different types of epithelial metaplasia such as apocrine, squamous metaplasia and mesenchymal conversion of epithelial cells are described in detail in **Chapter 3**.

In **Chapters 4 to 6** we discuss practical issues. **Chapter 4** is related to the assessment of radiologic abnormalities with minimally invasive biopsies. In principle, a definite diagnosis of malignancy or benignity should be made preoperatively whenever possible. Thus minimally invasive procedures such as needle biopsies have become important tools in making specific morphologic diagnoses and in correlating morphology with mammographic and clinical findings. This is mainly due to the rapid progress in radiology and the widespread availability of stereotactic devices and biopsy instruments. In **Chapter 5** we discuss the newly introduced B-classification system of minimally invasive biopsies, which will help in interpreting such needle biopsies. This has recently been introduced in the United Kingdom and has now also been published by the European Commission (European Guidelines, 2006).

It is clear that accurate morphologic work-up of DCIS specimens, including the excision margins, is a prerequisite of good medical practice. Inking of specimen margins and systematic and oriented sampling of tissue for histological analysis are only valuable in the appropriate context of microcalcification. This is discussed in detail in **Chapter 6**.

In **Chapters 7 to 17**, the third part of this book, we address benign proliferative breast disease lesions. **Chapter 7** contains a general and mainly theoretical/conceptual approach to benign lesions. To verify the presence of usual ductal hyperplasia the pathologist has to be conceptually familiar with it (its cellular components, architecture, clinical implications etc.). As will be seen, with the exception of microglandular adenosis, all benign lesions display striking similarities to the cellular composition of normal breast epithelium. Although these benign lesions themselves may occasionally be the ground on which in situ malignancies develop, they cannot be regarded as obligate precursor lesions of noninvasive or even invasive carcinomas. **Chapters 8 to 16** are devoted to discussing the eight different categories of benign proliferative lesions that are currently recognized.

Chapters 17 to 21 once more return to the main topic of this book, discussing the currently recognized precursor lesions of ductal and lobular type. **Chapter 17** is theoretical/conceptual in its remit and should help readers to further understand these lesions in cell-biological terms. As we will see, most of these lesions are, in contrast to benign lesions, the result of a neoplastic transformation of Ck8/18+ cells of the normal breast epithelium. **Chapters 18 to 21** specifically address flat epithelial atypia, atypical ductal hyperplasia and ductal carcinoma in situ.

The following two chapters, **Chapters 22 and 23**, are devoted to cytopathology and risk assessment. Cytopathology is still employed as a diagnostic technique in some clinics.

A further major emphasis is the therapy of ductal carcinoma in situ, to which **Chapters 24 and 25** are exclusively devoted. An account of the management of other precursor lesions will be given in the corresponding chapters.

The last chapters, **Chapters 26 and 27**, summarize some molecular findings that are crucial to understanding benign proliferative breast disease lesions and breast cancer development.

The text contains an unavoidable element of repetition, due to the inevitable overlap of some material in topics dealt with in separate chapters. Furthermore, in writing the book it seemed desirable to repeatedly emphasize important points based on the novel conceptual approach, which many pathologists may not yet be familiar with.

Abbreviations

AAA	atypical apocrine adenosis
AAH	atypical apocrine hyperplasia
ABBi	advanced breast biopsy instrumentation
ABL	Abelson leukemia viral oncogene homologue
A-categories	action categories
ACR	American College of Radiology
ADH	atypical ductal hyperplasia
aFGF(R)	acidic fibroblastic growth factor (receptor)
ALH	atypical lobular hyperplasia
Alx-4	aristaless like homeobox 4
AMP	adenosine monophosphate
AMT	adenomyoepithelial tumor
ANDI	aberration of normal development and involution
AP1	activated protein 1
AR	absolute risk
AT(M)	(mutated) ataxia-telangiectasia gene
34βE12	cocktail of antibodies directed against high-molecular-weight keratins
B-categories	pathologic categories 1–5 in core biopsies
bcl2	b-cell lymphoma 2
BCT	breast-conserving therapy
BDA	blunt duct adenosis
BI-RADS	breast imaging reporting and data system (Bi-RADS 1–5)
BPBD	benign proliferative breast disease
BRCA1	breast cancer gene 1
BRCA2	breast cancer gene 2
CD34	cluster of differentiation 34
cdc	cyclin-dependent kinase
CGH	comparative genomic hybridization
CIS	carcinoma in-situ
CK	cytokeratin
CLIS	carcinoma lobulare in-situ
CSL	complex sclerosing lesion
Cy3	indocarbocyanine
DCIS	ductal carcinoma in situ
DIN	ductal intraepithelial neoplasia
DNA	deoxyribonucleic acid
E(R)	estrogen (receptor)
ECD	extra cellular domain
EGF	epidermal growth factor
EORTC	European Organization for Research and Treatment of Cancer

erbB	receptor tyrosine kinase of the epidermal growth factor receptor
ERE	estrogen receptor element
ESX	ETS domain transcription factor
ETS	avian erythroblastosis virus E26 oncogene homologue
EUSOMA	European Society of Mastology
EWGBSP	European Working Group for Breast Screening Pathology
FA	fibroadenoma
FCC	fibrocystic change
FDA	US Food and Drug Administration
FEA	flat epithelial atypia
FGF(R)	fibroblastic growth factor (receptor)
FISH	fluorescence in-situ hybridization
FITC	fluorescein isothyocyanate
FNA	fine-needle aspiration biopsy
GCDFP	gross cystic disease fluid protein
GFAP	glial fibrillary acid protein
GGF	glial growth factor
GRT	glandular replacement therapy
HCS	human chronic somatomammotropin
HER2/NEU	receptor tyrosine kinase of the epidermal growth factor receptor
HFF35	monoclonal antibody against sm-actin
HMW	high molecular weight
HPF	high power field
HRT	hormone replacement therapy
HUVEC	human umbilical vein endothelial cells
ICD	intracellular domain
IGF(R)	insulin-like growth factor (receptor)
JK	Janus kinase
kB	kilobyte
Ki67	Kiel 67 proliferation antigen
lg	low grade
LCIS	lobular carcinoma in-situ
LMW	low molecular weight
LN	lobular neoplasia
LOH	loss of heterozygosity
MAPK	mitosis-activating protein kinase
MAR	multiple aberration region
MB	megabyte
MC	microcalcification
MEK	see MAPK
MGA	microglandular adenosis

MIB	minimal invasive biopsy		RAS	Hawey rat sarcoma virus
Mib1	monoclonal antibody against Ki67		RBP	RNA-binding protein
MRI	magnetic resonance imaging		RNA	ribonucleic acid
MSI	microsatellite instability		RR	relative risk
			RS	radial scar
NCB	needle core biopsy			
NCK	noncatalytic region of tyrosine kinase		SA	sclerosing adenosis
NDF	new differentiation factor		SH	svc homologue
NHS	National Health Service		sm-actin	smooth-muscle actin
NSABP	National Surgical Adjuvant Breast and Bowel Project		SMM-hc	smooth-muscle myosin heavy chain
			SR	specimen radiography
			SSR	simple sequence repeat
OCH	oral contraceptive hormones		SVC	Rous sarcoma virus
OCI score	overall clinical and imaging evaluation score			
			TDLU	terminal duct lobular unit
			TGF	transforming growth factor
p53	p53 gene or protein		TNM	tumor, lymph, node, metastasis (staging)
p63	p63 gene or protein			
PAS	periodic acid Schiff			
PASH	pseudoangiomatous stromal hyperplasia		UDH	usual ductal hyperplasia
			UICC	Unio Internationalis Contra Cancrum (International Union against Cancer)
PCR	polymerase chain reaction			
PDGF(R)	platelet-derived growth factor (receptor)		US	ultrasound
PIP2	phosphoinositol phosphate 2		VANCB	vacuum-assisted needle core biopsy
PLC	phospholipase C		VNPI	van Nuys prognostic index
PPV	positive predictive value			
P(R)	progesterone (receptor)		WHO	World Health Organization

Credits

Nieschlag + Wentrup, Büro für Gestaltung, Muenster, Germany:
Figures 1.1, 1.3, 1.6, 1.11a–b, 1.12, 1.19, 2.2, 3.1, 3.2, 4.9, 7.4, 7.5, 7.6, 7.9, 7.10, 8.6, 8.7, 8.17, 9.3, 9.4, 11.2, 11.3, 13.2, 13.10, 13.11, 14.3, 14.6, 14.16, 17.3, 17.15, 17.23, 20.1, 20.7, 20.17

Susanne Adler, Luebeck, Germany:
Figures 4.1, 24.6, 24.12a

Content

Content

Content

1

THE NORMAL BREAST

WERNER BOECKER, STEFANIE WEIGEL, WALTER HEINDEL AND PETRA STUTE

The human breast consists of an elaborate **branching tree-like ductal system derived from lobules,** each containing a number of ductules (acini). The entire ductal lobular system is lined with epithelium. Hematoxylin-eosin staining shows that breast epithelial cells are arranged in two layers: the luminal glandular (inner) and the basal myoepithelial (outer) cell layer.

Recent studies suggest that **the epithelium harbors cells that function as progenitor cells** with the capability of differentiating into either glandular or myoepithelial cell lineages. In contrast to the myoepithelial layer, which is remarkably stable, glandular epithelium should be regarded as a highly immature, labile tissue.

During **organogenesis** ectodermally-derived 'stem cells' from the milk hill infiltrate and proliferate within the surrounding mesenchymal tissue. This 'physiological' ductal infiltration remains a key process at various stages of breast gland development. During this process, breast epithelium and mesenchyme interact with each other in response to a number of stimuli. Such cross-talk appears to be an important driver in breast development, and is currently a subject of intense investigation.

The data emerging from cell biological and embryological studies will not only provide a new basis for breast physiology; it will contribute to a better understanding of benign and malignant proliferative breast pathology.

The normal breast

◼ GENERAL TISSUE ORGANIZATION

The parenchyma of the breast is subdivided into anywhere from 15 to more than 40 lobes [1]. These lobes display a great variability in size, ranging from a few percent to more than 50% of the breast's volume. Most lobes form a complicated tree-like branching ductal system with lobular units supported by a fibro-fatty stroma. The nomenclature of the ductal lobular system applied in this book is introduced in the schematic drawing (Fig. 1.1). The terminal duct and its derivative lobule are often referred to as the **terminal duct lobular unit (TDLU)** [2–4]. The lobules form the secretory structures and thus represent the functional compartment of the breast. At the subgross and histological level individual lobules within the same breast, and even within the same lobe, display considerable morphological heterogeneity [4] (Fig. 1.2). Fully developed lobules of the resting breast contain about 40 to 80 ductules or acini.

No visible or palpable anatomical separation is evident between individual lobes. Rather, adjacent lobes or segments of branching ducts overlap in a haphazard fashion (Fig. 1.3). A further equally important finding is the existence of anastomosing channels between branches of the same and, even more significantly, between separate lobes [5]. These ductal anastomoses are located at various levels of the ductal system, but the anastomoses near the nipple may be of special importance for the spread of in situ lesions. Such channels provide routes for the dissemination of malignant cells within and across lobes or segments.

The **nipple and the areola** are covered by a stratified squamous epithelium, which is continuous with the most distal portion of the duct system. The lactiferous ducts of each lobe unite in the collecting ducts before opening on to the surface of the nipple via secretory pores. Directly under the surface of the nipple, the lactiferous duct is dilated to form the lactiferous sinus. The nipple stroma consists of collagenous

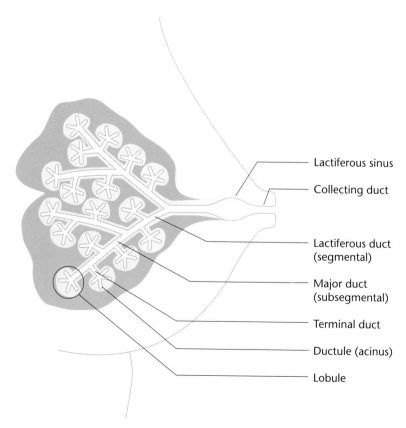

Lactiferous sinus

Collecting duct

Lactiferous duct (segmental)

Major duct (subsegmental)

Terminal duct

Ductule (acinus)

Lobule

Fig. 1.1 Schematic drawing of a lobe. The ductal lobular tree is enveloped by a specialized stroma.

tissue with circular and longitudinal bundles of smooth muscle around the ducts and occasional elastic tissue. A number of sebaceous and apocrine glands are present superficially underneath the surface.

Breast parenchyma consists of a luminal glandular (inner) layer, a basal myoepithelial (outer) cell layer and a basement membrane [6–13].

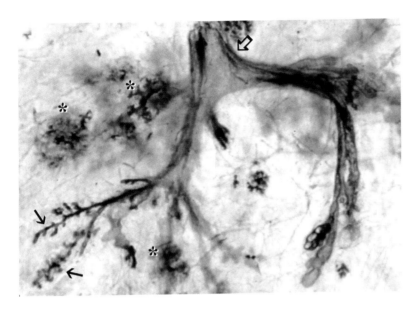

Fig. 1.2 Subgross view of the branching ductal system of a section of a lobe with regular branching of the major ducts. The lobules at the periphery are the secretory units of the breast. Note the great variability of the lobules, some of which are undifferentiated lobules (arrows; type 1) and some are differentiated lobules (asterisks; well-developed type 2 lobules according to Russo). The larger duct shows longitudinal infoldings (double arrow).

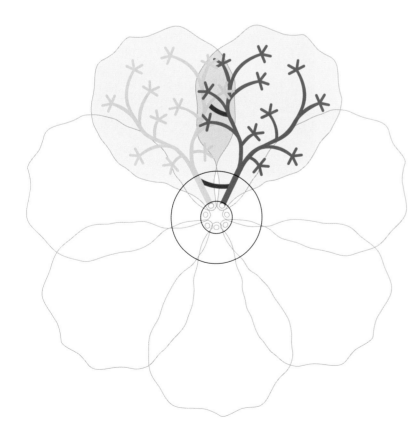

Fig. 1.3 Schematic drawing of the lobar architecture of the breast. Note that adjacent lobes overlap. Furthermore there are anastomosing channels between branching ducts of identical and different lobes (red). These may be routes of progression of in-situ carcinomas.

The normal breast consists of parenchyma and stroma. The latter is subdivided into specialized connective tissue surrounding ducts and lobules, dense interlobular fibrous stroma and adipose tissue (Fig. 1.4).

The luminal glandular cell layer tends to be rather more columnar in the large ducts and cuboidal in the smaller ones. In the resting adult female breast, the glandular cell layer of the lobules consists of cuboidal cells with deeply stained monomorphic nuclei (Fig. 1.5a). A basal myoepithelial cell layer usually surrounds and invests the epithelial cells. These cells seem to play a major role in safeguarding the architecture of the epithelial double layer and they may affect both growth and differentiation of luminal cells [14]. The histological appearance of the myoepithelial cells is more conspicuous in the ductal system, but more or less continuous throughout the ductal-lobular system (Fig. 1.5b–c). The ductal-lobular tree is surrounded by a basement membrane.

The whole ductal-lobular tree is enveloped by a **hormone-sensitive specialized stroma,** which is most

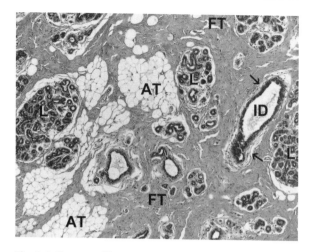

Fig. 1.4 The normal breast consists of parenchyma and stroma. The parenchyma is composed of the interlobular ducts (ID) and the terminal duct lobular units (L). The stroma is subdivided into specialized connective tissue, which surrounds ducts (arrows) and lobules. Dense interlobular fibrous (FT) and adipose tissue (AT).

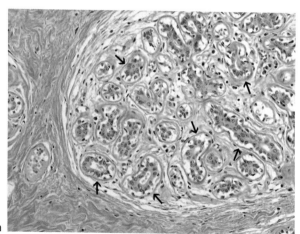

a

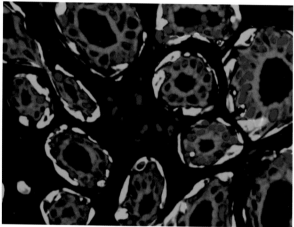

b

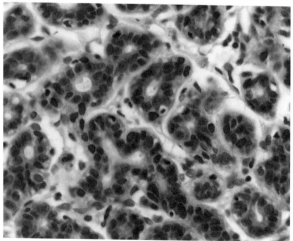

c

Fig. 1.5a–c Normal lobule.

1.5a Normal lobule at higher magnification. Note the characteristic loose stroma against the background of collagenous tissue. Glandular and myoepithelial cells surrounded by a basement membrane (arrows) can be easily identified. Occasional lymphocytes are seen in the specialized stroma.

1.5b Double immunolabeling of acinar structures of a lobule for sm-actin (green signal) and cytokeratins 8/18 (red signal). The acinar structures display the typical architecture with luminal glandular cells expressing Ck8/18 and myoepithelial cells expressing sm-actin.

1.5c Immunostaining for the myoepithelial marker p63. Many myoepithelial cells express p63 in their nuclei.

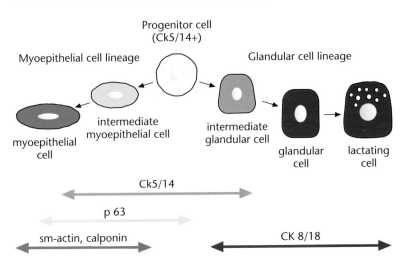

Fig. 1.6 Progenitor cell model of normal human breast epithelium. Progenitor cells of the breast epithelium give rise to both the glandular and myoepithelial cell lineages. The progenitor cell and its progeny are phenotypically characterized by specific expression of cytokeratins and/or sm-actin.

prominent in the lobules. In the vicinity of the ducts, it only consists of a cuff of loose, slightly cellular, vascularized connective tissue. The specialized stroma of the lobules is much more distinctive and can be clearly separated from the fibrous interlobular stroma. The alcian blue-positive lobular stroma contains a network of fibroblasts in contrast to the dense interlobular connective tissue [15]. Lobular stroma also harbors a fair number of lymphocytes and occasional histiocytes, plasma cells and mast cells [16]. Furthermore, in contrast to the lobules, the ductal system is invested by elastic fibers, which are absent in the TDLUs.

■ A NEW APPROACH TO EPITHELIAL TISSUE ■ REGENERATION AND DIFFERENTIATION

Although a host of experimental data suggests the existence of a self-renewing mammary adult stem cell within the epithelium [17–21], over the last decades the lack of specific cell markers has prevented any significant progress in the field [17, 18].

Recently, phenotypic characterization of breast epithelial cells using high molecular weight cytokeratins 5/14 and lineage-specific markers such as cytokeratins 8/18 and sm-actin has provided further evidence of the existence of common progenitor cells.

■ The epithelium of the resting human breast contains Ck5/14+ cells that differentiate into either Ck8/18+ glandular cells or sm-actin+ myoepithelial cells (Fig. 1.6).

Using double immunofluorescence techniques, a distinct subpopulation of cells within the breast epithelium can be demonstrated that fulfills the criteria of epithelial progenitor cells. These Ck5/14+ cells differentiate into lineage-specific intermediate glandular (Ck5/14+ and Ck8/18+) or intermediate myoepithelial cells (Ck 5/14+ and sm-actin+) before maturing into 'differentiated' glandular (Ck8/18+) or myoepithelial cells (sm-actin+) (Figs 1.7–1.9). During the lineage-specific differentiation process, expression of Ck5/14 gradually decreases, while expression of Ck8/18 (glandular lineage) or sm-actin (myoepithelial lineage) gradually

Tab. 1.1 Normal breast

Epithelium	The breast epithelium consists of a double layer of glandular and myoepithelial cells. Ck5/14+ progenitor cells give rise to glandular (Ck8/18+) and myoepithelial (sm-actin) progeny through transitory cells (Ck5/14+ and Ck8/18+ or Ck 5/14+ and sm-actin+). The glandular cells are constantly renewed. Myoepithelial cells, in contrast, represent a stable, mitotically less active cell pool.
Functional organization	Functionally, the breast epithelium is divided into the lobular and ductal system. Under the synergenic action of lactogenic hormones, the cells of the lobules differentiate into Ck8/18+ secretory end cells. Immature glandular epithelium, however, persists in ducts, as well as terminal ducts, even during pregnancy and lactation.
Post-weaning involution	Post-weaning the lactating cells undergo apoptosis to be replaced by a resting glandular epithelium. We hypothesize that progenitor cells in intralobular terminal ducts may play a key role in this process.

1 The normal breast

increases. This indicates that commitment to one lineage involves suppression of the other.

Based on these findings, the authors proposed a cell biological concept as depicted in the above schematic drawing (Fig. 1.6) [22, 23]. Recently Dontu et al. [24] provided further support for this model by showing that cultured human epithelium contains Ck5+ cells, which have the capacity for self-renewal and, equally important, generate both epithelial cell lineages. Thus the model includes the following subsets of cells.

Progenitor cells characterized by extensive expression of high molecular weight cytokeratins 5 and 14.

Intermediate glandular cells characterized by expression of both Ck5/14 and Ck8/18. These cells represent a transitory stage. As yet, we are unsure whether these cells are already fully committed to their glandular lineage differentiation or whether they may have the plasticity to return to the progenitor cell state.

'Differentiated' glandular cells characterized by expression of cytokeratins 8/18 [25–29]. It should be borne

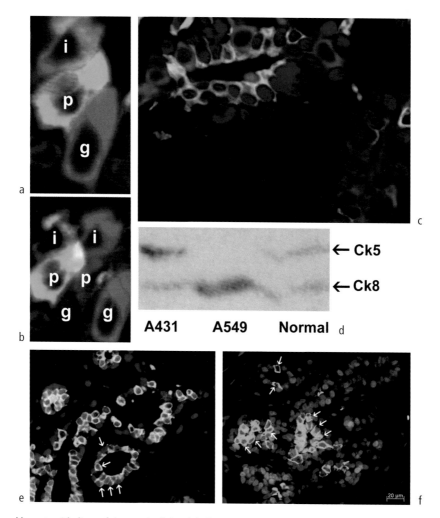

Fig. 1.7a–f Normal breast epithelium of the terminal duct lobular unit.
1.7a Breast ductule at high magnification. Double immunolabeling for Ck5 (green signal for FITC) and Ck8/18 (red signal for Cy3).
1.7b Cells from a ductule as in 1.7a with a 57-pixel shift of Ck8/18 (red component) to the right, revealing a progenitor cell (p) expressing only Ck5 (green signal), intermediate glandular cells (i) with co-expression of Ck5 and Ck8/18 (hybrid signal), and a differentiated glandular cell (g) expressing only Ck8/18 (red signal).
1.7c Immunophenotypic heterogeneity of luminal epithelial cells. Double immunolabeling of two acini for Ck5 (green signal) and Ck8/18 (red signal). Note the scarcity of differentiated glandular cells expressing Ck8/18 (red signal).
1.7d Western blotting immunoreaction with Ck5 and Ck8 antibodies of total cellular proteins from micro-dissected lobular cells (normal) and of two well-known cell lines (A413 and A 549). As expected, a clear-cut Ck5 and Ck8 band can be obtained by protein extraction of normal epithelial cells.
1.7e Most of the Ck8/18+ cells express estrogen receptor α; however, there are a few Ck8/18+ cells that lack this receptor (arrows). Double immunolabeling for Ck8/18 and estrogen receptor.
1.7f In contrast, Ck5+ cells are usually estrogen receptor α negative (arrows). Double staining for Ck14 and estrogen receptor α.

It is assumed that, after weaning, the secretory cells undergo apoptosis and must be replaced [51]. In the human this process of remodeling, known as 'involution', is associated with gradual reduction of the lobular parenchyma. At the cellular level, the secretory epithelium is then replaced by an immature glandular epithelium. At the time of writing, the exact mechanism of this process remained unknown. The most probable explanations are that immature glandular cells may escape the apoptotic process and gradually replace the lactating cells or, alternatively, that glandular precursor cells of the terminal ducts might contribute to such a replacement process. The former hypothesis is in line with recent observations in mice which demonstrate that, in multiparous animals, differentiated cells in ducts bypass apoptosis during postparous involution before serving as lobular progenitors [52]. The latter assumption would imply a migration of glandular precursor cells from the intralobular part of terminal ducts to the acini of the lobules. Although an analogous process has been established for regeneration in colonic crypts [53], until now it has never been considered with respect to breast epithelium.

It appears that the lobular myoepithelial framework in this postparous involution process is largely

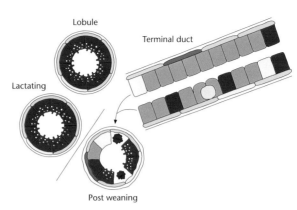

Fig. 1.11b Hypothetical remodeling process of the lactating breast epithelium after weaning. We hypothesize that under the effects of hormones of pregnancy/lactation, nearly all luminal cells of the lobule differentiate into Ck8/18+ secretory end cells. However, Ck5/14+ progenitor cells along with their progenies prevail in the terminal ducts. After weaning, the apoptotic secretory cells could be gradually replaced by glandular progenitor cells from the terminal ducts.

preserved and plays a key role in the remodeling process.

The epithelial tissue of the resting breast is constantly renewed during menstrual cycles.

In order to safeguard the integrity of TDLUs in resting breast epithelium during menstrual cycles, loss of cells must be compensated by replacement of equivalent cells with an identical phenotype. Several studies have shown that a peak of proliferation in the luteal phase is followed by a peak of apoptosis at the onset of the menstrual phase [54–62]. Theoretically, such replacement may be achieved by mitoses within a population of differentiated cells. Alternatively there may be de novo replacement through selective differentiation following mitotic proliferation of progenitor cells or partially differentiated cells. The resting breast epithelium shows marked differences in the proliferative capacity of the glandular and myoepithelial cell lineage. Whereas the cells of the glandular cell lineage show remarkable proliferative activity [63], mitotic activity of the myoepithelial cell lineage seems to be absent or extremely low (Fig. 1.12) [64, 65]. It is therefore possible that the glandular cells of the resting breast play the main role in physiologic regeneration. Furthermore, this data suggests that the myoepithelial cell lineage is much more stable than its labile glandular equivalent. This may, to a certain extent, explain why breast tumors are usually glandular in phenotype, and rarely myoepithelial.

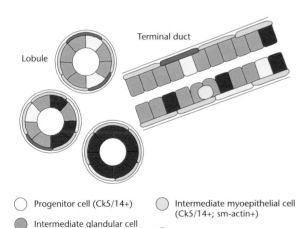

○ Progenitor cell (Ck5/14+)

◐ Intermediate glandular cell (Ck5/14+; Ck8/18+)

● Glandular cell (Ck8/18+)

◔ Intermediate myoepithelial cell (Ck5/14+; sm-actin+)

● Myoepithelial end cell (sm-actin+)

Fig. 1.11a Architectural organization of human resting breast epithelium. The epithelium of the resting breast is immature and dynamic. Ck5/14+ progenitor cells are observed in the luminal epithelium of both the terminal duct and lobules. They give rise to intermediate and differentiated glandular cells. The differentiation state of the glandular lineage varies greatly between acini. The outer layer consists mainly of intermediate myoepithelial cells and contains few differentiated cells. The location of stem cells is currently unclear; there is, however, some circumstantial evidence that they may be located in the terminal ducts (blue).

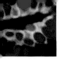

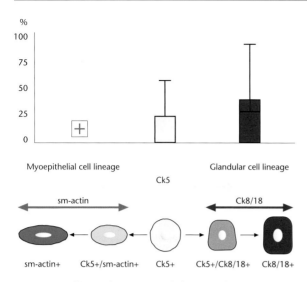

Fig. 1.12 Differential MIB1 growth fraction of normal breast epithelium (see text).

ARE ADULT BREAST STEM CELLS CK5/14+ CELLS?

Adult stem cells, according to the current definition, exhibit two properties:
1. the ability of self-renewal; and
2. the ability to give rise to differentiated end cells [17, 19, 66–69].

The existence of epithelial stem cells in the breast can no longer be denied [14, 17, 52, 69–72]. Such a stem cell concept is in line with evidence from the transplantation of mouse mammary epithelium into cleared mammary fat pads of syngeneic or athymic nude mice [17, 19–21]. Transplants were capable of developing into an entire new gland [17, 18]. Even a single cell has the potential to form a complete mammary gland [18]. Furthermore, there is sound evidence that the mature glandular and myoepithelial progeny have a common origin in Ck5/14+ cells, which thus represent the earliest recognizable common precursors [22]. Cultures of human breast epithelium provided evidence that Ck5+ cells are capable of self-replication and bilineage differentiation, which would make them stem cells according to the above definition [24]. We are, nevertheless, still unsure where the stem cells are localized.

Theories on hierarchies in cell growth of other organs [73, 74], the analogies to Ck5+ cells in the prostate and parotid gland and the data from proliferation studies [63] allow us to hypothesize that several cell populations representing different stages of differentiation must be involved in the regeneration of breast epithelium:

1. a slowly cycling adult stem cell pool, probably Ck5+ cells;
2. a pool of proliferative glandular cells at various stages of differentiation, that constitute an amplifying compartment;
3. myoepithelial lineage-specific precursor cells and a larger pool of more mature transitory cells that have mainly lost the capacity to divide; and
4. differentiated end cells in both cell lineages that do not divide and are finally lost.

Based on this concept, our current hypothesis is that only few of the Ck5/14+ cells in the resting breast epithelium may belong to a slowly cycling cell pool. Given the clonality of TDLUs [72, 75] it is tempting to speculate that one or several TDLUs may have or share such cells, and that these are located in the terminal ducts of TDLUs rather than in the lobules themselves. The relative contribution of these cells to the maintenance of breast epithelium under physiological conditions is unclear. As discussed in the previous paragraph it may well be that Ck8/18+ glandular cells readily replicate and the 'stem cell' compartment is not activated under normal conditions. Most Ck5/14+ cells in breast epithelium co-express Ck8/18 and thus seem to be lineage-specific precursors and transitory cells. Even differentiated Ck8/18+ glandular cells in resting breast epithelium represent a transitory, mitotically active stage, the final stages of the differentiation process being lactating glandular cells. Having lost its proliferative potential, it is this cell type which must be regarded as differentiated end cell.

IMAGING

MAMMOGRAPHY

Specialized X-ray mammography equipment and modified digital processing based on quality control guidelines are the gold standards in breast screening and diagnostic examination [76, 77]. However, digital mammography has recently been subjected to increasingly critical scrutiny. Although it still suffers from limited spatial resolution in comparison with conventional mammography, it is expected to replace the screen film technique in the future [78, 79].

Before maturity, the undeveloped breast parenchyma can be seen as a bud-like central density with a ground-glass appearance. Until the age of 30, development of the gland results in an increasing ramification of the ductal system. The combination of parenchyma and connective tissue creates an effect of density [80]. The radiographic appearance of the parenchyma varies individually in form, size and composition and is age-dependent. After the age of thirty, involutional changes of the parenchyma and the interlobular stroma set in. Mammographic changes in the menopause are, however, far more significant than those which are purely age related [81]. Changes occurring in the menopause include: reduction in the area of radiographically dense tissue, an increase in the area of radiolucent tissue, and a percentage decrease in density. Various radiological classifications have been formulated. The Tabár classification, for instance, is based on anatomic mammographic patterns, resulting from three-dimensional histopathologic-mammographic comparisons [82]. In 1998 the American College of Radiology (ACR) suggested a now internationally accepted classification of four patterns, representing a gradation in parenchymal opacity:

- (ACR 4) extremely dense (Fig. 1.13a);
- (ACR 3) heterogeneously dense (Fig. 1.13b);
- (ACR 2) fibroglandular (Fig. 1.13d); and
- (ACR 1) almost entirely fatty (Fig. 1.13c).

Breast density is an important predictor of mammographic accuracy [83]. While mammography provides a sensitivity of almost 100% in the fatty breast, sensitivity decreases significantly in the dense and very dense breast. Whereas tumors with micro-calcifications are still quite reliably identified, those without micro-calcifications may be obscured by dense breast tissue. Unless subtle architectural distortion, asymmetry, or some change with time attracts the mammographer's attention, tumors that exhibit the same radiodensity as the surrounding dense breast tissue are invisible. Although radiologically dense breast tissue is associated with an increased risk of breast cancer [84], the basis of this association remains unclear. In order to demonstrate the entire breast tissue including part of the pectoral muscle a two-view technique is generally employed, encompassing the cranial-caudal and the oblique medio-lateral views.

In the normal breast, the dominant part of the parenchyma is mainly located in the periphery of the upper outer quadrant. Adipose tissue that appears round or bent in shape is interposed. Fibrous bands, the Cooper's ligaments, which attach the breast tissue to the skin, are often seen as a thin line in the pre-pectoral and subcutaneous fat (Fig. 1.13c). Normal ducts are not visible except in the space behind the areola as a stripe-like opacity [80]. Physiologically, the premenstrual breast is less radiolucent than the postmenstrual one as a result of water retention and dilatation of the acini combined with increased blood circulation. It is often sensitive to pressure [85].

During involution, the acini become smaller and the reduction of the stroma results in a substitution of fat tissue. The parenchyma becomes more transparent; however, in one third of the tissue, stromal involution remains incomplete. The remains of the mammary parenchyma, the fibrous bands and the vessels can all be seen. The central ducts may also dilate. Involution starts medially and ends in the upper outer quadrant [80].

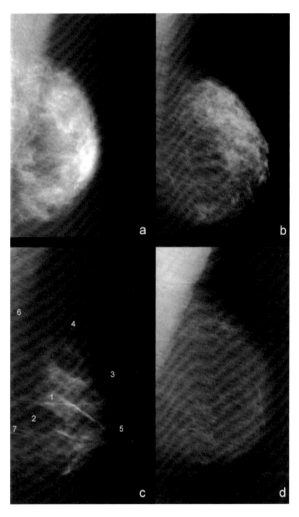

Fig. 1.13a–d Normal mammograms (screen-film mammography, oblique view). Radiographic density classified using the American College of Radiology (ACR) criteria.
1.13a Extremely dense pattern (ACR 4), typical during adolescence and early stage after maturity.
1.13b Heterogeneously dense pattern (ACR 3).
1.13c An almost entirely fatty pattern (ACR 1) is observed after menopause associated with an increase in sensitivity and specificity.
The parenchyma (1) is depicted as a summation of glandular components and connective tissue. Lucent fatty tissue (2) is interposed. Cooper's ligaments (3), skin (4), nipple (5), blood vessels (6) and pectoral muscle (7) can be distinguished.
1.13d Scattered fibroglandular tissue (ACR 2). The density decreases after maturity, but the range varies widely in individuals between the age of 30 to 50.

1 The normal breast

ULTRASOUND

High-resolution ultrasound (US) is required when imaging the breast [86, 87]. During prepuberty and puberty the mammary ducts and the connective tissue are depicted as a homogeneous structure surrounded by a thin seam of lucent fatty tissue. Echogenicity is low due to connective tissue containing immature parenchyma. The breast can appear as a nodule and should not be erroneously diagnosed as a tumor (Fig. 1.14). The juvenile gland is still hypoechoic, similar in appearance to fat. After maturity, in contrast to mammography, the highly echoic stroma can be separated from less echoic areas of adenosis and fibrosis. The use of both ultrasound and mammography to image opaque tissue therefore has a high diagnostic value [88]. Ductal-lobular tissue can also be visualized (Fig. 1.15). Owing to the orientation of the ducts and periductal fibrous tissue, reflection or absorption results in a shadow behind the areola which can impair assessment. After involution, the substitution of fat tissue leads to a hypoechoic pattern. The remaining mammary parenchyma is intermediately to highly echoic (Fig. 1.16) [89]. As most tumors are of low echogenicity, similar to fat, the sensitivity of ultrasound decreases after involution.

MAGNETIC RESONANCE IMAGING

In magnetic resonance mammography, the breast is usually imaged using gradient echo sequences, depicting the whole breast in a series of slices of less than four millimeters in thickness [90, 91]. In T1-weighted images, fat is depicted as a high signal, and the glandular tissue, the ducts and the connective tissue, as a low signal (Fig. 1.17a). Standardized intravenous application of an extracellular paramagnetic contrast agent followed by repetitive measurements of five to eight sequences, each taking less than two minutes, provides information on tissue enhancement in relation to time as a parameter of vascularization and permeability. Fat, glandular tissue and stroma are not normally enhanced. Vessels and, in approximately half of the studies, the nipples demonstrate an increasing signal (Fig. 1.17b) [92]. Patchy enhanced areas may be seen inter- and intra-individually, especially in younger women. These may be pronounced in the second half of the cycle and during menstruation, but usually lack an anatomic correlation. The most suitable time for imaging is therefore the second week of the cycle [93, 94].

The use of magnetic resonance imaging as a supplement to mammography and ultrasound may help to raise diagnostic confidence due to the technique's high sensitivity to solid lesions [92].

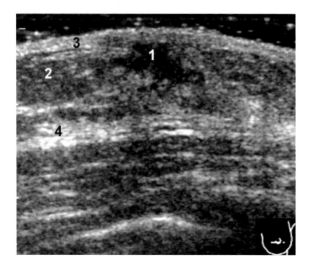

Fig. 1.14 Normal transversal sonogram before maturity (12 MHz). During puberty the central parenchyma (1) is hypoechoic, appearing as a nodule surrounded by fatty tissue (2). Skin (3) and breast muscle (4) are also shown.

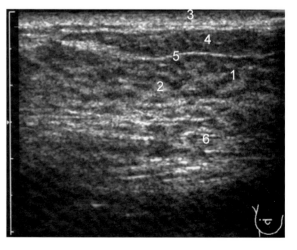

Fig. 1.15 Normal transversal sonogram after maturity (12 MHz). With a high-frequency probe the TDLU (1) is nodular and hypoechoic. The stroma (2) is hyperechoic. Skin (3), subcutaneous fat (4), the anterior fascia (5) and breast muscle (6) are shown.

12

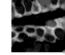

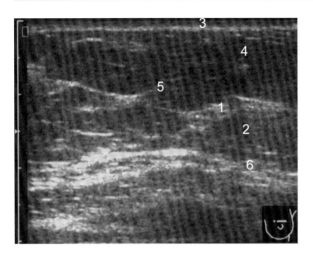

Fig. 1.16 Normal transversal sonogram after involution (12 MHz). Residual stroma is strongly hyperechoic (1). The parenchyma has been substituted by fat tissue with a hypoechoic appearance (2). Skin (3), subcutaneous fat (4), Cooper's ligaments (5) and breast muscle (6) can be seen.

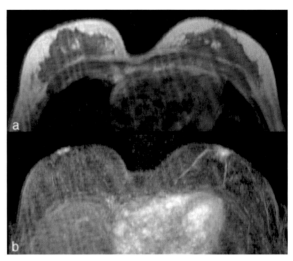

Fig. 1.17a–b An axial T1-weighted MR image (a) shows the parenchyma as a low signal, with the surrounding fat as a high signal.
Axial subtraction image (post-contrast minus pre-contrast, b) depicts an enhancement of vessels and the nipple. Normally the parenchyma is not enhanced. Circulating contrast agent is shown in the chambers of the heart.

IMMUNOHISTOCHEMISTRY

The majority of cells located in the inner layer of the ductal lobular system expresses glandular cytokeratins 8/18, while most myoepithelial cells situated in the outer layer characteristically express p63 and the functional proteins smooth-muscle actin and calponin (Fig. 1.6, Table 1.2). Cytokeratin 5/14 staining decorates most luminal and basal cells of the ductal system, including the cells of the terminal ducts, whereas the staining reaction of the luminal cells of the lobules depends on the degree of glandular differentiation

(Fig. 1.18a). Differentiated glandular cells and myoepithelial end cells express lineage-specific markers but not Ck5/14 (Figs 1.5b, 1.8, 1.9).

In the **luminal (glandular) layer** other markers have been detected, such as the human milk fat globule membrane proteins sialomycin [95, 96] and alpha-lactalbumin [97], and epithelial membrane antigen [98]. The luminal cell compartment is immunoreactive for bcl2, estrogen receptors, progesterone receptors and Ki67 [99].

The **basal (myoepithelial) layer** is immunoreactive for p63, smooth muscle contractile proteins [100–103], maspin [104], p63 [105–108], oxytocin [109,

Tab. 1.2 Immunophenotypic profile of normal epithelial cells in the breast

	Lobules		Ducts and terminal ducts	
	Luminal	Basal	Luminal	Basal
Low molecular weight cytokeratins 8/18	+++	(–)	+++	(–)
High molecular weight cytokeratins 5/14	+++ to (–)[1]	+ (+)	++ (+)[2]	++
Myoepithelial markers (p63, sm-actin, calponin)	(–)	+ (+)	(–)	++
Estrogen/progesterone receptors	+ (+)	(–)	+ (+)	(–)

[1] Luminal cells of lobules vary from +++ in nearly all lobular luminal cells to absence (–) of Ck5/14+ cells, depending on the differentiation status of the lobular cells (see text).
[2] Luminal cells of ducts and terminal ducts are usually positive (see text).

110], vimentin, beta-4 integrin and Galla [111–114, 99, 25], but negative for bcl-2 and both estrogen and progesterone receptors. In addition, basal cells express collagen type IV, heparansulfate proteoglycan and fibronectin [115], laminin receptors [116], metalloproteinases such as stromelysin, gelatinase and MMP 19 [117–119], and protease inhibitors such as inhibitors of metalloproteinase-1, protease nexin II, alpha-1 antitrypsin, and maspin [120]. Maspin, a member of the serpin family of serine proteinases, has been shown to function as tumor suppressant [104, 121, 122]. Myoepithelial cells have only limited proliferation potential. It should be borne in mind that S-100 positivity in breast tissue does not exclusively indicate myoepithelial differentiation, as has been suggested by several authors [123–126]. Some glandular cells, such as cells of microglandular adenosis, may show S-100 positivity [127–131].

A **basal lamina** is seen at the interface between parenchyma and stroma. It represents a lattice-like scaffolding containing collagen IV [128–130], V-laminin, entactin, proteoglycans and fibronectin among other substances. This structure is subject to constant remodeling.

Studies in rodents have revealed that the basement membrane is produced by stromal and myoepithelial cells [132, 133], whereas myoepithelial cells are responsible for its degradation [131,134]. Several metalloproteinases and their inhibitors seem to be involved in this process [134–137].

■ ESTROGEN RECEPTORS

Estrogen is considered to play a major role in promoting the proliferation of the normal breast. Most of the effects of estrogens are mediated by nuclear receptor proteins [138]. Two estrogen receptors (ER) have been identified: ERα [139, 140] and ERβ [141]. The ERβ protein is highly homologous to the ERα protein, but its gene transactivation properties are different. Both ERα and ERβ bind specifically to estrogen response elements (ERE) and activate ERE-containing promoters in response to 17β-estradiol (E2). At AP-1 and SP-1 sites, however, ERα and ERβ can have opposing effects [142].

In the mammary gland, both estrogen receptor subtypes have been found in epithelial cells of alveoli and ducts as well as in stromal cells [143]. However, their presence and cellular distribution is distinct. ERβ is constantly present in about 70% of epithelial cell nuclei. The percentage of ERα-positive nuclei varies according to the developmental and functional state of the mammary gland. Prior to puberty, ERα-positive cells account for 40% and co-expressing cells for 25% of epithelial cells [144]. Attempts to gauge the influence of hormonal changes during the menstrual cycle on the expression of estrogen receptors in the breast have yielded inconsistent results [145–147]. However, mRNA expression of ERα has been found to be higher in the luteal than in the follicular phase [148]. During

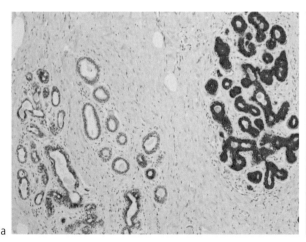
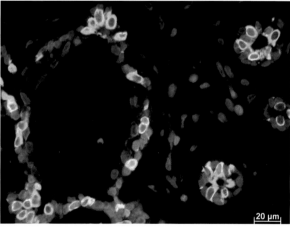

a   b

Fig. 1.18a–b Immunostaining of normal resting epithelium for Ck5 and estrogen receptor α.
1.18a Ck5/6 immunostaining of normal resting breast epithelium. In this figure the lobule in the right field contains Ck5+ ductules, indicating progenitor and/or intermediate cells. This staining pattern is in stark contrast to the staining intensity in the two lobules in the left field with no or only few Ck5+ cells, indicating that these lobules contain mostly differentiated cells expressing either Ck8/18 (luminal cells) or sm-actin (basal cells). Thus Ck5/14 immunohistochemistry enables a rough estimate of the differentiation status of the epithelium.
1.18b Immunostaining of normal resting breast epithelium for estrogen receptor α (red signal), showing intensive staining of nuclei only in CK8/18+ luminal cells (green signal). It should be acknowledged that the staining pattern depends on the differentiation status of the glandular cells (compare Fig. 1.1).

pregnancy, mRNA expression of ERα [148] as well as its protein [144] are low and only few cells express both ERs. Lactation is associated with induction of ERα, resulting in as much as 70% of positive nuclei. Here, co-expression of both receptor subtypes is found in up to 60% of epithelial cells. After lactation, however, ERα-expression again decreases, and co-localization of the two estrogen receptors is rare [144]. Expression of progesterone receptor (PR), a protein indicative of functional ERα [149], has been shown to be high during pregnancy and postlactation and low during lactation. There are several alternative explanations for estrogen insensitivity of cells despite the presence of ERα, such as limiting concentrations of co-activators or excessive amounts of co-repressors [150] as well as the presence of ERβ isoforms [151, 152].

Two distinct types of responses to E2 have been proposed: a direct effect on ERα-containing cells that occurs at low E2 concentrations and results in induction of the progesterone receptor (PR) and differentiation of the epithelium, and, at high E2 concentrations, an indirect action via ER-containing stromal cells, which induce the production of growth factors to cause replication of epithelial cells [153]. Surprisingly, approximately 60–70% of proliferating cells in normal breast tissue contain neither ERα nor ERβ [144, 154, 155] suggesting that, in normal breast tissue, ER-positive cells seem to act as sensor cells for circulating or local E2 concentrations, whereas proliferating cells apparently function as effector cells in terms of estrogen-stimulated mitogenesis [156].

The impact of E2 on epithelial proliferation has been studied using normal human breast tissue xenografted into athymic nude mice and then exposed to E2 at follicular and luteal phase serum concentrations, as well as concentrations approaching those seen in pregnancy. A dose response effect could be demonstrated between E2 treatment and epithelial proliferation, reaching a plateau, however, above serum E2 levels of 1500 pmol/l [154, 157]. These findings are supported by several in vivo studies in humans reporting higher proliferation indices during the luteal phase [57, 62, 147, 158, 159]. After the menopause, proliferation in normal breast tissue decreases, whereas the number of ERα-positive cells increases. Consequently, the proportion of dual-expressing cells in morphologically normal breast tissue is enhanced postmenopausally [160].

◼ MOLECULAR ALTERATIONS

In the current debate on breast cancer development the presence of genetic alterations is usually interpreted as an indicator of malignancy. Over the past few years, however, 'loss of heterozygosity' (LOH) was found in normal breast lobules adjacent to and even 'distant' from synchronous human breast cancer [161]. Furthermore, Lakhani and his co-workers detected such alterations in myoepithelial as well as luminal cells, indicating that these changes may even occur in common precursor cells [162, 163]. Moreover, Moinfar and colleagues [164] observed the incidence of concurrent and independent genetic changes in normal stromal cells and in parenchymal cells adjacent to or distant from foci of DCIS or invasive carcinoma.

In normal breast tissue, loss of heterozygosity (LOH) seems to be a random event for most genetic loci analyzed. However, it has become obvious that the incidence of genetic alteration varies significantly. Whereas such changes are rather infrequent in breast lobules originating from tissue removed for cosmetic reasons, the incidence of genetic alterations was significantly higher in apparently normal breast tissue taken from patients with biopsy-proven atypical hyperplasia or invasive breast cancer [165]. One article even demonstrated that LOH in normal lobular units is predictive of local recurrence [166–168]. It remains an open question to what extent 'malignancy-associated changes' described by means of elaborate morphometric techniques mirror those genetic changes [169, 170].

Several studies revealed distinct gene amplifications of sequences regulating the transcription of the epidermal growth factor receptor (EGFR) gene in morphologically unaltered breast tissue. These alterations were found to be correlated to tumor recurrence rates [171]. Little is known about the forces that might preclude such a development. In order to address this question in the future, comparing genetic alterations in normal breast tissue and the respective malignant lesions will be essential [172, 165]. At present, the distribution of genetically altered TDLUs in human breast tissue allows different interpretations. The tree-like, anatomic organization of the human breast with multiple patches of per se clonal cell groups on a microscopic level [71, 75, 163] might be seen as a result of genetic alterations occurring at an early stage during organogenesis. Another explanation could be a type of 'field cancerization/genetic field' [173–175]. The definition of multiple patches or fields might further explain the existence of genetically unrelated multifocal breast cancers [180] or unrelated tumor clones in DCIS [181] and invasive breast cancer [182, 183].

◼ EMBRYOLOGY AND BREAST DEVELOPMENT

The fundamental mechanisms in the evolutionary developmental biology of the breast (Fig. 1.19) –

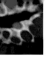

morphologically, genetically, functionally, and at the cell biological level – are currently under intense investigation [17, 19, 60, 67 – 70, 184 – 192].

Organogenesis of the breast, in principle, is a process that involves complex glandular/myoepithelial and connective tissue differentiation. Physiological invasion with epithelial outgrowth and stromal growth and differentiation in response to soluble and solid phase stimuli are key processes at various stages in the development of the breast. Cross-talk between developing breast epithelium and mesenchyme appears to be the most important driver in this process. [155, 184, 193 – 197].

The **embryonic phase** consists of two stages:

1. Formation of the final mammary anlage in the region of the thorax (**milk hill stage**) associated with underlying mesenchymal condensation around the milk hill [198 – 201]. Following this, ectodermally derived 'cells' from the milk hill infiltrate and proliferate within the surrounding mesenchymal tissue to form primitive solid buds (**budding stage**).
2. Dichotomous branching (**branching stage**) resulting in solid epithelial symmetric or asymmetric ramifications. This is associated with a distinct period of proliferation of both epithelial and mesenchymal structures, morphogenesis and glandular differentiation. Canalization of the primitive tubular buds occurs with formation of glandular and myoepithelial cells to form the rudimentary gland of the neonate.

In the monkey, myoepithelial cells seem to be the first to differentiate from Ck5/14+ cells, before the development of glandular cells (Figs 1.20a – f). Colostrum is secreted under the influence of maternal and placental steroids and of prolactin. Simultaneously, specific connective tissue of the nipple develops to form an everted nipple.

From birth to puberty, the gland remains rudimentary and relatively growth-quiescent. The most dramatic developmental changes can be seen in puberty – between the ages of ten and twelve years. There is an enhanced phase of proliferation and differentiation, and the rudimentary breast tissue begins to grow with physiological invasion and branching of the primitive ducts. Collagenous fibrous tissue from the reticular dermis extends into the breast to encompass the parenchyma. Periductal and lobular connective tissue give rise to hormone-sensitive specialized stroma. Simultaneously, fibrous cells differentiate into fat cells.

As a consequence of lateral sprouting (cleavage) of the end buds, approximately ten ductules or alveoli develop to form an undifferentiated lobule (virginal or lobule, type 1 according to Russo [60]). Further sprouting leads to differentiated lobules of the resting breast with considerable increase in the number of alveoli to about forty to eighty. This causes an increase in lobular size, although the individual alveoli are smaller than in undifferentiated lobules. In parous premenopausal women differentiated lobules predominate, while in nulliparous and involuted parous postmenopausal women undifferentiated lobules prevail [60].

CELLULAR DIFFERENTIATION AND MOLECULAR BIOLOGY

During breast organogenesis, basal cells of the primitive milk hill proliferate, invade the underlying mesenchymal tissue, differentiate, and interact with cells as well as the connective tissue, which also shows a characteristic pattern of growth and differentiation [202 – 205, 199]. The result of this process is the formation of a breast-specific spatial arrangement of parenchyma, specialized fibrous connective tissue and fat. One of the most important features of this process appears to be the differentiation of epithelial precursor cells into both glandular and myoepithelial lineages.

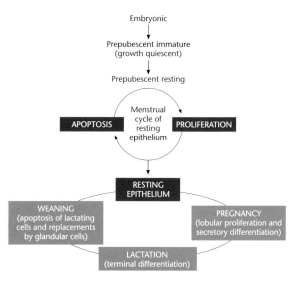

Fig. 1.19 Phases of breast gland development and cyclical renewal of the breast epithelium. Organogenesis can be divided into an embryonic and a postpubertal linear progression to the resting human breast. With each menstrual cycle the resting breast undergoes a cyclical process of proliferation and apoptosis. During pregnancy and lactation there is intense proliferation and growth of the lobular tissue with terminal differentiation of the luminal cells to become functionally mature secretory lactating cells. With weaning, the secretory cells undergo apoptosis. The apoptotic cells are replaced by an immature glandular epithelium. This process is associated with a remodeling of the breast back to its resting stage, known as involution.

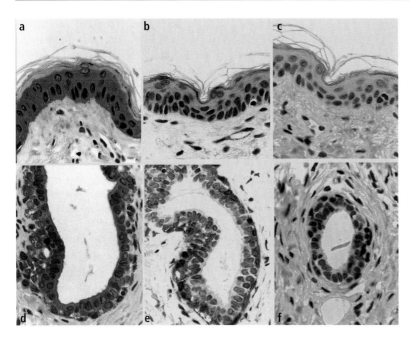

Fig. 1.20a–f Neonate female mammary gland of a monkey.
1.20a–c Nipple skin of the neonate.

1.20d–f Rudimentary gland of the neonate immunostained for Ck5 (a, d), sm-actin (b, e) and Ck8/18 (c, f). The primitive glands only contain Ck5+ luminal cells and basal cells co-expressing sm-actin.

Virtually nothing is known about how these different cell lineages are established. However, it seems likely that Ck5/14+ cells are involved in this process. This hypothesis is in line with the findings of Rudland, who provided evidence that undifferentiated 'cap cells' of terminal buds of the developing human breast show transitional forms of both luminal and myoepithelial cells [203]. Later on, these cells appear to acquire the function of adult breast progenitor cells and thus remain an important cellular constituent of the mature breast parenchyma throughout life [22].

Experimental data, mainly obtained from studies of ductal-lobular development and differentiation in the mouse, suggests that a variety of finely balanced mammotrophic hormones (estrogen), growth factors (TGF-α, TGF-β, FGF-family, Wnt gene family) and local cell-cell and cell-extracellular matrix interactions seem to mediate the initial complex organogenetic process [206–219]. Furthermore, the basement membrane [220, 221] and matrix metalloproteinases seem to play a key role in both developmental stages and in adult cycling and remodeling of the normal breast tissue [131, 134–136, 222–228]. During puberty, growth again occurs by extension of the cell population at the tips of the invading ductal net. As can be concluded from experimental data and localization studies, the pubertal processes appear to evolve under hormonal regulation (estrogen, progesterone, glucocorticoids, pituitary growth hormones). Local changes are caused by a number of stimulatory or inhibitory growth factors and basal membrane constituents with paracrine, juxtacrine or autocrine function. Local factors positively influencing ductal growth include IGF-I [184, 185] FGF1 and 2 [211] HGF, EGF and amphiregulin [229] as well as factors of the TGF-α family [209, 210]. In contrast, TGF-β inhibits growth and differentiation [212, 217, 230–232]. It has also been shown that FGF1 and 2 stimulate neo-vascularization during ductal growth [198, 211]. Localization of growth factors has been extensively studied over the last years, and parenchymal as well as stromal cells have been found to produce local factors which are partly deposited in the extracellular matrix (for an overview see [202]).

HOMEOBOX GENES IN MAMMARY GLAND DEVELOPMENT

Cellular differentiation (whereby cells subtly become committed to developmental glandular and myoepithelial cell lineages), their spatial pattern, and their relation to mesenchymal tissues are controlled by regulatory molecules and their genes. Such homeobox genes are active in a spatial and temporal manner [233]. Morphogenesis is, in all likelihood, controlled by activating or deactivating specific sets of homeobox genes. Thus, in the mouse, in-situ hybridization of breast tissue has shown that a number of homeobox genes (Alx-4, Msx-1, Msx-2, Hoxb-7, Hox-b9, Hoxd-4, Hoxd-9, Hoxd-10 and others) are differentially expressed at particular stages of mammary gland differentiation. Most likely these genes are therefore required for regulation of cell proliferation, the rate of apoptosis, cell motility, invasion of surrounding tissue

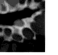

and neo-vascularization [233]. All of these processes are prerequisites for an appropriate breast identity, form and function [233].

PREGNANCY AND LACTATION

In pregnancy and lactation the gland undergoes a series of highly orchestrated changes starting with lobular growth. The glandular cells then display an irreversible, terminal differentiation with the formation of secretory cells [234].

A variety of hormones such as estrogen, progesterone, placental lactogen, human chorionic somatomammotropin (HCS), prolactin, and glucocorticosteroids influence this process [229, 235], with a progressive increase of parenchyma and coincidental decrease in fibrofatty tissue [200, 234, 236]. This process is most pronounced in the second and third trimesters of pregnancy. Proliferative activity is highest during the first twenty weeks of gestation, as can be shown by the MIB1 proliferation index. Microscopically, there is an increase in the number and size of lobules. The lobular epithelium is enlarged with cytoplasmic vacuolization and prominent nucleoli [97], while myoepithelial cells become less prominent and elongated.

In the second half of gestation, there is an increasing functional differentiation of the lobular epithelium associated with secretory and lactational changes [237]. In H&E sections, the epithelium now shows a vacuolated appearance with accumulation of fat droplets in the cytoplasm (Fig. 1.21a).

Contrary to the resting gland, Ck5/14+ progenitor cells are no longer present in the functional glandular compartment of the lobules [22]. Attenuated myoepithelial cells are also inconspicuous. In the terminal ducts, however, progenitor cells are still present.

The endocrine control of milk formation requires – after priming by estrogen, progesterone and other hormones – lactogenic hormones such as prolactin, glucocorticoids, insulin and thyroxin. It seems that the removal of the inhibitory effect of estrogen and progesterone on prolactin plays a major role in galactopoiesis. Under their influence, secretory material accumulates in the cytoplasm of lobular cells and in the lumen of dilated acini and ducts.

Upon weaning, a process of involution destroys the majority of the secretory epithelium with regression and remodeling of the breast. The lobular cells are pushed into programmed cell death (apoptosis), eliminated and replaced by resting epithelium.

The involution of the parenchyma takes place over a period of about three to four months, with a decrease in the number and size of lobules. As discussed above, it seems likely that some form of apoptosis of the secretory cells, and enzymatic degradation of the basement membrane by myoepithelial cells and macrophages both play a major role in this process [238–241]. Although it is obvious that this process is induced by hormonal alterations in combination with local cellular effects, the exact mechanisms involved are so far only poorly understood [239]. Furthermore, there is experimental evidence that metalloproteinase enzymes such as gelatinase A [134, 135], stromelysin 1 [134, 135, 242] and interstitial collagenase [242]

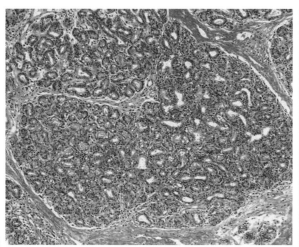
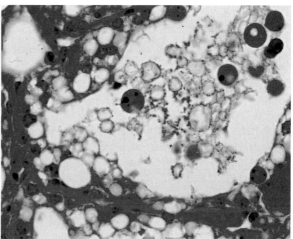

a   b

Fig. 1.21a–b Lactating breast.
1.21a Breast epithelium in late human pregnancy. Note the enlarged lobules with sparse interlobular connective tissue.
1.21b Early postlactational lobular involution in mouse mammary gland. Higher magnification of an acinus showing apoptotic bodies in the lumen as well as one in the epithelial lining of an acinus. Such an intense reaction is never seen in human post-weaning involution.

might play a role in the degradation process. The epithelial lining of lobules is more attenuated with degeneration and desquamation of apoptotic bodies into dilated lumina (Fig. 1.21b). The lobules are infiltrated by lymphocytes, plasma cells and macrophages. With lobular regression and involution there is an increase in fat and fibrovascular tissue. Some lobules are completely replaced by fibrous tissue. This process varies in degree from one area to another, making heterogeneity between different lobules more pronounced. Battersby and Anderson [243] describe the irregular lobular shape, angulated pyknotic ductular remnants and a crenulated basement membrane as typical features indicating recent pregnancy.

Compared to the mouse, in which the process of dismantling after weaning is more or less complete with loss of lobular structures, there are clear differences in the human breast. The process of remodeling (involution) after weaning in the human breast is characterized by a gradual loss of lactating cells with replacement of these cells by resting luminal epithelium. At the time of writing, the origin of cells that repopulate the luminal epithelium of the lobules was not yet identified [244]. However, based on data from our double immunofluorescence experiments, it seems that the apoptotic glandular cells are replaced in time by glandular precursor cells. As discussed above, cells of the terminal ducts probably replace the lobular luminal epithelium (Fig. 1.11). Thus the coordinated activity of apoptosis, protease-mediated remodeling by myoepithelial cells and histiocytes, and the replacement of the apoptotic secretory cells by glandular cells seem to play an important role in postlactational in-

volution. The result is a reduction in both, the size and probably also the number of lobules.

POSTMENOPAUSAL INVOLUTION

Following the menopause, involution involving the parenchyma and the connective tissue occurs [4, 245, 246]. However, this post-menopausal atrophy happens in a heterogeneous fashion, with individual lobules remaining unaffected or even hyperplastic. Some experts in the field believe that persistence of mature lobules within the postmenopausal breast must be taken as a sign of abnormality [4]. In addition, lobules may even show some degree of acinar dilation and the formation of microcysts.

The most characteristic feature of this process is the diminution of parenchymal structures. The number of lobular units is reduced to about one third of the number present in the reproductive years [247], while much of the main duct system is preserved (Figs 1.22a–c). Lobular involution is characterized by atrophy of the ductular epithelium to an attenuated inner cell layer and by transformation of the loose connective tissue into fibrous tissue [4, 245]. In contrast, the basal lamina around the lobular ductules (acini) thickens and fades into the surrounding ordinary background stroma. Glandular cells are then lost while the myoepithelial cells persist. Finally, myoepithelial cells diminish and lobules are reduced to remnants of hyaline nodules. In addition to this, ductules and acini ducts gradually disappear, and connective tissue, and in some cases even the lobular stroma, are reduced and replaced by adipose tissue.

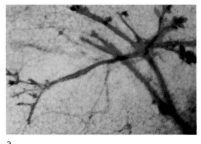 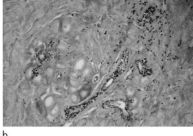 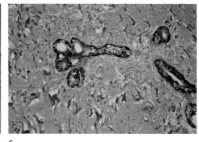

a   b   c

Fig. 1.22a–c Menopausal involution.
1.22a Submicroscopy showing an atrophic ductal-lobular system with involuted lobules.
1.22b Histology showing a small extra-lobular duct and an atrophic lobule with hyaline conversion of the specialized lobular tissue. The hyalinization of the lobule is mainly due to the extreme thickening of basement membranes of the acini, the outlines of which are clearly seen.
1.22c Ck5 immunohistochemistry of an involuted lobule. Note the intermediate myoepithelial cells in the outer layer and glandular precursor cells in the inner layer.

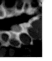

1 The normal breast

REFERENCES

1. Cowie AT. Proceedings: Overview of the mammary gland. J Invest Dermatol 1974;63:2–9.
2. Faverly D, Holland R, Burgers L. An original stereomicroscopic analysis of the mammary glandular tree. Virchows Arch A Pathol Anat Histopathol 1992;421:115–9.
3. Moffat DF, Going JJ. Three dimensional anatomy of complete duct systems in human breast: pathological and developmental implications. J Clin Pathol 1996;49:48–52.
4. Wellings SR, Jensen HM, Marcum RG. An atlas of subgross pathology of the human breast with special reference to possible precancerous lesions. J Natl Cancer Inst 1975;55:231–73.
5. Ohtake T, Abe R, Kimijima I, et al. Intraductal extension of primary invasive breast carcinoma treated by breast-conservative surgery. Computer graphic three-dimensional reconstruction of the mammary duct-lobular systems [see comments]. Cancer 1995;76:32–45.
6. Bargmann W, Fleischhauer K, Knoop A. Über die Morphologie der Milchsekretion. Zugleich eine Kritik am Schema der Sekretionsmorphologie. Z Zellforsch 1961;53:545–56.
7. Ozzello L. Ultrastructure of the human mammary gland. In: Pathology Annual. New York: Meredith Corporation; 1971. p.1–59.
8. Ozzello L. Ultrastructure of the human mammary gland. Pathol Annu 1971;6:1–59.
9. Spratt JS. Anatomy of the breast. Major Probl Clin Surg 1979;5:1–13.
10. Stirling JW, Chandler JA. The fine structure of the normal, resting terminal ductal-lobular unit of the female breast. Virchows Arch A Pathol Anat Histol 1976;372:205–26.
11. Stirling JW, Chandler JA. Ultrastructural studies of the female breast: I. 9 + 0 cilia in myoepithelial cells. Anat Rec 1976;186:413–6.
12. Stirling JW, Chandler JA. The fine structure of ducts and subareolar ducts in the resting gland of the female breast. Virchows Arch A Pathol Anat Histol 1977;373:119–32.
13. Gusterson B, Shipley J, Crew J. Application of molecular genetics and cytogenetics to breast cancer and soft tissue sarcomas. Ann Oncol 1994;5 Suppl 4:17–23.
14. Deugnier MA, Teuliere J, Faraldo MM, Thiery JP, Glukhova MA. The importance of being a myoepithelial cell. Breast Cancer Res 2002;4:224–30.
15. Azzopardi JG. Problems in Breast Pathology. 1st ed. London: W.B. Saunders; 1979.
16. Lwin KY, Zuccarini O, Sloane JP, Beverley PC. An immunohistological study of leukocyte localization in benign and malignant breast tissue. Int J Cancer 1985;36:433–8.
17. Smith GH, Medina D. A morphologically distinct candidate for an epithelial stem cell in mouse mammary gland. J Cell Sci 1988;90:173–83.
18. Williams JM, Daniel CW. Mammary ductal elongation: differentiation of myoepithelium and basal lamina during branching morphogenesis. Dev Biol 1983;97:274–90.
19. Daniel CW, Church K. Chromosome numbers of normal and preneoplastic mouse mammary tissues grown in vivo after monolayer culture. J Natl Cancer Inst 1968;40:1293–301.
20. Daniel CW, Young LJ. Influence of cell division on an aging process. Life span of mouse mammary epithelium during serial propagation in vivo. Exp Cell Res 1971;65:27–32.
21. Hayflick L, Moorhead PS. The serial cultivation of human diploid cell strains. Exp Cell Res 1961;25:585–621.
22. Boecker W, Moll R, Poremba C, et al. Common Adult Stem Cells in the Human Breast Give Rise to Glandular and Myoepithelial Cell Lineages: A New Cell Biological Concept. Lab Invest 2002;82:737–46.
23. Boecker W, Moll R, Dervan P, et al. Usual ductal hyperplasia of the breast is a committed stem (progenitor) cell lesion distinct from atypical ductal hyperplasia and ductal carcinoma in-situ. J Pathol 2002;198:458–67.
24. Dontu G, El Ashry D, Wicha MS. Breast cancer, stem/progenitor cells and the estrogen receptor. Trends Endocrinol Metab 2004;15:193–7.
25. Taylor PJ, Stampfer M, Bartek J, et al. Keratin expression in human mammary epithelial cells cultured from normal and malignant tissue: relation to in vivo phenotypes and influence of medium. J Cell Sci 1989;94:403–13.
26. Moll R, Franke WW, Schiller DL, Geiger B, Krepler R. The catalog of human cytokeratins: patterns of expression in normal epithelia, tumors and cultured cells. Cell 1982;31:11–24.
27. Böcker WJ, Bier B, Freytag G, et al. An immunohistochemical study of the breast using antibodies to basal and luminal keratins, alpha-smooth muscle actin, vimentin, collagen IV and laminin. Part I: normal breast and benign proliferative lesions. Virchows Archiv A 1992;421:315–22.
28. Böcker WJ, Bier B, Freytag G, et al. An immunohistochemical study of the breast using antibodies to basal and luminal keratins, alpha-smooth muscle actin, vimentin, collagen IV and laminin. Part II: Epitheliosis and ductal carcinoma in-situ. Virchows Archiv A 1992;421:323–30.
29. Jarasch E-D, Nagle RB, Kaufmann M, Maurer C, Böcker WJ. Differential Diagnosis of Benign Epithelial Proliferations and Carcinomas of the Breast Using Antibodies to Cytokeratins. Hum Pathol 1988;19:276–89.
30. Frid MG, Shekhonin BV, Koteliansky VE, Glukhova MA. Phenotypic changes of human smooth muscle cells during development: late expression of heavy caldesmon and calponin. Dev Biol 1992;153:185–93.
31. Lazard D, Sastre X, Frid MG, et al. Expression of smooth muscle-specific proteins in myoepithelium and stromal myofibroblasts of normal and malignant human breast tissue. Proc Natl Acad Sci U S A 1993;90:999–1003.
32. Longtine JA, Pinkus GS, Fujiwara K, Corson JM. Immunohistochemical localization of smooth muscle myosin in normal human tissues. J Histochem Cytochem 1985;33:179–84.
33. Eddinger TJ, Murphy RA. Developmental changes in actin and myosin heavy chain isoform expression in smooth muscle. Arch Biochem Biophys 1991;284:232–7.

34. Frid MG, Printesva OY, Chiavegato A, et al. Myosin heavy-chain isoform composition and distribution in developing and adult human aortic smooth muscle. J Vasc Res 1993;30:279–92.

35. Miano JM, Cserjesi P, Ligon KL, Periasamy M, Olson EN. Smooth muscle myosin heavy chain exclusively marks the smooth muscle lineage during mouse embryogenesis. Circ Res 1994;75:803–12.

36. Bussolati G, Alfani V, Weber K, Osborn M. Immunocytochemical detection of actin on fixed and embedded tissues: its potential use in routine pathology. J Histochem Cytochem 1980;28:169–73.

37. Gugliotta P, Sapino A, Macri L, et al. Specific demonstration of myoepithelial cells by anti-alpha smooth muscle actin antibody. J Histochem Cytochem 1988;36:659–63.

38. Foster CS, Dodson A, Karavana V, Smith PH, Ke Y. Prostatic stem cells. J Pathol 2002;197:551–65.

39. Bonkhoff H. Role of the basal cells in premalignant changes of the human prostate: a stem cell concept for the development of prostate cancer. Eur Urol 1996;30:201–5.

40. Wernert N, Seitz G, Achtstatter T. Immunohistochemical investigation of different cytokeratins and vimentin in the prostate from the fetal period up to adulthood and in prostate carcinoma. Pathol Res Pract 1987;182:617–26.

41. Verhagen AP, Ramaekers FC, Aalders TW, et al. Colocalization of basal and luminal cell-type cytokeratins in human prostate cancer. Cancer Res 1992;52:6182–7.

42. Hennighausen L, Robinson GW. Think globally, act locally: the making of a mouse mammary gland. Genes Dev 1998;12:449–55.

43. Horseman ND, Zhao W, Montecino-Rodriguez E, et al. Defective mammopoiesis, but normal hematopoiesis, in mice with a targeted disruption of the prolactin gene. EMBO J 1997;16:6926–35.

44. Ormandy CJ, Camus A, Barra J, et al. Null mutation of the prolactin receptor gene produces multiple reproductive defects in the mouse. Genes Dev 1997;11:167–78.

45. Liu X, Robinson GW, Wagner KU, et al. Stat5a is mandatory for adult mammary gland development and lactogenesis. Genes Dev 1997;11:179–86.

46. Miyoshi K, Shillingford JM, Smith GH, et al. Signal transducer and activator of transcription (Stat) 5 controls the proliferation and differentiation of mammary alveolar epithelium. J Cell Biol 2001;155:531–42.

47. Stocklin E, Wissler M, Gouilleux F, Groner B. Functional interactions between Stat5 and the glucocorticoid receptor. Nature 1996;383:726–8.

48. Wyszomierski SL, Rosen JM. Cooperative effects of STAT5 (signal transducer and activator of transcription 5) and C/EBPbeta (CCAAT/enhancer-binding protein-beta) on beta-casein gene transcription are mediated by the glucocorticoid receptor. Mol Endocrinol 2001;15:228–40.

49. Neville MC. Physiology of lactation. Clin Perinatol 1999;26:251–79, v.

50. Hennighausen L, Robinson GW. Signaling pathways in mammary gland development. Dev Cell 2001;1:467–75.

51. Lund LR, Romer J, Thomasset N, et al. Two distinct phases of apoptosis in mammary gland involution: proteinase-independent and -dependent pathways. Development 1996;122:181–93.

52. Wagner KU, Boulanger CA, Henry MD, et al. An adjunct mammary epithelial cell population in parous females: its role in functional adaptation and tissue renewal. Development 2002;129:1377–86.

53. Potten CS, Loeffler M. Stem cells: attributes, cycles, spirals, pitfalls and uncertainties. Lessons for and from the crypt. Development 1990;110:1001–20.

54. Potten CS, Watson RJ, Williams GT, et al. The effect of age and menstrual cycle upon proliferative activity of the normal human breast. Br J Cancer 1988;58:163–70.

55. Meyer JS. Cell proliferation in normal human breast ducts, fibroadenomas, and other ductal hyperplasias measured by nuclear labelling with tritiated thymidine. Hum Pathol 1977;8:67–81.

56. Anderson TJ, Battersby S, King RJ, McPherson K, Going JJ. Oral contraceptive use influences resting breast proliferation. Hum Pathol 1989;20:1139–44.

57. Going JJ, Anderson TJ, Battersby S, MacIntyre CC. Proliferative and secretory activity in human breast during natural and artificial menstrual cycles. Am J Pathol 1988;130:193–204.

58. Hayward JL, Parks AG. Alterations in the microanatomy of the breast as a result of changes in the hormonal environment. In: Currie AR, editor. Endocrine Aspects of Breast Cancer. Edinburgh: Churchill Livingstone; 1958. p.133–4.

59. Vogel PM, Georgiade NG, Fetter BF, Vogel FS, McCarty-KS J. The correlation of histologic changes in the human breast with the menstrual cycle. Am J Pathol 1981;104:23–34.

60. Russo J, Calaf G, Roi L, Russo IH. Influence of age and gland topography on cell kinetics of normal human breast tissue. J Natl Cancer Inst 1987;78:413–8.

61. Anderson TJ, Ferguson DJ, Raab GM. Cell turnover in the "resting" human breast: influence of parity, contraceptive pill, age and laterality. Br J Cancer 1982;46:376–82.

62. Longacre TA, Bartow SA. A correlative morphologic study of human breast and endometrium in the menstrual cycle. Am J Surg Pathol 1986;10:382–93.

63. Bankfalvi A, Ludwig A, de Hesselle B, et al. Different proliferative activity of the glandular and myoepithelial lineages in benign proliferative and early malignant breast diseases. Mod Pathol 2004;17:1051–61.

64. Joshi K, Smith JA, Perusinghe N, Monoghan P. Cell proliferation in the human mammary epithelium. Differential contribution by epithelial and myoepithelial cells. Am J Pathol 1986;124:199–206.

65. Lakhani SR, O'Hare MJ, Monaghan P, Winehouse J, Gazet JC. Malignant myoepithelioma (myoepithelial carcinoma) of the breast: a detailed cytokeratin study. J Clin Pathol 1995;48:164–7.

66. Kordon EC, Smith GH. An entire functional mammary gland may comprise the progeny from a single cell. Development 1998;125:1921–30.

67. Slack JM. Stem cells in epithelial tissues. Science 2000;287:1431–3.

68. Watt FM, Hogan BL. Out of Eden: stem cells and their niches. Science 2000;287:1427–30.

69. Smith GH, Chepko G. Mammary epithelial stem cells. Microsc Res Tech 2001;52:190–203.

70. Stingl J, Eaves CJ, Zandieh I, Emerman JT. Characterization of bipotent mammary epithelial progenitor cells in normal adult human breast tissue. Breast Cancer Res Treat 2001;67:93–109.

71. Tsai YC, Lu Y, Nichols PW, et al. Contiguous patches of normal human mammary epithelium derived from a single stem cell: implications for breast carcinogenesis. Cancer Res 1996;56:402–4.

72. Lakhani SR, Slack DN, Hamoudi RA, Collins N, Stratton MR. Detection of Allelic Imbalance Indicates That a Proportion of Mammary Hyperplasia of Usual Type Are Clonal, Neoplastic Proliferations. Lab Invest 1996;74:129–35.

73. Bonnet D. Haematopoietic stem cells. J Pathol 2002;197:430–40.

74. Brittan M, Wright NA. Gastrointestinal stem cells. J Path 2002;197:492–509.

75. Diallo R, Schaefer KL, Poremba C, et al. Monoclonality in normal epithelium and in hyperplastic and neoplastic lesions of the breast. J Pathol 2001;193:27–32.

76. Perry N, Broeders M, de Wolf C, Törnberg S. European guidelines for quality assurance in mammography screening. 3rd ed. Office for Official Publications of the European Communities; 2001.

77. Hendrick RE, Klabunde C, Grivegnee A, Pou G, Ballard-Barbash R. Technical quality control practices in mammography screening programs in 22 countries. Int J Qual Health Care 2002;14:219–26.

78. Shah AJ, Wang J, Yamada T, Fajardo LL. Digital mammography: a review of technical development and clinical applications. Clin Breast Cancer 2003;4:63–70.

79. Lewin JM, D'Orsi CJ, Hendrick RE, et al. Clinical comparison of full-field digital mammography and screen-film mammography for detection of breast cancer. AJR Am J Roentgenol 2002;179:671–7.

80. Heywang-Köbrunner S, Schreer I. Bildgebende Mammadiagnostik. Georg Thieme Verlag; 1996.

81. Boyd N, Martin L, Stone J, et al. A longitudinal study of the effects of menopause on mammographic features. Cancer Epidemiol Biomarkers Prev 2002;11:1048–53.

82. Gram IT, Funkhouser E, Tabar L. The Tabar classification of mammographic parenchymal patterns. Eur J Radiol 1997;24:131–6.

83. Mandelson MT, Oestreicher N, Porter PL, et al. Breast density as a predictor of mammographic detection: comparison of interval- and screen-detected cancers. J Natl Cancer Inst 2000;92:1081–7.

84. Boyd NF, Stone J, Martin LJ, et al. The association of breast mitogens with mammographic densities. Br J Cancer 2002;87:876–82.

85. Ursin G, Parisky YR, Pike MC, Spicer DV. Mammographic density changes during the menstrual cycle. Cancer Epidemiol Biomarkers Prev 2001;10:141–2.

86. AIUM standard for the performance of breast ultrasound examination J Ultrasound Med 2003;22:109–14.

87. Madjar H, Rickard M, Jellins J, Otto R. IBUS guidelines for the ultrasonic examination of the breast. IBUS International Faculty. International Breast Ultrasound School. Eur J Ultrasound 1999;9:99–102.

88. Kolb TM, Lichy J, Newhouse JH. Comparison of the performance of screening mammography, physical examination, and breast US and evaluation of factors that influence them: an analysis of 27,825 patient evaluations. Radiology 2002;225:165–75.

89. Friedrich M. Lehratlas der Mammasonographie. Darmstadt: Wissenschaftliche Verlagsgesellschaft; 1999.

90. Schnall MD. Breast MR imaging. Radiol Clin North Am 2003;41:43–50.

91. Kneeshaw PJ, Turnbull LW, Drew PJ. Current applications and future direction of MR mammography. Br J Cancer 2003;88:4–10.

92. Fischer U. Lehratlas der MR-Mammographie. Stuttgart: Georg Thieme Verlag; 2000.

93. Muller-Schimpfle M, Ohmenhauser K, Stoll P, Dietz K, Claussen CD. Menstrual cycle and age: influence on parenchymal contrast medium enhancement in MR imaging of the breast. Radiology 1997;203:145–9.

94. Kuhl CK, Bieling HB, Gieseke J, et al. Healthy premenopausal breast parenchyma in dynamic contrast-enhanced MR imaging of the breast: normal contrast medium enhancement and cyclical-phase dependency. Radiology 1997;203:137–44.

95. McIlhinney RA, Patel S, Gore ME. Monoclonal antibodies recognizing epitopes carried on both glycolipids and glycoproteins of the human milk fat globule membrane. Biochem J 1985;227:155–62.

96. Taylor-Papadimitriou J, Lane EJ, Chang SE. Cell lineages and interactions in neoplastic expression in the human breast. In: Rich MA, Hager J, Furmanski M, editors. Understanding Breast Cancer. New York: Marcel Dekker; 1983. p.215.

97. Bailey AJ, Sloane JP, Trickey BS, Ormerod MG. An immunocytochemical study of alpha-lactalbumin in human breast tissue. J Pathol 1982;137:13–23.

98. Sloane JP, Ormerod MG. Distribution of epithelial membrane antigen in normal and neoplastic tissues and it value in diagnostic tumor pathology. Cancer 1981;47:1786–95.

99. Petersen OW, van-Deurs B. Preservation of defined phenotypic traits in short-term cultured human breast carcinoma derived epithelial cells. Cancer Res 1987;47:856–66.

100. Sonnenberg A, Daams H, Van der Valk MA, Hilkens J, Hilgers J. Development of mouse mammary gland: identification of stages in differentiation of luminal and myoepithelial cells using monoclonal antibodies and polyvalent antiserum against keratin. J Histochem Cytochem 1986;34:1037–46.

101. Taylor-Papadimitriou J, Lane EB. Keratin expression in the mammary gland. In: Neville MC, Daniel CW, editors. The Mammary Gland. Development, Regulation and Function. New York and London: Plenum Press; 1987. p.191–215.

102. Daniel CW, Strickland P, Friedmann Y. Expression and functional role of E- and P-cadherins in mouse mammary ductal morphogenesis and growth. Dev Biol 1995;169:511–9.

103. Deugnier MA, Moiseyeva EP, Thiery JP, Glukhova M. Myoepithelial cell differentiation in the developing mammary gland: progressive acquisition of smooth muscle phenotype. Dev Dyn 1995;204:107–17.

104. Zou Z, Anisowicz A, Hendrix MJ, et al. Maspin, a serpin with tumor-suppressing activity in human mammary epithelial cells. Science 1994;263:526–9.

105. Nylander K, Vojtesek B, Nenutil R, et al. Differential expression of p63 isoforms in normal tissues and neoplastic cells. J Pathol 2002;198:417–27.

106. Reis-Filho JS, Milanezi F, Amendoeira I, Albergaria A, Schmitt FC. Distribution of p63, a novel myoepithelial marker, in fine-needle aspiration biopsies of the breast: an analysis of 82 samples. Cancer 2003; 99:172–9.

107. Di Como CJ, Urist MJ, Babayan I, et al. p63 expression profiles in human normal and tumor tissues. Clin Cancer Res 2002;8:494–501.

108. Werling RW, Hwang H, Yaziji H, Gown AM. Immunohistochemical distinction of invasive from noninvasive breast lesions: a comparative study of p63 versus calponin and smooth muscle myosin heavy chain. Am J Surg Pathol 2003;27:82–90.

109. Jenkins JS, Nussey SS. The role of oxytocin: present concepts. Clin Endocrinol (Oxf) 1991;34:515–25.

110. Soloff MS, Chakraborty J, Sadhukhan P, et al. Purification and characterization of mammary myoepithelial and secretory cells from the lactating rat. Endocrinology 1980;106:887–97.

111. Bartek J, Bartkova J, Taylor PJ. Keratin 19 expression in the adult and developing human mammary gland. Histochem J 1990;22:537–44.

112. Gomm JJ, Browne PJ, Coope RC, et al. Isolation of pure populations of epithelial and myoepithelial cells from the normal human mammary gland using immunomagnetic separation with Dynabeads. Anal Biochem 1995;226:91–9.

113. Guelstein VI, Tchypysheva TA, Ermilova VD, et al. Monoclonal antibody mapping of keratins 8 and 17 and of vimentin in normal human mammary gland, benign tumors, dysplasias and breast cancer. Int J Cancer 1988;42:147–53.

114. Mork C, van-Deurs B, Petersen OW. Regulation of vimentin expression in cultured human mammary epithelial cells. Differentiation 1990;43:146–56.

115. Nerlich AG, Lebeau A, Hagedorn HG, Sauer U, Schleicher ED. Morphological aspects of altered basement membrane metabolism in invasive carcinomas of the breast and the larynx. Anticancer Res 1998;18: 3515–20.

116. Viacava P, Naccarato AG, Collecchi P, et al. The spectrum of 67-kD laminin receptor expression in breast carcinoma progression. J Pathol 1997;182:36–44.

117. Djonov V, Hogger K, Sedlacek R, Laissue J, Draeger A. MMP-19: cellular localization of a novel metalloproteinase within normal breast tissue and mammary gland tumours. J Pathol 2001;195:147–55.

118. Rudolph-Owen LA, Matrisian LM. Matrix metalloproteinases in remodeling of the normal and neoplastic mammary gland. J Mammary Gland Biol Neoplasia 1998;3:177–89.

119. Kolb C, Mauch S, Peter HH, Krawinkel U, Sedlacek R. The matrix metalloproteinase RASI-1 is expressed in synovial blood vessels of a rheumatoid arthritis patient. Immunol Lett 1997;57:83–8.

120. Sternlicht MD, Kedeshian P, Shao ZM, Safarians S, Barsky SH. The human myoepithelial cell is a natural tumor suppressor. Clin Cancer Res 1997;3:1949–58.

121. Xiao G, Liu YE, Gentz R, et al. Suppression of breast cancer growth and metastasis by a serpin myoepithelium-derived serine proteinase inhibitor expressed in the mammary myoepithelial cells. Proc Natl Acad Sci U S A 1999;96:3700–5.

122. Streuli CH. Maspin is a tumour suppressor that inhibits breast cancer tumour metastasis in vivo. Breast Cancer Res 2002;4:137–40.

123. Yaziji H, Gown AM, Sneige N. Detection of stromal invasion in breast cancer: the myoepithelial markers. Adv Anat Pathol 2000;7:100–9.

124. Gottlieb C, Raju U, Greenwald KA. Myoepithelial cells in the differential diagnosis of complex benign and malignant breast lesions: an immunohistochemical study. Mod Pathol 1990;3:135–40.

125. Heatley M, Maxwell P, Whiteside C, Toner P. Cytokeratin intermediate filament expression in benign and malignant breast disease. J Clin Pathol 1995;48:26–32.

126. Joshi MG, Lee AK, Pedersen CA, et al. The role of immunocytochemical markers in the differential diagnosis of proliferative and neoplastic lesions of the breast. Mod Pathol 1996;9:57–62.

127. Viña M, Wells CA. Clear cell metaplasia of the breast: a lesion showing eccrine differentiation. Histopathol 1989;15:85–92.

128. Rasbridge SA, Millis RR. Carcinoma in-situ involving sclerosing adenosis: a mimic of invasive breast carcinoma [see comments]. Histopathol 1995;27:269–73.

129. Bose S, Lesser ML, Norton L, Rosen PP. Immunophenotype of intraductal carcinoma. Arch Pathol Lab Med 1996;120:81–5.

130. Takasaki T, Akiba S, Sagara Y, Yoshida H. Histological and biological characteristics of microinvasion in mammary carcinomas < or = 2 cm in diameter. Pathol Int 1998;48:800–5.

131. Monteagudo C, Merino MJ, San-Juan J, Liotta LA, Stetler SW. Immunohistochemical distribution of type IV collagenase in normal, benign, and malignant breast tissue. Am J Pathol 1990;136:585–92.

132. Warburton MJ, Ormerod EJ, Monaghan P, Ferns S, Rudland PS. Characterization of a myoepithelial cell line derived from a neonatal rat mammary gland. J Cell Biol 1981;91:827–36.

133. Keely PJ, Wu JE, Santoro SA. The spatial and temporal expression of the alpha 2 beta 1 integrin and its ligands, collagen I, collagen IV, and laminin, suggest important roles in mouse mammary morphogenesis. Differentiation 1995;59:1–13.

134. Dickson SR, Warburton MJ. Enhanced synthesis of gelatinase and stromelysin by myoepithelial cells during involution of the rat mammary gland. J Histochem Cytochem 1992;40:697–703.

135. Talhouk RS, Bissell MJ, Werb Z. Coordinated expression of extracellular matrix-degrading proteinases and their inhibitors regulates mammary epithelial function during involution. J Cell Biol 1992;118:1271–82.

136. Li F, Strange R, Friis RR, et al. Expression of stromelysin-1 and TIMP-1 in the involuting mammary

gland and in early invasive tumors of the mouse. Int J Cancer 1994;59:560–8.

137. Andersson LM, Dundas SR, O'Hare MJ, Gusterson BA, Warburton MJ. Synthesis of gelatinases by rat mammary epithelial and myoepithelial cell lines. Exp Cell Res 1994;212:389–92.

138. Nilsson S, Makela S, Treuter E, et al. Mechanisms of estrogen action. Physiol Rev 2001;81:1535–65.

139. Green S, Walter P, Kumar V, et al. Human oestrogen receptor cDNA: sequence, expression and homology to v-erb-A. Nature 1986;320:134–9.

140. Greene GL, Gilna P, Waterfield M, et al. Sequence and expression of human estrogen receptor complementary DNA. Science 1986;231:1150–4.

141. Kuiper GG, Enmark E, Pelto-Huikko M, Nilsson S, Gustafsson JA. Cloning of a novel receptor expressed in rat prostate and ovary. Proc Natl Acad Sci U S A 1996;93:5925–30.

142. Pettersson K, Gustafsson JA. Role of estrogen receptor beta in estrogen action. Annu Rev Physiol 2001;63:165–92.

143. Pelletier G, El Alfy M. Immunocytochemical localization of estrogen receptors alpha and beta in the human reproductive organs. J Clin Endocrinol Metab 2000;85:4835–40.

144. Saji S, Jensen EV, Nilsson S, et al. Estrogen receptors alpha and beta in the rodent mammary gland. Proc Natl Acad Sci U S A 2000;97:337–42.

145. Battersby S, Robertson BJ, Anderson TJ, King RJ, McPherson K. Influence of menstrual cycle, parity and oral contraceptive use on steroid hormone receptors in normal breast. Br J Cancer 1992;65:601–7.

146. Ricketts D, Turnbull L, Ryall G, et al. Estrogen and progesterone receptors in the normal female breast. Cancer Res 1991;51:1817–22.

147. Soderqvist G, von Schoultz B, Tani E, Skoog L. Estrogen and progesterone receptor content in breast epithelial cells from healthy women during the menstrual cycle. Am J Obstet Gynecol 1993;168:874–9.

148. Boyd M, Hildebrandt RH, Bartow SA. Expression of the estrogen receptor gene in developing and adult human breast. Breast Cancer Res Treat 1996;37:243–51.

149. Barnes DM. Progress in Pathology. Vol. vol. 2, Edinburgh: Churchill Livingstone; 1995.

150. Horwitz KB, Jackson TA, Bain DL, et al. Nuclear receptor coactivators and corepressors. Mol Endocrinol 1996;10:1167–77.

151. Dotzlaw H, Leygue E, Watson PH, Murphy LC. Expression of estrogen receptor-beta in human breast tumors. J Clin Endocrinol Metab 1997;82:2371–4.

152. Ogawa S, Inoue S, Watanabe T, et al. Molecular cloning and characterization of human estrogen receptor betacx: a potential inhibitor ofestrogen action in human. Nucleic Acids Res 1998;26:3505–12.

153. Wiesen JF, Young P, Werb Z, Cunha GR. Signaling through the stromal epidermal growth factor receptor is necessary for mammary ductal development. Development 1999;126:335–44.

154. Clarke RB, Howell A, Potten CS, Anderson E. Dissociation between steroid receptor expression and cell

proliferation in the human breast. Cancer Res 1997;57:4987–91.

155. Russo J, Ao X, Grill C, Russo IH. Pattern of distribution of cells positive for estrogen receptor alpha and progesterone receptor in relation to proliferating cells in the mammary gland. Breast Cancer Res Treat 1999;53:217–27.

156. Gustafsson JA, Warner M. Estrogen receptor beta in the breast: role in estrogen responsiveness and development of breast cancer. J Steroid Biochem Mol Biol 2000;74:245–8.

157. Laidlaw IJ, Clarke RB, Howell A, et al. The proliferation of normal human breast tissue implanted into athymic nude mice is stimulated by estrogen but not progesterone. Endocrinology 1995;136:164–71.

158. Chang KJ, Lee TT, Linares-Cruz G, Fournier S, de Lignieres B. Influences of percutaneous administration of estradiol and progesterone on human breast epithelial cell cycle in vivo. Fertil Steril 1995;63:785–91.

159. Ferguson DJ, Anderson TJ. Morphological evaluation of cell turnover in relation to the menstrual cycle in the "resting" human breast. Br J Cancer 1981;44:177–81.

160. Shoker BS, Jarvis C, Clarke RB, et al. Estrogen receptor-positive proliferating cells in the normal and precancerous breast. Am J Pathol 1999;155:1811–5.

161. Deng G, Lu Y, Zlotnikov G, Thor AD, Smith HS. Loss of heterozygosity in normal tissue adjacent to breast carcinomas. Science 1996;274:2057–9.

162. Lakhani SR, Chaggar R, Davies S, et al. Genetic alterations in 'normal' luminal and myoepithelial cells of the breast. J Pathol 1999;189:496–503.

163. Novelli M, Cossu A, Oukrif D, et al. X-inactivation patch size in human female tissue confounds the assessment of tumor clonality. Proc Natl Acad Sci U S A 2003;100:3311–4.

164. Moinfar F, Man YG, Arnould L, et al. Concurrent and independent genetic alterations in the stromal and epithelial cells of mammary carcinoma: implications for tumorigenesis. Cancer Res 2000;60:2562–6.

165. Larson PS, de las MA, Cupples LA, Huang K, Rosenberg CL. Genetically abnormal clones in histologically normal breast tissue. Am J Pathol 1998;152:1591–8.

166. Euhus DM, Cler L, Shivapurkar N, et al. Loss of heterozygosity in benign breast epithelium in relation to breast cancer risk. J Natl Cancer Inst 2002;94:858–60.

167. Li Z, Meng ZH, Chandrasekaran R, et al. Biallelic inactivation of the thyroid hormone receptor beta1 gene in early stage breast cancer. Cancer Res 2002;62:1939–43.

168. Li Z, Moore DH, Meng ZH, et al. Increased risk of local recurrence is associated with allelic loss in normal lobules of breast cancer patients. Cancer Res 2002;62:1000–3.

169. Zucca MP, Larson PS, Rosenberg CL, de las MA. Lack of correlation between morphometric analysis and presence of microsatellite alterations in proliferative ductal lesions of the breast. Anal Quant Cytol Histol 1999;21:369–73.

170. Poulin N, Susnik B, Guillaud M, et al. Histometric texture analysis of DNA in thin sections from breast

biopsies. Application to the detection of malignancy-associated changes in carcinoma in-situ. Anal Quant Cytol Histol 1995;17:291–9.

171. Tidow N, Boecker A, Schmidt H, et al. Distinct amplification of an untranslated regulatory sequence in the egfr gene contributes to early steps in breast cancer development. Cancer Res 2003;63:1172–8.

172. Charafe-Jauffret E, Moulin JF, Ginestier C, et al. Loss of heterozygosity at microsatellite markers from region p11–21 of chromosome 8 in microdissected breast tumor but not in peritumoral cells. Int J Oncol 2002;21:989–96.

173. Slaughter DP, Southwick HW, Smequal W. Field cancerization in oral stratified squamous epithelium. Cancer 1953;6:963–8.

174. Braakhuis BJ, Tabor MP, Kummer JA, Leemans CR, Brakenhoff RH. A genetic explanation of Slaughter's concept of field cancerization: evidence and clinical implications. Cancer Res 2003;63:1727–30.

175. Boecker W, Buerger H, Schmitz K, et al. Ductal epithelial proliferations of the breast: a biological continuum? Comparative genomic hybridisation and high-molecular-weight cytokeratin expression patterns. J Path 2001;195:415–21.

176. Muthuswamy SK, Li D, Lelievre S, Bissell MJ, Brugge JS. ErbB2, but not ErbB1, reinitiates proliferation and induces luminal repopulation in epithelial acini. Nat Cell Biol 2001;3:785–92.

177. Umbricht CB, Evron E, Gabrielson E, et al. Hypermethylation of 14–3–3 sigma (stratifin) is an early event in breast cancer. Oncogene 2001;20:3348–53.

178. Hassan HI, Walker RA. Decreased apoptosis in non-involved tissue from cancer-containing breasts. J Pathol 1998;184:258–64.

179. O'Connell P, Pekkel V, Fuqua SA, et al. Analysis of loss of heterozygosity in 399 premalignant breast lesions at 15 genetic loci. J Natl Cancer Inst 1998;90:697–703.

180. Dawson PJ, Baekey PA, Clark RA. Mechanisms of multifocal breast cancer: an immunocytochemical study. Hum Pathol 1995;26:965–9.

181. Fujii H, Marsh C, Cairns P, Sidransky D, Gabrielson E. Genetic divergence in the clonal evolution of breast cancer. Cancer Res 1996;56:1493–7.

182. Teixeira MR, Pandis N, Bardi G, et al. Clonal heterogeneity in breast cancer: karyotypic comparisons of multiple intra- and extra-tumorous samples from 3 patients. Int J Cancer 1995;63:63–8.

183. Going JJ, Stuart RC, Downie M, Fletcher-Monaghan AJ, Keith WN. 'Senescence-associated' beta-galactosidase activity in the upper gastrointestinal tract. J Pathol 2002;196:394–400.

184. Daniel CW, Silberstein GB. Developmental biology of the mammary gland. In: Neville MC, Daniel CW, editors. The Mammary Gland. 1st ed. New York: Plenum Press; 1987. p.3–36.

185. Sakakura T, Kusano I, Kusakabe M, Inaguma Y, Nishizuka Y. Biology of mammary fat pad in fetal mouse: capacity to support development of various fetal epithelia in vivo. Development 1987;100:421–30.

186. Chepko G, Smith GH. Three division-competent, structurally-distinct cell populations contribute to murine mammary epithelial renewal. Tissue Cell 1997;29: 239–53.

187. Friedman LS, Szabo CI, Ostermeyer EA, et al. Novel Inherited Mutations and Variable Expressivity of BRCA1 Alleles, Including the Founder Mutation 185delAG in Ashkenazi Jewish Families. Am J Hum Gen 1995;57:1284–97.

188. Trosko JE. Cloning of human stem cells: some broad scientific and philosophical issues. J Lab Clin Med 2000;135:432–6.

189. Dulbecco R, Henahan M, Armstrong B. Cell types and morphogenesis in the mammary gland. Proc Natl Acad Sci U S A 1982;79:7346–50.

190. Ferguson DJ. Intraepithelial lymphocytes and macrophages in the breast. Virchows Arch 1985;407:369–78.

191. Pechoux C, Gudjonsson T, Ronnov-Jessen L, Bissell MJ, Petersen OW. Human mammary luminal epithelial cells contain progenitors to myoepithelial cells. Dev Biol 1999;206:88–99.

192. Deugnier MA, Faraldo MM, Rousselle P, Thiery JP, Glukhova MA. Cell-extracellular matrix interactions and EGF are important regulators of the basal mammary epithelial cell phenotype. J Cell Sci 1999; 112 (Pt 7):1035–44.

193. Russo J, Russo IH. Development of human mammary gland. In: Neville MC, Daniel CW, editors. Mammary gland development regulation and function. New York: Plenum Press; 1987. p.67.

194. Russo IH, Russo J. Role of hormones in mammary cancer initiation and progression. J Mammary Gland Biol Neoplasia 1998;3:49–61.

195. Brisken C, Park S, Vass T, et al. A paracrine role for the epithelial progesterone receptor in mammary gland development. Proc Natl Acad Sci U S A 1998;95: 5076–81.

196. Zeps N, Bentel JM, Papadimitriou JM, D'Antuono MF, Dawkins HJ. Estrogen receptor-negative epithelial cells in mouse mammary gland development and growth. Differentiation 1998;62:221–6.

197. Dickson RB, Lippman ME. Growth regulation of normal and malignant breast epithelium. In: Bland KI, Copeland EM, editors. The breast. Philadelphia: WB Saunders; 1998. p.518.

198. Hamilton NJ, Boyd JD, Mossman HW. Human embryology. Cambridge (UK): Heffer; 1968.

199. Hughes ESR. Development of the mammary gland. Ann Roy Coll Surg Eng 1950;6:99.

200. Dawson EK. A histological study of the normal mamma in relation to tumour growth. I. Early development to maturity. Edinb Med J 1934;653.

201. Dabelow A. Milchdrüse. In: Bargmann W, editor. Handbuch der Mikroskopischen Anatomie des Menschen. Berlin: Springer-Verlag; 1957.

202. Dickson RB, Russo J. Biochemical Control of Breast Development. In: Harris JR, Lippman ME, Morrow M, Kent Osborne C, editors. Diseases of the Breast. 2 nd ed ed. Philadelphia: Lippincott Williams & Wilkins; 2001. p.15–31.

203. Rudland PS. Histochemical organization and cellular composition of ductal buds in developing human breast: evidence of cytochemical intermediates

between epithelial and myoepithelial cells. J Histochem Cytochem 1991;39:1471–84.

204. Osin PP, Anbazhagan R, Bartkova J, Nathan B, Gusterson BA. Breast development gives insights into breast disease. Histopathol 1998;33:275–83.

205. Anbazhagan R, Bartek J, Monaghan P, Gusterson BA. Growth and development of the human infant breast. Am J Anat 1991;192:407–17.

206. Osborne MP, Osborne M. Breast Anatomy and Development. In: Harris JR, editor. Diseases of the Breast. 2nd ed. Philadelphia: Lippincott, Williams & Wilkins; 2000. p.1–13.

207. Sutherland RL, Prall OW, Watts CK, Musgrove EA. Estrogen and progestin regulation of cell cycle progression. J Mammary Gland Biol Neoplasia 1998;3:63–72.

208. Medina D. The mammary gland: a unique organ for the study of development and tumorigenesis. J Mammary Gland Biol Neoplasia 1996;1:5–19.

209. Snedeker SM, Brown CF, DiAugustine RP. Expression and functional properties of transforming growth factor alpha and epidermal growth factor during mouse mammary gland ductal morphogenesis. Proc Natl Acad Sci U S A 1991;88:276–80.

210. Liscia DS, Merlo G, Ciardiello F, et al. Transforming growth factor-alpha messenger RNA localization in the developing adult rat and human mammary gland by in-situ hybridization. Dev Biol 1990;140:123–31.

211. Jackson D, Bresnick J, Dickson C. A role for fibroblast growth factor signaling in the lobuloalveolar development of the mammary gland. J Mammary Gland Biol Neoplasia 1997;2:385–92.

212. Daniel CW, Robinson S, Silberstein GB. The role of TGF-beta in patterning and growth of the mammary ductal tree. J Mammary Gland Biol Neoplasia 1996;1:331–41.

213. Nusse R, Varmus HE. Wnt genes. Cell 1992;69: 1073–87.

214. Coleman S, Silberstein GB, Daniel CW. Ductal morphogenesis in the mouse mammary gland: evidence supporting a role for epidermal growth factor. Dev Biol 1988;127:304–15.

215. Vonderhaar BK. Local effects of EGF, alpha-TGF, and EGF-like growth factors on lobuloalveolar development of the mouse mammary gland in vivo. J Cell Physiol 1987;132:581–4.

216. Matsui Y, Halter SA, Holt JT, Hogan BL, Coffey RJ. Development of mammary hyperplasia and neoplasia in MMTV-TGF alpha transgenic mice. Cell 1990;61:1147–55.

217. Pierce-DF J, Johnson MD, Matsui Y, et al. Inhibition of mammary duct development but not alveolar outgrowth during pregnancy in transgenic mice expressing active TGF-beta 1. Genes Dev 1993;7:2308–17.

218. Gavin BJ, McMahon AP. Differential regulation of the Wnt gene family during pregnancy and lactation suggests a role in postnatal development of the mammary gland. Mol Cell Biol 1992;12:2418–23.

219. Buhler TA, Dale TC, Kieback C, Humphreys RC, Rosen JM. Localization and quantification of Wnt-2 gene expression in mouse mammary development. Dev Biol 1993;155:87–96.

220. Petersen OW, Ronnov-Jessen L, Howlett AR, Bissell MJ. Interaction with basement membrane serves to rapidly distinguish growth and differentiation pattern of normal and malignant human breast epithelial cells. Proc Natl Acad Sci U S A 1992;89:9064–8.

221. Gudjonsson T, Ronnov-Jessen L, Villadsen R, et al. Normal and tumor-derived myoepithelial cells differ in their ability to interact with luminal breast epithelial cells for polarity and basement membrane deposition. J Cell Sci 2002;115:39–50.

222. Witty JP, Wright JH, Matrisian LM. Matrix metalloproteinases are expressed during ductal and alveolar mammary morphogenesis, and misregulation of stromelysin-1 in transgenic mice induces unscheduled alveolar development. Mol Biol Cell 1995;6:1287–303.

223. Sympson CJ, Talhouk RS, Alexander CM, et al. Targeted expression of stromelysin-1 in mammary gland provides evidence for a role of proteinases in branching morphogenesis and the requirement for an intact basement membrane for tissue-specific gene expression. J Cell Biol 1994;125:681–93.

224. Wilson CL, Heppner KJ, Rudolph LA, Matrisian LM. The metalloproteinase matrilysin is preferentially expressed by epithelial cells in a tissue-restricted pattern in the mouse. Mol Biol Cell 1995;6:851–69.

225. Wilson CL, Matrisian LM. Matrilysin: an epithelial matrix metalloproteinase with potentially novel functions. Int J Biochem Cell Biol 1996;28:123–36.

226. Pullan S, Wilson J, Metcalfe A, et al. Requirement of basement membrane for the suppression of programmed cell death in mammary epithelium. J Cell Sci 1996;109 (Pt 3):631–42.

227. Alexander CM, Howard EW, Bissell MJ, Werb Z. Rescue of mammary epithelial cell apoptosis and entactin degradation by a tissue inhibitor of metalloproteinases-1 transgene. J Cell Biol 1996;135:1669–77.

228. Rudolph-Owen LA, Cannon P, Matrisian LM. Overexpression of the matrix metalloproteinase matrilysin results in premature mammary gland differentiation and male infertility. Mol Biol Cell 1998;9:421–35.

229. Kenney NJ, Smith GH, Maroulakou IG, et al. Detection of amphiregulin and Cripto-1 in mammary tumors from transgenic mice. Mol Carcinog 1996;15:44–56.

230. Jhappan C, Geiser AG, Kordon EC, et al. Targeting expression of a transforming growth factor beta 1 transgene to the pregnant mammary gland inhibits alveolar development and lactation. EMBO J 1993;12: 1835–45.

231. Koli KM, Ramsey TT, Ko Y, et al. Blockade of transforming growth factor-beta signaling does not abrogate antiestrogen-induced growth inhibition of human breast carcinoma cells. J Biol Chem 1997;272:8296–302.

232. Reiss M, Barcellos-Hoff MH. Transforming growth factor-beta in breast cancer: a working hypothesis. Breast Cancer Res Treat 1997;45:81–95.

233. Lewis MT. Homeobox genes in mammary gland development and neoplasia. Breast Cancer Res 2000;2: 158–69.

234. Salazar H, Tobon H, Josimovich JB. Developmental, gestational and postgestional modifications of the human breast. Clinical Obstetrics and Gynecology 1975;18:113–37.

235. Coleman-Krnacik S, Rosen JM. Differential temporal and spatial gene expression of fibroblast growth factor family members during mouse mammary gland development. Mol Endocrinol 1994;8:218–29.

236. Vorherr H. Factors influencing fetal growth. Am J Obstet Gynecol 1982;142:577–88.

237. Battersby S, Anderson TJ. Proliferative and secretory activity in the pregnant and lactating human breast. Virchows Archiv A 1988;413:189–96.

238. Lascelles AK, Lee CS. Involution of the mammary gland. In: Larson BE, editor. Lactation. A comprehensive treatise. New York: Academic Press; 1978.

239. Strange R, Li F, Saurer S, Burkhardt A, Friis RR. Apoptotic cell death and tissue remodelling during mouse mammary gland involution. Development 1992;115:49–58.

240. Anderson TJ. Classifying benign breast changes [letter]. Lancet 1988;1:240–1.

241. Benaud C, Dickson RB, Thompson EW. Roles of the matrix metalloproteinases in mammary gland development and cancer. Breast Cancer Res Treat 1998;50:97–116.

242. Lefebvre O, Wolf C, Limacher JM, et al. The breast cancer-associated stromelysin-3 gene is expressed during mouse mammary gland apoptosis. J Cell Biol 1992;119:997–1002.

243. Battersby S, Anderson TJ. Histological changes in breast tissue that characterize recent pregnancy. Histopathol 1989;15:415–33.

244. Howard BA, Gusterson BA. Human breast development. J Mammary Gland Biol Neoplasia 2000;5:119–37.

245. Hutson SW, Cowen PN, Bird CC. Morphometric studies of age related changes in normal human breast and their significance for evolution of mammary cancer. J Clin Pathol 1985;38:281–7.

246. Prechtel K. Mastopathie und altersabhängige Brustdrüsenveränderungen. Fortschr Med 1971;89:1312–5.

247. Haagensen CD. Anatomy of the Mammary Glands. In: Haagensen CD, editor. Diseases of the Breast. 3rd ed. Philadelphia: Saunders; 1986. p.1–46.

Content

2

FIBROCYSTIC CHANGE AND MISCELLANEOUS 'NON-NEOPLASTIC' EPITHELIAL AND STROMAL LESIONS

WERNER BOECKER, SYLVIA HEYWANG-KOEBRUNNER, STEFANIE WEIGEL AND WALTER HEINDEL

The breast is subject to constant developmental and cyclical changes. Orchestrated by complex hormonal interactions, such changes ensure that even 'normal' breast tissue displays a histological spectrum of considerable width. This chapter is dedicated to those lesions which have mostly come to be regarded as physiological variants of normal breast morphology, in particular fibrocystic change. In addition, we discuss a number of miscellaneous non-neoplastic epithelial and/or mesenchymal lesions of the breast.

Fibrocystic change is the term commonly used to refer to alterations characterized by cyst formation, often with apocrine change, fibrosis, blunt duct adenosis and mild usual ductal hyperplasia. It is important to realize that only the lobular units are affected, with dilatation and confluence of lobular ductules and unfolding of lobules. Fibrocystic change is the most common disorder of the breast in women between the ages of 20 and 45. Most authors agree that there is no evidence that fibrocystic change, as such, is usually associated with an increased breast cancer risk.

Miscellaneous 'non-neoplastic' epithelial and stromal lesions. Upon histological examination, a great number of other clinically and prognostically irrelevant lesions may be detected in breast tissue. Most of these are generally conceived of as aberrations of normal development and involution (ANDI). Examples include lactational (pregnancy-like) change, myoepithelial hyperplasia, blunt duct adenosis, and mild forms of epithelial ductal hyperplasia. Collagenous spherulosis and a number of stromal lesions have also been included in this chapter. **A clear distinction must be made between these lesions and benign proliferative breast disease:** the latter is associated with an increased breast cancer risk.

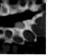

Fibrocystic change

■ DEFINITION

Fibrocystic change includes gross and/or microscopic cysts (Fig. 2.1), apocrine metaplasia, fibrosis, blunt duct adenosis and minor degrees of sclerosing adenosis and epithelial hyperplasia [1–5]. In recent times several terms have been applied to the complex of fibrocystic change such as cystic or fibrocystic disease, chronic cystic mastitis, mazoplasia, fibrous mastopathy, fibroadenosis cystica, mammary dysplasia, Reclus' disease and Schimmelbusch's disease. It must be acknowledged that many of these terms were used to include other proliferative epithelial changes such as adenosis, fibroadenoma and ductal hyperplasia. An important step has been made by realizing that the presence and type of epithelial proliferation determine the risk of subsequent carcinoma rather than fibrocystic disease per se. A detailed review on this subject is given in the publication by Love et al. [4]. The term 'fibrocystic disease' was abandoned in favor of 'fibrocystic change', as defined above at the consensus meeting in New York in 1985 [6].

■ CONCEPTUAL APPROACH

Cystic change is an alteration of lobules [5]. Three-dimensional studies of sections with fibrocystic change have established that the cysts gradually develop by dilatation and coalescence of ductules with unfolding of the terminal duct lobular units (Fig. 2.2). There is, however, controversy as to the mechanisms that govern this process [5, 7–11].

Most experts in the field agree that fibrocystic change is the result of an exaggerated process of involution or mechanical obstruction of ductules, caused by overgrowth of fibrous tissue. Persistence of secretory activity of apocrine cells leads to the formation of cysts. On the other hand cysts may contain multilayered and even papillary epithelium, indicative of a proliferative process [12].

There is evidence that endogenous and exogenous factors may play a role [13, 14]. Interestingly, patients with fibrocystic change often show a relative excess of estrogen over progesterone, and hormonal imbalances must therefore be taken into account [15–17]. This is in line with reports according to which the use of oral contraceptives decreases the risk of fibrocystic change owing to their potential to

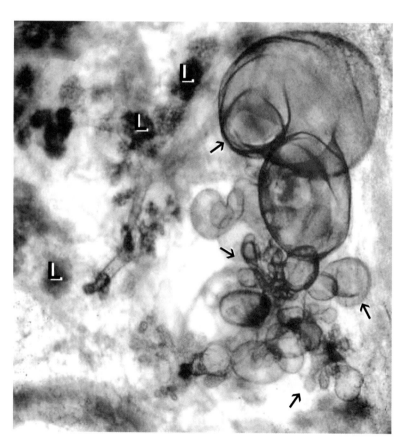

Fig. 2.1 Submacroscopy of an area with fibrocystic change. The affected TDLUs are distended and increased to several times the size of normal lobules. Compare the fibrocystic changes in the right field (arrows) with the normal lobules (L) in the left field.

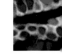

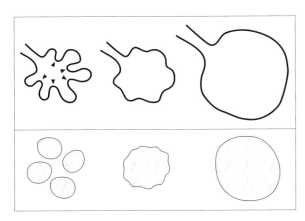

Fig. 2.2 Wellings et al. showed that unfolding of lobules represents the main process in fibrocystic change, as depicted in this figure.

adjust hormonal imbalances. Other hormonal abnormalities that have been implied include hyperprolactinemia and increased thyroid hormone activity [18]. The cellular composition of the epithelial structures in fibrocystic change is reminiscent of normal breast epithelium (see Chapter 1). One of the most characteristic findings is apocrine change of the cells lining the cysts. Several proteins known as gross cystic disease fluid proteins (GCDFP) have been found in cystic fluid, in particular types 15 and 24. These proteins were shown to be specifically expressed in apocrine epithelium [19, 20], (for details see Chapter 3).

Several reports claim a positive association of fibrocystic change with excess consumption of tea, coffee, chocolates and certain cola drinks [21, 22]. However, this has not been confirmed in other studies [23, 24].

■ CLINICAL FEATURES AND IMAGING

CLINICAL FEATURES

Fibrocystic change occurs with great frequency in the general population [25], both in clinically normal breasts (~ 50%) [25, 26] and in cancer-bearing breasts (~ 25 to 40%) [27]. It is rare below the age of thirty [26]. Fibrocystic change usually affects both breasts with formation of palpable nodularity in the breast tissue. Occasionally, the process is more localized, producing a clinically detectable lump. When symptomatic, patients complain of breast pain, tenderness or swelling with multiple nodules and possible palpable lumps or cysts in both breasts. Symptomatic women may also complain of menstrual abnormalities, and they usually do not take oral contraceptives. With menopause and involution the symptoms may subside.

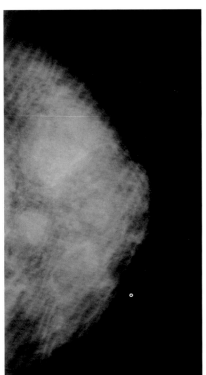

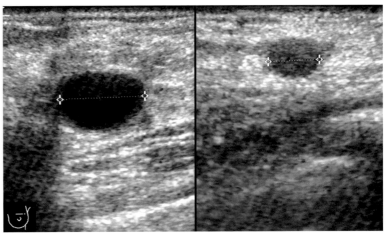

Fig. 2.3a – b Fibrocystic change.
2.3a Mammogram showing a dense background and several dense round masses with well-defined margins.
2.3b Breast ultrasound image of the same patient as in 2.3a. The ultrasound image shows an anechoic mass with acoustic distal enhancement due to a simple cyst (left) (BI-RADS 2). An adjacent mass (right) is depicted with internal echoes, representing a complicated cyst as a result of hemorrhage. Such cysts are difficult to distinguish from a solid lesion (BI-RADS 3).

2 Fibrocystic change and miscellaneous 'non-neoplastic' epithelial and stromal lesions

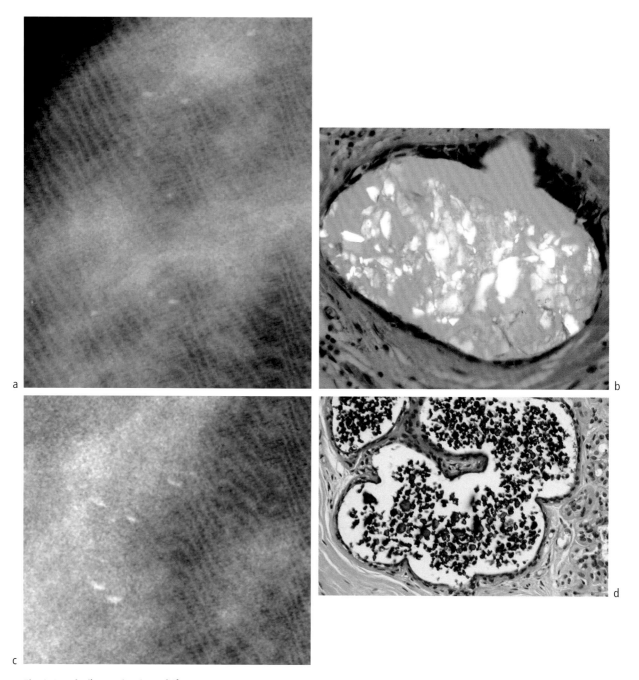

Fig. 2.4a – d Fibrocystic microcalcifications.
2.4a This figure shows low-density, round-shaped, coarse microcalcifications of diffuse pattern. In the absence of features such as pleomorphism or branching this aspect is essentially benign or, at worst, indicative of low-risk calcifications. These calcifications were classified as BI-RADS 2.
2.4b Histology of an H&E stained section. This cyst contains many calcium oxalate crystals (wedellite). These calcifications present as transparent, amber-colored material on H&E sections. They are birefringent and can therefore be identified under polarized light.
2.4c Magnification of a lateral view showing microcalcifications with a 'teacup' appearance due to sedimentation of calcificated particles within cysts.
2.4d Histology of a cyst containing small dense hematoxyphilic lamellar calcifications. The calcified material may sediment onto the floor of the cyst to produce the 'teacup' calcification pattern seen in Figure 2.4c.

Whether fibrocystic change is a marker of elevated cancer risk has been addressed in a number of publications [2–4, 28–33]. Haagensen's and Page's results [28, 30] suggest that macroscopic cysts and papillary apocrine cysts may be associated with a slightly increased risk of cancer (twice the average incidence). The currently prevailing view shared by most experts in the field is that neither fibrocystic nor apocrine change have any significant impact on cancer risk.

IMAGING

MAMMOGRAPHY

Mammograms and ultrasound scans of fibrocystic change are characterized by cysts, densities and/or microcalcifications. Generalized fibrocystic change appears as nodular thickening of breast tissue. The appearance of calcifications may show the classic 'teacup' phenomenon (see above). Mammographically, cysts are round or ovoid masses, usually with low to intermediate density. There is usually no tissue reaction surrounding the cysts (Fig. 2.3a). Cysts cannot be distinguished from solid masses on mammography. Benign cystic changes may be associated with microcalcifications. The following features are indicative of benign change.

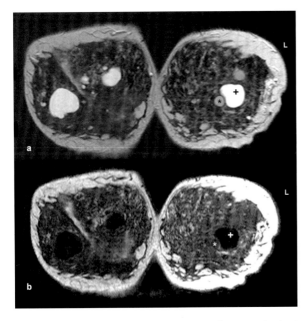

Fig. 2.5a–b Coronal magnetic resonance images obtained from a patient with proven cysts on ultrasound. The uncomplicated cyst (+) shows a hyperintense signal on T2-weighted sequences (2.5a) and a hypointense signal on T1-weighted images (2.5b). The complicated cyst (*) is depicted as an intermediate signal on both sequences due to its higher protein content. No enhancement was present in the dynamic study.

- Granular calcifications, which are symmetrically distributed and scattered. On mammography they have a coarse, irregular pattern and show low to medium density (Fig. 2.4a–b). These calcifications represent calcium oxalate deposits.
- Fine, punctate or round calcifications with medium to high density indicating lobular calcifications. Usually, these are densely packed calcifications arranged in a rosette-like fashion. The calcifications represent calcium phosphate deposits. Contrary to their ductal counterparts, lobular microcalcifications are not indicative of malignancy; however, well-differentiated in-situ carcinomas usually display patterns of calcification identical to benign changes.
- 'Teacup' calcifications representing lakes of sedimented calcium deposits within cysts. On the cranio-caudal mammographic view these calcifications appear as indistinct amorphous 'lakes' of calcium, mostly 0.5–3 mm in size. They are diagnosed on the 90% lateral view, where the typical 'teacup' sign is visible (Fig. 2.4c–d). The lower portion of the cyst is filled with dense calcium and thus sharply outlined with a convex lower margin. As a result of calcium sedimentation within the cysts a horizontal apical surface is produced, which corresponds to fluid with differing concentration of milk of calcium. Identification of such 'teacup' calcifications indicates benign changes, provided that no additional suspicious calcifications are observed.

ULTRASOUND

Ultrasound is the most important modality in assessing a cyst. Ultrasound of cysts shows well-defined anechoic masses with through transition of sound causing increased echogenicity of the posterior tissue (Fig. 2.3b). Echoes within the cysts can be due to blood clots, increased protein content as a result of inflammation or tumor formation.

MAGNETIC RESONANCE IMAGING

Cystic changes are well-circumscribed lesions of high signal intensity on T2-weighted sequences and of low signal intensity on T1-weighted images. The signal intensity can increase due to a high protein content or hemorrhage (Fig. 2.5a–b). Associated enhancement may be seen in combination with inflammatory conditions. Due to the accuracy of ultrasound in assessing cystic change, magnetic resonance is not used routinely.

■ PATHOLOGY

MACROSCOPY

The cut surface of fibrocystic change is characterized by cysts of varying size filled with straw-colored to dark brown fluid (Fig. 2.6). Due to their appearance the larger cysts are known as 'blue-dome' cysts. The cysts sit in a fibrofatty to fibrous tissue.

HISTOLOGY

The hallmarks of fibrocystic change are:
1. cysts of varying size,
2. apocrine metaplasia and hyperplasia,
3. fibrosis,
4. blunt duct adenosis and its variants and/or minor forms of hyperplasia.

Cysts are the most common feature of fibrocystic change found in patients presenting with a breast lump. Cysts often occur in clusters (Fig. 2.7) and can measure up to several centimeters. Cystic fluid contains a group of proteins (gross cystic disease fluid proteins, GCDFPs [34]), electrolytes and immunoglobulins. Smaller cysts coalesce to form larger cysts. Cysts of 1–2 mm in diameter have cuboidal or typical apocrine glandular epithelium and an outer layer of myoepithelium, while larger cysts are often lined by an attenuated and flattened epithelium and myoepithelium. In H&E sections the myoepithelium may be missing, but can usually be demonstrated in sm-actin immunostains. Occasionally, only a single cell layer is found or the epithelium may be completely missing.

Apocrine metaplasia is frequently found in fibrocystic change [35] (Fig. 2.8a–b, see Chapter 4). Generally, apocrine metaplasia is seen in a lobular cluster of cystic ductules similar to blunt duct adenosis. The cells may be moderately pleomorphic and may even show micropapillary or small papillary tufts [30] (papillary apocrine change). Although the nuclei are usually large, they are monomorphic and normochromatic and contain a single uniform nucleolus. The association of these cells with normal cells in adjacent epithelial structures helps the pathologist avoid categorizing these cells as malignant.

Although **fibrosis and hyalinization** of tissue are features often associated with fibrocystic change they show considerable variations in intensity.

Calcifications are occasionally seen, which are of two types: those composed of calcium phosphate and those of calcium oxalate (wedellite). The first are non-crystalline, non-birefringent, densely hematoxyphilic, and round to ovoid deposits, which are easily recognized on H&E sections. The individual deposit

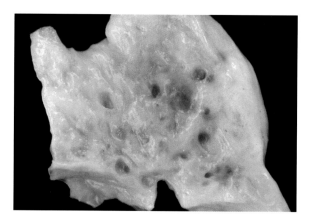

Fig. 2.6 Fibrocystic change in an excision biopsy. Cysts are surrounded by fibrosis of the stroma. Note the blue color of some of the cysts.

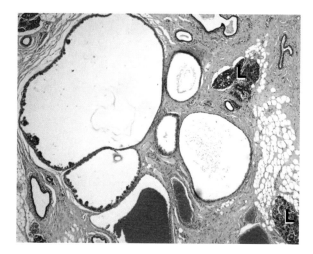

Fig. 2.7 Low power view of fibrocystic change with several distended TDLUs which are lined in part by apocrine, in part by flat epithelium. The specialized stroma turned fibrotic and is indistinguishable from normal interlobular stroma. On the right normal lobules (L) and an interlobular duct.

may be of small size so that calcifications are only identified mammographically when present in clusters or as calcified contents in the cyst fluid (Fig. 2.4c–d). The latter is rarely encountered in breast pathology and consists of amber material easily missed on H&E sections. However, wedellite appears as large, angulated, birefringent crystals in polarized light. It is nearly always associated with benign disease and is typically found in apocrine cysts [36].

Blunt duct adenosis and minor forms of proliferative lesions such as sclerosing adenosis and mild ductal hyperplasia are a common finding in fibrocystic change. From the available data we conclude that these changes are not associated with an increased risk of developing breast carcinoma.

Sometimes, **tension cysts** evolve in the process of fibrocystic change. They are defined as apocrine cysts

Tab. 2.1 Distinguishing features of fibrocystic change and periductal mastitis/duct ectasia

	Fibrocystic change	Duct ectasia
Definition	Disease of the terminal duct lobular units characterized by cystic transformation and confluence of ductules with an unfolding process of the lobular structures.	Chronic inflammatory disease of ducts, mainly major subareolar ducts, usually with a segmental centrifugal spread.
Pathology	Lobules with small cystic ductules usually found in clusters. Later cysts coalesce to form larger cysts associated with an unfolding process with flattening of the epithelium. Inflammatory reaction only when cysts rupture.	Severe periductal inflammation with lymphocytes, plasma cells and macrophages around non-dilated ducts. Granulomatous reaction with giant cells not uncommon. Later, duct fibrosis and hyalinosis with duct dilation or obliteration of ducts by fibrous plugs. Calcification of duct walls common. Lumen contains macrophages and cell debris.
Epithelial composition	Typical apocrine metaplasia with attenuated appearance as the cysts enlarge. Outer myoepithelial cells attenuated.	Normal duct epithelium. May be destroyed by inflammatory process. Occasionally squamous metaplasia. Myoepithelial cells inconspicuous.
Clinical presentation	Involves periphery of parenchymal tree. Palpable nodularity of both breasts, occasionally localized lumps. Tenderness and swelling in some cases. No nipple discharge.	Nipple inversion, mass formation. Involves mainly subareolar ducts. Nipple discharge.
Radiology	Cysts present as round or oval masses. Typical ultrasound with anechoic mass(es) with posterior acoustic enhancement. Benign calcifications, e. g. 'teacup' calcifications.	Tubular radio-opaque retroalveolar structures, microcalcifications (ring or tubular etc.). On ultrasound, dilated ducts with anechoic fluid or echogenic debris.

Modified according to Table 5-1 in: *Problems in Breast Pathology* by JG Azzopardi (1979), pp 58–59.

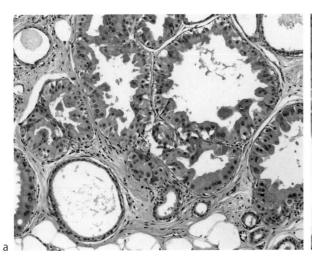
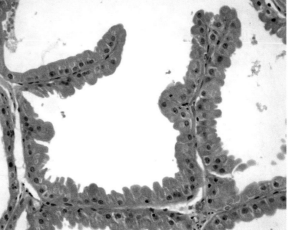

a b

Fig. 2.8a–b Fibrocystic change with typical apocrine metaplasia.
2.8a Lobular cluster of cystic ductules lined by micropapillary apocrine benign epithelium characterized by its granular, deeply eosinophilic cytoplasm. Note the flattened apocrine epithelial cells at the periphery.
2.8b Higher magnification showing the typical cytological features of apocrine cells with abundant eosinophilic granular cytoplasm. Note the regular spacing of the nuclei.

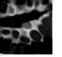

containing fluid under pressure, often with rupture and inflammation [5]. Clinically, ruptured cysts present as a painful and tender lump. Tension cysts usually have a highly attenuated, barely visible apocrine epithelial lining and a fibrous capsule. Often the lining is detached. The lumen may contain foam cells. If ruptured, the cyst shows an inflammatory infiltrate containing neutrophils, foamy histiocytes, lymphocytes and plasma cells. The extrusion of particulate matter such as crystalline may elicit a strong histiocytic inflammatory reaction including foreign body giant cells.

■ INTERPRETATION OF CORE AND ■ VACUUM-ASSISTED BIOPSIES

Histologically, lesions of fibrocystic change are easy to diagnose. They must be classified as B2 lesions. The differential diagnosis includes cystic hypersecretory hyperplasia, mucocele-like lesions (see below) and flat epithelial atypia (see Chapter 18). It is important not to over-diagnose papillary apocrine proliferations as atypical (see Chapter 19).

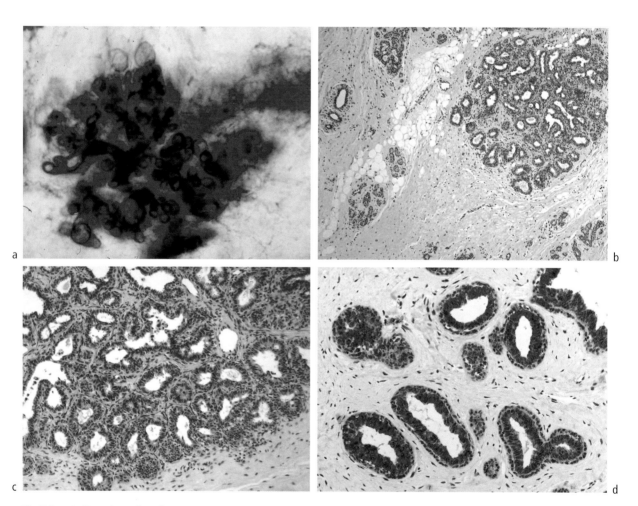

Fig. 2.9a–g Blunt duct adenosis.
2.9a Submacroscopic view of an adenotic lobule with organoid architecture. The number and size of the acinar structures are increased.
2.9b Low power view showing an enlarged lobule with an increase in the number of ductules (acini) compared with normal lobules in the left field.
2.9c High power view of the adenotic lobule shown in Figure 2.9b highlights a disorderly luminal epithelium with some epithelial tufting. These features distinguish blunt duct adenosis from flat epithelial atypia, which is usually characterized by a monotonous atypical epithelium.
2.9d Ck5 immunohistochemistry. Part of the adenotic lobule, showing intense but heterogeneous staining of the epithelium with Ck5, a characteristic feature of benign epithelium.
Continuation

Miscellaneous 'non-neoplastic' epithelial and stromal lesions

DEFINITION

This section describes a variety of epithelial lesions and some stromal alterations. Most of these lesions in themselves are benign and do not bear an increased breast cancer risk. However, lesions such as cystic hypersecretory hyperplasia and mucocele-like lesions have to be examined very carefully to exclude any associated malignancy.

CONCEPTUAL APPROACH

Some miscellaneous 'non-neoplastic' epithelial lesions are currently regarded as variations of normal development and involution of the breast (aberration of normal development and involution = ANDI) [7]. Examples include blunt duct adenosis, mild ductal hyperplasia, tiny microscopic lesions of sclerosing adenosis and fibroadenomatoid lesions, small microscopic acinar cysts, fibro-nodular densities, lactational or apocrine change and myoepithelial hyperplasia. At both ends of the spectrum, several of these lesions merge into the appearances of either normal structures of the breast parenchyma or their classic pathological counterparts [5].

Most non-neoplastic epithelial lesions show the same cellular constituents as normal breast epithelium. On a cellular level some of these lesions are reminiscent of simple organoid hyperplastic lesions of breast parenchyma such as blunt duct adenosis or myoepitheliosis. Other lesions can be categorized as glandular metaplasias and are described in more detail in Chapter 4. The nature of collagenous spherulosis is currently poorly understood, yet its similarity with adenoid-cystic carcinoma is striking (see below and Chapter 20).

The exact etiology and nature of pseudo-angiomatous hyperplasia are still unknown.

CLINICAL FINDINGS AND IMAGING

Most of those lesions have no specific characteristics. Cystic hypersecretory hyperplasia, mucocele-like lesions and pseudo-angiomatous hyperplasia, however, may present as palpable tumors or be found on mammography and ultrasound as ill-defined masses.

PATHOLOGY

MACROSCOPY

The macroscopic appearance of most of these lesions is non-specific. Excised tissue often appears quite normal or may contain ill-defined areas of indurated gray-white tissue as seen in fibrocystic change [37–39].

Grossly cystic hypersecretory hyperplasia and mucocele-like lesions are characterized by an aggregation of cystic spaces and a certain degree of fibrosis. The cysts are filled with serous fluid or mucin.

HISTOLOGY

EPITHELIAL LESIONS
BLUNT DUCT ADENOSIS
This name was originally proposed by Foote and Stewart [33]. Blunt duct adenosis is characterized by a numerical increase of individual ductules within single lobules, lined by altered glandular and myoepithelial cells [5, 40]. The lobular architecture is retained and there is usually some dilatation of the ductules. Based on their glandular appearance several forms of blunt duct adenosis can be distinguished:

1. The first form shows overall lobular architecture of the lesions at low magnification with enlarged ductular spaces containing a hypertrophic glandular-myoepithelial cell layer (Fig. 2.9a–g) [5]. The glandular cells display Ck5/14 mosaicism similar in appearance to usual ductal hyperplasia (Fig. 2.9d). Transitions to micropapillary epithelial proliferations may be seen. Most authors agree that these lesions are not associated with an increased risk of malignancy [41].

2. The second form displays a glandular layer with a monotonous appearance, referred to in the literature as 'cylinder cell change without atypia' [42–47]. The glandular cells usually display columnar cell morphology with evenly spaced, oval, darkly stained nuclei (Fig. 2.9e–f). Other features may include increased cytoplasm and apical snouts. The glandular cells express Ck8/18, but lack Ck5/14 (Fig. 2.9g). Recently the EC Working Group on Breast Screening Pathology recommended classifying such lesions as fibrocystic change (Wells CA et al., European Guidelines for Quality Assurance in Mammography Screening – Fourth Edition, Office for Official Publications of the European Communities [in press]).

3. The third form is characterized by apocrine change (compare Fig. 2.8). These lesions usually contain a lobular cluster of cysts lined by non-malignant apocrine cells with micropapillary tufts or even

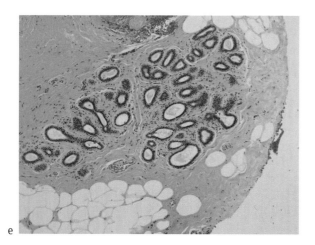

e

papillary structures, which clearly indicate a proliferative process. Although several molecular studies have provided data suggesting a clonal proliferation of apocrine cells (for details see Chapters 4 and 9) there is currently no evidence that patients with such lesions are at an increased risk for development of carcinoma. We therefore include these lesions in the category of blunt duct adenosis and classify them as blunt duct adenosis, apocrine type.

All forms of blunt duct adenosis lesions must be distinguished from flat epithelial atypia/atypical ductal hyperplasia and other unrelated lesions such as cystic hypersecretory hyperplasia and mucocele-like lesions. [48].

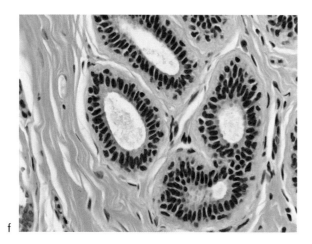

f

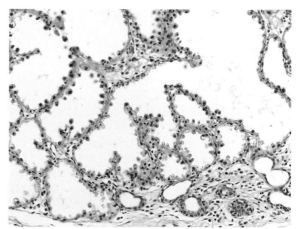

Fig. 2.10 Focal lactational change with enlarged, distended acini in an overall enlarged lobule.

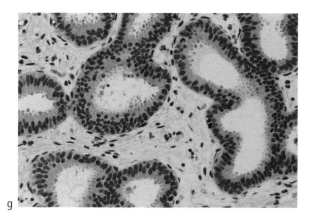

g

Fig. 2.9a–g Blunt duct adenosis.
2.9e Blunt duct adenosis demonstrating cylinder cell change without atypia. Adenotic lobule with enlarged, cystically dilated ductules, which are lined by a monomorphic epithelium with oval, hyperchromatic nuclei.
2.9f High magnification of the lesion shown in Figure 2.9e highlighting the monotonous cylinder cell change. The nuclei are deeply stained, slightly enlarged and usually oval. Such cellular monotony suggests clonal cell growth, but there is no evidence that such lesions are associated with an increased cancer risk.
2.9g Cylinder cell change is negative to Ck5 immunostaining.

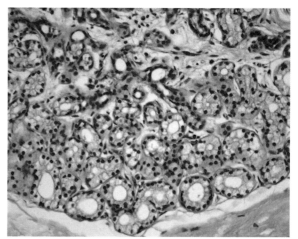

Fig. 2.11 Clear cell change. The normal glandular cells of this lobule are replaced by pale, finely granular cells. Note some normal glandular cells in the upper part of the figure.

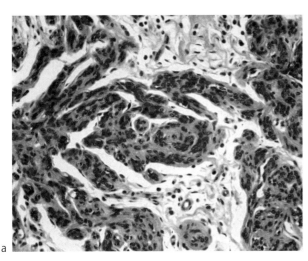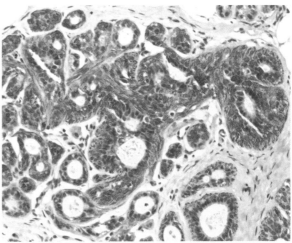

a   b

Fig. 2.12a – b Myoepithelial hyperplasia (myoepitheliosis).
2.12a Several lobules with preserved architecture showing an increased number of myoepithelial cells surrounding the somewhat flattened glandular epithelium.
2.12b Sm-actin immunohistochemistry showing the heavily stained hyperplastic myoepithelial cells in contrast to the normal myoepithelial layer of some acini at the bottom of the figure.

ISOLATED LACTATIONAL LOBULES
(FOCAL LACTATIONAL CHANGE, PREGNANCY-LIKE CHANGE)
Secretory activity is a physiological process during pregnancy. However, these changes may be found focally in otherwise resting breasts (Fig. 2.10) (see Chapter 3) [49, 50].

CLEAR CELL CHANGE
Clear cell change refers to a lesion characterized by lobular cells with a clear or pale, finely granular cytoplasm (Fig. 2.11) (see Chapter 4) [51].

APOCRINE METAPLASIA
Apocrine change as mentioned before may also be found in normal lobules.

MYOEPITHELIAL HYPERPLASIA (MYOEPITHELIOSIS)
Myoepithelial hyperplasia (myoepitheliosis) is occasionally seen in otherwise normal breast tissue. The lobular architecture is preserved with an increase in myoepithelial cells surrounding normal or atrophic acinar structures (Fig. 2.12). The myoepithelial cells can easily be identified in H&E sections or, even better, by their strong immunoreactivity to myoepithelial markers such as smooth muscle actin, calponin or p63 (Fig. 2.12b). In exceptionally rare cases they may give rise to nodular growth patterns around involved glandular structures. Tavassoli regards these changes as lesions at the lower end of the spectrum of adenomyoepithelial lesions [52]. It should be noted that these lesions do not bear any cancer risk. Due to their organoid architecture, we regard them as a physiological variant rather than a pre-neoplastic condition.

COLLAGENOUS SPHERULOSIS
Collagenous spherulosis is a far more complex lesion than myoepitheliosis. It is a rare, usually incidental microscopic finding in biopsy or mastectomy specimens observed in association with other benign proliferative processes such as sclerosing adenosis, radial scar and ductal papillomas [53 – 55]. The distended glandular structures contain a proliferation of basaloid/modified myoepithelial cells with secondary lumina that are filled with acellular, eosinophilic, hyaline and sometimes fibrillar spherules (Fig. 2.13a – b). The latter contain basement membrane material such as collagen IV and laminin [54], elastin, and acidic mucin. The spherules are alcianophilic and/or PAS-positive [56]. Cells surrounding the spherules appear to be myoepithelial cells, as they express sm-actin (Fig. 2.13d) and frequently cytokeratin 5/14. Double-immunofluorescence studies have revealed that, in addition to myoepithelial cells, Ck5/14+ and Ck8/18+ glandular cells are involved in collagenous spherulosis (Fig. 2.13c – e). The lesions therefore display the same characteristic bilinear differentiation as adenoid cystic carcinoma. Nuclear pleomorphism is usually mild and mitotic figures are absent. In view of the hyaline spherules and the cellular constituents, Clement et al. [53] as early as 1987 discussed the striking similarity with adenoid cystic carcinoma. Hence collagenous spherulosis may be conceived of as unusual form of hyperplasia or even in-situ neoplasia. In a clinical context, however, it has a benign connotation. It is therefore of vital importance to distinguish between collagenous spherulosis, the rare malignant adenoid cystic carcinoma [53, 57]

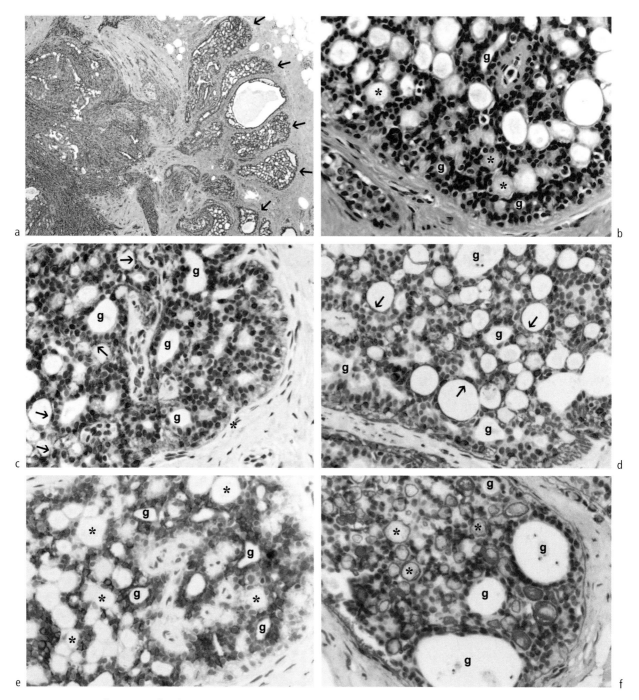

Fig. 2.13a–e Collagenous spherulosis.

2.13a Lower power magnification of a complex sclerosing lesion with several ductules in the right field, showing the typical aspect of collagenous spherulosis (arrows).

2.13b Higher magnification of the collagenous spherulosis highlights the hyaline spherules surrounded by basaloid/myoepithelial cells (asterisks) and the glandular spaces (g).

2.13c Immunostaining for Ck5/14 shows that the cells of the immediate surrounding of the spherules express Ck5/14 (arrows) as do the myoepithelial cells surrounding the whole lesion (asterisk).

2.13d Immunostaining for sm-actin. The cells surrounding the spherules also express sm-actin indicating myoepithelial differentiation (compare Fig. 2.15c). The cells lining glandular spaces are Ck5/14– cells and show glandular differentiation.

2.13e Immunostaining for Ck8/18. Note that the cells that lack expression of sm-actin do express Ck8/18 and vice versa. Glandular cells form well-defined glandular spaces (g). The hyaline spherules (asterisk) and their myoepithelical lining are Ck8/18–.

2.13f Immunostaining for collagen IV, highlighting the basement membrane nature of the hyaline spherules (asterisks). Glandular spaces (g).

and ductal carcinoma in-situ (signet-ring cell type) [56, 58].

Mucocele-like lesions

Mucocele-like lesions are rare multicystic irregular masses, which may present mammographically as a multinodular mass with or without microcalcifications ('teacup' microcalcifications). Macroscopically the lesions may mimic mucinous carcinoma. Histologically the lesions consist of multiple aggregated cysts separated by fibrous stroma. The cysts are lined with an inconspicuous flat to cuboidal epithelium and filled with mucin (Fig. 2.14a). A characteristic feature of these lesions is the extrusion of mucin into adjacent tissue [59] with a lymphocytic and/or histiocytic inflammatory response (Fig. 2.14b).

As these lesions often harbor atypical epithelial proliferations of ductal-type or even invasive breast cancer, they must be sampled and examined very carefully [59–61]. Data from several case reports strongly

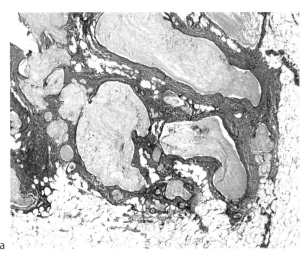
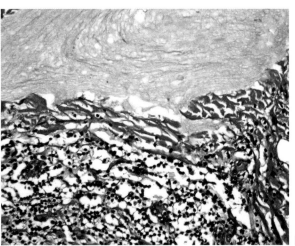

a

b

Fig. 2.14a–b Mucocele-like lesion.
2.14a Low power view of a mucocele-like lesion. Multiple aggregated cysts are filled with mucin and separated by fibrous stroma. The stroma contains lymphocytic infiltrates.
2.14b Higher power view of a mucocele-like lesion with extrusion of mucin into the adjacent tissue and a reactive inflammatory response. In this area the epithelial lining is lost. In core biopsies this lesion may mislead to a diagnosis of mucinous carcinoma.

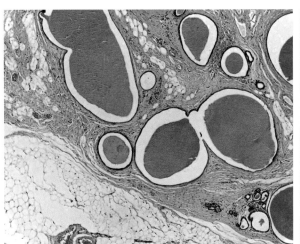
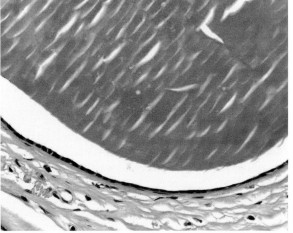

a

b

Fig. 2.15a–b Cystic hypersecretory hyperplasia.
2.15a Low power view of cystic hypersecretory hyperplasia. This also presents as a cystic mass, the result of aggregation of cysts filled with eosinophilic colloid-like material showing a striking similarity to thyroid colloid.
2.15b Higher power view of cystic hypersecretory hyperplasia. This cyst shows the typical aspect of colloid-like material and is lined by a bland flattened epithelium.

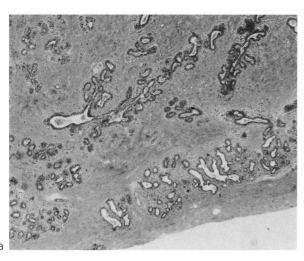
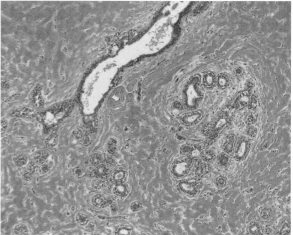

a   b

Fig. 2.16a–b Hamartoma.
2.16a Low power view of a hamartoma with ductal lobular elements in a dense fibrous stroma.
2.16b Higher power view with a smaller duct and lobules. Note the prominent pseudo-angiomatous hyperplasia of the stroma.

supports the hypothesis that a continuum of mucinous lesions exists: from benign changes through those of ADH/DCIS and finally to invasive mucinous carcinoma. Complete excision of such lesions is therefore recommended. Patients should be followed up closely.

CYSTIC HYPERSECRETORY HYPERPLASIA

This lesion presents mammographically as a multinodular cystic mass. Macroscopically it is characterized by an aggregate of cysts separated by fibrous tissue walls (Fig. 2.15a). The cysts are usually filled with colloid-like secretion which bears a striking resemblance to thyroid colloid. If the lesions exclusively contain a bland flattened epithelium, they are referred to as cystic hypersecretory hyperplasia (Fig. 2.15b). As malignancy in such lesions may be very focal, complete excision and extensive sampling are mandatory (see Chapter 20).

HAMARTOMA

Hamartoma usually presents as a macroscopically well-circumscribed, non-encapsulated mass consisting of normal epithelial and stromal breast tissue [62–66]. The ductal and lobular elements can be readily seen, although in some cases the stroma may be dense without distorting the ductal-lobular tree (Fig. 2.16a–b). Epithelial changes include cystic and apocrine change and usual ductal hyperplasia [61]. Pseudo-angiomatous hyperplasia may be prominent in hamartomas [61]. Stromal metaplasia such as smooth-muscle and cartilage differentiation has been observed in hamartomas [61, 67, 68].

GYNECOMASTIA-LIKE LESION

Rare changes in the female breast which, on histological examination, exclusively consist of tissue resembling that normally found in male gynecomastia have been described. The changes may be observed as a component of juvenile fibroadenoma [69] or mammary hamartoma, associated with juvenile hypertrophy [70], with fibrocystic change [71] or as a clinically palpable or mammographically detectable mass [71, 72]. The age of patients ranges from 19 to 60 years with an average age of 40.7 [71, 72]. The mass lesions ranged from 1 to a maximum of 5 cm. Histologically, the lesions contain ductular proliferations

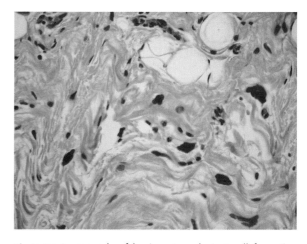

Fig. 2.17 An example of benign stromal giant cell formation with only few giant cells. These may be much more numerous and should not be mistaken for malignancy.

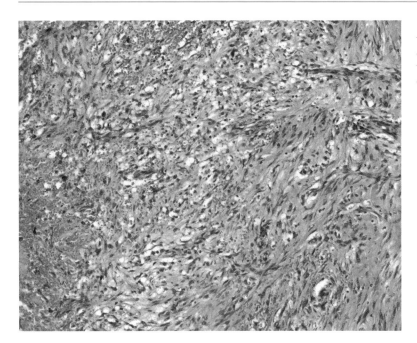

usually with epithelial hyperplasia and a periductular stroma with increased cellularity. The pathogenesis of this lesion is currently unknown.

STROMAL LESIONS

STROMAL GIANT CELLS

Stromal giant cells may be found incidentally in otherwise normal breast tissue [73–75]. Histologically, these fibroblast-derived cells are scattered randomly throughout the stroma. Their scant cytoplasm contains several nuclei which vary in size and shape (Fig. 2.17). Immunohistochemistry shows that the cells strongly express vimentin. They are regarded as a reactive and degenerate stromal response. It is important not to misdiagnose these changes as neoplastic.

REACTIVE SPINDLE CELL NODULES

These are small lesions elicited after fine needle or core biopsy procedures and characterized by a proliferation of spindle cells in a myxoid edematous stroma with delicate collagen and thin-walled blood vessels [76, 77]. The spindle cells have abundant cytoplasm and ovoid elongated nuclei (Fig. 2.18). Nuclear atypia is mild and mitotic figures are rare. The cells are immunoreactive for vimentin and sm-actin. Extravasated blood or hemosiderin-laden macrophages are seen in the lesion. An inflammatory reaction is always observed. The differential diagnosis includes other spindle cell lesions. The small size of these lesions, presence of a needle tract and their composition are clues leading to the correct diagnosis.

PSEUDO-ANGIOMATOUS HYPERPLASIA

This peculiar stromal lesion, first described by Vuitch in 1986 [78], consists of anastomosing empty channels lined by slender spindle cells with interweaving bundles of hyalinized collagen. The lesions are reminiscent of vascular proliferation. Pseudo-angiomatous hyperplasia was primarily diagnosed in women with palpable lesions [78, 79]. In a subsequent study comprising 2,000 consecutive surgical specimens of breast tissue, small histological lesions were found in 46 (23%) of the cases, usually in association with benign proliferative lesions. The lesions can be found both in intralobular tissue as well as between lobes. In Powell's series [80] the age of women affected ranged from 14 to 67 years, the size of the palpable lesions from 12 to 120 mm.

The lesions are easily identified, even at low power, and consist of spindle-shaped cells that are arranged in a pseudo-angiomatous pattern (Fig. 2.19a–c). The cells immunostain for vimentin, sm-actin, but not for factor VIII and CD34 [80]. As some of these lesions also stain for estrogen and progesterone receptors, it has been suggested that growth stimulation of stromal cells in estrogen-primed tissue may be a contributing factor [78, 81].

AMYLOIDOSIS

Localized amyloidosis is a rare lesion that may form a mass simulating a neoplasm, usually in elderly women [82–88]. Macroscopically the affected tissue is hardened and waxy. Histologically the homogeneous, eosinophilic amyloid can be affirmed by Congo red staining or by immunostaining for amyloid protein.

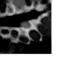

■ INTERPRETATION OF CORE AND
■ VACUUM-ASSISTED BIOPSIES

Biopsies containing these lesions are usually classified as B2. However, biopsies containing cystic hyper-secretory or mucocele-like lesions should be classified as B3 or even B4, depending on the type of epithelial lining. Spindle cell lesions may pose a diagnostic problem. This will be discussed in more detail in Chapter 14.

Differential diagnosis

EXAMPLES

FIBROCYSTIC CHANGE VS. PERIDUCTAL (PLASMA CELL) MASTITIS

Periductal mastitis is a chronic inflammatory process (Table 2.1, for details see Chapter 16) which usually involves the major subareolar ducts. It is characterized by a periductal inflammatory infiltration with histio-cytes, lymphocytes and plasma cells around non-dilated ducts in younger women, and duct ectasia with

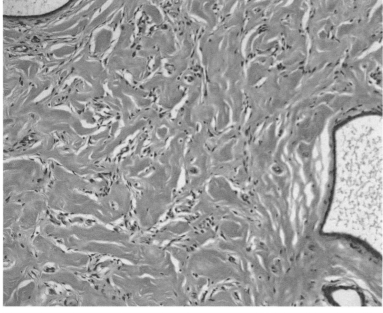

a

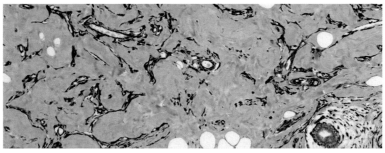

b

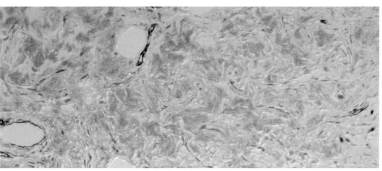

c

Fig. 2.19a–c Pseudo-angiomatous hyper-plasia.
2.19a Typical pattern showing dense hyaline stroma with spindle cells that are arranged in a pseudo-angiomatous pattern resembling small capillaries.

2.19b Immunostaining for vimentin dis-plays an intense reaction of the pseudo-vascular stromal cells.

2.19c Immunostaining for endothelial markers such as CD34 shows a negative reaction, which rules out a possible en-dothelial nature of these cells.

intense fibrosis/hyalinosis and dilation of ducts in older patients [89–93]. In some cases the inflammatory process may even lead to an obliteration of the ductal lumen [94]. The ductal lumen contains inspissated secretory material and foamy histiocytes [5, 95]. Post-menopausally, duct ectasia is usually detected mammographically due to the presence of calcifications. They may exhibit a high density with ring or tubular form, oval spherical shapes with central lucency and needle-like forms with a branching pattern [96, 97]. The clinical symptoms comprise nipple discharge, retraction, eczema-like reactions and even mass formation and coarse calcifications, which is why periductal mastitis may be mistaken for breast carcinoma.

Fibrocystic change must be distinguished from periductal mastitis and, as the process becomes burnt out, duct ectasia. Important distinguishing features are the location of the process – duct ectasia usually affects major ducts near the nipple, while fibrocystic disease is located in the periphery of the parenchymal tree –, the presence of apocrine metaplasia, which is usually found in cystic change but seldom in duct ectasia, and, last but not least, the presence of elastic tissue found in duct ectasia but not in fibrocystic change. In addition to this, mammographic calcifications usually help to distinguish both diseases. The clinical symptoms of duct ectasia are usually those of nipple discharge and, sometimes, of nipple inversion, usually not found in fibrocystic change. Inflammatory reactions in fibrocystic disease are only found in ruptured tension cysts leading to granulation tissue and fibrosis [5].

APOCRINE CYSTS VS. GALACTOCELE

A galactocele is defined as a cystic structure containing milk-like fluid occurring after abrupt termination of breast-feeding. It is excessively rare and there are only anecdotic reports in the literature [5]. Histologically, these cysts cannot be distinguished from their counterparts in fibrocystic change. The flat cuboidal epithelium may contain cytoplasmic vacuoles due to fat accumulation and may even show apocrine change [98]. Ultrastructurally, these cells may exhibit an abundance of cytoplasmic organelles [99].

Blunt duct adenosis vs. flat epithelial atypia (Chapter 18)
Apocrine change vs. atypical apocrine proliferations (Chapters 19 and 20)
Mucocele-like lesion vs. mucocele-like DCIS (Chapter 20)
Cystic secretory hyperplasia vs. cystic secretory DCIS (Chapter 20)
Stromal tumors vs. adenomyoepithelial tumors (Chapter 14)
Spindle cell lesions (Chapter 14)

REFERENCES

1. Huseby RA, Thomas LB. Histological and histochemical alterations in normal breast tissues of patients with advanced breast cancer being treated with estrogenic hormones. Cancer 1954;145:54–74.
2. Consensus Meeting: Is "fibrocystic disease" of the breast precancerous? Arch Pathol Lab Med 2003;110:171–3.
3. Hutter RV. Goodbye to "Fibrocystic Disease". N Engl J Med 1985;312:179–81.
4. Love SM, Gelman RS, Silen W. Sounding Board: Fibrocystic "Disease" of the Breast – A Nondisease? N Engl J Med 1982;307:1010–4.
5. Azzopardi JG. Problems in Breast Pathology. 1st ed. London: W.B. Saunders; 1979.
6. Hutter RVP. Consensus meeting. Is fibrocystic disease of the breast precancerous. Arch Pathol 1986;110:171–3.
7. Hughes LE, Mansel RE, Webster DJT. Aberrations of normal development and involution (andi): a new perspective on pathogenesis and nomenclature of benign breast disorders. Lancet 1987;1316–9.
8. Hayward JL, Parks AG. Alterations in the microanatomy of the breast as a result of changes in the hormonal environment. In: Currie AR, editor. Endocrine Aspects of Breast Cancer. Edinburgh: Churchill Livingstone; 1958. p.133–4.
9. Vilanova JR, Simon R, Alvarez J, Rivera-Pomar JM. Early apocrine change in hyperplastic cystic diseasse. Histopathol 1983;7:693–8.
10. Wellings SR, Jensen HM, Marcum RG. An atlas of subgross pathology of the human breast with special reference to possible precancerous lesions. J Natl Cancer Inst 1975;55:231–73.
11. Tanaka Y, Oota K. A stereomicroscopic study of the mastopathic human breast. I. Three-dimensional structures of abnormal duct evolution and their histologic entity. Virchows Arch A Pathol Pathol Anat 1970;349:195–214.
12. Sloane JP. Non-neoplastic epithelial changes. In: Biopsy Pathology of the Breast. 2nd ed. London: Arnold; 2001. p.79–100.
13. Berkowitz GS, Kelsey JL, LiVolsi VA, et al. Oral contraceptive use and fibrocystic breast disease among pre- and postmenopausal women. Am J Epidemiol 1984;120:87–96.
14. Walsh PV, Bulbrook RD, Stell PM, et al. Serum Progesterone Concentration During the Luteal Phase in Women with Benign Breast Disease. Eur J Cancer Clin Oncol 1984;20:1339–43.
15. Geschickter CF. Diseases of the Breast. Diagnosis-Pathology-Treatment. 2nd ed. Philadelphia: JB Lippincott; 1945.
16. Kier LC, Kickey RC, Keettel WC, et al. Endocrine relationships in benign lesions of the breast. Ann Surg 1952;135:669–71.
17. Sitruk-Ware R, Sterkers N, Mauvais-Jarvis P. Benign Breast Disease I: Hormonal Investigation. Obstetrics and Gynecology 1979;53:457–60.
18. Drukker BH, deMendonca WC. Fibrocystic change and fibrocystic disease of the breast. Obstet Gynecol Clin North Am 1987;14:685–702.

45

19. Mazoujian G, Pinkus GS, Davis S, Haagensen DE, Jr. Immunohistochemistry of a gross cystic disease fluid protein (GCDFP-15) of the breast. A marker of apocrine epithelium and breast carcinomas with apocrine features. Am J Pathol 1983;110:105–12.

20. Wick MR, Lillemoe TJ, Copland GT, et al. Gross Cystic Disease Fluid Protein-15 as a Marker for Breast Cancer: Immunohistochemical Analysis of 690 Human Neoplasms and Comparison with Alpha-Lactabulmin. Hum Pathol 1989;20:281–7.

21. Minton JP, Foecking MK, Webster DJ, Matthews RH. Caffeine, cyclic nucleotides, and breast disease. Surgery 1979;86:105–9.

22. Boyle CA, Berkowitz GS, LiVolsi VA, et al. Caffeine consumption and fibrocystic breast disease: a case-control epidemiologic study. J Natl Cancer Inst 1984;72:1015–9.

23. Allen SS, Froberg DG. The effect of decreased caffeine consumption on benign proliferative breast disease: a randomized clinical trial. Surgery 1987;101:720–30.

24. Lubin F, Ron E, Wax Y, et al. A case-control study of caffeine and methylxanthines in benign breast disease. JAMA 1985;253:2388–92.

25. Frantz VK, Pickren JW, Melcher GW, Auchincloss H. Incidence of Chronic Cystic Disease in so-called "normal breasts": A Study Based on 225 Postmortem Examinations. Cancer 1951;4:762–83.

26. Bartow SA, Pathak DR, Black WC, Key CR, Teaf SR. Prevalence of benign, atypical, and malignant breast lesions in populations at different risk for breast cancer. A forensic autopsy study. Cancer 1987;60:2751–60.

27. Silverberg SG, Chitale AR, Levitt SH. Prognostic implications of fibrocystic dysplasia in breast removed for mammary carcinoma. Cancer 1972;29:574–80.

28. Haagensen CD. The relationship of gross cystic disease of the breast and carcinoma. Ann Surg 1977;185:375–6.

29. Page DL, Dupont WD. Are Breast Cysts a Premalignant Marker? Eur J Cancer Clin Oncol 1986;22:635–6.

30. Page DL, Vander Zwaag R, Rogers LW, et al. Relation Between Component Parts of Fibrocystic Disease Complex and Breast Cancer. J Natl Cancer Inst 1978;61:1055–60.

31. Geschickter CF. The early literature of chronic cystic mastitis. Bull Inst Hist Med 1939;2:249–57.

32. Dawson EK. Sweat gland carcinoma of the breast. Edinb Med J 1932;39:409–38.

33. Foote FW, Stewart FW. Comparative studies of cancerous versus non-cancerous breasts. Basic morphologic characteristics. Ann Surg 1945;121:6–53.

34. Pearlman WH, Gueriguian JL, Sawyer ME. A specific progesterone-binding component of human breast cyst fluid. J Biol Chem 1973;248:5736–41.

35. Ahmed A. Apocrine metaplasia in cystic hyperplastic mastopathy. Histochemical and ultrastructural observations. J Pathol 1975;115:211–4.

36. Gonzalez JE, Caldwell RG, Valaitis J. Calcium oxalate crystals in the breast. Pathology and significance. Am J Surg Pathol 1991;15:586–91.

37. Weidner N. Benign breast lesions that mimic malignant tumors: analysis of five distinct lesions. Semin Diagn Pathol 1990;7:90–101.

38. Tavassoli FA. Fibrocystic changes. In: Tavassoli FA, editor. Pathology of the Breast. 2nd ed. Stanford, Connecticut: Appleton & Lange; 1999. p.115–21.

39. Azzopardi JG. Cystic Disease: Duct Ectasia: Fat Necrosis: 'Fibrous Disease of the Breast'. In: Bennington JL, editor. Problems in Breast Pathology. London, Philadelphia, Toronto: W.B. Saunders Company Ltd.; 1979. p.57–91.

40. Bussolati G, Tavassoli FA, Nielsen BB, Ellis IO, MacGrogan G. Benign epithelial proliferations. In: Tavassoli FA, Devillee P, editors. Tumours of the Breast and Female Genital Organs. Lyon: IARC Press; 2003. p.81–5.

41. Black MM, Barclay TH, Cutler SJ, Hankey BF, Asire AJ. Association of atypical characteristics of benign breast lesions with subsequent risk of breast cancer. Cancer 1972;29:338–43.

42. Fraser JL, Raza S, Chorny K, Connolly JL, Schnitt SJ. Columnar alteration with prominent apical snouts and secretions: a spectrum of changes frequently present in breast biopsies performed for microcalcifications. Am J Surg Pathol 1998;22:1521–7.

43. Fraser JL, Raza S, Chorny K, Connolly JL, Schnitt SJ. Immunophenotype of columnar alteration with prominent apical snouts and secretions (CAPSS) [abstract]. Lab Invest 2000;80:21A.

44. Nasser SM. Columnar cell lesions: current classification and controversies. Semin Diagn Pathol 2004;21:18–24.

45. Schnitt SJ. Columnar cell lesions of the breast: pathological features and clinical significance. Current Diagnostic Pathology 2004;10:193–203.

46. Rosen PP. Adenosis and Microglandular Adenosis. In: Rosen's Breast Pathology. 2nd ed. Philadelphia: Lippincott Williams & Wilkins; 2001. p.139–63.

47. Chinyama CN. Columnar Cell Lesions. In: Benign Breast Diseases. Berlin, Heidelberg, New York, Hong Kong, London, Milan, Paris, Tokyo: Springer; 2004. p.107–19.

48. Bonser GM, Dossett JA, Jull W. Human and Experimental Breast Cancer. London: Pitman Medical; 1961.

49. Mills SE, Fechner RE. Focal pregnancy-like change of the breast. Diagn Gynecol Obstet 1980;2:67–70.

50. Tavassoli FA, Tien Yeh I. Lactational and Clear Cell Changes of the Breast in Nonlactating, nonpregnant women. Am J Clin Pathol 1987;87:23–9.

51. Barwick KW, Kashgarian M, Rosen PP. "Clear-cell" change within duct and lobular epithelium of the human breast. Pathol Annu 1982;17:319–28.

52. Tavassoli FA. Pathology of the Breast. 2nd ed. Norwalk: Appleton and Lange; 1999.

53. Clement PB, Young RH, Azzopardi JG. Collagenous Spherulosis of the Breast. Am J Surg Pathol 1987;11:411–7.

54. Wells CA, Wells CW, Yeomans P, et al. Spherical connective tissue inclusions in epithelial hyperplasia of the breast ("collagenous spherulosis"). J Clin Pathol 1990;43:905–8.

55. Grignon DJ, Ro JY, Mackay BN, Ordonez NG, Ayala AG. Collagenous spherulosis of the breast. Immunohistochemical and ultrastructural studies. Am J Clin Pathol 1989;91:386–92.

56. Elston CW, Ellis IO. The Breast. 1st ed. Edinburgh: Harcourt Brace and Company Ltd; 1998.

57. Tyler X, Coghill SB. Fine needle aspiration cytology of collagenous spherulosis of the breast. Cytopathology 1991;2:159–62.

58. Fisher ER, Brown R. Intraductal signet ring carcinoma. A hitherto undescribed form of intraductal carcinoma of the breast. Cancer 1985;55:2533–7.

59. Chinyama CN, Davies JD. Mammary mucinous lesions: congeners, prevalence and important pathological associations. Histopathol 1996;29:533–9.

60. Komaki K, Sakamoto G, Sugano H, et al. The morphologic feature of mucus leakage appearing in low papillary carcinoma of the breast. Hum Pathol 1991;22:231–6.

61. Fisher CJ, Millis RR. A mucocele-like tumour of the breast associated with both atypical ductal hyperplasia and mucoid carcinoma. Histopathol 1992;21:69–71.

62. Arrigoni MG, Dockerty MB, Judd ES. The identification and treatment of mammary hamartoma. Surg Gynecol Obstet 1971;133:577–82.

63. Linell F, Östberg G, Söderström J, et al. Breast Hamartomas. An Important Entity in Mammary Pathology. Virchows Arch A 1979;383:253–64.

64. Sloane JP. Biopsy Pathology of the Breast. Vol. 24, 2nd edition ed. London: Arnold; 2001.

65. Jones MW, Norris HJ, Wargotz ES. Hamartomas of the breast. Surg Gynecol Obstet 1991;173:54–6.

66. Fisher CJ, Hanby AM, Robinson L, Millis RR. Mammary hamartoma – a review of 35 cases. Histopathol 1992;20:99–106.

67. Davies JD, Riddell RH. Muscular hamartomas of the breast. J Pathol 1973;111:209–11.

68. Oberman HA. Hamartomas and hamartoma variants of the breast. Semin Diagn Pathol 1989;6:135–45.

69. Millis RR, Hanby AM, Girling AC. The breast. In: Sternberg SS, editor. Diagnostic Surgical Pathology. 3rd ed. Philadelphia: Lippincott Williams & Wilkins; 1999. p.365–6.

70. Tavassoli FA. Hamartoma and Choristoma. In: Pathology of the Breast. Stanford, Connecticut: Appleton & Lange; 1999. p.168–71.

71. Kang Y, Wile M, Schinella R. Gynecomastia-like changes of the female breast. Arch Pathol Lab Med 2001;125:506–9.

72. Umlas J. Gynecomastia-like lesions in the female breast. Arch Pathol Lab Med 2000;124:844–7.

73. Rosen PP. Multinucleated mammary stromal giant cells: a benign lesion that simulates invasive carcinoma. Cancer 1979;44:1305–8.

74. Abdul-Karim FW, Cohen RE. Atypical stromal cells of lower female genital tract. Histopathol 1990;17:249–53.

75. Campbell AP. Multinucleated stromal giant cells in adolescent gynaecomastia. J Clin Pathol 1992;45:443–4.

76. Brogi E. Benign and malignant spindle cell lesions of the breast. Semin Diagn Pathol 2004;21:57–64.

77. Gobbi H, Tse G, Page DL, et al. Reactive spindle cell nodules of the breast after core biopsy or fine-needle aspiration. Am J Clin Pathol 2000;113:288–94.

78. Vuitch MF, Rosen PP, Erlandson RA. Pseudoangiomatous hyperplasia of mammary stroma. Hum Pathol 1986;17:185–91.

79. Ibrahim RE, Sciotto CG, Weidner N. Pseudoangiomatous hyperplasia of mammary stroma. Some observations regarding its clinicopathologic spectrum. Cancer 1989;63:1154–60.

80. Powell CM, Cranor ML, Rosen PP. Pseudoangiomatous stromal hyperplasia (PASH). A mammary stromal tumor with myofibroblastic differentiation. Am J Surg Pathol 1995;19:270–7.

81. Anderson C, Ricci A, Jr., Pedersen CA, Cartun RW. Immunocytochemical analysis of estrogen and progesterone receptors in benign stromal lesions of the breast. Evidence for hormonal etiology in pseudoangiomatous hyperplasia of mammary stroma. Am J Surg Pathol 1991;15:145–9.

82. Fernandez BB, Hernandez FJ. Amyloid tumor of the breast. Arch Pathol 1973;95:102–5.

83. Lipper S, Kahn LB. Amyloid tumor. A clinicopathologic study of four cases. Am J Surg Pathol 1978;2:141–5.

84. McMahon RF, Waldron D, Given HF, Connolly CE. Localised amyloid tumour of breast – a case report. Ir J Med Sci 1984;153:323–4.

85. Lew W, Seymour AE. Primary amyloid tumor of the breast. Case report and literature review. Acta Cytol 1985;29:7–11.

86. Cheung PS, Yan KW, Alagaratnam TT, Collins RJ. Bilateral amyloid tumours of the breast. Aust N Z J Surg 1986;56:375–7.

87. Silverman JF, Dabbs DJ, Norris HT, et al. Localized primary (AL) amyloid tumor of the breast. Cytologic, histologic, immunocytochemical and ultrastructural observations. Am J Surg Pathol 1986;10:539–45.

88. Walker AN, Fechner RE, Callicott JH, Jr. Amyloid tumor of the breast. Diagn Gynecol Obstet 1982;4:339–41.

89. Dixon JM, Anderson TJ, Lumsden AB, et al. Mammary duct ectasia. Br J Surg 1983;70:601–3.

90. Dixon JM. Periductal mastitis/duct ectasia. World J Surg 1989;13:715–20.

91. Dixon JM, Ravisekar O, Chetty U, Anderson TJ. Periductal mastitis and duct ectasia: different conditions with different aetiologies. Br J Surg 1996;83:820–2.

92. Bonser GM, Dossett JA, Jull JW. Duct ectasia in the human breast. In: Human and experimental breast cancer. London: Pitman Medical Publishing; 1961. p.237–65.

93. Bässler R. Mastopathie. In: Remmele W, editor. Pathologie 3 – Urogenitalorgane, Mamma, Endokrine Organe, Kinderpathologie, Bewegungsapparat (außer Muskulatur), Haut. Berlin, Heidelberg, New York, Tokyo: Springer; 1984. p.333–41.

94. Payne RL, Strauss AF, Glasser RD. Mastitis obliterans. Surgery 1943;14:719–27.

95. Davies JD. Neural invasion in benign mammary dysplasia. J Path 1973;109:225–31.

96. Sweeney DJ, Wylie EJ. Mammographic appearances of mammary duct ectasia that mimic carcinoma in a screening programme. Australas Radiol 1995;39:18–23.

97. Tabár L, Dean PB. Circumscribed lesions; calcifications. In: Teaching atlas of mammorgaphy. Stuttgart, New York: Georg Thieme Verlag; 1985. p.18, 172–210.

98. Rosen PP. Rosen's Breast Pathology. 2nd ed. Philadelphia: Lippincott Williams & Wilkins; 2001.

99. Ironside JW, Guthrie W. The galactocoele: a light- and electronmicroscopic study. Histopathol 1985;9:457–67.

Content

3

METAPLASTIC CHANGES AND THEIR NEOPLASTIC COUNTERPARTS

WERNER BOECKER AND HERMANN HERBST

Metaplasias of breast tissue comprise a heterogeneous group of cellular changes seen in the normal breast and in a wide spectrum of benign and malignant breast lesions. The term 'metaplasia' refers to a change in which a specific differentiated epithelial or mesenchymal cell type is replaced by another differentiated cell type. The pathogenesis of most metaplasias of breast lesions is poorly understood.

According to the currently prevailing concept, metaplasia is caused by genetic reprogramming of cells as a result of external disturbance in the cells' environment. This type of metaplasia is regarded as an adaptive process seen, for example, in the change of glandular cells to squamous epithelium in infarcted papillomas. Interestingly, similar histological changes can be observed in malignant breast neoplasias. It must be assumed that, in contrast to adaptive metaplasia, such neoplastic metaplasia may be caused by different pathogenetic mechanisms such as gene mutations, which involve or influence the 'phenotype' genes.

These metaplasias include:

1. **Metaplasia developing from Ck8/18+ glandular breast epithelium.** Apocrine and lactational changes are the primary and most common types. Other benign glandular metaplasias include clear cell change and oncocytic metaplasia. Malignant counterparts of these are found in non-invasive and invasive cancers.

2. **Metaplasias that are derived from Ck5/14+ cells.** In these metaplastic changes, Ck5/14+ precursor cells differentiate along a new pathway of either epithelial or mesenchymal phenotype. Examples are squamous cell change and lesions with chondromyxoid and osseous matrix formation. In contrast to the salivary glands, this type of metaplasia is rarely observed in the breast.

3. **Metaplasias originating from stromal cells** represent a third group. These may, for example, be transformed into smooth muscle cells. Such mesenchymal metaplasias are observed in the stromal part of fibroepithelial tumors and rare heterologous primary breast sarcomas.

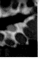

Metaplastic changes and their neoplastic counterparts

■ DEFINITION

The term metaplasia (Greek: *metaplasis* – reconstruction, transformation) is used to refer to a process of transformation in which one differentiated epithelial or mesenchymal cell type is replaced by another differentiated cell type. According to their suggested pathogenetic mechanisms two different types of metaplasia should be distinguished:

- Adaptive and benign metaplasia: The prototype of metaplasia is glandular to squamous cell change, which occurs as a result of an adaptive response to stimuli from the cells' environment, such as chronic irritation. This is, for example, observed in squamous metaplasia, in periductal mastitis or in infarcted papilloma. The breast epithelium, however, is subject to a variety of other benign metaplastic changes including apocrine or oncocytic change, the pathogenetic mechanisms of which are currently unknown.
- Neoplastic metaplasia: In a number of benign and malignant breast tumors similar transformations can be observed, which both morphologically and functionally show striking similarities with adaptive metaplasias. In contrast to cells of typical breast tumors which closely mimic comparable normal cellular phenotypes, such metaplastic cells can differentiate to heterologous elements usually not seen in the breast.

Metaplasias are usually classified according to their acquired form of altered differentiation. In this chapter we follow this rule, but in addition we also attempt to classify metaplasias according to their suggested cell of origin by analyzing the component cells of metaplastic lesions. This provides a more accurate basis for explaining and understanding this group of disorders.

Using these defining features, the following three groups of metaplasias will be distinguished in this book:

1. The most important and largest group of metaplasias involve the **Ck8/18+ glandular breast epithelium** from which apocrine and oncocytic metaplasia, lactational (pregnancy-like) and clear-cell change take their origin. The mechanisms that cause these changes are currently unknown. Most of these glandular metaplasias are benign changes which can occur in different breast lesions. Some of them have malignant counterparts.

2. A different, smaller group of **metaplasias is derived from Ck5/14+ cells**. These include epithelial metaplasias such as squamous cell change and special types of mesenchymal conversions with formation of chondroid or osteoid tissue. Adaptive squamous cell metaplasia is a common finding in the uterine cervix and in the respiratory tract, where columnar cells are replaced by squamous cells. In breast tissue they are rarely seen as, for example, in mastitis and infarcted papillomas. Their neoplastic counterpart is squamous cell differentiation in primary breast tumors such as syringomatous, adenosquamous tumors and squamous cell carcinoma of the breast. Particular metaplasias derived from Ck5/14+ cells involving mesenchymal conversion are characterized by the formation of chondroid and osseous tissue. This type of metaplasia only occurs as neoplastic metaplasia as, for example, in pleomorphic adenomas and metaplastic carcinomas.

3. A **third type of metaplasia** involves the formation of heterologous tissue elements **primarily of mesenchymal cell origin.** Examples are smooth muscle-cell change in the stroma of fibroepithelial lesions or bone formation in primary osteosarcomas.

Transdifferentiation is defined as change of one mature differentiated tissue into another and is exceptionally rare. A change, for example, from glandular to myoepithelial or even mesenchymal cells has been described in vitro, but to the authors' best knowledge has not been proven in human breast tissue.

While apocrine metaplasia and lactational change are a common finding in breast pathology, all other types of metaplasia are extremely rare. The neoplastic counterparts of epithelial and mesenchymal metaplastic changes can be seen in a variety of unusual benign and malignant tumors.

■ CONCEPTUAL APPROACH

It is commonly held that adaptive metaplasia is caused by reprogramming of precursor cells, which, as a result, differentiate along a new pathway. Theoretically the process of reprogramming might be triggered by changes in the concentration of physiologically active tissue factors such as cytokines, growth factors and extracellular matrix components in the cells' environment. Such changes may occur in response to stress such as infarction or chronic irritation (chronic inflammatory disease). These external tissue factors then induce specific transcription factors within the cell, leading to an activation of phenotype-specific differentiation genes and the formation of specific cellular lineages. These changes thus are adaptive reactions of cells to changes and can be theoretically reversible.

It must be assumed that metaplasias seen in neoplastic tissues might be caused by different pathogenetic mechanisms. Thus they may be the result of mutational alterations which influence or even involve specific phenotypic genes. It must, however, be acknowledged that, from a cellular point of view, adaptive and neoplastic metaplasias have many features in common. Both display a proliferation of a specific cell type which differentiates along certain pathways.

In breast tissue, metaplastic change may occur in epithelial or mesenchymal cells. Hypothetical candidates are epithelial precursor cells, glandular cells and mesenchymal cells present in connective tissue. Pechoux and his group [3] have shown that in vitro mammary-derived epithelial cells demonstrate considerable phenotypic plasticity with trans-differentiation of 'luminal' to myoepithelial cells. However, the metaplastic potential of breast cells in vivo seems to be limited [4].

Some possible lines of differentiation are outlined in Figs 3.1 and 3.2 and discussed in the following paragraphs.

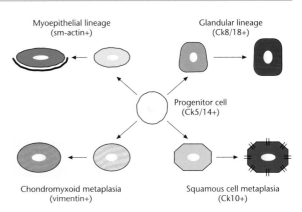

Fig. 3.2 Differentiation pathways for Ck5/14+ progenitor cells. Normal differentiation and heterologous epithelial and mesenchymal metaplasia. Heterologous metaplasias such as chondromyxoid and squamous cell metaplasia are derived from Ck5/14+ cells.

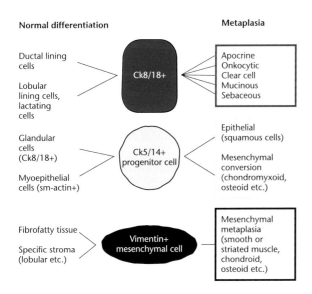

Fig. 3.1 Possible lines of metaplastic development and their hypothetical cells of origin compared to physiological differentiation.

EPITHELIAL METAPLASIA MAY ORIGINATE IN CK8/18+ OR CK5/14+ GLANDULAR EPITHELIAL CELLS

■ In normal breast tissue, **glandular cells** can undergo a number of cellular changes, in which a new cellular appearance is achieved. This seems to be the case when normal glandular cells are replaced by apoc-

rine, oncocytic, clear, mucinous, or goblet cells or when they undergo lactational changes. In special situations these changes may be associated with cellular growth and hyperplasia. Some of these metaplastic changes may be observed in malignancies. The hypothesis that these cells derive from glandular cells is substantiated by immunohistological data, revealing that these metaplastic cells express Ck8/18, but not Ck5/14 or myoepithelial markers. This would indicate that such metaplasias are unlikely to have arisen from Ck5/14+ or myoepithelial cells. It must be borne in mind that Ck8/18+ cells of the normal resting breast are still transitory cells with considerable growth and differentiation potential. They do not become terminally differentiated until they are exposed to the hormonal environment accompanying pregnancy and lactation.

■ **Squamous cell metaplasia** is another prototypic metaplasia. It can occur as adaptive or neoplastic change. The view currently held that squamous metaplasia arises from myoepithelial cells [5, 6] is conceptually problematic, as myoepithelial cells are mature, differentiated cells. It is therefore more attractive to assume the involvement of a Ck5/14+ precursor in this process. Recent data supports this view. Thus squamous cell differentiation is usually observed in lesions in which Ck5/14+ cell growth plays a major role. In areas of displaced normal breast epithelium or in papillomas with infarction, Ck5/14+ cells regenerate and produce squamous epithelium, whereas glandular cells seem to be more fragile and unable to survive (Fig. 3.3). In a number of rare tumors such as syringomatous, adenomyoepithelial and adenosquamous lesions of the breast Ck5/14+ cells prevail, and these tumors tend to un-

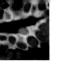
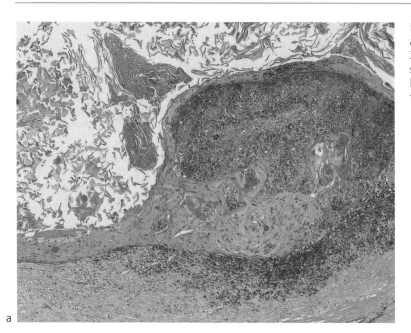

a

Fig. 3.3a–e Squamous cell metaplasia of a papilloma with hemorrhagic infarction. **3.3a** This conventional H&E-stained slide shows the area of squamous cell epithelium at the border of a hemorrhagic infarction of a papilloma. *Continuation*

dergo squamous cell change (for details see Chapter 14). The most convincing data concerning the pathogenesis of squamous cell metaplasia in breast epithelium comes from double immunofluorescence experiments, showing intense staining reactions for Ck5/14 with transition to keratinization and expression of Ck10/11 (Fig. 3.3). It is important to emphasize that the basal keratinocyte-type cytokeratins 5 and 14 are constitutive components of normal basal (reserve) cells of the bronchial and endocervical epithelia, which are better known to give rise to squamous metaplasia and squamous cell carcinomas [7–12]. Moreover, it has been shown that these basal cells are related to the basal cells of squamous epithelia as both contain well-developed hemidesmosomes [13, 14]. Ck10/11 staining, which seems to correlate to the maturation and keratinization of cells [15], can be observed in maturing, keratinizing cells and in horn pearls. Even in morphologically less differentiated primary squamous cell carcinoma of the breast, for example, Ck10/11 can be detected in individual cells undergoing keratinization. Several reports also demonstrate cytokeratins 6 and 16 in squamous cell carcinomas of different origin, making them another possible marker for squamous cell differentiation [9, 16]. The simple epithelial Ck8/18 may be detected focally and in heterogeneous distribution, usually at low levels. On the other hand, Ck7 and Ck20 were not detected in any of the cases seen by the authors. On the whole, the data on squamous cell metaplasia and primary tumors with squamous differentiation is in line with observations of similar phenomena at other sites,

which consistently show the prevalence of the above-mentioned cytokeratins, regardless of their origin and degree of differentiation [17–23]. In contrast, cells expressing sm-actin or any other specific myoepithelial marker do not occur within these lesions. Any possibility that this type of metaplasia arises in myoepithelial cells can therefore be ruled out. Thus we conclude that squamous cell metaplasia in breast epithelium is derived from Ck5/14+ cells.

■ **Conversion of Ck5/14+ precursor cells to connective tissue** with or without matrix formation is an even more intriguing concept. This process is nearly exclusively seen in neoplasia. It is based on the observation that Ck5/14+ epithelial tumors may transform into areas with mesenchymal appearance with heterologous chondroid or osseous matrix. Pleomorphic adenomas and a number of metaplastic carcinomas may show such changes. The specific feature of the mesenchymal cell population in those lesions is their capacity to form an extracellular matrix (Fig. 3.4a–c). According to the conventional view, these changes originate from epithelial or myoepithelial cells [24]. Double immunofluorescence experiments, however, highlight the true nature of such a transition process, confirming that such mesenchymal differentiation originates from Ck5/14+ and their progeny. The factors leading to the production of the heterologous extracellular matrix in these lesions are unknown. To assume that this type of epithelial-mesenchymal conversion represents a specific form of metaplasia may seem surprising from a cell biological point of view. However, given

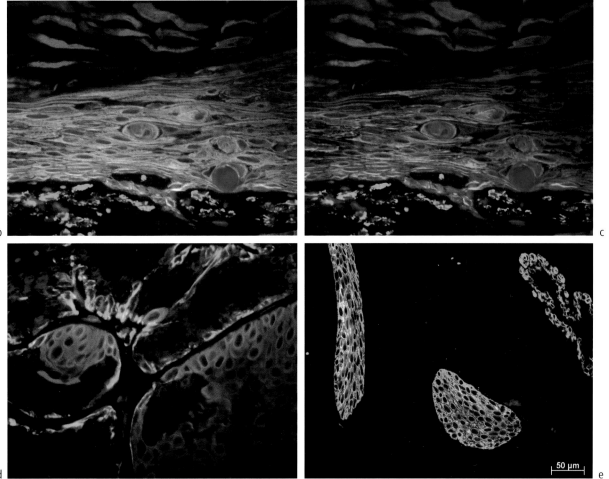

Fig. 3.3a–e Squamous cell metaplasia of a papilloma with hemorrhagic infarction.

3.3b Triple staining for sm-actin (green), Ck5 (red) and Ck10 (violet), showing the transition of proliferating Ck5+ cells to keratinized cells in the lumen of this lesion. The sm-actin+ myofibroblasts in the vicinity are not involved in this process.

3.3c Double staining for Ck5 and sm-actin (green signal) an Ck10 (violet signal) showing that the metaplastic cells express Ck5 and Ck10.

3.3d This figure was taken close to the area shown above. It displays early proliferative changes of Ck5+ cells (red signal) in persisting papillary structures. Ck 5+ cells are the hypothetical cells of origin for squamous cell differentiation of dislodged cells. They seem capable of surviving and responding to the environmental stress by proliferation and squamous cell differentiation. This seems therefore to be an adaptive process similar to squamous cell metaplasia in the uterine cervix. Sm-actin (green signal).

3.3e Neoplastic squamous cell change in an adenosquamous carcinoma of the breast. Double staining for Ck5/6 (green signal) and Ck10 (red signal). Note that all the cells of the tumor in this field express Ck5/6, whereas only the cells in the central portion express Ck10 indicating squamous differentiation. In contrast, a normal interlobular duct stains only for Ck5/6 in the basal layer.

that the myoepithelial cell as the progeny of the Ck5/14+ progenitor cell is physiologically involved in the formation and turnover of extracellular matrix, namely basement membrane material [25], the assumption that Ck5/14+ cells might be causative in mesenchymal transformation suggests itself. Thus slight alterations of the cell-specific protein expression pattern in transformed basal cells and their progeny may induce a change in the type of extracellular matrix produced. This view is supported by immunohistochemical findings in pleomorphic adenomas of the salivary gland and in metaplastic carcinomas of the breast. Such tumors not only contain cells that express Ck5/14; they also display direct transitions from Ck5/14+ tumor cells to vimentin-positive cells within matrix-producing tumors. Interestingly, such tumors may also display a differentiation of Ck5/14+ cells to Ck8/18+ glandular cells or, within the same tumor, to squamous cells. This is in agreement with the literature on metaplastic carcinoma,

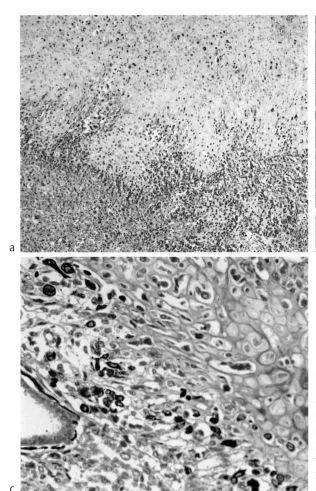

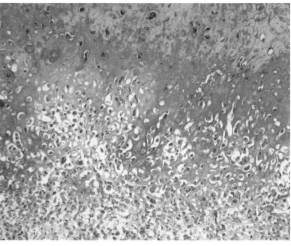

Fig. 3.4a–c Chondroid metaplasia in a metaplastic carcinoma.
3.4a H&E section of an undifferentiated sarcomatoid tumor with transformation to chondroid metaplasia in the lower field.
3.4b Same case with alcian-blue staining, clearly showing the chondroid matrix.
3.4c Ck5/6 immunohistochemistry. The common denominator of these lesions is the presence of a Ck5/6+ cell population in various stages of transition to vimentin-positive mesenchymal elements and matrix production.

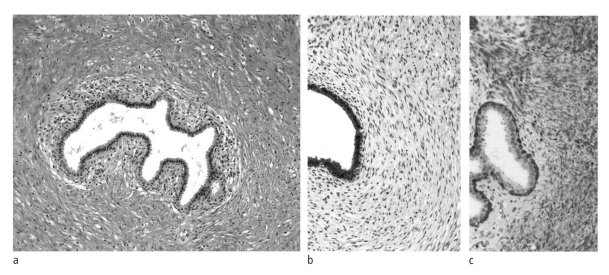

Fig. 3.5a–c Smooth-muscle metaplasia in a fibroadenoma.
3.5a H&E section of a glandular structure surrounded by stromal tissue showing spindling of cells in the outer zones.
3.5b Ck5/6 immunohistochemistry. The epithelial cells of the gland stain for Ck5/6, but there is no staining of the stromal cells, indicating that the latter are mesenchymal in mature.
3.5c Sm-actin immunohistochemistry shows expression of this antigen in many tumor cells, which is indicative of a transition of stromal cells to smooth-muscle cells.

according to which the lesions show transitions from high grade, non-specific ductal-type carcinomas to matrix-producing tumors [26–29]. It should be borne in mind that spindle-cell carcinoma in itself is often classified as a metaplastic carcinoma in the literature [30–34]. Such classification is, however, incorrect considering the strict sense of the term 'metaplasia' (see also Chapter 14).

■ Several types of **connective tissue metaplasias deriving from mesenchymal cells** have been described in different parts of the body [35]. Their common precursors are cells with the morphology of fibroblasts. Smooth-muscle, bone and cartilage formation are most often the result of such metaplastic changes. They are occasionally seen in fibroepithelial lesions in which the tumor contains large amounts of mesenchymal tissue. Thus the stroma of fibroadenomas and phyllodes tumors may show a pattern of smooth muscle-cell metaplasia (Fig. 3.5 a–c) [36–38] or, more rarely, a chondroid or osseous differentiation. Furthermore, malignant phyllodes tumors may display heterologous mesenchymal elements [38–47]. Primary rhabdomyosarcoma, chondrosarcoma or osteosarcoma of the breast are also typical examples of the vastly heterologous differentiation potential of mesenchymal stromal cells [24, 48].

■ CLINICAL FEATURES AND IMAGING

With the exception of common apocrine metaplasia these changes are only detected in approximately one to four percent of breast biopsies [48–53]. They may be observed in normal breast tissue and in benign proliferative breast disease. Most experts in the field are convinced that none of those metaplasias are associated with an increased cancer risk, nor do the changes show any specific clinical features and imaging. The age of patients ranges from twenty-eight to eighty-two [54, 55].

In exceptional cases in-situ or invasive breast cancer may evolve in these lesions [56–58]. Neoplastic metaplasias are, however, extremely rare. The underlying type of tumor determines the clinical features and imaging.

■ PATHOLOGY

MACROSCOPY

The macroscopic appearance is not specific [54–56, 59].

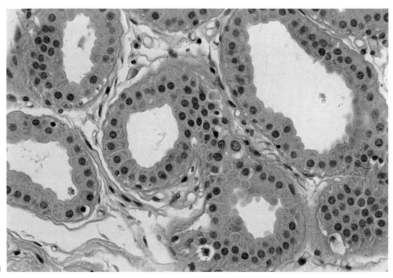
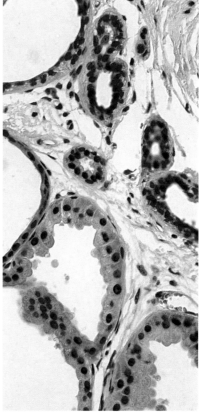

a

b

Fig. 3.6 a–f Apocrine metaplasia.
3.6a H&E section of a lobule with typical apocrine metaplasia. The cells display abundant eosinophilic granular cytoplasm in which the nuclei are usually localized at the base of the cells. The nuclei may show some polymorphism and prominent nucleoli, which should not lead to a mistaken diagnosis of malignancy.
3.6b Immunohistochemistry showing expression of androgen receptor in a number of apocrine cells. These cells were estrogen receptor-negative. *Continuation*

HISTOLOGY

METAPLASIAS FROM CK8/18+ CELLS

APOCRINE METAPLASIA

The prototypic appearance of apocrine cell change is characterized by the abundant granular eosinophilic cytoplasm and large nuclei (Fig. 3.6a) [50–53, 60]. Electron microscopy shows a large amount of mitochondria and basal membrane foldings [61–64]. Sometimes luminal projections may be seen. The apical cytoplasm may contain small periodic acid-Schiff (PAS)-positive and diastase-resistant granules. In addition, yellow-brown lipofuscin granules or, rarely, iron pigment may be present [65, 66]. Occasionally, these cells may display a vesicular (clear cell) transformation of parts or of their entire cytoplasm, probably due to a swelling of cytoplasmic organelles (Fig. 3.6). The nuclei of apocrine cells may be large with prominent nucleoli. Apocrine cells express androgen receptors (Fig. 3.6f), but usually no estrogen and progesterone receptors [67]. In the largest series of 102 benign and malignant apocrine lesions investigated so far, androgen receptors were identified by immunohistochemistry in 94% of benign and 72% of malignant apocrine lesions, whereas the estrogen and progesterone receptor status was negative in 98% of cases [68]. An important marker of apocrine differentiation is the 15 kDa glycoprotein of cystic breast disease (GCDFP-15) [69] (Fig. 3.6e), which has been shown to be identical with prolactin-inducible protein (PIP) [70, 71] The gene coding for this protein is localized in the long arm of chromosome 7 [72–76]. Apocrine cells may form small papillary or even more complex proliferations. Wellings and Alpers [52, 77] included papillary apocrine metaplasia as a risk factor for subsequent development of breast carcinoma, but since this feature is such a common finding, its usefulness in determining the risk for individual patients is limited.

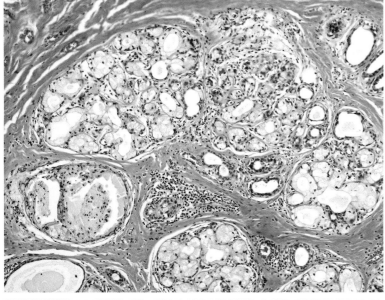

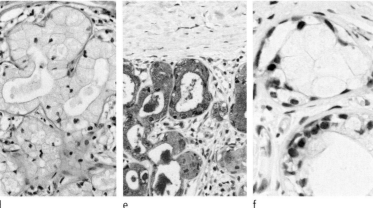

Fig. 3.6 a–f Apocrine metaplasia.
3.6c Apocrine change with clear cell transformation due to swelling of cytoplasmic organelles in an area of several TDLUs with apocrine metaplasia.

3.6d The clear cells often retain the granularity of the cytoplasm.
3.6e Immunostaining for GCDFP-15 protein showing intense staining of these cells.
3.6f Immunostaining for adrenogen receptor shows nuclear staining.

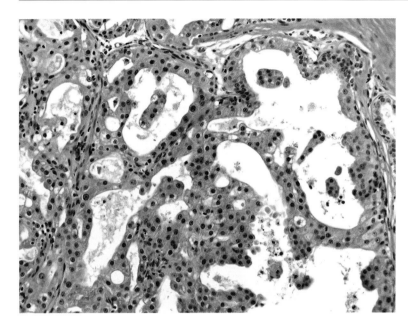

Fig. 3.7 Ductal carcinoma in-situ, apocrine type. This apocrine proliferation classifies as atypical due to its complex and rigid growth pattern. The neoplastic cells often display a pink and less granular cytoplasm compared to benign apocrine cell change. Nearly all nuclei are relatively small with subtle nucleoli so that this lesion would classify as a non-high grade lesion.

APOCRINE HYPERPLASIA

Pure apocrine hyperplasia retains the characteristics of orderly growth and regularity of benign apocrine epithelium [78]. Apocrine changes in benign proliferative lesions such as sclerosing adenosis, usual ductal hyperplasia, papillomas and fibroadenomas [79, 49, 80] are usually focal. However, apocrine changes in sclerosing lesions sometimes display cellular and architectural abnormalities that may be misdiagnosed as malignancy [80]. These changes must be distinguished from apocrine neoplasia (Fig. 3.7), which either reveals the characteristic growth patterns of in-situ carcinoma with a more complex architecture or an overtly malignant cellular phenotype. This will be discussed in Chapters 19 and 20.

ONCOCYTIC METAPLASIA

Care must also be taken not to mistake apocrine metaplasia for oncocytic metaplasia [81, 82]. Both apocrine and oncocytic cells have abundant eosinophilic granular cytoplasm at light-microscopic level. Oncocytes, however, lack the immunohistochemical features described above (GCDFP-15 protein, androgen receptor), show an increased number of regularly dispersed mitochondria within the cytoplasm and, in some cases, estrogen and progesterone-receptor positivity.

LACTATIONAL CHANGE

Lactational change (focal lactational change, pregnancy-like change) may occur in normal breast lobules, as well as benign and malignant breast lesions. As secretory activity is a physiological process

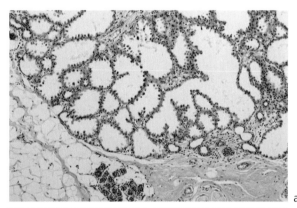

a

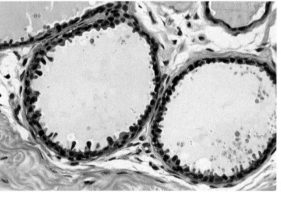

b

Fig. 3.8a–b Lactational lobule.
3.8a The lobular cells lining the dilated acini show a swollen or vacuolated cytoplasm with irregular apical outlines.
3.8b Higher magnification of another case showing a lactational lobule with prominent apocrine snouting and displacement of nuclei towards the luminal border. The hyperchromatic nuclei show some irregularities. This should not be mistaken for flat epithelial atypia.

during lactation, it is not a metaplasia in the strict sense. Secretory change may be found in otherwise resting breasts or in elderly patients, who might not even have experienced pregnancy [83, 84]. Usually, one or several lobules are affected. Partial lobular involvement is not uncommon. The acini are dilated, although there is no or very little secreted material in their lumina (Fig. 3.8a). The lobular cells show a swollen or vacuolated cytoplasm with irregular apical outlines. The nuclei are irregular in size or pyknotic and may be located in apical blebs of cytoplasm with

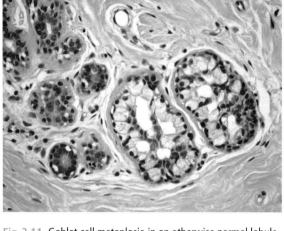

Fig. 3.11 Goblet cell metaplasia in an otherwise normal lobule.

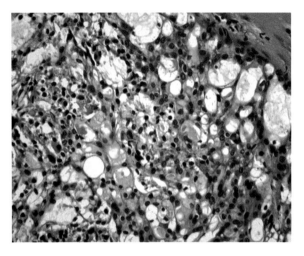

Fig. 3.9 Secretory carcinoma. The cells show a striking vacuolation of the cytoplasm and eosinophilic pink secretion into the lumina.

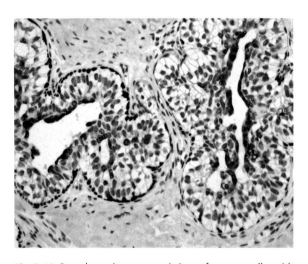

Fig. 3.10 Ductal carcinoma, consisting of tumor cells with clear cytoplasm. Ck5-immunostaining highlights the luminal displacement of normal cells and the positive staining of the myoepithelial cell layer. The tumor is composed of one cell type with clear cytoplasm and enlarged nuclei. All glandular metaplasias are characterized by a negative reaction for Ck5/14.

the appearance of hobnail cells (Fig. 3.8). It has been shown that exogenous hormones (estrogen, stilbestrol [85, 63, 86], conjugated estrogens [84]) and other drugs such as digitalis, dilantin, reserpine [86] and thioridazine [87] may play a role in inducing these changes. Some of them act by increasing pituitary prolactin secretion. In addition, a selective increase in sensitivity to hormonal stimulation may play a role [88]. A special type of 'secretory change' is seen in secretory tumors (Fig. 3.9). Such changes may be observed in lesions such as fibroadenoma, adenoma, or even infiltrating carcinoma.

CLEAR CELL CHANGE

Clear cell change is defined by clearing of cell cytoplasm in hematoxylin-eosin stained sections. It is a rare, incidental finding in breast biopsies [77, 89]. This metaplasia is known to be benign and has no connotation of pre-malignancy. The lesion is characterized by cells with a clear vacuolated or granular cytoplasm and central, small nuclei in single lobules or terminal ducts. The basic structure of the lobules is preserved, but they may become enlarged as the clear cells outsize the original ones. The finding of alcianophilic granules and the cytoplasmic positivity for S-100 have prompted Viña and Wells [77] to suggest a relationship to sweat gland epithelium. Clear cells are easily confused with myoepithelial cells or histiocytes. They can be distinguished from myoepithelial cells by their luminal position and their immunoreactivity with antibodies against glandular cytokeratins 8/18, whereas they fail to react to sm-actin or basal-type cytokeratins. The etiology of clear-cell change is unknown although an association with steroid and psychotropic drug therapy has been suggested. Clear cells may also occur in fibrocystic change and benign and malignant breast lesions (Fig. 3.10).

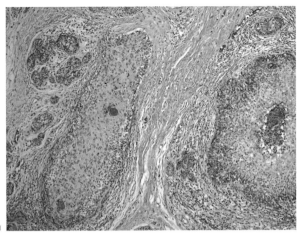

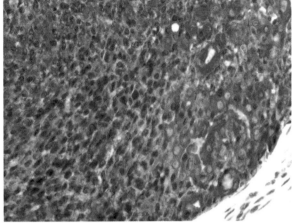

a

b

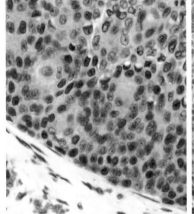

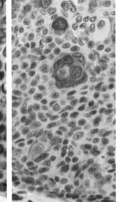

c

d

Fig. 3.12a–d Ductal carcinoma in-situ with squamous cell differentiation.
3.12a Low power view of a ductal carcinoma in-situ, squamous cell type. In this case the squamous differentiation is easily recognized by the presence of horn pearls in the left field.
3.12b Ck5/6-immunostaining highlights this lesion as one being composed exclusively of Ck5+ progenitor cells and Ck6 squamous cells, since Ck6, not found in normal breast epithelium, is a marker of squamous cell differentiation.
3.12c Immunostaining for p63 highlights the more immature cells.
3.12d Ck10-immunostaining specifically highlights the keratinized cells.

MUCINOUS CHANGE AND GOBLET CELL METAPLASIA

Very rare findings include true-type mucinous metaplasia and goblet cell metaplasia. These are easily recognizable (Fig. 3.11) and rarely cause diagnostic difficulties.

METAPLASIAS DERIVED FROM CK5/14+ CELLS

SQUAMOUS CELL METAPLASIA

Squamous cell change is easily recognized by its typical squamous cell appearance in more differentiated tissues. As described in the preceding paragraph, squamous cell metaplasia takes its origin from Ck5/14+ progenitor cells. Fully developed keratinization with horn pearls is the exception. Less well-differentiated areas show a solid pattern and stain for Ck10/11 in areas of keratinocytic differentiation. Furthermore squamous cell change always stains intensely for Ck5/14. In the authors' experience, p63-reactivity is observed in immature cells of squamous metaplasia and of squamous cell tumors. Ck8/18 may be expressed focally.

Squamous cell differentiation may be observed in the epithelium of infarcted papilloma (Fig. 3.3), adenoma of the nipple and fibroadenoma [90, 48]. Furthermore, it may be found in areas of dislodged regenerative epithelium at biopsy or needle track sites, in areas of inflammation [91, 92] or following trauma [93]. These metaplasias are neither frequent in benign breast lesions [91, 93] nor in breast cancer. In contrast, squamous differentiation in adenomyoepithelial tumors is observed in about a quarter of cases, often with single cell keratinization which may require Ck10/11 immunohistochemistry to be detected. Squamous differentiation may be seen in non-invasive (Fig. 3.12) and invasive carcinoma. These carcinomas are usually poorly differentiated with a greater degree of cellular polymorphism, higher nuclear to-cytoplasmic ratios and more frequent mitoses with individually keratinized, dyskeratotic cells, recognizable by their densely eosinophilic cytoplasm and occurring singly or in small clusters. This diagnosis should not be made using light microscopy in the absence of some evidence of squamous cell differentiation. In difficult lesions, Ck5/6 and Ck10/11 immunostaining is of great help. It is also a constitutive feature of syringomatous and adenosquamous tumors, but these lesions often contain clearly recognizable intercellular bridges and well-shaped horn pearls [94–96, 28, 97, 90, 99–107].

MESENCHYMAL METAPLASIA DERIVED FROM CK5/14+ CELLS

Chondroid and osseous metaplasia is defined as the formation of chondroid or osseous tissue. As discussed above, it arises from Ck5/14+ progenitor cells of the breast epithelium. The rare pleomorphic adenoma of the breast is an example of a benign chondromyxoid metaplasia. Metaplastic carcinomas with chondroid and osseous metaplasias may be their malignant counterpart, in which Ck5/14+ cells differentiate to vimentin-positive mesenchymal cells with matrix formation (Fig. 3.4). Mesenchymal metaplasia derived from stromal cells can usually be distinguished from Ck5/14+ progenitor cell-derived metaplasia by Ck5/14 immunohistochemistry, which shows at least a focal expression of these high molecular weight cytokeratins in the latter condition.

MESENCHYMAL METAPLASIA DERIVED FROM STROMAL CELLS

Stroma cell-derived mesenchymal metaplasia is thought to be caused by heterologous mesenchymal differentiation. Chondroid, osseous, and leiomyomatous metaplasia has been observed in benign lesions, in particular fibroadenomas and malignant phyllodes tumors [45–47]. These lesions do not usually express Ck5/14.

■ INTERPRETATION OF CORE AND ■ VACUUM-ASSISTED BIOPSIES

Diagnosis of metaplastic change is often easy. A diagnosis of benign apocrine metaplasia in fibrocystic change, for example, is readily made. However, as is evident from the descriptions of the histology of various types of breast metaplasias and the lesions in which they may occur, overall features of the lesions must be taken into consideration. Even then, it may still prove difficult reaching a definitive diagnosis in particular cases. Thus a malignant phyllodes tumor with leiomyomatous metaplasia cannot be distinguished from an adenomyoepithelial lesion in hematoxylin-eosin stained sections. The use of Ck5/14, Ck8/18 and sm-actin, however, often enables a more precise definition of the broader context in which metaplastic changes must be considered (compare Figs. 3.13 and 3.14). Assessment of malignant potential may be particularly problematic. The whole range of benign and malignant lesions (B2 to B5) must be taken into account. This will be discussed in the corresponding chapters.

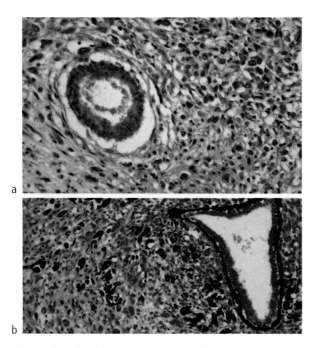

Fig. 3.13a–b Malignant adenomyoepithelial tumor.
3.13a H&E section mainly showing a spindle cell lesion with malignant nuclear features and a glandular structure.
3.13b Immunostaining for Ck5 highlights the presence of many Ck5+ cells. These tumors also stain for Ck8/18 and myoepithelial markers such as sm-actin, calponin, p63.

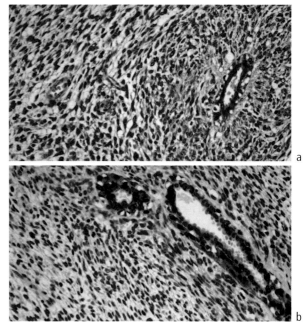

Fig. 3.14a–b Malignant phyllodes tumor.
3.14a H&E section with a similar appearance to the tumor in 3.14b.
3.14b Immunostaining for Ck5. Note the lack of Ck5 expression in the stromal compartment.

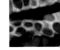
DIFFERENTIAL DIAGNOSIS

Benign glandular metaplasia vs. malignant counterparts (Chapter 20)

Metaplasia derived from Ck5+ cells (Chapters 9, 10, 12, 15, 16, 21)

Metaplasia derived from stromal cells (Chapters 15, 16)

REFERENCES

1. Lugo M, Putong PB. Metaplasia. An overview. Arch Pathol Lab Med 1984;108:185–9.
2. Tosh D, Slack JM. How cells change their phenotype. Nat Rev Mol Cell Biol 2002;3:187–94.
3. Pechoux C, Gudjonsson T, Ronnov-Jessen L, Bissell MJ, Petersen OW. Human mammary luminal epithelial cells contain progenitors to myoepithelial cells. Dev Biol 1999;206:88–99.
4. Boecker W, Moll R, Poremba C, et al. Common Adult Stem Cells in the Human Breast Give Rise to Glandular and Myoepithelial Cell Lineages: A New Cell Biological Concept. Lab Invest 2002;82:737–46.
5. Raju GC. The histological and immunohistochemical evidence of squamous metaplasia from the myoepithelial cells in the breast. Histopathol 1990;17:272–5.
6. Reddick RL, Jennette JC, Askin FB. Squamous metaplasia of the breast. An ultrastructural and immunologic evaluation. Am J Clin Pathol 1985;84:530–3.
7. Blobel GA, Moll R, Franke WW, Vogt-Moykopf I. Cytokeratins in normal lung and lung carcinomas. I. Adenocarcinomas, squamous cell carcinomas and cultured cell lines. Virchows Arch B Cell Pathol Incl Mol Pathol 1984;45:407–29.
8. Broers JL, Ramaekers FC, Rot MK, et al. Cytokeratins in different types of human lung cancer as monitored by chain-specific monoclonal antibodies. Cancer Res 1988;48:3221–9.
9. Leube RE, Rustad TJ. Squamous cell metaplasia in the human lung: molecular characteristics of epithelial stratification. Virchows Arch B Cell Pathol Incl Mol Pathol 1991;61:227–53.
10. Gigi-Leitner O, Geiger B, Levy R, Czernobilsky B. Cytokeratin expression in squamous metaplasia of the human uterine cervix. Differentiation 1986;31:191–205.
11. Weikel W, Wagner R, Moll R. Characterization of subcolumnar reserve cells and other epithelia of human uterine cervix. Demonstration of diverse cytokeratin polypeptides in reserve cells. Virchows Arch B Cell Pathol Incl Mol Pathol 1987;54:98–110.
12. Smedts F, Ramaekers F, Troyanovsky S, et al. Basal-cell keratins in cervical reserve cells and a comparison to their expression in cervical intraepithelial neoplasia. Am J Pathol 1992;140:601–12.
13. Gould PR, Barter RA, Papadimitriou JM. An ultrastructural, cytochemical, and autoradiographic study of the mucous membrane of the human cervical canal with reference to subcolumnar basal cells. Am J Pathol 1979;95:1–16.
14. McDowell EM, Combs JW, Newkirk C. A quantitative light and electron microscopic study of hamster tracheal epithelium with special attention to so-called intermediate cells. Exp Lung Res 1983;4:205–26.
15. Moll R. Cytokeratins as markers of differentiation in the diagnosis of epithelial tumors. Subcell Biochem 1998;31205–62:-62.
16. Stoler A, Kopan R, Duvic M, Fuchs E. Use of monospecific antisera and cRNA probes to localize the major changes in keratin expression during normal and abnormal epidermal differentiation. J Cell Biol 1988;107:427–46.
17. Schaafsma HE, Ramaekers FC. Cytokeratin subtyping in normal and neoplastic epithelium: basic principles and diagnostic applications. Pathol Annu 1994;29 Pt 1:21–62.
18. Moll R, Zimbelmann R, Goldschmidt MD, et al. The human gene encoding cytokeratin 20 and its expression during fetal development and in gastrointestinal carcinomas. Differentiation 1993;53:75–93.
19. Ivanyi D, Groeneveld E, Van Doornewaard G, Mooi WJ, Hageman PC. Keratin subtypes in carcinomas of the uterine cervix: implications for histogenesis and differential diagnosis. Cancer Res 1990;50:5143–52.
20. Heyden A, Huitfeldt HS, Koppang HS, et al. Cytokeratins as epithelial differentiation markers in premalignant and malignant oral lesions. J Oral Pathol Med 1992;21:7–11.
21. Takahashi H, Shikata N, Senzaki H, Shintaku M, Tsubura A. Immunohistochemical staining patterns of keratins in normal oesophageal epithelium and carcinoma of the oesophagus. Histopathol 1995;26:45–50.
22. Su L, Morgan PR, Lane EB. Keratin 14 and 19 expression in normal, dysplastic and malignant oral epithelia. A study using in-situ hybridization and immunohistochemistry. J Oral Pathol Med 1996;25:293–301.
23. Balm AJ, Hageman PC, van Doornewaard MH, Groeneveld EM, Ivanyi D. Cytokeratin 18 expression in squamous cell carcinoma of the head and neck. Eur Arch Otorhinolaryngol 1996;253:227–33.
24. Tavassoli FA. Pathology of the Breast. 2nd ed. Norwalk: Appleton and Lange; 1999.
25. Deugnier MA, Teuliere J, Faraldo MM, Thiery JP, Glukhova MA. The importance of being a myoepithelial cell. Breast Cancer Res 2002;4:224–30.
26. Wargotz ES, Norris HJ. Metaplastic carcinomas of the breast. I. Matrix-producing carcinoma. Hum Pathol 1989;20:628–35.
27. Wargotz ES, Norris HJ. Metaplastic carcinomas of the breast. III. Carcinosarcoma. Cancer 1989;64:1490–9.
28. Wargotz ES, Norris HJ. Metaplastic carcinomas of the breast. IV. Squamous cell carcinoma of ductal origin. Cancer 1990;65:272–6.
29. Wargotz ES, Norris HJ. Metaplastic carcinomas of the breast: V. Metaplastic carcinoma with osteoclastic giant cells. Hum Pathol 1990;21:1142–50.
30. Bauer TW, Rostock RA, Eggleston JC, Baral E. Spindle cell carcinoma of the breast: four cases and review of the literature. Hum Pathol 1984;15:147–52.

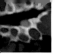

31. Wargotz ES, Deos PH, Norris HJ. Metaplastic carcinomas of the breast. II. Spindle cell carcinoma. Hum Pathol 1989;20:732–40.

32. Ruffolo EF, Maluf HM, Koerner FC. Spindle cell endocrine carcinoma of the mammary gland. Virchows Arch 1996;428:319–24.

33. Gersell DJ, Katzenstein AL. Spindle cell carcinoma of the breast. A clinocopathologic and ultrastructural study. Hum Pathol 1981;12:550–61.

34. Huvos AG, Lucas JC, Jr., Foote FW, Jr. Metaplastic breast carcinoma. Rare form of mammary cancer. N Y State J Med 1973;73:1078–82.

35. Slack JMW. Metaplasia. In: McGee JO, Isaacson PG, Wright NA, editors. Oxford Textbook of Pathology. Oxford, New York, Tokyo: Oxford University Press; 1992. p.565–8.

36. Davies JD, Riddell RH. Muscular hamartomas of the breast. J Pathol 1973;111:209–11.

37. Mackenzie DH. A fibro-adenoma of the breast with smooth muscle. J Pathol Bacteriol 1968;96:231–2.

38. Norris HJ, Taylor HB. Relationship of Histologic Features to Behavior of Cystosarcoma Phyllodes. Analysis of Ninety-four Cases. Cancer 1967;20:2090–9.

39. Beltaos E, Banerjee TK. Chondrosarcoma of the breast. Report of two cases. Am J Clin Pathol 1979;71:345–9.

40. Pietruszka M, Barnes L. Cystosarcoma Phyllodes. A Clinicopathologic Analysis of 42 Cases. Cancer 1978; 41:1974–83.

41. Qizilbash AH. Cystosarcoma phyllodes with liposarcomatous stroma. Am J Clin Pathol 1976;65:321–7.

42. Smith BH, Taylor HB. The occurence of bone and cartilage in mammary tumors. Am J Clin Pathol 2002;51:610–8.

43. Jernstrom P, Lindberg L, Meland ON. Osteogenic sarcoma of the mammary gland. Am J Clin Pathol 1963;40:521–6.

44. Oberman HA. Sarcomas of the Breast. Cancer 1965; 18:1233–43.

45. Grimes MM. Cystosarcoma phyllodes of the breast: histologic features, flow cytometric analysis, and clinical correlations. Mod Pathol 1992;5:232–9.

46. Gisser SD, Toker C. Chondroblastic sarcoma of the breast. Mt Sinai J Med 1975;42:232–5.

47. Anani PA, Baumann RP. Osteosarcoma of the breast. Virchows Arch A Pathol Pathol Anat 1972;357:213–8.

48. Rosen PP. Rosen's Breast Pathology. 2nd ed. Philadelphia: Lippincott Williams & Wilkins; 2001.

49. Simpson JF, Page DL, Dupont WD. Apocrine adenosis – mimic of mammary carcinoma. Surg Pathol 1990;3: 289–99.

50. Cowan DF, Herbert TA. Involution of the breast in women aged 50 to 104 years: A histopathologic study of 102 cases. Surg Pathol 1989;2:323–33.

51. Frantz VK, Pickren JW, Melcher GW, Auchincloss H. Incidence of Chronic Cystic Disease in so-called "normal breasts": A Study Based on 225 Postmortem Examinations. Cancer 1951;4:762–83.

52. Wellings SR, Alpers CE. Apocrine Cystic Metaplasia: Subgross Pathology and Prevalence in Cancer-associated vesus Random Autopsy Breasts. Hum Pathol 1987; 18:381–6.

53. Sloss PT, Bennett WA, Clagett OT. Incidence in normal breasts of features associated with chronic cystic mastitis. Am J Pathol 1957;33:1181–91.

54. Rosen PP. Microglandular adenosis. A benign lesion simulating invasive mammary carcinoma. Am J Surg Pathol 1983;7:137–44.

55. Tavassoli FA, Norris HJ. Microglandular adenosis of the breast. A clinicopathologic study of 11 cases with ultrastructural observations. Am J Surg Pathol 1983; 7:731–7.

56. James BA, Cranor ML, Rosen PP. Carcinoma of the breast arising in microglandular adenosis. Am J Clin Pathol 1993;100:507–13.

57. Nielsen BB, Holm-Nielsen P, Kiear HR. Microglandular adenosis of the breast concomitant with secretory carcinoma. Path Res Pract 1993;189:769.

58. Koenig C, Dadmanesh F, Bratthauer GL, Tavassoli FA. Carcinoma Arising in Microglandular Adenosis: An Immunohistochemical Analysis of 20 Intraepithelial and Invasive Neoplasms. Int J Surg Pathol 2000;8:303–15.

59. Weidner N. Benign breast lesions that mimic malignant tumors: analysis of five distinct lesions. Semin Diagn Pathol 1990;7:90–101.

60. Bartow SA, Pathak DR, Black WC, Key CR, Teaf SR. Prevalence of benign, atypical, and malignant breast lesions in populations at different risk for breast cancer. A forensic autopsy study. Cancer 1987;60:2751–60.

61. Archer F, Omar M. The fine structure of fibro-adenoma of the human breast. J Pathol 1969;99:113–7.

62. Ahmed A. Apocrine metaplasia in cystic hyperplastic mastopathy. Histochemical and ultrastructural observations. J Pathol 1975;115:211–4.

63. Pier WJJ, Garancis JC, Kuzma JF. The ultrastructure of apocrine cells in intracystic papilloma and fibrocystic disease of the breast. Arch Pathol 1970;89:446–52.

64. Ozzello L. Ultrastructure of the human mammary gland. In: Pathology Annual. New York: Meredith Corporation; 1971. p.1–59.

65. Azzopardi JG. Problems in Breast Pathology. 1st ed. London: W.B. Saunders; 1979.

66. Bonser GM, Dossett JA, Jull W. Human and Experimental Breast Cancer. London: Pitman Medical; 1961.

67. Gatalica Z. Immunohistochemical analysis of apocrine breast lesions. Consistent over-expression of androgen receptor accompanied by the loss of estrogen and progesterone receptors in apocrine metaplasia and apocrine carcinoma in-situ. Pathol Res Pract 1997; 193:753–8.

68. Tavassoli FA, Purcell CL, Bratthauer GL. Androgen receptor positivity along with loss of bcl-2, ER and PR expression in benign and malignant apocrine lesions of the breast. Implications for therapy. Breast 1996;2:1–10.

69. Haagensen DE, Jr., Mazoujian G, Dilley WG, et al. Breast gross cystic disease fluid analysis. I. Isolation and radioimmunoassay for a major component protein. J Natl Cancer Inst 1979;62:239–47.

70. Pagani A, Sapino A, Eusebi V, Bergnolo P, Bussolati G. PIP/GCDFP-15 gene expression and apocrine differentiation in carcinomas of the breast. Virchows Arch 1994; 425:459–65.

71. Eusebi V, Betts C, Haagensen DE, et al. Apocrine Differentiation in Lobular Carcinoma of the Breast: A Morphologic, Immunologic, and Ultrastructural Study. Hum Pathol 1984;15:134–40.

72. Murphy LC, Lee-Wing M, Goldenberg GJ, Shiu RP. Expression of the gene encoding a prolactin-inducible protein by human breast cancers in vivo: correlation with steroid receptor status. Cancer Res 1987;47:4160–4.

73. Murphy LC, Murphy LJ, Tsuyuki D, Duckworth ML, Shiu RP. Cloning and characterization of a cDNA encoding a highly conserved, putative calcium binding protein, identified by an anti-prolactin receptor antiserum. J Biol Chem 1988;263:2397–401.

74. Myal Y, Gregory C, Wang H, Hamerton JL, Shiu RP. The gene for prolactin-inducible protein (PIP), uniquely expressed in exocrine organs, maps to chromosome 7. Somat Cell Mol Genet 1989;15:265–70.

75. Myal Y, Robinson DB, Iwasiow B, et al. The prolactin-inducible protein (PIP/GCDFP-15) gene: cloning, structure and regulation. Mol Cell Endocrinol 1991;80:165–75.

76. Shiu RP, Myal Y, Robinson DB, et al. The prolactin-inducible protein/gross cystic disease fluid protein (PIP/GCDFP-15): genetic analysis and hormonal regulation of gene expression. In: Dogliotti L, Sapino A, Bussolati G, editors. Breast cancer: biological and clinical progress. Boston: Kluwer Academic; 1992. p. 93–101.

77. Viña M, Wells CA. Clear cell metaplasia of the breast: a lesion showing eccrine differentiation. Histopathol 1989;15:85–92.

78. Raju U, Zarbo RJ, Kubus J, Schultz DS. The Histologic Spectrum of Apocrine Breast Proliferations: A Comparative Study of Morphology and DNA Content by Image Analysis. Hum Pathol 1993;24:173–81.

79. Bussolati G, Cattani MG, Gugliotta P, Patriarca E, Eusebi V. Morphologic and Functioanl Aspects of Apocrine Metaplasia in Dysplastic and Neoplastic Breast Tissue. Ann NY Acad Sci 1986;464:262–74.

80. Carter DJ, Rosen PP. Atypical Apocrine Metaplasia in Sclerosing Lesions of the Breast: A Study of 51 Patients. Mod Pathol 1991;4:1–5.

81. Hamperl H. [Oncocytes and hyaline inclusions in the human breast]. Virchows Arch B Cell Pathol 1972;10:88–92.

82. Damiani S, Eusebi V, Losi L, D'Adda T, Rosai J. Oncocytic carcinoma (malignant oncocytoma) of the breast. Am J Surg Pathol 1998;22:221–30.

83. Mills SE, Fechner RE. Focal pregnancy-like change of the breast. Diagn Gynecol Obstet 1980;2:67–70.

84. Tavassoli FA, Tien Yeh I. Lactational and Clear Cell Changes of the Breast in nonlactating, nonpregnant women. Am J Clin Pathol 1987;87:23–9.

85. Huseby RA, Thomas LB. Histological and histochemical alterations in normal breast tissues of patients with advanced breast cancer being treated with estrogenic hormones. Cancer 1954;145:54–74.

86. Wellings SR, Jensen HM, Marcum RG. An atlas of subgross pathology of the human breast with special reference to possible precancerous lesions. J Natl Cancer Inst 1975;55:231–73.

87. Hooper JHJr, Welch VC, Shackelford RT. Abnormal lactation associated with tranquilizing drug therapy. JAMA 1961;178:506–7.

88. Kiaer HW, Andersen JA. Focal pregnancy-like changes in the breast. Acta path microbiol scand A 1977;85:931–41.

89. Barwick KW, Kashgarian M, Rosen PP. "Clear-cell" change within duct and lobular epithelium of the human breast. Pathol Annu 1982;17:319–28.

90. Cornog JL, Mobini J, Steiger E, Enterline HT. Squamous carcinoma of the breast. Am J Clin Pathol 1971;55:410–7.

91. Habif DV, Perzin KH, Lipton R, Lattes R. Subareolar abscess associated with squamous metaplasia of lactiferous ducts. Am J Surg 1970;119:523–6.

92. Gottfried MR. Extensive squamous metaplasia in gynecomastia. Arch Pathol Lab Med 1986;110:971–3.

93. Hurt MA, Diaz-Arias AA, Rosenholtz MJ, Havey AD, Stephenson HE, Jr. Posttraumatic lobular squamous metaplasia of breast. An unusual pseudocarcinomatous metaplasia resembling squamous (necrotizing) sialometaplasia of the salivary gland. Mod Pathol 1988;1:385–90.

94. Eggers JW, Chesney TM. Squamous cell carcinoma of the breast: a clinicopathologic analysis of eight cases and review of the literature. Hum Pathol 1984;15:526–31.

95. Drudis T, Arroyo C, Van Hoeven K, Cordon-Cardo C, Rosen PP. The pathology of low grade adenosquamous carcinoma of the breast. An immunohistochemical study. Pathol Annu 1994;29 (Pt 2):181–97.

96. Foschini MP, Fulcheri E, Baracchini P, et al. Squamous cell carcinoma with prominent myxoid stroma. Hum Pathol 1990;21:859–65.

97. Bogomoletz WV. Pure squamous cell carcinoma of the breast. Arch Pathol Lab Med 1982;106:57–9.

98. Chen KT. Fine needle aspiration cytology of squamous cell carcinoma of the breast. Acta Cytol 1990;34:664–8.

99. Dalla PP, Parenti A. Squamous breast cancer: report of two cases and review of the literature. Appl Pathol 1983;1:14–24.

100. Eusebi V, Lamovec J, Cattani MG, Fedeli F, Millis RR. Acantholytic variant of squamous-cell carcinoma of the breast. Am J Surg Pathol 1986;10:855–61.

101. Foot NC, Moore SW. A fatal case of deep-seated epidermoid carcinoma of the breast with widespread metastasis. Am J Cancer 1938;34:226–33.

102. Harrington SW, Miller JM. Intramammary squamous cell carcinoma. Proc Mayo Clin 1939;14:487.

103. Harris M. Spindle cell squamous carcinoma: ultrastructural observations. Histopathol 1982;6:197–210.

104. Hasleton PS, Misch KA, Vasudev KS, George D. Squamous carcinoma of the breast. J Clin Pathol 1978;31:116–24.

105. Jones EL. Primary squamous-cell carcinoma of breast with pseudosarcomatous stroma. J Pathol 1969;97:383–5.

106. Tashjian J, Kuni CC, Bohn LE. Primary squamous cell carcinoma of the breast: mammographic findings. Can Assoc Radiol J 1989;40:228–9.

107. Toikkanen S. Primary squamous cell carcinoma of the breast. Cancer 1981;48:1629–32.

Content

4

PERCUTANEOUS BREAST BIOPSY

ROBIN WILSON AND ANDREW EVANS

Preneoplastic breast pathology has no specific clinical or imaging features. **The clinical, mammographic and ultrasound features of benign epithelial proliferations and malignant change are often indistinguishable.** Preneoplastic breast pathology is associated with a spectrum of clinical signs and symptoms and a wide variety of imaging features. **Microcalcification** is the single most common abnormality on imaging that causes diagnostic difficulty [77]. In the absence of reliable imaging or clinical features to differentiate benign from malignant processes in the breast, biopsy is required to provide definitive diagnoses. **Percutaneous needle biopsy** is the preferred method as a clearly benign result obviates the need for an open surgical procedure, while an unequivocal malignant result facilitates definitive treatment without the need for prior diagnostic surgical open biopsy. The technique is now routinely used both in correctly identifying benign disease and in pre-operative diagnosis and preliminary staging of breast cancer [1–5, 53, 62]. **Liberal use of needle biopsy ensures that benign processes are accurately diagnosed, giving patients reassurance on the nature of their condition as well as avoiding unnecessary further investigations such as surgery.** Having to carry out an open surgical biopsy for diagnosis should be regarded as a failure of the diagnostic process [1].

Fundamental to the modern approach to breast diagnosis is the application of the **'triple test'** – the combination of clinical assessment, imaging (usually mammography and/or ultrasound) and percutaneous needle biopsy. The triple test ensures optimum sensitivity and specificity of the diagnostic process. This triple approach to breast diagnosis is best provided by breast dedicated specialists working together as a team. Such a **multidisciplinary team** should jointly review breast biopsy results in context with clinical and imaging findings before determining the correct course of action and future management, such as whether to proceed to further needle biopsy or open surgical biopsy [1, 32, 67].

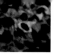

Percutaneous breast biopsy

GUIDANCE TECHNIQUES FOR NEEDLE BIOPSY

Mammographic screening and the use of imaging to diagnose symptomatic breast problems have now become routine. As a result, an increasing proportion of breast problems are clinically occult. This has necessitated the development of sophisticated image-guided needle biopsy techniques (Fig. 4.1). However, these techniques are equally applicable to palpable breast abnormalities, providing more accurate sampling with significantly improved sensitivity, specificity and positive predictive values for disease than are achievable with traditional freehand needle biopsy techniques [1, 55].

Ultrasound guidance – less costly and easier to perform than other image-guided techniques [1, 39] – is the technique of choice. Ultrasound provides real time visualization of the biopsy procedure and visual confirmation of adequate sampling. Approximately 80% of all breast abnormalities are clearly visible and amenable to biopsy using ultrasound. Biopsies of abnormalities which cannot be adequately visualized using ultrasound must be performed using stereotactic X-ray guidance.

The negative predictive value of combined normal mammography and normal ultrasound is extremely high: where there is a clinically palpable abnormality and mammography and ultrasound are entirely normal, the likelihood of malignancy is low (< 1%) [78]. However, in these circumstances it may be considered prudent to carry out freehand biopsy to exclude the occasional diffuse malignant process, such as classical lobular carcinoma or low grade ductal carcinoma in-situ, which may be occult on both mammography and ultrasound.

Some breast abnormalities are only identifiable on magnetic resonance (MR) imaging, but this technique, although highly sensitive for breast pathology, has a relatively low specificity. In these circumstances MR-guided biopsy may be the only method for achieving an accurate diagnosis. However, the equipment required for MR-guided needle biopsy is not currently widely available.

NEEDLE BIOPSY METHODS

Current methods available for breast diagnosis include:
- fine needle aspiration for cytology,
- automated needle core biopsy for histology,
- vacuum assisted mammotomy,
- open surgical biopsy.

While open surgical biopsy represents the 'gold standard' for breast diagnosis, using modern needle biopsy techniques it is possible to make an accurate diagnosis without resorting to this invasive procedure. This applies to both palpable and impalpable breast lesions. There is no necessity to surgically excise a breast abnormality because it happens to be palpable when needle biopsy has shown it to be definitively benign.

There has been much debate over recent years about the comparative benefits of fine needle aspiration for cytology and automated core biopsy. The relative attributes of both techniques are listed in Tables 4.1 and 4.2.

Advantages	Quick to carry out and relatively inexpensive. Immediate reporting possible. Multiple sampling possible. Readily usable for very small lesions.
Disadvantages	Success relies greatly on the expertise of the operator. Requires specialist cytopathological expertise. High inadequate sample rates. Limitation for sampling certain pathological lesions such as DCIS and lobular carcinoma. Significant false negative and false positive rates. Difficulty in reliably distinguishing types of benign pathology and in-situ from invasive malignancy.

Tab. 4.1 Advantages and disadvantages of fine needle aspiration

Advantages	Less dependent on the expertise of the operator. Higher sensitivity and specificity (particularly for the causes of microcalcification and lobular invasive carcinoma). False positive results very rare. Definitive diagnosis of benign lesions. Can distinguish between in-situ and invasive malignancy.
Disadvantages	More expensive than FNA. Immediate reporting not easily available.

Tab. 4.2 Advantages and disadvantages of automated core biopsy

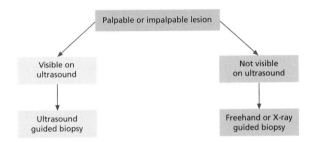

Fig. 4.1 A simple algorithm for choosing how to carry out breast biopsy.

It is possible to achieve discrimination between benign and malignant processes with fine needle aspiration (FNA) for cytology, but differentiation of significant from non-significant benign processes is difficult relying on cytological features alone. Effective pathological assessment of preneoplastic breast processes is much better achieved using needle biopsy techniques that provide material suitable for histological and immunohistochemical assessment [6, 10, 13, 30, 48]. There have been a large number of studies of the comparative performance of FNA versus automated core biopsy in the diagnosis of breast disease, and the vast majority of these conclude that automated core biopsy provides significantly better results [50, 79, 80]. Fourteen gauge 20 mm throw automated core biopsy provides significantly better sensitivity, specificity and positive predictive value for both benign and malignant diseases than do smaller core needles and FNA for cytology. In stereotactic biopsy and sampling of microcalcifications, the results of core biopsy are significantly better than those of FNA [79]. Comparisons of the effectiveness of these two techniques based on the analyses of Britton are shown in Tables 4.3 and 4.4 [79].

LARGER CORE BIOPSY TECHNIQUES

Recognition that a significant proportion of breast lesions cannot be accurately diagnosed using fine needle aspiration or conventional automated core biopsy led in the 1990s to the development of larger core techniques. The main reason for failure to achieve an accurate diagnosis is sampling error or failure to achieve sufficient representative material. The theory behind the development of very large core devices is that the retrieval of significantly larger volumes of tissue will lead to more accurate diagnosis. Very large single core biopsy techniques such as Advanced Breast Biopsy Instrumentation (ABBI™) and SiteSelect™, both of which have to be used using a prone biopsy table, had some clinical exposure in the late 1990s. However, these techniques have not proven to offer any significant advantages and are associated with significant failure rates and more complications than other techniques. They are therefore no longer recommended for routine use [66, 82, 81].

Vacuum assisted mammotomy has proven to be a very successful technique for both ultrasound and X-ray guided biopsy, using both upright and prone table devices to improve the accuracy of diagnoses of borderline breast lesions and of lesions at sites in the breast difficult to biopsy using other techniques [7, 8, 12, 14–20, 26–29, 31, 60]. Overall, vacuum assisted mammotomy has been shown to understage both in-situ and invasive cancer approximately half as often as conventional core biopsy: approximately 20% in core biopsy compared to 10% in vacuum assisted mammotomy [33–36]. The vacuum technique also has a higher sensitivity as it facilitates sampling of lesions that are difficult to biopsy using either FNA or core biopsy, either because of their small size or their site in the breast (such as immediately behind the nipple or close to the chest wall). A major added advantage of vacuum assisted mammotomy over core biopsy is that it provides multiple contiguous core samples rather than samples obtained from random areas of the tissue being targeted. This means that the pathologist can be more confident that the tissue samples are representative of the actual histology present at the target site.

Core biopsy or vacuum assisted mammotomy are now the recommended techniques for all calcifications and mammographic architectural distortions [48, 61, 63, 71, 72]. For calcifications it is imperative that there is proof of accurate sampling; all core samples of breast tissue containing calcification must be examined by specimen radiography (Fig. 4.3b). If calcification is not demonstrated on the core specimen radiograph and the histology is benign, then management cannot be based on this result as there is a high risk of sampling error. In this case the procedure must either be repeated or an open surgical biopsy must be performed.

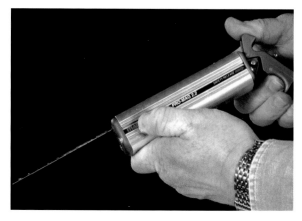

Fig. 4.2 An example of an automated needle core biopsy device.

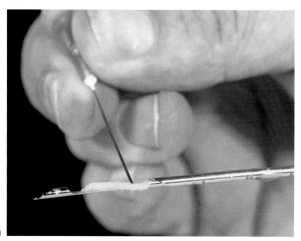

a

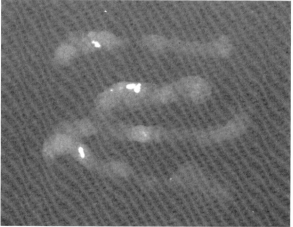

b

Fig. 4.3a – b
4.3a Core specimen contained in the sampling chamber of a 14 gauge core needle.
4.3b A specimen radiograph demonstrating microcalcifications in the core samples.

BIOPSY PERFORMANCE

FINE NEEDLE ASPIRATION FOR CYTOLOGY

A detailed account of the techniques used in fine needle aspiration can be found in the literature [50]. A variety of different techniques exist using 22 to 24 French gauge needles with or without suction. The most widely employed technique uses a 23 gauge needle with a small amount of suction applied using a 10 cm syringe. The needle is passed through the abnormality rapidly, using the bevel of the needle to shear off representative cellular and stromal material. Samples can either be prepared on cytology slides or the content of the needle washed out into an appropriate buffer solution. Smearing on a slide is the more

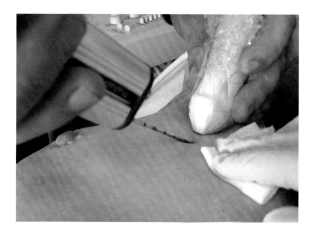

Fig. 4.4 A 14 gauge automated core needle being positioned for sampling a lesion in the upper breast under ultrasound guidance.

widely used technique, with the smear either air-dried or wet fixed. Air-drying is the most commonly used technique.

One of the advantages of fine needle aspiration for cytology is that the smears can be stained, immediately examined by a cytopathologist and assessed for adequacy, providing an immediate diagnosis. In most circumstances it is not possible to differentiate between invasive and noninvasive carcinoma, and there is a significant overlap in the diagnosis of the various epithelial hyperplasias and low grade carcinoma. False positive and false negative results are more commonly reported with FNA than with other techniques. To satisfactorily obtain a sample using fine needle aspiration an adequate yield of benign epithelial cells must be achieved. If insufficient epithelial material is obtained, an inadequate diagnosis has to be given. Inadequate aspiration is one of the commonest reasons for the lower sensitivity of the FNA technique. FNA is not recommended for sampling mammographic microcalcifications, architectural distortions or if there is a clinical suspicion of lobular carcinoma. In each case, FNA is significantly less sensitive than other techniques.

AUTOMATED CORE BIOPSY

Automated core biopsy is currently the technique of first choice for the majority of breast biopsies [1]. Fourteen gauge, rather than 16 or 18 gauge needles, provide consistently better results, yielding approximately 17 mg of tissue per core specimen [68–70, 85]. Core biopsy provides material that can be used in histological assessment. This is a significant benefit over fine needle aspiration and allows for more confident and more reliable definition between normal, benign and malignant epithelial and stromal processes (Figs 4.2–4.4).

As core samples must be obtained through the lesion, the needle must be positioned in such a way to achieve this. Core biopsy is ideal for either ultrasound or a stereotactic-guided biopsy and is also widely used for freehand biopsy of the breast. It is important that the result of the core biopsy is always correlated with the clinical and imaging findings. For instance, if ultrasound or mammography reveals an abnormal mass but the core biopsy report is of normal breast tissue, then this should not be regarded as a satisfactory sample. Similarly, it is not uncommon for calcification to be seen on histology when it was not apparent on the specimen radiograph. It is important not to regard this calcification as representative of the mammographic calcification that led to the biopsy being carried out. Histological calcification is frequently of a size too small to be visible on mammography. When there is no representative calcification on specimen radiography

Tab. 4.3 Comparative performance of FNA versus core biopsy carried out under ultrasound guidance [79]

	FNA [%]	Core biopsy [%]
Absolute sensitivity	83	97
Complete sensitivity	95	98.5
Specificity	84	99
PPV (Cat 5)	98	100
False positive	1.4	0
Inadequate	12.8	0.05
Inadequate for Ca	2.1	0

Tab. 4.4 Comparative performance of FNA versus core biopsy carried out under stereotactic guidance [79]

	FNA [%]	Core biopsy [%]
Absolute sensitivity	62	91
Complete sensitivity	83	95
Specificity	86	98
PPV (Cat 5)	99	99
False positive	0.5	0.4
Inadequate	6.4	1.0
Inadequate for Ca	5.0	1.5

and the histology is reported to contain calcification that is associated with benign disease, the biopsy must be regarded as unrepresentative and either repeated or a surgical excision performed [1, 72].

Core biopsy has the advantage of being able to demonstrate the presence of invasive disease. Since core biopsy represents piecemeal sampling, however, the sole presence of ductal carcinoma in-situ (DCIS) does not mean that invasive disease is not also present. In up to 40% of patients with DCIS demonstrated on core biopsy of microcalcifications, invasive disease will be identified at subsequent surgery [34]. Where invasive disease is present in these circumstances, core biopsy can be expected to provide this diagnosis in approximately 55% of cases. Because of this and other limitations of core biopsy, larger core techniques such as vacuum assisted mammotomy are being increasingly used.

REASONS FOR FAILURE OF AUTOMATED CONVENTIONAL CORE BIOPSY

Conventional core biopsy obtains separate noncontiguous cores of tissue that are usually sufficient in volume and architectural information to allow for accurate pathological assessment [48, 49, 57]. The most common reason for failure to achieve accurate diagnosis with conventional automated core biopsy is a borderline pathological condition where the pathologist requires a larger volume of tissue than can be obtained by conventional core biopsy to assess the true nature of the pathological process [9, 11]. These include conditions such as radial scar, papillary lesion, mucocele-like lesion, differentiation of low grade ductal carcinoma in-situ from epithelial proliferation with atypia (ADH) and the detection of invasive disease associated with in-situ carcinoma [37, 38, 45–49, 52, 54, 56, 84].

Another common reason for failure to retrieve any or sufficient representative cellular material is difficulty in accurately targeting the abnormality due to its small size or inaccessible site in the breast. For successful core biopsy the needle must pass directly through the tissue containing the calcifications at the correct depth. With both upright and prone biopsy devices, successful core biopsy can prove to be difficult or impossible in a proportion of cases because the cluster of calcifications is very small or is at a site difficult to access due to its position in the breast or the habitus of the patient. Vacuum assisted mammotomy is ideal in these circumstances as this technique only requires the sampling probe to be placed close to, rather than through, the area to be sampled. The vacuum and ability to sample tissue in a particular direction allows tissue in an otherwise inaccessible site to be sampled, for instance at the chest wall and immediately behind the nipple. Using a lateral approach, vacuum assisted mammotomy can also be used to obtain tissue from breasts that are too thin to sample when compressed using the conventional perpendicular approach [58, 64, 65].

Not infrequently, sampling difficulty is caused by the breast tissue itself being too tough to advance the core needle through to the area being targeted. To overcome this problem a radiofrequency 'cutting' core device (SenoCore™) or vacuum mammotomy introducer (EasyGuide™) can be used to cut a path to the target using cutting diathermy.

NUMBER OF SAMPLES FOR CORE BIOPSY

Satisfactory sampling using needle techniques requires retrieval of sufficient material to allow the pathologist to provide an accurate diagnosis [51, 74–76]. For ultrasound guided core biopsy this may simply be a single core. By knowing on ultrasound that the needle has passed through the center of the abnormality and looking at the sample with the naked eye it is usually possible to tell if a satisfactory sample has been obtained. It is unnecessary to prescribe multiple cores as a matter of routine. The number of core specimens obtained should reflect the nature of the abnormality being sampled. Where there is a suspicion of carcinoma it is normally recommended that a minimum of two core specimens are obtained for ultrasound guided biopsy.

X-ray guided needle biopsy (stereotaxis) is used for abnormalities that are impalpable and either difficult to define or invisible on ultrasound. These abnormalities are, by their very nature, more difficult to sample, and it is recommended that a minimum of five core specimens are obtained. It is not necessary when sampling calcifications to remove all of the calcifications in the breast; it is sufficient just to obtain sufficient material for accurate diagnosis. For microcalcifications, this is usually achieved by ensuring that calcification is present in at least three separate cores, and/or that five separate flecks of calcification are retrieved from the area of suspicion. Routine removal of more than 20 separate core specimens or attempting complete removal of the whole imaging abnormality may be considered where previous biopsy has shown atypical features or diagnostic uncertainty is predicted. In these circumstances, complete excision by the VAM technique has been shown to significantly reduce the

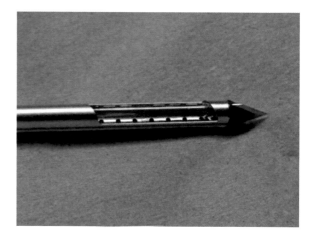

Fig. 4.5 8 gauge Mammotome™ probe sampling chamber. Note the cutting blade incorporated into the probe tip to assist placement.

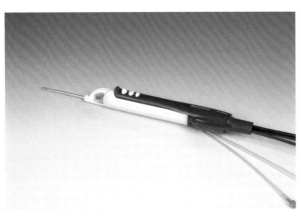

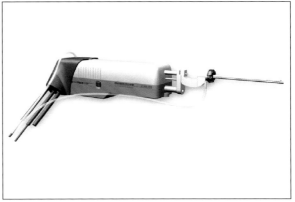

a   b

Fig. 4.6a–b Mammotome™ biopsy devices.
4.6a Hand-held Mammotome™ biopsy device for ultrasound guided breast biopsy.
4.6b The Mammotome ST™ for stereotactic breast biopsy using a prone table or upright X-ray system.

discordance between needle core sample histology and subsequent histology of the excised surgical specimen (0.2% compared to 2.5%) [87]. For mammographic architectural distortions a minimum of ten core specimens are recommended, because of the difficulties of accurate diagnosis of epithelial changes often associated with radial scar/complex sclerosing lesions [9, 83]. In these circumstances 8 or 11 gauge vacuum assisted mammotomy is often preferred [83, 84, 87].

Where there is significant diagnostic uncertainty or complete excision of the abnormality is desirable, 8 gauge vacuum assisted mammotomy can be used to obtain even larger tissue samples [86] (Fig. 4.5). Each core achieved with this type of probe yields approximately 300 mg of tissue. The 8 gauge Mammotome™ is preferred for therapeutic removal of breast lesions such as fibroadenoma and benign papillary lesions [86]. For papillary lesions, vacuum assisted mammotomy can be used for complete excision; when the histology of the excision cores shows only benign papillary changes with no evidence of any epithelial atypia, surgical excision is not required. However, if there is any evidence of atypia, surgical excision should be recommended [56]. Similarly, when histology shows a radial scar/complex sclerosing lesion, extensive sampling can be achieved with 8 gauge VAM and, provided there is no evidence of epithelial atypia, surgical excision can be safely avoided. At present, attempted therapeutic removal of malignant processes using vacuum assisted mammotomy is not recommended as ascertainment of complete excision is not possible.

A few breast lesions are only visible on MR, and must therefore be localized and biopsied under MR guidance. A number of different approaches have been developed for this procedure using both closed and open magnets. FNA, core biopsy and vacuum assisted mammotomy are suitable for MR guided sampling [88].

VACUUM ASSISTED MAMMOTOMY

A number of different vacuum assisted mammotomy devices are currently available. These include Mammotome™ (Breast Care, Ethicon Endosurgery) (Fig. 4.6a–b), SenoCor 360 (SenoRx Inc.) (Fig. 4.7) and VacuFlash (Biomed.-Instrumente und Produkte [BIP] GmbH). The SenoCor 360 and VacuFlash are designed as diagnostic techniques with the needle having to be removed from the breast to retrieve each core sample, and they are therefore less adaptable for multiple contiguous sampling or piecemeal percutaneous needle excision. The Mammotome™ (Breast Care Ethicon Endosurgery) probe is the most widely used, and there are extensive reports in the literature

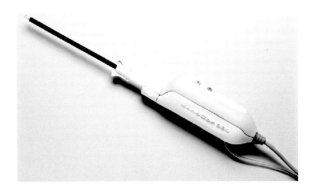

Fig. 4.7 The SenoCor 360 vacuum assisted biopsy device incorporating a radiofrequency cutting tip for easy placement of the needle in the breast.

about its efficacy. These devices use the principle of a vacuum applied along a double lumen needle to both obtain and retrieve multiple contiguous core samples without the need to remove the needle from the breast for each core specimen. Core size can be 14, 11 or 8 gauge delivering specimens of average weight of 35, 100 and 300 mg respectively (Fig. 4.8). This compares to only 17 mg for the average automated 14 gauge core biopsy.

The principles of how the vacuum assisted mammotomy technique works are shown below (Fig. 4.9). The Mammotome™ probe consists of three main parts:

1. an outer double lumen probe with a lower section through which suction is applied and an upper sampling chamber,
2. a hollow rotating motorized cutting trocar, and
3. an inner specimen retrieval suction trocar.

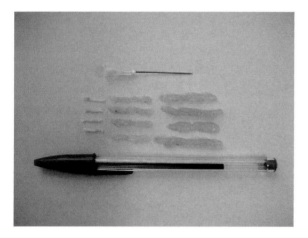

Fig. 4.8 Comparison of core biopsy tissue sample sizes (on the left a 14 gauge automated core [17 mg], in the center an 11 gauge mammotomy [100 mg] and on the right an 8 gauge mammotomy [300 mg]).

The system is computer controlled for ease of use, with the sampling sequences preprogrammed by the user. Once placed in the breast, tissue is sucked into the stationary upper sample chamber and the motorized hollow rotating inner cutting trocar separates the specimen. This is then retrieved from the sample site by withdrawing the trocar while applying suction through an inner second trocar. The biopsy probe remains in the breast throughout the sampling process, and multiple radial contiguous core samples can be obtained by rotating the whole probe around the biopsy site. Because there is no forward throw action, sampling of lesions that are small, superficial or close to the chest wall can be easily achieved. Vacuum assisted mammotomy is therefore to be preferred

where larger tissue samples are required, when conventional core biopsy has failed to provide a definitive diagnosis, for some very small lesions and for lesions at sites difficult to target with conventional automated core.

Vacuum assisted mammotomy is very well tolerated by patients, and, despite the needle size, many patients prefer this procedure to automated core biopsy, particularly for stereotactic X-ray guided biopsy. With automated core biopsy the noise of the gun firing and the shock wave that this causes in the breast along with the need to remove and reinsert the device for each sample cause anxiety and distress despite reassurance and prior warning. Anxiety caused by the sampling technique itself is significantly less with the mammotomy technique; there is no loud noise when the sample is obtained and retrieved by the relatively slowly forward and backward rotating cutting inner trocar and the device remains in the breast while multiple specimens are obtained.

Vacuum assisted mammotomy retrieves much larger volumes of tissue using a rotating cutting trocar, and for this reason it is important and necessary to use more local anesthesia than is usually needed for automated core biopsy. Local anesthetic should be injected into the skin and deeply into the breast tissue around the target area. Local anesthetic combined with adrenaline to promote vasoconstriction is recommended for infiltration of the breast tissue around the biopsy site. The adrenaline-induced vasoconstriction prolongs the anesthetic effect, allows for larger doses of anesthetic to be used and reduces local hematoma formation. The vacuum itself also appears to assist hemostasis and should be used to aspirate any bleeding during the sampling procedure. Volumes of 15 to 25 ml of local anesthetic are usually sufficient, and volumes approaching the upper safe dose limit are virtually never required. Local anesthetic without adrenaline may be preferred for the skin and in patients who have contraindications to the use of adrenaline. Longer acting local anesthetic may also be used around the biopsy site. However, there are no comparative studies to show that this more complicated local anesthetic regime provides any less patient morbidity than the use of a single local anesthetic preparation.

As with all biopsy techniques, the patient should be fully informed verbally and with written instructions about why the procedure is taking place, what it involves, what they will experience during the biopsy, how long it will take, what they will need to do afterwards and where they will receive the result.

When the biopsy needle is removed from the breast, local compression is applied directly over the biopsy site as firmly as the patient can tolerate for 10 to 15 minutes. The skin entry site is then closed with an

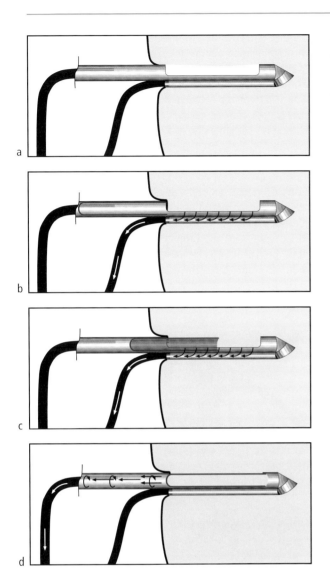

a

b

c

d

e

Fig. 4.9a–e Diagrammatic representation of the principle of vacuum assisted mammotomy.

4.9a Stereotactic or ultrasound guidance used to position the probe.

4.9b Tissue is gently vacuum aspirated into the aperture.

4.9c The rotating cutter is advanced forward, cutting and capturing a specimen.

4.9d After the cutter has reached its full forward position, rotation and vacuum cease.

4.9e The cutter is withdrawn, transporting the specimen to the tissue collection chamber while the outer probe remains in the breast.

adhesive strip or skin adhesive. Aftercare is the same as for automated core biopsy but it is advisable to also apply folded swabs directly over the biopsy site with a secure skin dressing held in place by a wrap round bandage. To reduce local hematoma formation and the risk of delayed bleeding following vacuum assisted mammotomy, patients should be advised not to undertake any vigorous exercise for at least 24 hours.

INDICATIONS FOR VACUUM ASSISTED MAMMOTOMY

Mammotomy, with its ability to sample larger volumes of breast tissue, has been shown to be more reliable in confirming that no frankly malignant change is present in association with conditions such as radial scar and atypical ductal hyperplasia. However, despite the wider sampling achievable by mammotomy, until studies show that this technique is completely reliable in excluding associated malignancy, caution should be used, and surgical excision is recommended where any doubt exists about the nature of the abnormality.

The scar tissue around the surgical site in the conserved breast, particularly following radiotherapy, can be extremely fibrous and difficult to biopsy by conventional means when recurrence of malignancy is suspected. The mammotomy device with its motorized cutting trocar can be used to successfully obtain sufficient tissue to achieve a reliable diagnosis.

For malignant lesions, where ascertaining excision margins is fundamental to confirming adequate treatment, mammotomy must not be considered a therapeutic procedure. Orientation of the piecemeal cores of tissue is difficult, and it is impossible to ascertain with any degree of certainty whether adequate clearance of excision margins has been obtained. However, for some benign lesions, such as fibroadenoma, mammotomy can be used for therapeutic excision. Ultrasound guidance is ideal for this procedure, which is significantly more cost effective and associated with less morbidity than surgical excision.

Indications for stereotactic vacuum assisted mammotomy:

1. Very small cluster of microcalcifications that is likely to be difficult to sample with core biopsy.
2. Cluster of calcifications at a site difficult to access with core biopsy.
3. Conventional core biopsy has failed to provide sufficient material for diagnosis.
4. Indeterminate pathology where it is likely that larger tissues volumes will be required for diagnosis.

Vacuum assisted mammotomy will understage disease less than half as often as conventional core biopsy. The difference is particularly marked in the understaging of ductal carcinoma in-situ (DCIS).

Vacuum assisted mammotomy is ideal for sampling calcifications associated with papillary lesions as it allows for the whole lesion to be excised. Papillary lesions are often reported as indeterminate by pathologists. Thus removal of the whole lesion along with a rim of surrounding normal tissue and histological confirmation that the lesion is entirely benign can be achieved without the need for surgical biopsy.

Indications for ultrasound guided mammotome biopsy include:
1. Mammographically detected architectural distortion visible on ultrasound (differentiation of radial scar from malignant disease).
2. Focal and suspicious microcalcifications visible on ultrasound.
3. Lesions too small for conventional core biopsy.
4. Lesions too superficial or deep in the breast for conventional core biopsy.
5. Previous failed conventional core biopsy.
6. Further evaluation of core or fine needle aspiration showing suspicious changes of uncertain malignant potential (such as atypical ductal hyperplasia or lobular carcinoma in-situ or radial scar).
7. Diagnosis of recurrent disease in patients treated by conservation surgery.
8. Abnormalities where wide sampling is considered important (such as mammographic asymmetric density with a nonspecific ultrasound correlate).
9. Removal of benign lesions such as fibroadenoma as an alternative to surgery.

The main advantages of vacuum assisted mammotomy compared to automated core biopsy are that it requires only a single pass of the probe into the breast to obtain multiple cores of tissue, the cores are contiguous and circumferential, and the tissue volume removed is considerably larger. VAM is also associated with significantly less morbidity than core biopsy – most women who have experienced both profess to proffer mammotomy. The main comparative disadvantages are its increased comparative cost and that the procedure takes significantly longer to perform.

ULTRASOUND GUIDED MAMMOTOMY

The various hand-held vacuum assisted mammotomy devices currently available are easy to use and are effective and accurate methods for retrieving larger volumes of tissue from ultrasound visible abnormalities [16, 59] (Figs 4.6a and 4.7). An initial ultrasound scan is carried out to identify the best direction for access to the abnormality. Local anesthetic is injected into the skin, the breast tissue down to the lesion and liberally inferior to and around the lesion itself. The local anesthetic needle is used to identify the best direction and angle in which to insert the mammotomy

needle. The needle, or introducing trocar, is placed through a small (2 mm) skin incision under direct real time ultrasound vision so that the biopsy chamber lies immediately behind or through the lesion (Fig. 4.10). The relationship between the sampling chamber and the lesion can be easily identified on the scan by manually moving the cutting trocar. Samples are obtained by incremental rotating of the probe through various angles through 180 degrees around the 12 o'clock neutral position (Fig. 4.11). The number of samples taken depends on the type and size of the abnormality. A metal marker clip or gel pellets can be placed through the probe or introducer for future identification of the biopsy site. In a few cases there may be difficulty in advancing the probe to the required site through dense uncompressed breast

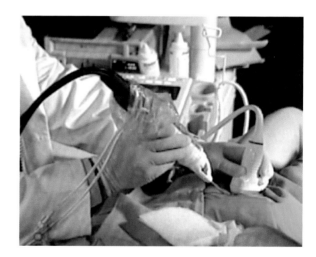

Fig. 4.10 Placement of the Mammotome HH™ probe under direct ultrasound guidance.

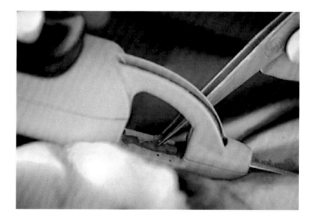

Fig. 4.11 Retrieval of the core specimen from the Mammotome HH™ biopsy probe.

tissue. In these circumstances forming a track for the probe with the local anesthetic injection is usually effective. Alternatively a radiofrequency outer sheath (EasyGuide™) can be placed for the Mammotome™ probe to be passed through to the biopsy site. As the patient is lying supine, the procedure is well tolerated. Hematoma is kept to a minimum because the breast is not under compression and intermittent suction is applied through the probe at the biopsy site.

X-RAY STEREOTACTIC GUIDED MAMMOTOMY

The techniques for prone table and upright vacuum assisted mammotomy are very similar to those for conventional automated core biopsy. Special attachments are needed for the probe guides, and all manufacturers can provide these (Figs 4.12 and 4.13). The localization software for the equipment must also be amended to allow for accurate placement of the probe. The depth of passage is calculated as for core biopsy such that the center of the sampling chamber corresponds to the point target selected on the stereoscopic images. Vacuum assisted mammotomy has been performed more widely on prone table devices, but it is also easy to perform this technique on upright stereotactic devices using the Breast Care Ethicon Endosurgery Mammotome ST device. This has been designed for both prone and upright use. In the upright position a lateral approach is preferred for most procedures as the probe is inserted along the long axis of the compressed breast. With this approach the compressed thickness of the breast is not a factor – with a vertical approach the compressed breast cannot be less than 30 mm or the sampling chamber will not be wholly within the breast and the vacuum will not function correctly. The lateral approach also allows for easier access to lesions lying superficially, close behind the nipple and close to the chest wall. These are all sites that can be difficult to target with core biopsy either with upright or prone biopsy tables.

When there is a possibility that the whole of the abnormality may have been removed by the needle biopsy procedure, it is prudent to place a marker at the biopsy site to facilitate localization of the biopsy at a future date. A small metal clip (Micromark™) or series of gel pellets (Gel Mark Ultra™) can be placed down the needle or introducer to mark the biopsy site after ultrasound or stereotactic biopsy. The metal clip is usually too small to reliably identify on ultrasound and stereotactic relocalization is required. The gel marker has the advantage of being visible on ultrasound for at least four weeks after the biopsy [23–25].

Some concern has been expressed about possible long-term changes to the breast structure shown on mammography as a result of mammotomy but this has not been shown to be a particular problem. Immediate

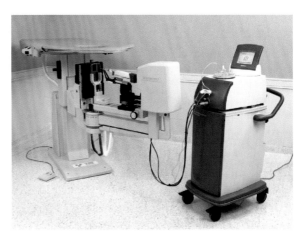

Fig. 4.12 Mammotome ST™ driver and probe shown set up for use with a prone biopsy table.

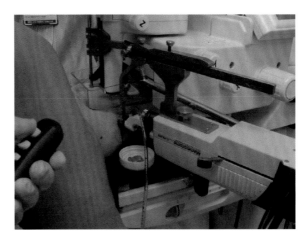

Fig. 4.13 The Mammotome ST™ in use with an upright digital stereotactic mammography system.

sequelae, including air at the biopsy site and visible hematoma, are common: occurring in around two thirds of cases. These changes, however, resolve quickly leaving no long-term mammographic interpretation problems [41]. Similarly, displacement of viable malignant cells by the vacuum assisted technique is not thought to pose a significant problem [40, 42–44].

Significant acute complications, mainly bleeding and hematoma that require intervention, are equally uncommon: vacuum assisted mammotomy and core biopsy occur in approximately 0.15% of cases [44]. Bruising following mammotomy is common for both procedures. The contraindications to vacuum assisted mammotomy are the same as those for conventional automated core biopsy.

■ SUMMARY

- The aim of percutaneous needle biopsy of the breast is to achieve as near as possible 100% diagnostic success without resort to open surgical biopsy.
- Both palpable and impalpable breast lesions can be more accurately and reliably biopsied under image guidance.
- Automated core biopsy is a technique that is reliable, cost effective and accurate and is preferred to fine needle aspiration for cytology in most circumstances.
- For image guided biopsy, ultrasound should be the guidance technique of first choice.
- Digital stereotactic core biopsy should only be used for impalpable lesions which are not visible on ultrasound.
- Vacuum assisted mammotomy is a highly effective method for providing larger volumes of breast tissue, facilitating very accurate breast diagnosis and often avoiding the need for open surgical biopsy. It is particularly effective in providing more reliable diagnosis in borderline pathology such as papillary lesions, mucinous lesions and radial scar.
- Stereotactic guided mammotomy is particularly effective for small clusters of indeterminate microcalcifications and calcifications in sites difficult to access with core biopsy.
- Mammotomy is an effective and well tolerated device for solving problems in breast diagnosis and can also be used to completely excise benign lesions.

REFERENCES

1. Teh WL, Evans AJ, Wilson ARM. Definitive Non-Surgical Breast Diagnosis: The Role of The Radiologist. Clinical Radiology 1998;24:1–9.
2. Parker SH, Burbank F, Jackman J, Aucreman CJ, Cardenosa G, Clink TM, et al. Percutaneous Large-Core Breast Biopsy: A Multi-institutional Study. Radiology 1994;3(2):359–63.
3. Vargas HI, Agbunag RV, Khaikhali I. State of the Art of Minimally Invasive Breast Biopsy: Principles and Practice. Breast Cancer 2000;7(4):370–9.
4. Russin LD. New Directions in Breast Biopsy: Review of Current Minimally Invasive Methods and Presentation of a New Coaxial Technique. Semin Ultrasound CT MR 2000;21(5):395–403.
5. Parker SH, Burbank F. A Practical Approach to Minimally Invasive Breast Biopsy. Radiology 1996;200:11–20.
6. Darling ML, Smith DN, Lester SC, Kaelin C, Selland DL, Denison CM, et al. Atypical Ductal Hyperplasia and Ductal Carcinoma In-Situ as Revealed by Large- Core Needle Breast Biopsy: Results of Surgical Excision. American Journal of Roentgenology 2000;175(5):1341–6.
7. Heywang-Kobrunner SH, Schaumloffel U, Viehweg P, Hofer H, Buchmann J, Lampe D. Minimally Invasive Stereotaxic Vacuum Core Breast Biopsy. European Radiology 1998;8(3):377–85.
8. Liberman L, Dershaw DD, Rosen PP, Morris EA, Abramson AF, Borgen PI. Percutaneous Removal of Malignant Mammographic Lesions at Stereotactic Vacuum-Assisted Biopsy. Radiology 1998;206(3):711–5.
9. Michell MJ, Andrews DA, Humphreys Sea. Results of 14 Gauge Biopsy of Architectural Distortion Stellate Lesions Using a Dedicated Prone Biopsy System. The Breast 1996;5:442.
10. Jackman RJ, Nowels KW, Shepard MJ, Finkelstein SI, Marzoni F, Jr. Stereotactic large-core needle biopsy of 450 nonpalpable breast lesions with surgical correlation in lesions with cancer or atypical hyperplasia. Radiology 1994;193(1):91–5.
11. Liberman L, Cohen MA, Dershaw DD, et al. Atypical ductal hyperplasia diagnosed at stereotaxic core biopsy of breast lesions: an indication for surgical biopsy. American Journal of Roentgenology 1995; 164: 1111–3.
12. Jackman RJ, Burbank F, Parker SH, al e. Atypical Ductal Hyperplasia Diagnosed at Stereotactic Breast Biopsy: Improved Reliability with 14-Guage, Directional, Vacuum-Assisted Biopsy. Radiology 1997;204:485–8.
13. Reynolds HE. Core biopsy of challenging benign breast conditions: a comprehensive literature review. American Journal of Roentgenology 2000;174:1245–50.
14. Brem RF, Schoonjans JM, Sanow L, Gatewood OM. Reliability of Histologic Diagnosis of Breast Cancer with Stereotactic Vacuum-Assisted Biopsy. Am Surg 2001;67(4):388–92.
15. Gajdos C, Levy M, Herman Z, Herman G, Bleiweiss IJ, Tartter PI. Complete Removal of Nonpalpable Breast Malignancies with a Stereotactic Percutaneous Vacuum-Assisted Biopsy Instrument. J Am Coll Surg 1999; 189(3):237–40.
16. Parker SH, Klaus AJ, McWey PJ, Schilling KJ, Cupples TE, Duchesne N, et al. Sonographically Guided Directional Vacuum-Assisted Breast Biopsy Using a Handheld Device. American Journal of Roentgenology 2001;177(2):405–8.
17. Parker SH, Dennis MA, Stavros AT, Johnson KK. A New Breast Biopsy Technique. Journal of Diagnostic Medical Sonography 1996;12:113–8.
18. Parker SH, Jobe WE, Dennis MA, al e. US-Guided Automated Large-Core Breast Biopsy. Radiology 1997; 187:507–11.
19. Parker SH, Klaus AJ. Performing a Breast Biopsy with a Directional, Vacuum-Assisted Biopsy Instrument. Radiographics 1997;17(5):1233–52.
20. Brem RF, Schoonjans JM, Goodman SN, Nolten A, Askin FB, Gatewood OM. Nonpalpable Breast Cancer: Percutaneous Diagnosis with 11-Gauge and 8-Gauge Stereotactic Vacuum-Assisted Biopsy Devices. Radiology 2001;219(3):793–6.
21. Brem RF, Schoonjans JM. Local Anesthesia in Stereotactic, Vacuum-Assisted Breast Biopsy. Breast 2001; 7(1):72–3.
22. Melotti MK, Berg WA. Core Needle Breast Biopsy in Patients Undergoing Anticoagulation Therapy: Prelimi-

nary Results. American Journal of Roentgenology 2000;174(1):245–9.

23. Liberman L, Dershaw DD, Morris EA, Abramson AF, Thornton CM, Rosen PP. Clip Placement after Stereotactic Vacuum-Assisted Breast Biopsy. Radiology 1997;205(2):417–22.

24. Burbank F, Forcier N. Tissue Marking Clip for Stereotactic Breast Biopsy: Initial Placement Accuracy, Long-Term Stability, and Usefulnes as a Guide for Wire Localisation. Radiology 1997;205(2):407–15.

25. Parker SH, Kaske TI, Gerharter JE, Dennis MA, Chavez JL. Placement accuracy and ultrasonographic visulaization of a new percutaneous breast biopsy marker. Radiology (supplement) 2001;221 (P):431.

26. Philpotts LE, Shaheen NA, Carter D, Lange RC, Lee CH. Comparison of Re-biopsy Rates After Stereotactic Core Needle Biopsy of the Breast with 11-Gauge Vacuum Suction Probe Versus 14-Gauge needle and Automatic Gun. American Journal of Roentgenology 1999;172(3):683–7.

27. Liberman L, Gougoutas CA, Zakowski MF, LaTrenta LR, Abramson AF, Morris EA, et al. Calcifications Highly Suggestive of Malignancy: Comparison of Breast Biopsy Methods. American Journal of Roentgenology 2001;177(1):165–72.

28. Reynolds HE, Poon CM, Goulet RJ, Lazaridis CL. Biopsy of Breast Microcalcifications Using an 11-Gauge Directional Vacuum-Assisted Device. American Journal of Roentgenology 1998;171(3):611–3.

29. Liberman L, Smolkin JH, Dershaw DD, Morris EA, Abramson AF, Rosen PP. Calcification Retrieval at Stereotactic, 11-Gauge, Directional, Vacuum-Assisted Breast Biopsy. Radiology 1998;208(1):251–60.

30. Philpotts LE, Lee CH, Horvath LJ, Lange RC, Carter D, Tocino I. Underestimation of Breast Cancer with 11-Gauge Vacuum Suction Biopsy. American Journal of Roentgenology 2000;175(4):1047–50.

31. Cangiarella J, Gross J, Symmans WF, Waisman J, Petersen B, D'Angelo D, et al. The Incidence of Positive Margins with Breast Conserving Therapy Following Mammotome Biopsy for Microcalcification. J Surg Oncol 2000;74(4):263–6.

32. Liberman L. Clinical Management Issues in Percutaneous Core Breast Biopsy. Radiol Clin North Am 2000;38(4):791–807.

33. Won B, Reynolds HE, Lazaridis CL, P. JV. Stereotactic Biopsy of Ductal Carcinoma In-Situ of the Breast Using an 11-Gauge Vacuum-Assisted Device: Persistent Underestimation of Disease. American Journal of Roentgenology 1999;173(1):227–9.

34. Lee CH, Carter D, Philpotts LE, Couce ME, Horvath LJ, Lange RC, et al. Ductal Carcinoma In-Situ Diagnosed with Stereotactic Core Needle Biopsy: Can Invasion be Predicted? Radiology 2000;217(2):466–70.

35. Jackman RJ, Burbank F, Parker SH, Evans II WP, Lechner MC, Richardson TR, et al. Stereotactic breast biopsy of non-palpable lesions: determinants of ductal carcinoma in-situ underestimation rates. Radiology 2001;218(2):497–502.

36. Brem R, Berndt V, Sanow L, Gatewood D. Atypical Ductal Hyperplasia: Histological Underestimation of Carcinoma in Tissue Harvested from Impalpable Breast Lesions Using 11-Guage Stereotactically Guided Directional Vacuum-Assisted Biopsy. American Journal of Roentgenology 1999;172:1405–7.

37. Guenin MA. Benign Intraductal Papilloma: Diagnosis and Removal at Stereotactic Vacuum-Assisted Directional Biopsy Guided by Galactography. Radiology 2001;218(2):576–9.

38. Dennis MA, Parker S, Kaske TI, Stavros AT, Camp J. Incidental Treatment of Nipple Discharge Caused by Benign Intraductal Papilloma Through Diagnostic Mammotome Biopsy. American Journal of Roentgenology 2000;174(5):1263–8.

39. Wilson ARM, Teh W. Mini Symposium: Imaging of the breast. Ultrasound of the breast. Imaging 1998;9:169–85.

40. Simon JR, Kalbhen CL, Cooper RA, Flisak ME. Accuracy and Complication Rates of US-Guided Vacuum-Assisted Core Breast Biopsy: Initial Results. Radiology 2000;215(3):694–7.

41. Lamm RL, Jackman RJ. Mammographic Abnormalities Caused by Percutaneous Stereotactic Biopsy of Histologically Benign Lesions Evident on Follow-Up Mammograms. American Journal of Roentgenology 2000;174(3):753–6.

42. Diaz LK, Wiley EL, Venta LA. Are malignant cells displaced by large-gauge needle core biopsy of the breast? American Journal of Roengenology 1999;173:1303–13.

43. Liberman L, Vuolo M, Dershaw DD, Morris EA, Abramson AF, LaTrenta LR, et al. Epithelial Displacement After Stereotactic 11-Gauge Directional Vacuum-Assisted Breast Biopsy. American Journal of Roentgenology 1999;172(3):677–81.

44. Lai JT, Burrowes P, MacGregor JH. Vacuum-Assisted Large-Core Breast Biopsy: Complications and Their Incidence. Can Assoc Radiol J 2000;51(4):232–6.

45. Liberman L, Drotman M, Morris EA, LaTrenta LR, Abramson AF, Zakowski MF, et al. Imaging-Histologic Discordance at Percutaneous Breast Biopsy. Cancer 2000;89(12)(2538–46).

46. Mercado CL, Hamele-Bena D, Singer C, Koenigsberg T, Pile-Spellman E, Higgins H, Smith SJ. Papillary Lesions of the Breast: Evaluation with Stereotactic Directional Vacuum-assisted Biopsy. Radiology 2001;221:650–655.

47. Jackman RJ, Birdwell RL, Ikeda DM. Atypical Ductal Hyperplasia: Can some lesions be defined after stereotactic 11-gauge vacuum assisted biopsy, eliminating the recommendation for surgical excision? Radiology 2002;224:548–554.

48. Brenner RJ, Bassett LW, Fajardo LL, Dershaw DD, Evans WP, Hunt R, et al. Stereotactic Core Needle Breast Biopsy: A multi-institutional Prospective Trial. Radiology 2001; 218:866–872.

49. Philpotts LE, Shaheen NA, Jain KS, Carter D and Lee CH. Uncommon High Risk Lesions of the Breast Diagnosed at Stereotactic Core Needle. Radiology 2000; 216:831–837.

50. Pisano ED, Fajardo LL, Caudry DJ, Sneige N, Frable WJ, Berg WA, Et al. Fine needle aspiration biopsy of non-palpable breast lesions in a multicentre clinical trial: Results from the Radiologic Diagnostic Oncology Group. Radiology 2001; 219:785–792.

51. Fishman JE, Milikowski C, Ramsinghani R, Velasquez MV and Aviram G. US-Guided Core-Needle Biopsy of the Breast: How many specimens are necessary? Radiology 2003; 226:779–782.

52. DiPiro PJ, Gulizia JA, Lester SC and Meyer JE. Mammographic and Sonographic Appearances of Nodular Adenosis. American Journal of Roentgenology 2000;175: 31–34

53. Liberman L, Goodstine SL, Dershaw D, Morris EA, LaTrenta LR, Abramson AF and Van Zee KJ. One operation after percutaneous diagnosis of non-palpable breast cancer: Frequency and associated factors. American Journal of Roentgenology 178:673–679

54. Kushwa AC, O'Toole M, Sneige N, Stelling CB and Dryden MJ. Mammographic pathological correlation of apocrine metaplasia diagnosed using vacuum assisted stereotactic core needle biopsy: Our 4-year experience. American Journal of Roentgenology 180:795–798.

55. Liberman L, Ernberg LA, Heerdt A, Zakowski MF, Morris EA, La Trenta LR, et al. Palpable breast masses: Is there a role for percutaneous images guided core biopsy? American Journal of Roentgenology 175: 779–787.

56. Rosen EL, Bently RC, Baker JA, Scott Soo. Imaging-guided core needle biopsy of papillary lesions of the breast. American Journal of Roentgenology 179:1185–1192.

57. Margolin FR, Leung JWT, Jacobs RP, Benny SR. Percu-taneous imaging guided core breast biopsy: 5 Years experience in a community hospital. American Journal of Roentgenology 177: 559–564.

58. Wunderbladinger P, Wolf G, Turetschek K and Helbich TH. Comparison of sitting versus prone position for stereotactic large-core breast biopsy in surgically proven lesions. American Journal of Roentgenology 178: 1221–1225.

59. Scott Soo M, Baker JA, Rosen EL and Vo TT. Sono-graphically guided biopsy of suspicious microcalcifica-tions of the breast: A pilot study. American Journal of Roentgenology 178: 107–1015.

60. Laura Liberman and Michelle P. Sama. Cost effective-ness of stereotactic 11-gauge directional vacuum assis-tant breast biopsy. American Journal of Roentgenology 175:53–58.

61. Rodenfield Darling ML, Smith DN, Lester SC, Kaelin C, Selland DG, Denison CM, et al. Atypical ductal hyperplasia and ductal carcinoma in-situ as revealed by large core needle breast biopsy: Results of surgical excision. American Journal of Roentgenology 175 1341–1346.

62. Roger J. Jackman and Francis A. Marzoni. Stereotactic histologic biopsy with patients prone: Technical feasi-bility in 98% of mammographically detected lesions. American Journal of Roentgenology 180:785–794.

63. Becker L, Taves D, McCurdy L, Muscedere G, Karlik S and Ward S. Stereotactic core biopsy of breast micro-calcifications: Comparison of film versus digital mammography, both using an add-on unit. American Journal of Roentgenology 177:1451–1457.

64. Georgian-Smith D, D'Orsi C, Morris E, Clark Jnr CF, Liberty E and Lehman CD. Stereotactic biopsy of the breast using an upright unit, a vacuum-suction needle and a lateral arm support system. American Journal of Roentgenology 178:1017–1024.

65. GJ Welle, M Clark, S Loos, D Pauls, D Warden M Sheffield and C Parsells. Stereotactic breast biopsy: Recumbent biopsy using add-on upright equipment. American Journal of Roentgenology 175:59–63.

66. Ralph L Smathers. Advanced breast biopsy instrumental device: Percentages of lesion and surrounding tissue removed. American Journal of Roentgenology 175: 801–803.

67. Ellis IO, Galea MH, Locker A, Roebuck EJ, Elston CW, Blamey RW, Wilson ARM. Early experience in Breast Cancer Screening: emphasis on development of proto-cols for triple assessment. The Breast, 1993; 2: 148 153.

68. Krebs TL, Berg WE, Severson MJ, Magder LS, Gold-berg PA, Campassi C, et al. Large core biopsy guns: comparison for yield of breast tissue. Radiology 1996;200:365–8.

69. Nath ME, Robinson TM, Tobon H, Chough DM, Sumkin JH. Automated Large-Core Needle Biopsy of Surgicall Removed Breast Lesions: Comparison of Samples Obtained with 14-, 16- and 18-guage Needles. Radio-logy 1995;197:739–43.

70. Evans AJ, Whitlock JP, Burrell HC, Pinder SE, Ellis IO, Geraghty JG, et al. A comparison of 14 and 12 gauge needles for core biopsy of suspicous mammographic calcification. British Journal of Radiology 1999;72: 1152–4.

71. Whitlock JPL, Evans AJ, Burrell HC, Pinder SE, Ellis IO, Blamey RW, et al. Digitally acquired imaging improves upright stereotactic core biopsy of mammo-graphic microcalcifications. Clinical Radiology 2000; 55:374–7.

72. Liberman L, Evans III WP, Dershaw DD, Hann LE, Deutch BM, Abramson AF, et al. Radiography of micro-calcifications in stereotaxic mammary core biopsy speci-mens. Radiology 1994;190:223–5.

73. Moritz JD, Luftner-Nagel S, Westerhof JP, J.W. O, Grabbe E. Microcalcifications in breast core biopsy specimens: disappearance at radiography after storage in formaldehyde. Radiology 1996;200:361–3.

74. Brenner RJ, Fajardo L, Fisher PR, Dershaw DD, Evans WP, Bassett L, et al. Percutaneos Core Biopsy of the Breast: Effect of Operator Experience and Number of Samples on Diagnostic Accuracy. AJR 1996;166:341–6.

75. Rich PM, Michell MJ, Humphreys S, Howes GP, Nunnerley HB. Stereotactic 14G core biopsy of non-palpable breast cancer: what is the relationship between the number of core samples taken and the sensitivity for detection of malignancy? Clinical Radiology 1999;54:384–9.

76. Bagnall MJC, Evans AJ, Wilson ARM, Burrell HC, Pinder SE, Ellis IO. When have mammographic calcifi-cations been adequately sampled at needle core biopsy? Clinical Radiology 2000;55:548–53.

77. Burrell HC, Pinder S, Wilson ARM, Evans AJ, Yeoman LJ, Elston CW, Ellis IO. The positive predictive value of mammographic signs: a review of 425 non-palpable breast lesions. Clinical Radiology 1996; 51: 277–281

78. Lister D, Evans AJ, Burrell HC, Blamey RW, Robertson JFR, Pinder SE, Ellis IO, Elston CW, Kollias J, Wilson ARM. The accuracy of breast ultrasound in the evaluation of clinically benign discrete breast lumps. Clinical Radiology 1998; 53: 490–492.

79. Britton PD. Fine needle aspiration or core biopsy. The Breast 1999;8:1–4.

80. Britton PD, McCann J. Needle biopsy in the NHS breast screening programme 1996/7: how much and how accurate? The Breast 1999;8:5–11.

81. Ferzli G et al. Advanced Breast Biopsy Instrumentation (ABBI): A Critique. Journal of the American College of Surgery 1997; 185: 145–151.

82. Liberman L. Advanced Breast Biopsy Instrumentation (ABBI): Analysis of Published Experience. American Journal of Roengenology 1999; 172: 1413–1416.

83. Brenner RJ, Jackman RJ, Parker SH et al. Percutaneous Core Needle Biopsy of Radial Scars of the Breast: When is Excision Necessary? American Journal of Roengenology 2002; 179: 1179–1184.

84. Pfarl G, Helbich TH, Riedl CC et al. Stereotactic 11-Gauge Vacuum Assisted Breast Biopsy: A Validation Study. Amercian Journal of Roengenology 2002; 179: 1503–1507.

85. Liberman L. Percutaneous Image-Guided Core Breast Biopsy: State of the Art at the Millennium. American Journal of Roengenology 2000; 174: 1191–1199.

86. March DE, Coughlin BF, Barham RB et al. Breast Masses: Removal of All US Evidence during Biopsy by Using a Handheld Vacuum-assisted Device – Initial Experience. Radiology 2003; 227:

87. Liberman L, Kaplan JB, Morris EA et al. To Excise or To Sample the Mammographic Target: What is the Goal of Stereotactic 11-Gauge Vacuum Assisted Breast Biopsy. American Journal of Roengenology 2002; 179: 679–683

88. Kuhl CK et al. MR Imaging-guided Large-Core (14-Gauge) Needle Biopsy of Small Lesions Visible at Breast MR Imaging Alone. Radiology 2001; 220: 31–39.

Content

PATHOLOGIC DIAGNOSIS IN MINIMAL INVASIVE BIOPSY

THOMAS DECKER, WERNER BOECKER, UTE KETTRITZ, MONIKA RUHNKE, HEIKE JACOB, KRISZTINA ZELS, ELKE KEIL AND RAINER OBENAUS

Minimal invasive biopsy (MIB) performed as automated needle core biopsy (NCB) or vacuum-assisted needle core biopsy (VANCB) is now the method of choice for diagnostic assessment of mammographically detected breast lesions. Using stereotactic or ultrasound guidance, MIB allows harvesting of continuous tissue from almost all lesions independently of their localization. MIB therefore represents a valid alternative to open surgical biopsy (for details see Chapter 4).

Over the past decades fine needle aspiration (FNA) combined with clinical and radiological assessment has assured rapid, inexpensive and accurate diagnosis in symptomatic breast disease. However, a meta-analysis of data collected in the context of the FNA and MIB series published so far has revealed that MIB will eventually supersede FNA in diagnosing nonpalpable radiologic lesions due to its greater sensitivity and specificity [1]. Histologic examination in MIB facilitates diagnosis of benign lesions and, in the event of carcinoma, allows invasive growth, grade, and subtype of a given lesion to be assessed. It is therefore replacing FNA cytology as the diagnostic method of choice in palpable and mammographically detected breast lesions [2, 3].

The pathologist's task in MIB diagnostics has become much more complex and now goes beyond merely determining the malignant potential of a palpable lump. Instead, the pathologist is a fully authorized member of an interdisciplinary team responsible for the joint diagnosis and management of patients with breast lesions. With increasingly widespread use of high-quality breast imaging, the ratio of early node-negative cancers of up to 10 mm in diameter has steadily grown, especially in those countries where a population-based mammographic screening program has been implemented. The same holds true for mammographically detected ductal carcinoma in-situ (DCIS) verified by MIB diagnosis. Interestingly, more than half of these early lesions are now nonpalpable. Moreover, due to improvements in radiology, a considerably wider range of benign lesions can be detected, as a result of which morphology has become much more complex. Pathologists are therefore expected to draw up reports capable of reflecting the clinical implications of their findings and thus support treatment planning and management of breast patients.

Provided that an appropriate sample has been taken, benign lesions can clearly be diagnosed in MIB material, reducing the need for open surgery. Genuine false-negative rates of 0.3–1.2% [4, 5] and false-positive rates of 0.4% [6] confirm the reliability of MIB as a diagnostic method. In view of this data the threshold for proceeding to open surgical biopsy has risen in recent years. In our opinion, it should be set as high as possible.

Pathologic diagnosis in minimal invasive biopsy

■ QUALITY ASSURANCE

Continuous quality assurance (QA) must be guaranteed in MIB diagnostics. In the multidisciplinary setting of a screening assessment center or a breast unit, quality assurance in pathology is an integral part of the overall QA program and is mandatory for the entire multidisciplinary breast team. Multidisciplinary team meetings are therefore not only essential for the process of individually assessing patients; at the same time they form the basis of the QA program. The sensitivity and specificity of MIB cannot be calculated unless surgical procedures and follow-up data from patients with both benign and malignant lesions are subjected to constant quality assurance. The tools listed below may help in implementing an appropriate quality assurance program.

1. Protocol for handling and technical work-up of specimens.
2. Checklists for clinical data as well as for pathology reports.
3. Diagnostic categories for reporting results of imaging **(BI-RADS™)**, overall clinical and imaging evaluation **(OCI score)** and pathologic findings **(B categories)**.
4. Categories for correlating pathologic and radiologic results **(CO categories)**.
5. Categories for determining appropriate action **(A categories)** in decision-making in a multidisciplinary team.
6. Correlation of MIB results and results of surgical excisions.
7. Follow-up of patients with nonmalignant lesions.
8. Standardized statistics for calculating quality parameters.

Implementing and running a QA program requires considerable resources, both in terms of personnel and time. It is essential to individual patient care as well as to the technical improvement and enhancement of the skills of the pathologists involved. An audit of quality parameters defined within the program is an effective method of determining the quality of team performance. Within the framework of a population-based breast screening program, it enables an informed and qualified comparison of different screening areas and breast units [9].

■ REPORTING MIB PATHOLOGY

The MIB diagnosis detailed in the **pathology report** is the key element in decision-making by a multidisciplinary breast team to determining further appropriate action. This report should not only be precise and rapidly delivered; it must be conveyed in a clinically relevant and concise manner. The sections detailing with macroscopic and microscopic findings must contain all relevant information, including a competent and comprehensible interpretation for the clinician. Unnecessarily detailed descriptions lacking clinical consequences must be avoided.

Clinical information is of particular importance in the report. The histologic 'diagnosis' must be entered in a separate field of the report with its most important findings summarized at its start. It should also include a clear statement on the correlation between pathologic and radiologic findings. Even in cases of carcinoma, the pathologist should try to convey whether the pathology seen in the biopsy was the target of the image-guided lesion or whether a different coexisting lesion could have produced the main mammographic or sonographic finding.

The pathology report of MIB specimens brings the assessment process to a close. At its conclusion our team always makes recommendations for treatment based on the multidisciplinary in-house protocol of the unit, although this may not be applicable in every clinical setting. Any recommendations of the pathologist that are given verbally to the clinician must also be part of the written report. This is essential, especially in cases requiring re-biopsy either by MIB or by open surgical procedure.

The 'European Working Group for Breast Screening Pathology' (EWGBSP) was founded in 1993 and now operates within the 'Europe Against Cancer' program as one of the organizations of the 'European Breast Cancer Network'. To describe the results of the assessment process of MIB samples, the EWGBSP recommends a system – the **B categories** – for grouping biopsies into a finite number of diagnostic classes [7]. These categories allow the multidisciplinary breast team to make confident protocol-based decisions on whether to proceed to therapeutic surgery, re-biopsy, or to discharge and refer back to routine screening. B categories should be used for every pathology report in MIB (for details see below), independently of the possibility of a definitive diagnosis.

CLINICAL INFORMATION

Interpretation of clinically relevant core biopsies by the pathologist requires a thorough knowledge of the indication and the biopsy procedure of the target lesion. Detailed information concerning clinical presentation and imaging findings of the lesion should therefore be available to the pathologist. To document its impact on the final pathologic evaluation the most relevant clinical information should also be included in the pathology report.

The following minimal information should be included in the MIB request form submitted by the radiologist and/or clinician.

1. The patient's personal details (surname, forename, date of birth, hospital number etc.).
2. Site of the biopsy (laterality and quadrant).
3. Clinical findings, especially of palpation and inspection of skin and nipple, as well as family and past medical history, if relevant.
4. Type of imaging findings (mass, microcalcifications, architectural distortion) including a description (i. e. not solely the BI-RADS™ category).
5. Mammographically and/or sonographically determined size of the lesion.
6. Differential diagnosis by the radiologist and category according to the American College of Radiology Breast Imaging Reporting and Data System Atlas (BI-RADS™ Atlas) [8] or according to the R categories within the *European Guidelines for Quality Assurance in Mammography Screening* [7].
7. Overall clinical and imaging evaluation (for scoring see below).
8. Number of specimens obtained.
9. Presence or absence of microcalcifications in core biopsy specimen radiogram.

TECHNICAL PROCESSING

SPECIMEN RADIOGRAPHY

Specimen radiography is essential for all lesions containing calcifications. It can be used to decide whether all mammographically detected calcifications were appropriately sampled. In addition it enables the pathologist to identify those biopsy samples containing microcalcifications (Fig. 5.1). Depending on the presence or absence of calcifications, specimens should be placed in different cassettes and, if possible, submitted to the pathologist along with the specimen radiograph.

In rare cases, microcalcifications that are unequivocally removed using stereotactic vacuum-assisted biopsy devices cannot be detected on the initial specimen radiograph. In our experience one of the most important reasons for loss of microcalcifications when proceeding from biopsy to specimen radiography is rupture of microcysts (Fig. 5.2) and the ensuing aspiration of their liquid content, including microcalcification particles, into the debris canister of the device. In such specific circumstances, Friedman and colleagues recommend obtaining radiographs of all the debris in the canister to evaluate whether it contains sufficient diagnostic material to warrant its routine submission to pathology for histologic diagnosis [10] (for further details on loss of microcalcifications see Table 5.1).

HANDLING OF SPECIMENS

All tissues obtained should be submitted for microscopic examination. Specimens of needle core or vacuum-assisted biopsies should be placed in 4%

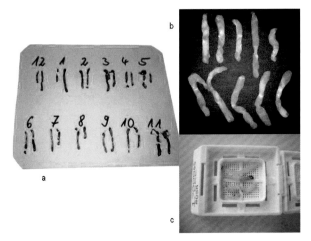

Fig. 5.1 a–c Biopsies obtained by vacuum-assisted MIB (a), a specimen radiogram (b) showing all biopsies containing microcalcifications, and a cassette with four cores (c).

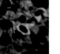

Tab. 5.1 Loss of microcalcifications

Reason	MC Detection SR	H	Appropriate action
MC missed by MIB	–	–	Re-MIB
Aspiration of MC during VACNB	–	–	Radiogram of aspirated debris
Fixation in glyoxal	+	–	Avoid glyoxal fixation
Eccentric superficial localization of MC	+	–	Carefully trim the very first level of paraffin blocks and avoid frozen sectioning

MC = microcalcification, VACNB = vacuum assisted core needle biopsy, SR = specimen radiogram, H = histology

neutral buffered formaldehyde immediately after harvesting. This is the responsibility of the performing radiologist. He or she must also label the tissue container and fill in the accompanying forms. In our team the radiologist places the specimens directly in tissue cassettes labeled with the ID number for the pathology laboratory (Fig. 5.1). Specimens from different locations must be placed in cassettes with different ID numbers.

The number of biopsy samples should be recorded. In general, a maximum of five biopsies can be placed in the same cassette. Whenever possible, the cores should be arranged in parallel arrays. Patients' details entered on the form must be rigorously cross-checked with the biopsy sample (see below for the minimal dataset).

The proposed fixative guarantees routine processing and allows a histologic diagnosis to be made within 24 hours. Only a single report exists on radiographic disappearance of microcalcifications in core biopsy specimens after prolonged immersion in aqueous fixative. However, we were able to detect microcalcifications both by specimen radiography and histologic investigation of cores obtained from mastectomy specimens up to 21 days after harvesting. Recently, data has been published on the influence of glyoxal, a

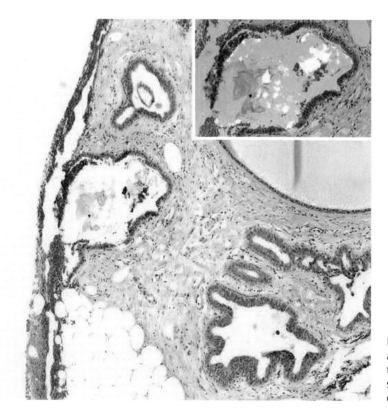

Fig. 5.2 Microcalcifications (calcium oxalate type) outside ruptured microcysts at the margin of the MIB specimen. The inset shows the result of polarization microscopy of the birefringent particles.

formalin-free aldehyde fixative, on microcalcification detection. Glyoxal was recommended to pathologists as an environment-friendly agent. It has been found, however, that glyoxal fixation tends to diminish the visibility of microcalcifications to the point of completely obscuring them and may therefore result in a lack of correlation with mammographic findings. The likely explanation for this phenomenon is that calcium is more soluble in glyoxal than in formalin [11] (for further details on loss of microcalcifications see Table 5.1).

GROSS PATHOLOGY IN MIB

Gross pathology of MIB specimens is only of limited value in establishing a final diagnosis. It may be helpful for the radiologist to decide whether the tissue obtained is representative and therefore sufficient for histopathologic diagnosis when diagnosing solid malignant tumors. The description by the pathologist should include the number of specimens and their maximum length. In addition, a short macroscopic description may help in avoiding errors in tissue identification in the pathology laboratory. The descrip-

tion should be restricted to three simple categories (predominantly fatty tissue, predominantly soft solid tissue and predominantly firm solid tissue).

HISTOLOGIC TECHNIQUE

Histologic sections in MIB diagnosis must be at least 4 μm thick and of high quality. At least three levels from each block should be taken in cases of masses or architectural distortions on imaging. If microcalcifications are seen, stepwise sections from at least four levels at 20 μm intervals should be taken. The very first slide should be seized to avoid loss of eccentrically located microcalcifications (Fig. 5.3). Additional levels may be needed (for instance in cases where the targeted microcalcifications are not found in the initial set of sections). In such situations it is advisable to prepare additional slides from every level at the onset, as immunostaining may be necessary later on in the process (for further reasons for loss of microcalcifications see Table 5.1).

Lesions such as atypical ductal hyperplasia, radial scar, and complex papillary proliferations may be extremely difficult to interpret in frozen section

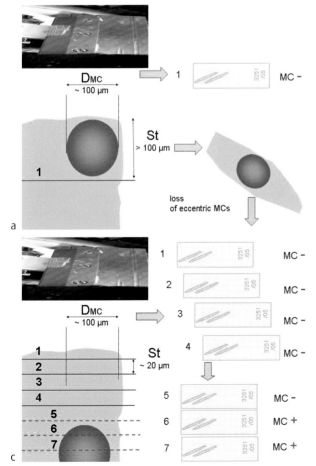

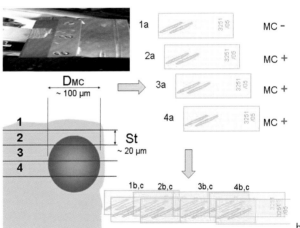

Fig 5.3a–c Stepwise sectioning of an MIB specimen with microcalcifications identified at radiography.
5.3a Loss of microcalcifications may, for example, occur by trimming the paraffin block deeper than 100 μm for the first slide.
5.3b Additional slides should be prepared for immunohistochemistry from each level (b, c).
5.3c When calcifications are not found in the initial sections, additional sections are needed until the calcified area is visible (MC = microcalcifications, D_{MC} = diameter of MC, St = step section interval, 1–7 = level numbers: a = first slides from each level, b and c = additional slides for immunohistochemistry).

preparations, and small foci of DCIS or microinvasive carcinoma may be lost or rendered uninterpretable as an artifact of freezing. Therefore frozen sections of nonpalpable microcalcifications are strongly discouraged, even in excisional biopsies [12–14]. Moreover, frozen sections should only be performed when the information obtained is necessary for immediate therapeutic decision-making, which is not the case in MIB. Finally, a precondition for the use of frozen sections is that sufficient residual tissue is present to establish a definite final diagnosis. This cannot be guaranteed in MIB. In view of the diagnostic advancements made in recent years, there is no doubt that preparation of frozen sections is not useful in MIB.

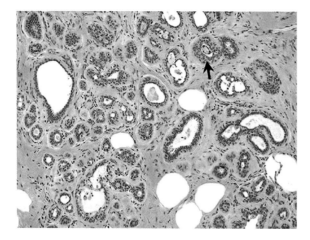

Fig. 5.4 Category B1: Blunt duct adenosis with microcalcification smaller than 100 μm.

■ ■ PATHOLOGY REPORTING CATEGORIES

The five category reporting system (see Table 5.2) was initially proposed by the UK National Coordinating Group for Breast Screening Pathology in its 1997 publication with the aim of collating basic data required for a standardized QA program [15]. The B category system was subsequently adopted and recommended by the EWGBSP [16]. The categories can be used for all types of nonpalpable and symptomatic lesions (microcalcifications, architectural deformities and mass lesions) and should also be used outside the screening setting. The B category system is exclusively based on histologic features of the sample, not on clinical or imaging characteristics. The definitions given below are in agreement with the fourth edition of the *European Guidelines for Quality Assurance in Mammography Screening* [9].

B1: NORMAL (BREAST) TISSUE/UNINTERPRETABLE

This category indicates either a core of normal tissue (with or without breast parenchyma) or of uninterpretable artifactual tissue. From a histopathologic point of view this means that no breast lesion can be detected. If microscopically circumscribed fibrocystic alterations are present, but there is doubt as to whether these are associated with any type of radiologic findings at all, these should be categorized as B1. Similarly, microcalcifications smaller than 80–100 μm in diameter should also be classified as B1 due to the fact that these are considered radiologically irrelevant (Fig. 5.4). As a rule this category implies an unsatisfactory biopsy, but in special constellations B1 biopsies with normal fatty or breast tissue may be consistent with a lipoma or hamartoma respectively. Therefore, when reporting a B1 category, the different tissues included in the specimen must be commented on.

B2: BENIGN LESION

This category indicates that the specimen contains a benign lesion. The spectrum of benign abnormalities includes benign tumors, proliferating breast lesions, and involutionary and reactive changes. Typical examples of B2 lesions include fibroadenoma, some (but not all!) papillary lesions (see below), ductal hyperplasia, sclerosing adenosis, fibrocystic change and cysts, duct ectasia, other inflammatory conditions, abscesses, and fat necrosis. Involutionary microcalcifications may be classified as B2 provided they are larger than 100 μm and, consequently, radiologically relevant. In some cases with very small areas of fibrocystic change or with minor involutionary calcifications, it may be difficult to determine whether a specific lesion is present. When in doubt, it may be more appropriate to classify such lesions as B1 rather than B2.

B3: LESION OF UNCERTAIN MALIGNANT POTENTIAL

This category indicates benign abnormal findings with an increased risk of synchronously associated malignancy. There are two different groups of B3 lesions:
1. lesions more often associated with malignancy, which, however, in the specific situation may be missed in the biopsy due to a sampling error; and
2. lesions in which, due to their heterogeneous composition, atypical or malignant proliferations may not be detected within the MIB specimens.

The first group includes lobular neoplasia (LN), atypical epithelial proliferations of ductal-type (Fig. 5.5) and atypical columnar cell lesions (columnar

Tab. 5.2 Reporting categories*

Category		Description
B1		Normal tissue/uninterpretable
B2		Benign lesion
B3		Lesion of uncertain malignant potential
B4		Lesion suspicious of malignancy
B5		Malignant lesion
	B5a	In-situ carcinoma
	B5b	Invasive carcinoma
	B5c	Invasive status not assessable
	B5d	Other malignancy

* EWGBSP 2005 [9]

cell change or hyperplasia with atypia = flat epithelial atypia [FEA]). Their association with DCIS or invasive carcinoma has been well documented. In general, it is not possible in MIB specimens to differentiate reliably between atypical ductal hyperplasia (ADH) (Fig. 5.5) and secondary lobular cancerization by DCIS of low or intermediate grade [17]. Even larger tissue volumes obtained by vacuum-assisted MIB rarely allow a definite diagnosis of ADH, for instance when a very tiny area of microcalcification was

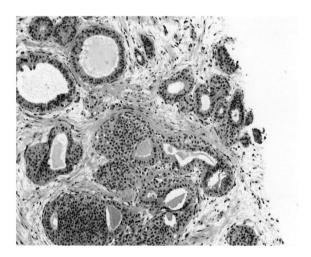

Fig. 5.5 Category B3: Lesions with increased risk of associated malignancy. Atypical proliferation of ductal-type. In general, MIB specimens do not enable a definitive diagnosis of ADH vs. non-high grade DCIS with secondary lobular involvement.

completely sampled, when there is no involvement of larger extralobular ducts or when the radiologic-pathologic correlation is absolutely sure [18–28]. Therefore, according to the EWGBSP guidelines [9] for such findings we recommend using the descriptive term 'atypical epithelial proliferation of ductal-type'. It should be borne in mind that all these lesions (LN, ADH and FEA) hardly ever produce characteristic findings on imaging. Therefore it must be assumed that the target was missed as a result of inadequate sampling. If these lesions are detected histologically in MIB as single abnormal findings associated with radiologically suspicious findings (BI-RADS™ 4 or 5, respectively), there is an urgent need for further diagnostic activity.

The lesions of the second group (papillary lesions, complex sclerosing lesions [CSL], phyllodes tumors without clear malignancy, mucocele-like lesions and cystic-hypersecretory lesions) may show intralesional heterogeneity. Due to the limited amount of tissue obtained by MIB, the area of malignancy may therefore have been missed. Consequently, findings within this subgroup need to be clarified according to a standardized protocol.

The majority of B3 lesions require surgical excision or re-MIB, but such cases must be discussed at a preoperative multidisciplinary meeting. The B3 category does not apply to so-called marker lesions such as usual ductal hyperplasia, which indicate an increased risk of developing subsequent carcinoma.

B4: LESION SUSPICIOUS OF MALIGNANCY

The B4 category is applied when findings are suggestive of invasive or intraductal malignancy, but preclude a definitive assessment. This may be due to two reasons.

1. The changes detected in the specimen are too small. When sufficient amounts of neoplastic epithelial proliferations of low and intermediate grade are found, a non-high grade DCIS should be diagnosed. However, the lesion should only be categorized as B5, if there is no doubt that the entire population of cells fulfills the criteria of malignancy. Care must be taken, if only part of a ductal space is seen containing highly atypical epithelial cells without necrosis, or if the epithelial cells show features of apocrine phenotype. Such lesions are more appropriately classified as B4. Furthermore, neoplastic cells contained within a blood clot adherent to the outer margin of the biopsy specimen (Fig. 5.6) or in necrotic material suggestive of comedonecrosis should be classified as B4. Due to their inherently different clinical implications, lobular intraepithelial neoplasia of classic type (formerly termed 'atypical lobular hyperplasia' or

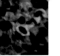

'lobular carcinoma in-situ') should not be classified as B4. However, more extensive lesions of lobular intraepithelial neoplasia, particularly of the pleomorphic subtype and with comedonecroses, may be indistinguishable from DCIS and should be classified as B4 (see Chapter 21).

2. The diagnostic evaluation of findings is limited by artifacts. Crushed or poorly fixed cores that probably contain carcinoma but cannot provide a definitive diagnosis are correctly categorized as B4.

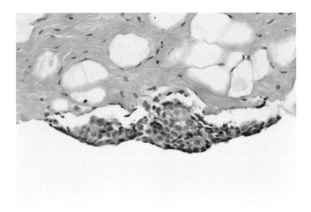

Fig. 5.6 Category B4: Neoplastic cells suggestive of DCIS, adherent to the outer margin of the biopsy specimen.

B5: MALIGNANT LESION

This category is appropriate for cases of unequivocal malignancy. Carcinomas should be subdivided into intraductal and invasive lesions by using the subcategories 5a or 5b respectively. In cases of invasive malignancy other than primary breast carcinoma (malignant phyllodes tumors, malignant lymphomas, sarcomas, metastases, etc.) subcategory 5d should be used. If there is uncertainty as to whether the carcinoma is intraductal or invasive, subcategory 5c is appropriate. Biopsies of skin for Paget's disease may also be recorded as nonoperative diagnostic procedures and can be classified accordingly as 5a. In general, lobular neoplasia is included in the B3 category as it does not have the same management implications as a diagnosis of DCIS or invasive malignancy. Nevertheless, pleomorphic variants or the exceptional combination of lobular neoplasia with comedonecrosis and wide distribution in the specimen via extension in multiple extralobular ducts may be classified as B5. It must be emphasized that the B categories do not represent a pathologic classification of breast lesions, but a code for the assessment of histopathologic status. They are therefore part of the minimum dataset in MIB (see

below) and serve the pathologist as a basis for discussing a problem within a multidisciplinary team meeting. The minimum dataset enables a multidisciplinary decision to be made on patient management, even if a definite diagnosis cannot be achieved.

PROBLEMS AND PITFALLS

Six groups of lesions pose a diagnostic problem in the pathologic assessment of MIB specimens: so-called borderline lesions, sclerosing lesions, papillary lesions, mucocele-like lesions, spindle cell lesions and some fibroepithelial lesions. Assessing the size of some lesions, usually small malignant lesions, may be nearly impossible due to the fragmentation of specimens obtained with vacuum-assisted core needle biopsy.

BORDERLINE LESIONS

These include the differential diagnoses of lobular vs. ductal in-situ lesions, ductal hyperplasia vs. neoplastic proliferation, atypical ductal hyperplasia vs. DCIS, and DCIS vs. microinvasive carcinoma. On occasion, reaching a final decision may be impossible, even after employing immunostaining techniques (see Chapter 20).

Focal lactational change, which may appear atypical with irregular, large, or pyknotic nuclei, may occasionally be mistaken for cancerization of lobules. Apocrine atypia, particularly in association with sclerosing adenosis (apocrine adenosis), may also be difficult to interpret in MIB. Large nuclei, often with prominent nucleoli, may be mistaken for DCIS if pleomorphism is also present. In some cases of proliferative apocrine change a definite diagnosis cannot be made, but such a process should be categorized as a B3 lesion of uncertain malignant potential. In cases with cytologic atypia and complex architectural patterns, a definite diagnosis of DCIS (B5a) is more appropriate.

Immunohistochemistry is essential to the differential diagnosis of hyperplastic and neoplastic ductal proliferations. Whenever the non-neoplastic nature of an epithelial proliferation in MIB is in doubt, Ck5/14 immunohistochemistry should be performed (for details see Chapters 8, 17, 19 and 20).

Ductal proliferations with cytomorphological and architectural characteristics of atypical ductal hyperplasia in MIB should be classified as atypical ductal proliferations: the main criterion of ADH – that it manifests as a very focal neoplastic process confined to single terminal duct lobular units – cannot be verified on MIB (see Chapter 20). For this reason the EWGBSP recommends using the term 'atypical epithelial proliferation of ductal-type' [9]. The appropriate category is thus B3. If the atypical ductal proliferation is found in interlobular ducts, the lesion is said to be 'suspicious of DCIS', and therefore, if detected in MIB, such a lesion should be categorized as B4. The reported risk of malignancy in cases where MIB samples contain an atypical epithelial proliferation varies from 18 to 83%. This data illustrates the difficulties of assessing epithelial proliferations in limited amounts of material [22, 29–32]. Thus, referral for excision is mandatory in these circumstances. However, if involvement of extralobular ducts seems obvious, a diagnosis of DCIS of low or intermediate grade is justified and the B5a category is appropriate.

Microinvasive carcinoma is by definition a predominantly intraductal carcinoma with a maximum invasion of 1 mm. This subgroup was integrated into the TNM system as pT1mic in 1997 [21, 33]. The definition is very strict and very few tumors fulfill the criteria.

For quality assurance purposes according to EU Guidelines, DCIS with microinvasion must be categorized as an in-situ carcinoma (B5a) rather than as an invasive cancer, while at the same time microinvasion must also be specified [9].

SCLEROSING LESIONS

Benign sclerosing lesions of the breast include sclerosing adenosis (SA), radial scar/complex sclerosing lesion (RS/CSL), sclerosing papillary lesions and, occasionally, adenomyoepithelial tumors. They may be problematic in MIB diagnosis. The main differential diagnosis is invasive carcinoma, especially of tubular type. The morphologic features of the sclerosing lesions and tubular carcinoma are discussed in Chapters 9, 10, 11 and 14 and are shown in Table 9.2.

RS/CSL has been reported in the older literature to harbor foci of atypical epithelial proliferations of ductal-type, DCIS or invasive malignancy respectively (see Chapter 10). Therefore, the recommendation is to classify these lesions as B3: 'lesion of uncertain malignant potential' [9].

PAPILLARY LESIONS

Potential pitfalls with papillary lesions in MIB result partly from sampling error and partly from architectural distortion or artifacts. Finding benign papillary structures in MIB does not rule out malignant change elsewhere in the lesion. For this reason, when benign papillary structures are identified, these findings must be placed in the B3 category: 'lesion of uncertain malignant potential'. In addition, local excision should be advised. Even in excision specimens, adequate sampling is required to exclude the presence of associ-

ated atypical ductal proliferations. Only in rare cases of small papillary lesions that are:
1. widely sampled by MIB; and
2. no longer detectable by imaging after the biopsy procedure;

can one make a diagnosis of benign papilloma without further diagnostic excision. A multidisciplinary team meeting is a prerequisite in dealing with such cases. On the other hand, atypical proliferations of ductal-type within a papillary lesion must be classified as B4 and an open diagnostic biopsy is indicated. Additionally, care must be taken not to overdiagnose malignancy, especially if tubular structures are found entrapped in sclerosed areas.

MUCOCELE-LIKE LESIONS

The main features of mucocele-like lesions are pseudocystic areas within the interstitium containing amorphous mucinous material that extrudes from cystically dilated ducts. These are lined by flat or cuboidal epithelium devoid of cellular atypia. Such characteristic features of benign mucocele-like lesions were originally described by Hamele-Bena et al. [34] and may be seen in association with a broad spectrum of lesions with mucin-distended ducts and varying degrees of epithelial proliferation or atypia [34–39]. In truth, such histologic characteristics cannot be utilized to safely distinguish between isolated benign mucocele-like lesions and their counterparts associated with malignant mucinous lesions (mucinous DCIS or invasive carcinoma), unless such malignancy is also seen in the sample. Although mucinous carcinoma could not be detected in a subgroup of screening-detected mucocele-like lesions, as published by Farshid et al. [40], statistically robust follow-up studies of large series capable of confirming that there is a lower risk of missed mucinous cancer are not yet available, even for microcalcification-associated mucocele-like lesions detected at screening. Therefore, at present, mucocele-like lesions must be categorized as B3 and discussed in the multidisciplinary team [9].

SPINDLE CELL PROLIFERATIONS

Spindle cell proliferations may also prove diagnostically difficult. Such proliferations may indicate different mesenchymal spindle cell tumors or a carcinoma with spindle cell elements. Most cases can be diagnosed correctly by immunohistochemistry (see Chapter 14). A small ratio of spindle cell lesions may represent reactive processes that are indistinguishable from tumors, even using immunohistochemistry. When a definitive histologic diagnosis cannot be made, the abnormality should be reported as a spindle cell lesion of uncertain origin and categorized as B3. In any case, spindle cell proliferations of all types must be discussed in a multidisciplinary meeting, in particular to ensure that any unknown trauma in the patient's history was taken into account.

FIBROEPITHELIAL TUMORS

The spectrum of fibroepithelial tumors ranges from benign cellular fibroadenoma to malignant phyllodes tumor (see Chapter 15).

Only clearly malignant phyllodes tumors should be categorized as B5d. Fibroepithelial lesions with cellular stroma, stromal overgrowth or some mitotic activity suggesting a phyllodes tumor should be reported as a 'fibroepithelial lesion suspicious of phyllodes tumor' and classified as B3 to avoid under-diagnosis. Even clear-cut phyllodes tumors with a benign appearance or borderline findings in MIB should be categorized as B3: a 'lesion of uncertain malignant potential'. Discussion at a multidisciplinary meeting will usually enable appropriate management.

SIZE ESTIMATION OF SMALL MALIGNANT LESIONS AFTER VACUUM-ASSISTED BIOPSY

Size measurement may be difficult after VACNB, especially in small lesions, as lesions of up to 20 mm may be completely removed but also simultaneously fragmented by the procedure. Sometimes the largest diameter of lesions along the longitudinal axis of the involved biopsy may help to obtain a rough estimate of their size. More often, however, the size can only be estimated by careful reconstruction. This naturally requires information on the orientation of every specimen. In combination with the exclusion of residual tumor in the surgical specimen, the upper size limit can thus at least be realistically gauged. This is important as two therapeutic decisions explicitly depend on tumor diameter. Firstly, according to the EUSOMA guidelines [41] axillary dissection, lymph node sampling or sentinel node biopsy should not be performed in invasive breast carcinomas of less than 2 mm and in tubular carcinomas of less than 10 mm. Secondly, the International Consensus Conference in St. Gallen stipulated that node-negative patients with G1 invasive cancers of less than 20 mm do not need adjuvant chemotherapy [42]. In addition, the pT categories for breast cancer as specified in the UICC TNM classification are defined according to tumor diameters: pT1mic up to 1 mm, pT1a up to 5 mm, pT1b up to 10 mm and pT1c up to 20 mm [43]. Even if this estimation technique is applied, the pathologist is not likely to come up with the exact measurements of tumor diameters required for assessing the limits

discussed above. Therefore, from the pathologist's point of view, VACNB of masses highly suspicious of malignancy should be avoided. In most cases, biopsies of such lesions can alternatively be performed by automated CNB without alteration of the outer contour of the invasive cancer.

THE MINIMUM DATASET

In countries with nationwide quality assurance programs it is widely recognized that the information included in breast cancer histopathology reports continues to vary considerably between different departments [44, 45]. The minimum dataset aims to standardize the quality of histopathology reporting. This idea is derived from the nationwide breast screening program of the UK National Health Service [15] and was adopted in 1996 by the European Working Group on Breast Screening Pathology [16].

Reporting MIB pathology on a standardized form makes it easier to ensure that all the necessary data has been included, agreed terminology and diagnostic criteria are observed, only data of clinical value is reported and the information is delivered consistently.

This dataset is the basis for radiologic-pathologic correlation, for choice of the individual patient's treatment and for counseling patients on prognosis. Moreover, it may be helpful for research and audit purposes: for monitoring specific patterns of cancer by cancer registries and for implementing quality assurance in screening programs.

In the Berlin-Buch breast unit, we use a checklist that includes clinical information, imaging results, pathologic data, the correlation established between radiology and pathology and, finally, the treatment option(s) suggested to the patient. The form is based on the multidisciplinary in-house protocol (the Berlin-Buch practice protocol), which in turn is modeled on the one proposed by the *European Guidelines for Quality Assurance in Mammography Screening* [9].

In 2001, Mathers et al. were able to demonstrate a general improvement in documentation of individual pathologic features (especially of microcalcification, ductal carcinoma in-situ, tumor grade, size and hormone receptor status) after introduction of a standard reporting proforma using the Royal College of Pathologist's minimum dataset for breast cancer histopathology reports and the national histopathology reporting form of the National Health Service (NHS) breast screening program [34, 46].

THE TEAM APPROACH IN MIB

The aim of diagnostic assessment of clinical or radiologic breast anomalies by minimal invasive biopsy technique (MIB) is to obtain a definitive diagnosis without delay in a multidisciplinary team approach. In addition to other key personnel such as the surgeon, radiologist, radiographer, and breast care nurse, the pathologist is an indispensable member of such a professional diagnostic breast team [47]. Pathologists need to be highly qualified and experienced in breast diseases as they are key players in interdisciplinary communication and decision-making. Each member of the team must be familiar with the most recent literature and state-of-the-art treatment options.

The aims of the team meeting after MIB are:
1. to correlate radiology and pathology;
2. to decide the final assessment outcome; and
3. to formulate a recommendation for the patient's management.

All recommendations concerning patient management require a consensus of all team members. The team meeting should therefore be held before treatment of the patient has been initiated.

RADIOLOGIC-PATHOLOGIC CORRELATION

In principle, correlation involves imaging and histopathologic results; pathologic investigation in MIB is effectively restricted to histopathology. Information from MIB specimens on the size and shape of the lesion from which the tissue has been sampled is impossible to obtain. This is exacerbated by the fact that, whereas virtually any lesion in breast pathology can occur in MIB, the specimens may deliver only a partial view of the lesion of interest. Abnormalities seen by the pathologist often represent a lesion but sometimes indicate only minimal nonpathologic tissue change without connection to the target of the MIB procedure. Deciding on the radiologic-pathologic correlation requires a good working knowledge of the basic terminology and features of diagnostic imaging on the part of the pathologist dealing with MIB. For basic information on lesions in diagnostic imaging (masses, asymmetries, architectural distortions and calcifications) see Chapters 2, 8–15.

MASSES

All lesions are characterized by different combinations of features (shape, margins, density, and size) associated with varying risks of malignancy. In addition, ultrasound techniques yield additional findings, which can be employed to better evaluate masses. The most important is the echogenicity of masses, which helps in preventing unnecessary biopsies of simple ductal cysts. The schematic drawing in Figure 5.7 shows some characteristic mass lesions with their pathologic counterpart. Masses with spiculated margins carry a much higher risk of malignancy than all other types. Spiculated masses account for about 14% of biopsied lesions, whereby about 81% of these are malignant [48].

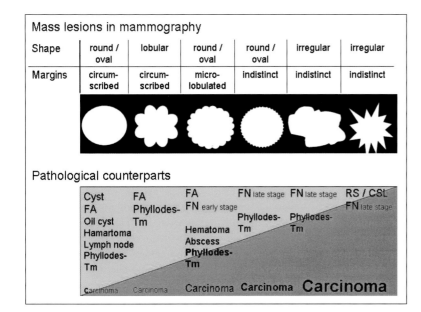

Fig. 5.7 Scheme of different mass lesions in imaging and their pathologic counterparts. Different combinations of shape and margins are not specific for a distinct pathologic diagnosis but predict the likelihood of carcinoma (FA = fibroadenoma, Tm = tumor, FN = fat necrosis, RS = radial scar, CSL = complex sclerosing lesion).

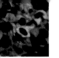
ASYMMETRIES

Although breast asymmetry, as detected in mammography, is likely to be a predictor of breast cancer [49], the overall positive predictive value of asymmetry found on mammography seems only to be low. Additional investigations have confirmed that, in particular in cases of visible ultrasound findings, MIB is indicated. Not surprisingly, fibrosis is a frequently observed feature on histological examination, especially when associated with palpable asymmetries. Focal fibrosis, periductal mastitis (duct ectasia) and sclerosing adenosis may therefore be found in MIB. Alternatively, findings may be consistent with the well-recognized, but ill-defined pattern of invasive lobular or lobular mixed types of carcinoma [50]. Even DCIS can cause asymmetries, as Sneige et al. were able to show in up to 16% of their symptomatic DCIS series [51].

ARCHITECTURAL DISTORTIONS

Lesions presenting mammographically with radiating spiculations and focal retraction or distortion at the edge of the parenchyma but without any definite mass are strongly suggestive of malignancy. Approximately 48–60% of architectural distortions biopsied are found to be breast carcinomas [52–55], and about 80% of those cancers are invasive [52]. It is estimated that 12–45% of breast carcinomas missed in mammographic screening are architectural distortions [56–58]. Recently, a growing number of studies have confirmed that MIB is accurate in differential diagnosis of architectural distortions. If targeting is accurate and the amount of tissue obtained sufficient, it is possible to distinguish distortions due to cancer from benign causes, which include radial scar/complex sclerosing lesion and sclerosing adenosis [59–62] (see below for further details on management).

CALCIFICATIONS

The main problem in the radiologic-pathologic correlation of microcalcifications is to categorize the different findings. Radiologically, microcalcifications are classified according to their size, shape, distribution, site and number (see below). From a pathologic perspective, classifications using chemical and optical properties, staining features, form, size and localization have been recommended. These classification schemes, however, cannot be reconciled. Therefore, after covering the physicochemical principles of calcifications in general, we try to describe them pathologically in terms of BI-RADS™ scores, the most commonly used classification for microcalcifications. Finally, we discuss different microcalcification findings with reference to their lobular and ductal origin.

PHYSICOCHEMICAL NATURE OF CALCIFICATIONS

Mammographically-detectable calcifications are calcium deposits caused by glandular secretory or necrotic cell material. The end products of these different pathogenetic processes do not, however, correspond to the two different chemical types of calcifications described by Frappart [63]. Type 1 is a rather rare finding [63–65], almost exclusively localized in (micro)cystic ductules. It contains a special subtype of calcium oxalate (wedellite), which is a very light, yellow, transparent crystalline material not easily visible in routine H&E-stained slides. Like many others, we have never detected type 1 calcifications within intraductal or invasive carcinomas [65, 66]; they are so rare as to be of minor diagnostic relevance. They cannot be visualized using the von Kossa stain and may therefore be overlooked. To detect this type of calcification, it is prudent to evaluate slides using polarization microscopy, where wedellite appears angulated and birefringent (Fig. 5.8a). Type 2 calcifications contain a subtype of calcium phosphate (hydroxyapatite), which is easily detected by conventional light microscopy as deep hematoxyphilic deposits of different shape. These are much more frequently detected in both secretory and necrobiotic material (Figs 5.8b–c). Radiologically, these microcalcifications are seen both within benign and malignant lesions. It has been suggested that those within benign lesions have a rather low density, whereas those within malignant ones show higher density on mammography.

RADIOLOGIC CATEGORIES OF CALCIFICATIONS AND RELATED HISTOPATHOLOGY

MACROCALCIFICATIONS

Calcifications larger than 2 mm in diameter are referred to as macrocalcifications, whereas those smaller than 1 mm are known as microcalcifications [67]. In general, macrocalcifications are exclusively associated with benign lesions of the breast such as fibroadenomas or fat necroses. The pathologist will therefore hardly ever see macrocalcifications in MIB. Consequently, there is no difficulty in correlating radiologic and pathologic findings.

MICROCALCIFICATIONS

Microcalcifications are associated with a broad spectrum of lesions. They are an important feature indicating underlying alterations of the breast tissue, yet their overall specificity is low [68]. According to a recent analysis only 30–40% of microcalcifications are produced by malignancies [69]. Even after categorizing microcalcifications according to their BI-RADS™ score [8], there is no category associated with a 100% rate of intraductal or invasive cancer

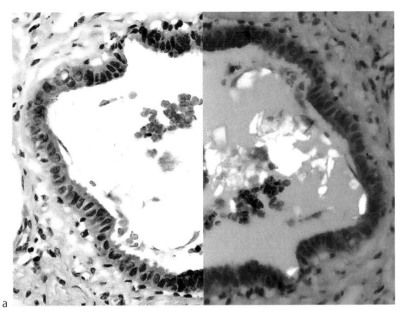

a

Fig. 5.8a – c Pathogenesis of microcalcifications.

5.8a Secretory-type calcium oxalate (wedellite).

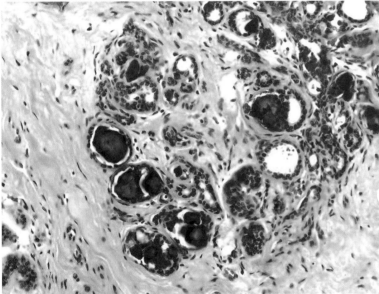

b

5.8b Secretory-type calcium phosphate.

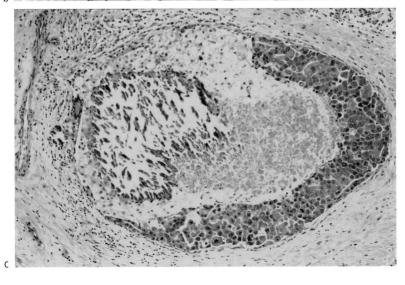

c

5.8c Comedo-type necrosis with dystrophic-type calcifications (calcium phosphate).

(BI-RADS™ score 4: 2–95%, BI-RADS™ score 5: > 95%). Moreover, there is some doubt about the upper limit of the malignancy rate in the BI-RADS™ 3 category in microcalcifications. Whereas in general, this rate should be lower than 2%, we could show a frequency of 19% malignancies in BI-RADS™ 3 microcalcification lesions [28].

According to the BI-RADS™ definition, the spectrum of microcalcifications includes benign, intermediate and probably malignant microcalcifications. In the event of **'typical benign' microcalcifications** MIB should be only performed in exceptional cases. Therefore skin and vascular microcalcifications as well as milk of calcium (from large cysts) will almost never be seen in MIB specimens. Indications for MIB in 'typical benign' microcalcifications include coarse microcalcifications of otherwise undetectable, very small and shrunken hyalinized fibroadenomas without the typical 'popcorn' appearance; spherical, thin, but relatively large microcalcifications of pseudo-cystic fat necrosis (oil cysts) without the characteristic 'eggshell' appearance; and large (approx. 1 mm), rod-like microcalcifications of duct ectasia/plasma cell mastitis when the involved areas are very small as a result of their ductal distribution. In our experience, the most frequently biopsied benign microcalcification findings are areas with punctate particles (less than 0.5 mm with smooth margins and lobular distribution) that have been recently detected or that have increased in size compared to earlier mammographic findings.

'Typical malignant' microcalcifications are, as a rule, smaller than 0.5 mm, but can range up to 0.9 mm in diameter. Three types of so-called malignant microcalcifications exist.

1. Fine linear, occasionally branching microcalcifications of the casting type, which are typically found in comedonecrosis of high grade DCIS. In our experience this radiologic pattern of microcalcification is highly specific for DCIS.
2. Pleomorphic microcalcifications varying extremely in form and size are frequently associated with necroses of comedo type, most often in DCIS of high and quite often of intermediate grade. Microcalcifications of this type may occasionally be seen in some cases of old hyalinized fibroadenomas as well as in old fat necroses.
3. Granular microcalcifications, which have irregular margins and a maximum diameter between that of pleomorphic malignant and punctate benign microcalcifications. 'Malignant' microcalcification of this type can be found in equal proportions in DCIS of high and of intermediate grade. However, even granular microcalcifications are unspecific. They can be found in microcystically dilated ductules in fibrocystic disease, most often associated with columnar cell lesions like blunt duct adenosis.

'Microcalcifications of intermediate concern' are also referred to as **'amorphous microcalcifications'** due to their indistinct margins. Their shape is round to flake-like, and their specificity is low: such microcalcifications can be found in DCIS (mostly in DCIS of low and intermediate grade) as well as in (sclerosing) adenoses, columnar cell lesions (with or without atypia) and, rarely, in usual ductal hyperplasia.

The distribution of all types of microcalcifications in the breast may, to a varying degree, be helpful in diagnostic analysis. Distribution patterns of microcalcifications provide the breast radiologist with a practical tool to summarize any suspicious facts in imaging. To a certain extent these well-defined patterns correlate with histopathologic findings. Unfortunately, multiple 'clustered' microcalcifications that mammographically appear to be arranged in a small area are histologically not always located exclusively in lobules and may also be seen in benign and malignant lesions. Therefore analysis of the distribution of microcalcifications should always encompass an assessment of the size and shape of the individual particles.

CORRELATION OF LOCALIZATION OF CALCIFICATIONS WITH RADIOLOGIC AND PATHOLOGIC FINDINGS

All microcalcifications develop in microscopically small cavities, mostly within, but sometimes outside, the glandular tree. In keeping with the principles of DCIS extension (see Chapters 20, 21), only intraductal – not lobular – microcalcifications are thought to represent intraductal carcinoma, whereas microcalcifications restricted to the lobules are almost always associated with benign lesions. Therefore, the specific distribution of particles may not only influence the diagnostic statement of the radiologist; it also helps the pathologist to search for specific microcalcifications in breast tissue as well as to evaluate them.

Both radiologists and pathologists should be familiar with microcalcifications of lobular and ductal-type (see Table 5.3 and Fig. 5.9).

LOBULAR MICROCALCIFICATIONS

In principle, lobular microcalcifications are detected in microcystic adenosis (most often in blunt duct adenosis) (Fig. 5.9a), sclerosing adenosis, involuted lobules and fibroadenomas. These microcalcifications are secretory calcium phosphate particles of lamellar structure. Their size and shape depend on the architectural alteration of the lobule (see Table 5.3). For example, microcalcifications in acini of involuted lobules are small, round and uniform, while their counterparts in sclerosing adenosis consist of fine to larger, round, comma-shaped or linear, slightly aniso-morphous particles according to the size of the ectatic ductules. Calcifications of 'ossifying' type are irregu-

Tab. 5.3 Local origin, pathology, and radiology of microcalcifications

Diagnosis	Origin	Type	Individual MC		MC Cluster	
			Size (µm)	Shape	Size (mm)	Shape
Involution	L	S	80–120	Round, smooth bordered	< 5	Round
BDA	L	S	80–300	Round, flattened, smooth bordered	< 7	Round/oval
SA	L	S	80–300	Round, linear, comma-shaped	< 7	Round/oval
FA	L	S	80–1,500	Round, corkscrew or popcorn shaped	Very small, up to 30	Round/oval
DCIS ig/lg	D	S	80–300	Round, smooth bordered	Up to 100	Triangular, angulated
Periductal mastitis	D	S	80–900	Linear, rod-like spindle shaped	Up to 100	Segmental
DCIS hg/ig	D	N	80–400	Coarse granular	Up to 100	Triangular, angulated, segmental
DCIS hg	D	N	100–900	Linear branching	Up to 100	Segmental, triangular, angulated

MC = microcalcification; BDA = blunt duct adenosis; SA = sclerosing adenosis; FA = fibroadenomas; DCIS = ductal carcinoma in-situ;
lg = low grade; ig = intermediate grade; hg = high grade; L = lobular; D = ductal; S = secretory; N = necrobiotic.

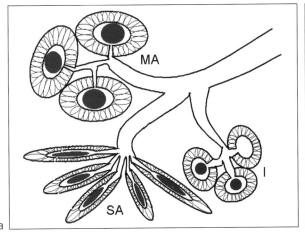
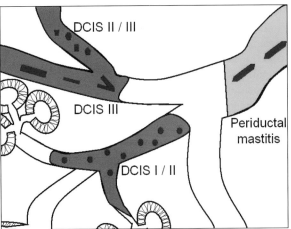

Fig. 5.9a–b Scheme illustrating different types of mammographic microcalcifications and their histopathologic counterparts.
5.9a Lobular microcalcifications. All lobular microcalcifications represent benign lesions. Their shape and size depend on the alteration of the lobular architecture (MA = blunt duct adenosis; SA = sclerosing adenosis; I = involuted lobule).
5.9b Ductal microcalcifications. Most ductal microcalcifications represent DCIS: Whereas high grade DCIS shows polymorphous linear or coarse crushed stone-like particles within necroses, low grade DCIS is associated with tiny lamellar spherical particle of secretory type. Intermediate grade DCIS may show both types. Periductal mastitis represents the exceptional benign variant of ductal micro-calcifications: needle shaped smooth particles oriented towards the nipple (DCIS I, II, III = low, intermediate, and high grade DCIS, respectively).

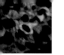

larly shaped, basophilic, often lamellar and surrounded by an eosinophilic matrix (Fig. 5.10). The term 'ossifying' was introduced by Rosen due to their resemblance to the matrix of an ossifying nodule [70]. However, this material does not contain osteocytes and is not lined by osteoblasts, nor is it birefringent on polarizing microscopy. Even though, in principle, ossifying calcifications are luminal and not interstitial [70, 71], we could neither find them as isolated free particles within the ductal lumen nor as intraepithelial microcalcifications completely surrounded by epithelium [70]. Rather, they were always detected beneath the epithelium, surrounded by a pinkish matrix. Based on such findings we interpret the matrix as a basement membrane-like product of the associated epithelia, although we have never been able to detect laminin or type 4 collagen within this material. As shown in Figure 5.10, after atrophy of the ductular wall, ossifying microcalcifications can be seen located in the interstitium. It seems that this process is responsible for a large number of breast microcalcifications described as 'primarily interstitial'. Microcalcifications of ossifying type are also typically associated with epithelia of columnar cell type. The spectrum includes simple columnar cell change, columnar cell hyperplasia, flat epithelial atypia, and low grade clinging carcinoma of columnar cell type (for the latter see 'Simultaneous lobular and ductal calcifications' below). In our experience, which is, moreover, shared by other authors [71], ossifying calcifications appear slightly polymorphous and densely clustered on mammography. Within microcysts they can agglomerate to form slightly polymorphic morula-like configurations, which may produce suspicious mammographic findings of 'amorphous' microcalcifications when the involved lobule is enlarged. The same type of microcalcification localized in larger ductal-lobular ('macro')cysts can be easily categorized as benign on two-view mammography, which is capable of detecting sedimentation of microcalcifications at the bottom of ductal-lobular units – the 'teacup' phenomenon [72]. This phenomenon is evident in a lateral or, less obviously, in an oblique view.

Ductal microcalcifications

Ductal microcalcifications may originate in subsegmental and segmental ducts containing DCIS, periductal mastitis, or papillomas (Figs 5.9b, 5.11). The morphology of individual particles of ductal microcalcifications covers a broad spectrum, ranging from small, round, lamellar and large, rod-like particles of the 'benign' type to granular, linear, moderately sized, 'malignant' microcalcifications, as described above. If arranged in a ductal pattern, granular and linear microcalcifications invariably consist of dystrophic calcium deposits exclusively located within comedonecroses,

which will generally be found in DCIS with equal proportions in high and intermediate grade lesions [13, 73] (Fig. 5.11).

Linear forms develop from tube-like arrangements of typical, symmetrically extended comedonecroses in the center of ducts, whereas granular microcalcifications will be found in smaller, more irregular necroses. This is also the reason why linear and branching microcalcifications are more often associated with DCIS of high grade [74,75] than other types. In extremely rare cases necrosis-associated microcalcifications can be seen in extensive lobular neoplasia with ductal involvement. In ductal hyperplasia this type of microcalcification is quite exceptional. The ductal variant of small, round, lamellar microcalcifications is much less frequent than its lobular counterpart. Like the latter, they represent calcium deposits within secretory material. In the case of DCIS they are produced by more differentiated tumor cells of low grade (more frequently) or intermediate grade DCIS [13, 76]. However, the histologic grade of DCIS cannot be accurately determined based on the pattern of microcalcifications as seen at mammography [77, 78]. Mixed, differentiated forms of DCIS ensure that detecting microcalcifications of both the lamellar secretory and of the dystrophic type in different areas of the same DCIS lesion is not unusual.

Another ductal form of microcalcification typically presents as monomorphous, linear, needle-shaped particles of high density, arranged in the direction of the nipple. These microcalcifications develop within abnormal secretory material in periductal mastitis (duct ectasia) [79]. However, the entire set of typical features – reminiscent of linear microcalcifications of ductal-type – may not be visible. In these cases, MIB is indicated for differential diagnostic purposes. In periductal mastitis (duct ectasia) inspissated microcalcifications are detected within retained abnormal secretory material and debris of ectatic ducts. In combination with periductal chronic inflammatory infiltrate and periductal sclerosis of varying intensity a definite diagnosis is nearly always possible. Problems may arise, however, if some atypical epithelia are detected in the periphery of intraluminal debris. Under these circumstances a DCIS cannot be excluded, and an excisional biopsy should be performed. In rare cases, DCIS may cause a 'secondary' chronic periductal mastitis.

Finally, microcalcifications in papillary lesions represent a further subgroup of the ductal-type. They may occur in sclerosing papillomas as pleomorphic, often shell-like particles arranged in round to oval, but sometimes even angular, clusters. In particular, smaller lesions present with clustered polymorphous calcifications without a definite mass or halo. Histologically, they are located within the mostly hyalinized,

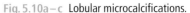

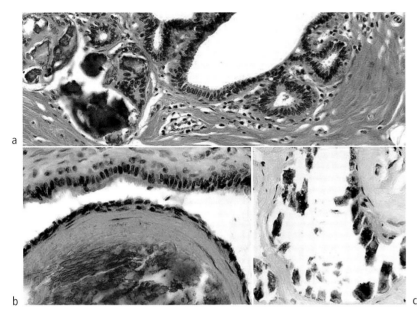

Fig. 5.10a–c Lobular microcalcifications.
5.10a Blunt duct adenosis – columnar cell change within adenosis.
5.10b Subepithelial microcalcifications, 'ossifying' type. This type is characteristically associated with columnar cell lesions and will be found in both benign and malignant variants.
5.10c After atrophy of the ductular wall, ossifying microcalcifications can be seen within the interstitium.

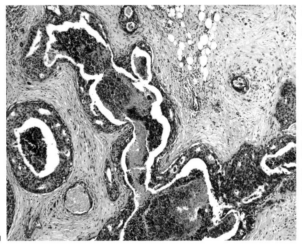

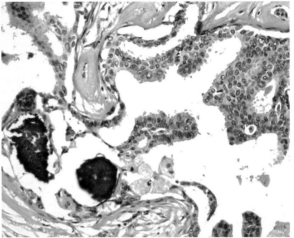

Fig. 5.11a–c Ductal microcalcifications.
5.11a High grade DCIS with dystrophic linear microcalcifications.
5.11b Intermediate grade DCIS with multiple lamellar spherical microcalcifications.

5.11c Periductal mastitis with needle shaped microcalcifications.

extracellular matrix of the stromal component. In a considerable number of cases, small and round microcalcifications, often arranged in angular clusters, may be associated with papillary lesions within prominent benign or malignant epithelial proliferations. In both hyperplasia and neoplasia the calcifications are of the secretory laminar type and localized within the intraepithelial sponge-like lumina. For the clinical relevance of histological MIB results see 'Pathology reporting categories' and 'Problems and pitfalls' above.

SIMULTANEOUS LOBULAR AND DUCTAL CALCIFICATIONS

Simultaneous lobular and ductal calcifications have also occasionally been described in the literature. They may be seen in the event of secondary lobular cancerization as well as in very rare cases of hyperparathyroidism. In our experience, columnar cell lesions associated with DCIS of low and intermediate grades are by far the most frequent variant of simultaneous lobular and ductal microcalcifications. As a rule, microcalcifications of ossifying type located within the lobules interspersed with blunt duct adenosis can be seen in combination with the ductal variant of secretory, small, round, lamellar microcalcifications in DCIS of low or intermediate grades. The radiologic counterparts are slight polymorphous microcalcifications arranged in clusters with some minimal protuberances. This mammographic constellation with slight irregularities in cluster form is typical of findings in population-based screening. The smaller the clusters, the more difficult the assessment of their shape. Clearly round or oval clusters are only associated with DCIS in exceptional cases and, as a rule, larger than their benign lobular counterpart (average diameter 7 mm compared to 2–5 mm).

MICROCALCIFICATIONS OUTSIDE OF LOBULES AND DUCTS

These microcalcifications are generally the so-called benign variant, easily identified by its location, and include vascular, cutaneous and foreign body calcifications, which are not biopsied.

Although in general associated with typical ring- or shell-shaped macrocalcifications and therefore easily diagnosed, fat necroses may present, at least in a small number of cases, as amorphous or even pleomorphic microcalcifications in an irregular, sometimes angulated arrangement. In a series of 114 cases of fat necrosis with abnormal mammograms the rate of suspicious microcalcifications was 3.9% [80]. They are invariably associated with the later stages of fat necrosis evolution. Mammographically, calcified lipid pseudocysts are spontaneously transformed into a cluster of suspicious microcalcifications [80,81]. If MIB is performed in these cases the pathologist will

detect irregularly shaped, large (mostly larger than 200 μm in diameter) microcalcifications of the calcium phosphate type. Another typical localization is within a lipophagic granuloma, which later on may lead to a fibrous connective tissue response, evolving a hard stellate scar with several calcification patterns [82]. In all these constellations detection of microcalcifications is essential to assure correlation with mammographically suspicious microcalcifications and to exclude an inflammatory reaction encompassing a carcinoma.

Mucocele-like lesions are another important example, especially when detected at screening; there are differences in the presentation of benign screening-detected and symptomatic mucocele-like lesions. Whereas symptomatic mucocele-like lesions and most mucinous carcinomas radiologically present as a mass, microcalcifications are the dominant radiologic abnormality in benign mucocele-like lesions detected at screening. Farshid et al. observed this constellation in 84.6% of cases [40]. Histologically prominent calcium phosphate microcalcifications of coarse granular shape can be detected in pools of mucin surrounded by a mainly histiocytic response within the interstitial tissue. These interstitial pools originate in focal ruptures of mucin-distended ducts in the vicinity, with at least a partially denuded epithelial lining. It must be borne in mind that, even in the absence of atypical epithelial proliferations, neither the imaging characteristics nor the histologic result of MIB of mucinous lesions are sufficient grounds for justifying a definitive exclusion of a malignant mucinous process (for further management see 'Problems and pitfalls' above).

DOCUMENTATION OF CORRELATION

To come to a final decision on management of a patient after an MIB-based diagnosis, imaging and clinical characteristics of the lesion targeted must be used as a surrogate for the macroscopic findings from a surgical specimen delivered to the pathologist. An overall clinical and imaging score scheme (**OCI score**) incorporating five categories is helpful in correlating findings (see Table 5.4). The Berlin-Buch team uses the following system.

The OCI score is a tool for monitoring the decision-making process within the team (see below). The first decision that needs to be taken is whether or not to proceed with MIB. In our clinic we feel that an OCI score of 3–5 requires a minimal invasive biopsy procedure (Fig. 5.12).

As described above, the B categories exclusively mirror the histologic findings of the core biopsies. The decision as to whether histology correlates with radiology can only be made in the multidisciplinary team (Fig. 5.13).

Tab. 5.4 Overall clinical and imaging (OCI) score scheme

Score	Description
OCI1	Normal
OCI2	Benign
OCI3	Indeterminate
OCI4	Probably malignant
OCI5	Definitely malignant

Tab. 5.5 Microcalcification categories (MC) as detected in histologic slides

Category	Description
MC1	Relevant* microcalcification detectable
MC2	No relevant* microcalcification detectable

* Only MC larger than 80–100 μm are considered radiologically relevant

In terms of microcalcifications, the findings of both the specimen radiogram/mammogram and the histologic sections are essential in deciding whether sampling of the lesion was adequate. Special care must be given if malignant microcalcification is suspected. If histology does not yield any positive finding, the procedure must be repeated or an open surgical biopsy performed. Therefore, before the detailed correlation of all findings can proceed, the team pathologist gives a separate statement regarding the microscopic detection of any calcification using two simple categories (Table 5.5). As a rule all needle MIB results must be discussed in depth, especially those not consistent with the OCI score scheme, until mutual agreement and a definite management decision are reached.

It is important to stress that, in addition to the histopathologic B category, a separate statement on the result of the correlation of pathologic and radiologic microcalcifications should be given. To specify this we use a correlation (CO) score (Table 5.6), which specifies the definitive result of the correlation of pathologic, radiologic and clinical findings must be specified.

Tab. 5.6 Correlation score (CO) for pathologic and radiologic findings

Category	Description
CO1	Definite correlation
CO2	Definite lack of correlation
CO3	Correlation uncertain

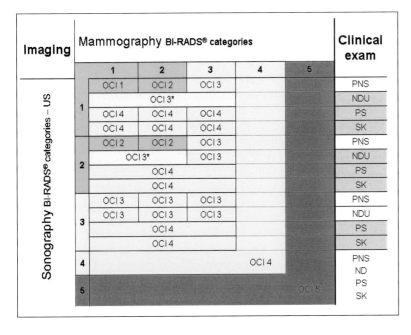

Fig 5.12 Overall clinical and imaging (OCI) score. Clinical and radiologic opinions must be documented before MIB. The most suspicious opinion is to be taken and results in the OCI score. Therefore, the impact of clinical findings depends on imaging results and may be decisive (gray table fields) or can be definitely neglected (white table fields) (OCI score = overall clinical imaging score, PNS = palpable non-suspicious, PS = palpable suspicious, NDU = nipple discharge unilateral, SK = skin symptoms).
OCI scores are used to decide on indication for MIB. OCI scores of 1 or 2 entail returning to routine screening, whereas MIB is mandatory in patients with OCI scores of 3 to 5. OCI 3* is, however, also an indication for galactography.

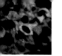

5 Pathologic diagnosis in minimal invasive biopsy

OUTCOME DECISION-MAKING

In general only two possible outcomes exist:
1. return to the routine screening program; and
2. refer for treatment.

Ideally, the outcome decision should be made according to a written protocol agreed by all team members. Deviations from the protocol should be allowed only after detailed discussion in the team and must be documented for audit purposes. So-called short-term recall is one of these deviations and generally not accepted as an outcome category. It should not be used as an alternative to proper assessment. This requires that the breast team including the pathologist act in a very responsible manner and that all MIB results be discussed in the context of the imaging and clinical findings during the multidisciplinary assessment meetings. Should an MIB result be inconsistent with the clinical/imaging opinion, a clear management decision must be reached (Fig. 5.13). After a decision has been made in terms of correlation of histology and pathology, the whole process is channeled into the appropriate action category (see Table 5.7 and Fig. 5.14). Finally, the conclusion reached on patient management should be reported. The latter is important not only for the individual patient, but also for assessing the performance parameters of the team.

The A (action) categories are grouped analogously to the B (histopathologic) categories in five hierarchical levels. However, for individual cases a given histopathologic B category can evolve into a different A category after additional information from the team meeting has been incorporated. For example, for the majority of cases categorized as B3 further clarification will take place and they can be categorized as A1 (re-MIB) or A2 (discharge). Some B3 cases must be classified as A4 due to a high suspicion of malignancy based on clinical and imaging data. Very few cases of uncertain histopathologic malignant potential but with a definite pathologic-radiologic correlation need to undergo early recall diagnostic imaging (A3) (see Figs 5.13a–d for information on the other categories). Using these tools it is possible to assess performance parameters relating to the pathology report alone or to the diagnostic achievement resulting from the team approach (see Chapter 6). In analogy to the B categories it is possible to evaluate the accuracy of the A classification with respect to diagnostic sensitivity and specificity, positive predictive value, false negative rate, false positive rate and inadequate rate [9]. When comparing these performance parameters for the A and B categories one should see significantly better results in the A category. This difference is a direct measure of the impact of the multidisciplinary team conference.

Some rules for deciding on outcome in standard situations after MIB may be helpful for teams in drawing up their protocol. In our experience it is easier handling the different combinations of the overall clinical and imaging opinion (OCI), the histopathologic category (B) and the correlation (CO) by using the scores mentioned above. Additionally, the resulting action after the team meeting (A) is also scored, as shown above.

The starting point of every structured team discussion is the question of correlation between imaging and histopathology. The three possible results have different consequences.
1. CO1: if a definite correlation between pathology and radiology is deemed to exist, the team may open the discussion for outcome decision-making, as described below.
2. CO2: if there is definitely no correlation between pathology and radiology, the results of the team discussion depend on the histopathology result. In the case of B4 and B5, the team may move on to decision-making as described below. In all B1 to B3 results the team must decide whether a repeated MIB procedure is promising or if there is an indication for an open surgical biopsy. The appropriate action category is A1 (see above).
3. CO3: if the radiologic-pathologic correlation is uncertain, the B categories once again become important. In B4 and B5 lesions a team decision is possible (see below). In B3 lesions only the combination with an overall clinical opinion of 'normal' or 'benign' (OCI1 or 2) allows a decision in favor of a category A2 action: discharge of the patient into regular screening. In B3 lesions combined with OCI3–5 scores as well as in all B1 and B2 lesions an uncertain correlation between imaging and

Tab. 5.7 Action categories

Category	Action	Assessment result
A1	Re-MIB/diagnostic excision	Not adequately sampled
A2	Discharge*	Benign
A3	Early recall	Uncertain biological potential
A4	Diagnostic excision/re-MIB	Suspicious of malignancy
A5	Refer for therapy	Malignant

* Alternative: nondiagnostic excision at the patient's request

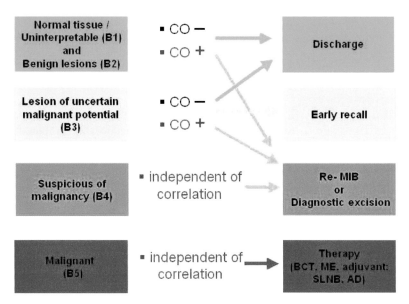

Fig. 5.13 Influence of radiologic-pathologic correlation on interpretation of B categories (CO– = no correlation, CO+ = definite correlation, BCT = breast conserving therapy, ME = mastectomy, SLNB = sentinel lymph node biopsy, AD = axillary dissection).

histopathology is not acceptable. The team must once more decide whether MIB should be repeated or an open biopsy performed (action category A1 or A4).

After solving all the problems pertaining to radiologic-pathologic correlation the team may move on and compare overall clinical opinion scores (OCI) with histopathologic B categories. In the context of this book, we will demonstrate this kind of decision-making from the pathologist's viewpoint starting with the B category (Figs 5.14a–d). Starting with the OCI score would be equally valid; it is of utmost importance, though, to combine both in the discussion to ensure an adequate outcome.

B1: NORMAL (BREAST) TISSUE/UNINTERPRETABLE

A result of 'normal tissue/uninterpretable' on MIB is acceptable when the indication for MIB was the result of an OCI2 (probably benign) lesion under the condition of a strict indication for MIB. Under those circumstances OCI2 applies to a clinical abnormality that is almost certainly benign if imaging is normal (in radiologically benign lesions without clinically suspicious findings MIB is not indicated). The resulting 'action' is to discharge the patient into routine screening (A2).

A B1 result is not acceptable in overall clinically indeterminate lesions (OCI3) and should be eliminated from the outcome discussion by forgoing radiologic-pathologic correlation (see above).

B2: BENIGN LESION

This category is the typical result of MIB of OCI2 lesions. Moreover, a result of B2 is required for all lesions with an indeterminate overall clinical opinion

score (OCI3), otherwise returning the patient to regular screening is not justified. In OCI2 and OCI3 lesions after MIB with a B2 assessment result, the final action category is A2: discharge of the patient. The same decision can be made in OCI4 cases only under the precondition of certain imaging/pathology correlation (CO1) – rather an exceptional situation. In most OCI4 and in all OCI5 situations, pathologic B2 results cannot be accepted (A4).

B3: LESION OF UNCERTAIN MALIGNANT POTENTIAL

B3 results do not automatically indicate the need for either repeated needle biopsy or open surgical biopsy. We comply with the procedure suggested by Ibrahim and co-workers who subdivided B3 lesions into two subcategories: one with a lesser, the other with a higher risk of associated malignancy [3]. For the reasons mentioned above, however, (see 'Reporting categories' and 'Problems and pitfalls', respectively) the two groups do not provide any clue as to the most reasonable action (A1, 2 or 3). Therefore, every case should be reviewed by the multidisciplinary team meeting, and a unanimous decision concerning management must be agreed. B3 cases are the main source of increases in the action categories A1, 2 and 4 after a multidisciplinary discussion, as control by early recall (A3) is an exception made only for a very small rate of B3/CO1 lesions. Regular follow-up (A2) may be appropriate for atypical lobular neoplasia (LN), atypical proliferation of ductal-type and columnar cell lesions with atypia when detected as incidental findings in association with a mass or calcification definitively identified as histologically benign by MIB. The same applies to very small papillary lesions or radial scars without residual imaging findings after MIB [83, 84]. A very small group of B3 lesions must be re-categorized as A4 after the team discussion, as a result of their highly suspicious overall clinical-imaging score (OCI4 or 5). Finally, the largest subgroup of B3 lesions represents lesions that are classified as 'not adequately sampled' (A1) after multidisciplinary discussion. We concur with Carder and colleagues [85] that, with an increasing number of target lesions for MIB, we are also noticing an increase in such B3 lesions. However, we are confident that the resulting diagnostic excisions can be reduced by proceeding to vacuum-assisted MIB after core needle MIB diagnosis of B3 lesions as complex sclerosing lesions and papillomas not associated with atypical epithelial proliferations. This was also recommended in the re-edition of the UK Clinical Guidelines for Breast Cancer Screening Assessment (p. 9) [86].

B4: LESION SUSPICIOUS OF MALIGNANCY

These results should lead the multidisciplinary team directly to an outcome decision, irrespective of the correlation with imaging. In general, the histopathologic B4 categories should result in an open surgical biopsy to obtain a definitive result. In exceptional

situations, such as inadequate sampling due to a reproducible failure during the MIB procedure, repeat MIB may be decided. The appropriate action category is A4.

B5: MALIGNANT LESION

Even in B5 results from MIB, the team must decide to refer the patient for therapeutic surgery (action category A5), regardless of the pathologic-radiologic correlation.

Obviously, in this outcome decision-making process in MIB the pathologist's task is not limited to interpreting the histological results for other team members. He or she must also take part in any joint decision on correlation with imaging leading to further action. Finally, the overall clinical opinion and the histological results must be carefully weighed against each other. The pathologist's contribution is not only the histopathologic result itself, but its interpretation in the overall context of treatment. Therefore, the final outcome depends on the pathologist's communicative skills and his or her ability to interact with other team members in an efficient way with the final aim of reaching a clear diagnosis.

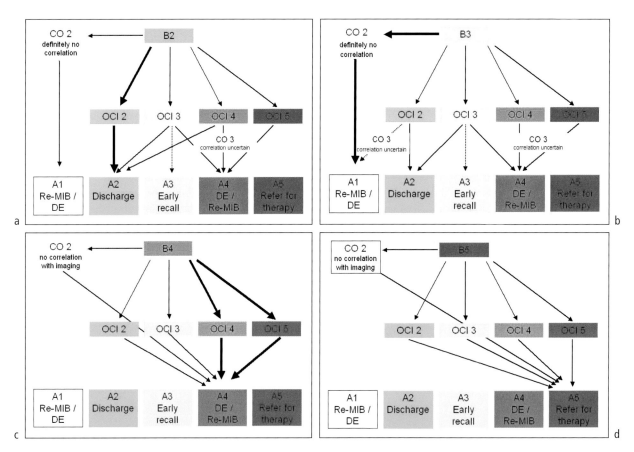

Fig. 5.14a–d Algorithm for outcome decision-making in the multidisciplinary team. For details see text (B = B category, OCI score = overall clinical imaging score, CO = correlation, A = action category).

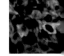
REFERENCES

1. Britton PD. Fine needle aspiration or core biopsy. Breast 1999;8:1–4.
2. Clarke D, Sudhakaran N, Gateley CA. Replace fine needle aspiration cytology with automated core biopsy in the triple assessment of breast cancer. Ann R Coll Surg Engl 2001;83:110–2.
3. Ibrahim AE, Bateman AC, Theaker JM, et al. The role and histological classification of needle core biopsy in comparison with fine needle aspiration cytology in the preoperative assessment of impalpable breast lesions. J Clin Pathol 2001;54:121–5.
4. Acheson MB, Patton RG, Howisey RL, et al. Three-to six-year followup for 379 benign image-guided large-core needle biopsies of nonpalpable breast abnormalities. J Am Coll Surg 2002;195:462–6.
5. Jackman RJ, Nowels KW, Rodriguez-Soto J, et al. Stereotactic, automated, large-core needle biopsy of nonpalpable breast lesions: false-negative and histologic underestimation rates after long-term follow-up. Radiology 1999;210:799–805.
6. White RR, Halperin TJ, Olson JA, Jr., et al. Impact of core-needle breast biopsy on the surgical management of mammographic abnormalities. Ann Surg 2001;233: 769–77.
7. Perry N, Broeders M, de Wolf C, Törnberg S. European guidelines for quality assurance in mammography screening. 3rd ed. Luxembourg: Office for Official Publications of the European Communities; 2001.
8. American College of Radiology. Illustrated breast imaging report and data system (BI-RADS). 3rd ed. Reston, VA.: American College of Radiology; 2003.
9. Wells CA, Amendoeira I, Apostolikas N, Bellocq JP et al. Quality assurance guidelines for pathology. In: Perry N, Broeders M, de Wolf C, editors. European Guidelines for Quality Assurance in Mammography Screening. 4th ed. Office for Official Publications of the European Communities; 2005.
10. Friedman PD, Sanders LM, Menendez C, Kalisher L, Petrillo G. Retrieval of lost microcalcifications during stereotactic vacuum-assisted core biopsy. AJR Am J Roentgenol 2003;180:275–80.
11. Umlas J, Tulecke M. The effects of glyoxal fixation on the histological evaluation of breast specimens. Hum Pathol 2004;35:1058–62.
12. Recommendations of the Association of Directors of Anatomic and Surgical Pathology. Part I. Immediate management of mammographically detected breast lesions Hum Pathol 1993;24:689–90.
13. Holland R, Hendriks JH. Microcalcifications associated with ductal carcinoma in-situ: mammographic-pathologic correlation. Semin Diagn Pathol 1994;11:181–92.
14. Fechner RE. Frozen section examination of breast biopsies. Practice parameter. Am J Clin Pathol 1995; 103:6–7.
15. National Coordinating Group for Breast Cancer Screening Pathology. Pathology reporting in breast cancer screening. Sheffield: 1997.
16. European guidelines for quality assurance in mammography screening Luxembourg: European Commission; 1996.
17. Goldstein NS, Martinez A, Vicini F, Stromberg J. The histology of radiation therapy effect on prostate adenocarcinoma as assessed by needle biopsy after brachytherapy boost. Correlation with biochemical failure. Am J Clin Pathol 1998;110:765–75.
18. Won B, Reynolds HE, Lazaridis CL, Jackson VP. Stereotactic biopsy of ductal carcinoma in-situ of the breast using an 11-gauge vacuum-assisted device: persistent underestimation of disease. AJR Am J Roentgenol 1999;173:227–9.
19. Liberman L, Smolkin JH, Dershaw DD, et al. Calcification retrieval at stereotactic, 11–gauge, directional, vacuum-assisted breast biopsy. Radiology 1998;208: 251–60.
20. Liberman L, Dershaw DD, Rosen PP, et al. Percutaneous removal of malignant mammographic lesions at stereotactic vacuum-assisted biopsy. Radiology 1998;206: 711–5.
21. Brem RF, Behrndt VS, Sanow L, Gatewood OM. Atypical ductal hyperplasia: histologic underestimation of carcinoma in tissue harvested from impalpable breast lesions using 11-gauge stereotactically guided directional vacuum-assisted biopsy. AJR Am J Roentgenol 1999;172:1405–7.
22. Darling ML, Smith DN, Lester SC, et al. Atypical ductal hyperplasia and ductal carcinoma in-situ as revealed by large-core needle breast biopsy: results of surgical excision. AJR Am J Roentgenol 2000;175:1341–6.
23. Sneige N, Lim SC, Whitman GJ, et al. Atypical ductal hyperplasia diagnosis by directional vacuum-assisted stereotactic biopsy of breast microcalcifications. Considerations for surgical excision. Am J Clin Pathol 2003;119:248–53.
24. Rao A, Parker S, Ratzer E, Stephens J, Fenoglio M. Atypical ductal hyperplasia of the breast diagnosed by 11-gauge directional vacuum-assisted biopsy. Am J Surg 2002;184:534–7.
25. Ely KA, Carter BA, Jensen RA, Simpson JF, Page DL. Core biopsy of the breast with atypical ductal hyperplasia: a probabilistic approach to reporting. Am J Surg Pathol 2001;25:1017–21.
26. Lim SC. Directional, vacuum-assisted stereotactic biopsy of non-palpable breast lesions with surgical correlation. Korean J Pathol 2004;36:314–22.
27. Gal-Gombos ED, Esserman LE, Said E. Accuracy of image-directed large core needle biopsy in atypical intraductal hyperplasia of the breast [abstract]. Breast J 2000;6:342.
28. Kettritz U, Morack G, Decker T. Stereotactic vacuum-assisted breast biopsies in 500 women with microcalcifications: radiological and pathological correlations. Eur J Radiol 2005;55:270–6.
29. Jackman RJ, Nowels KW, Shepard MJ, Finkelstein SI, Marzoni F-AJ. Stereotaxic large-core needle biopsy of 450 nonpalpable breast lesions with surgical correlation in lesions with cancer or atypical hyperplasia. Radiology 1994;193:91–5.
30. Liberman L, Cohen MA, Dershaw DD, et al. Atypical ductal hyperplasia diagnosed at stereotaxic core biopsy of breast lesions: an indication for surgical biopsy [see comments]. AJR Am J Roentgenol 1995;164:1111–3.

31. Brown TA, Wall JW, Christensen ED, et al. Atypical hyperplasia in the era of stereotactic core needle biopsy. J Surg Oncol 1998;67:168–73.
32. Philpotts LE, Lee CH, Horvath LJ, et al. Underestimation of breast cancer with II-gauge vacuum suction biopsy. AJR Am J Roentgenol 2000;175:1047–50.
33. Sobin LH, Wittekind CH. Breast tumours in TNM. New York: Wiley-Liss; 1997.
34. Hamele-Bena D, Cranor ML, Sciotto C, Erlandson R, Rosen PP. Uncommon Presentation of Mammary Myofibroblastoma. Mod Pathol 1996;9:786–90.
35. Chinyama CN, Davies JD. Mammary mucinous lesions: congeners, prevalence and important pathological associations. Histopathol 1996;29:533–9.
36. Rosen PP, Oberman HA. Tumors of the Mammary Gland. In: Armed Forces Institute of Pathology, editor. Atlas of Tumor Pathology. Washington, DC: 1993. p.350–2.
37. Wong NL, Wan SK. Comparative cytology of mucocelelike lesion and mucinous carcinoma of the breast in fine needle aspiration. Acta Cytol 2000;44:765–70.
38. Lee JS, Kim HS, Jung JJ, Lee MC. Mucocele-like tumor of the breast associated with ductal carcinoma in-situ and mucinous carcinoma : a case report. J Korean Med Sci 2001;16:516–8.
39. Renshaw AA. Can mucinous lesions of the breast be reliably diagnosed by core needle biopsy? Am J Clin Pathol 2002;118:82–4.
40. Farshid G, Pieterse S, King JM, Robinson J. Mucocele-like lesions of the breast: a benign cause for indeterminate or suspicious mammographic microcalcifications. Breast J 2005;11:15–22.
41. Rutgers EJ. Quality control in the locoregional treatment of breast cancer. Eur J Cancer 2001;37:447–53.
42. Goldhirsch A, Wood WC, Gelber RD, et al. Meeting highlights: updated international expert consensus on the primary therapy of early breast cancer. J Clin Oncol 2003;21:3357–65.
43. Sobin LH, Witteking CH. Breast tumors in TNM. 6th ed. New York: Wiley-Liss; 2002.
44. Dey P, Woodman CB, Gibbs A, Coyne J. Completeness of reporting on prognostic factors for breast cancer: a regional survey. J Clin Pathol 1997;50:829–31.
45. Harvey JM, Sterrett GF, Parsons RW, et al. Breast cancer in Western Australia in 1989: IV. Summary of histopathological assessment in 655 cases. Pathology 1995;27:12–7.
46. Mathers ME, Shrimankar J, Scott DJ, et al. The use of a standard proforma in breast cancer reporting. J Clin Pathol 2001;54:809–11.
47. Perry NM. Quality assurance in the diagnosis of breast disease. EUSOMA Working Party. Eur J Cancer 2001; 37:159–72.
48. Liberman L, Abramson AF, Squires FB, et al. The breast imaging reporting and data system: positive predictive value of mammographic features and final assessment categories. AJR Am J Roentgenol 1998;171:35–40.
49. Scutt D, Manning JT, Whitehouse GH, Leinster SJ, Massey CP. The relationship between breast asymmetry, breast size and the occurrence of breast cancer. Br J Radiol 1997;70:1017–21.
50. Krecke KN, Gisvold JJ. Invasive lobular carcinoma of the breast: mammographic findings and extent of disease at diagnosis in 184 patients. AJR Am J Roentgenol 1993;161:957–60.
51. Sneige N, McNeese MD, Atkinson EN, et al. Ductal carcinoma in-situ treated with lumpectomy and irradiation: histopathological analysis of 49 specimens with emphasis on risk factors and long term results. Hum Pathol 1995;26:642–9.
52. Orel SG, Kay N, Reynolds C, Sullivan DC. BI-RADS categorization as a predictor of malignancy. Radiology 1999;211:845–50.
53. Baker JA, Rosen EL, Lo JY, et al. Computer-aided detection (CAD) in screening mammography: sensitivity of commercial CAD systems for detecting architectural distortion. AJR Am J Roentgenol 2003;181:1083–8.
54. Liberman L, Sama MP. Cost-effectiveness of stereotactic 11-gauge directional vacuum-assisted breast biopsy. AJR Am J Roentgenol 2000;175:53–8.
55. Reynolds HE. Core needle biopsy of challenging benign breast conditions: a comprehensive literature review. AJR Am J Roentgenol 2000;174:1245–50.
56. Bird RE, Wallace TW, Yankaskas BC. Analysis of cancers missed at screening mammography. Radiology 1992;184:613–7.
57. Burrell HC, Sibbering DM, Wilson AR, et al. Screening interval breast cancers: mammographic features and prognosis factors. Radiology 1996;199:811–7.
58. Burrell HC, Evans AJ, Wilson AR, Pinder SE. False-negative breast screening assessment: what lessons can we learn? Clin Radiol 2001;56:385–8.
59. Sloane JP, Mayers MM. Carcinoma and atypical hyperplasia in radial scars and complex sclerosing lesions: importance of lesion size and patient age. Histopathol 1993;23:225–31.
60. Cawson JN, Malara F, Kavanagh A, et al. Fourteen-gauge needle core biopsy of mammographically evident radial scars: is excision necessary? Cancer 2003;97: 345–51.
61. Brenner RJ, Jackman RJ, Parker SH, et al. Percutaneous core needle biopsy of radial scars of the breast: when is excision necessary? AJR Am J Roentgenol 2002; 179:1179–84.
62. Kirwan SE, Denton ER, Nash RM, Humphreys S, Michell MJ. Multiple 14G stereotactic core biopsies in the diagnosis of mammographically detected stellate lesions of the breast. Clin Radiol 2000;55:763–6.
63. Frappart L, Boudeulle M, Boumendil J, et al. Structure and composition of microcalcifications in benign and malignant lesions of the breast: study by light microscopy, transmission and scanning electron microscopy, microprobe analysis, and X-ray diffraction. Hum Pathol 1984;15:880–9.
64. Gonzalez JE, Caldwell RG, Valaitis J. Calcium oxalate crystals in the breast. Pathology and significance. Am J Surg Pathol 1991;15:586–91.
65. Winston JS, Yeh IT, Evers K, Friedman AK. Calcium oxalate is associated with benign breast tissue. Can we avoid biopsy? Am J Clin Pathol 1993;100:488–92.
66. Going JJ, Anderson TJ, Crocker PR, Levison DA. Weddellite calcification in the breast: eighteen cases

with implications for breast cancer screening. Histopathol 1990;16:119–24.

67. Bun PA. Calcifications. In: Dronkers DJ, Hendricks JCL, Holland R, Rosenbusch G, editors. The practics of mammography. Stuttgart, New York: Georg Thieme; 2002. p.199–209.

68. Egan RL, McSweeney MB, Sewell CW. Intramammary calcifications without an associated mass in benign and malignant diseases. Radiology 1980;137:1–7.

69. Heywang-Köbrunner SH. Microcalcification. In: Diagnostic Breast Imaging. Stuttgart, New York: Thieme; 2001. p.434–52.

70. Rosen PP. Ductal hyperplasia. In: Rosen's Breast Pathology. Philadelphia: Lippincott-Raven; 2001. p.215–25.

71. Hoda SA, Gopalan A. Mammary calcifications of the ossifying type. Breast J 2003;9:129–30.

72. Lanyi M. [Differential diagnosis of the microcalcifications. The calcified mastopathic microcyst (author's transl)]. Radiologe 1977;17:217–8.

73. Evans A, Pinder S, Wilson R, et al. Ductal carcinoma in-situ of the breast: correlation between mammographic and pathologic findings. AJR Am J Roentgenol 1994;162:1307–11.

74. Hermann G, Keller RJ, Drossman S, et al. Mammographic pattern of microcalcifications in the preoperative diagnosis of comedo ductal carcinoma in-situ: histopathologic correlation. Can Assoc Radiol J 1999; 50:235–40.

75. Tan PH, Ho JT, Ng EH, et al. Pathologic-radiologic correlations in screen-detected ductal carcinoma in-situ of the breast: findings of the Singapore breast screening project. Int J Cancer 2000;90:231–6.

76. Foschini MP, Fornelli A, Peterse JL, Mignani S, Eusebi V. Microcalcifications in ductal carcinoma in-situ of the breast: histochemical and immunohistochemical study. Hum Pathol 1996;27:178–83.

77. Dinkel HP, Trusen A, Gassel AM, et al. Predictive value of galactographic patterns for benign and malignant neoplasms of the breast in patients with nipple discharge. Br J Radiol 2000;73:706–14.

78. Slanetz PJ, Giardino AA, Oyama T, et al. Mammographic appearance of ductal carcinoma in-situ does not reliably predict histologic subtype. Breast J 2001;7: 417–21.

79. Sweeney DJ, Wylie EJ. Mammographic appearances of mammary duct ectasia that mimic carcinoma in a screening programme. Australas Radiol 1995;39: 18–23.

80. Bilgen IG, Ustun EE, Memis A. Fat necrosis of the breast: clinical, mammographic and sonographic features. Eur J Radiol 2001;39:92–9.

81. Elorz M, Pina L, Bergaz F, et al. Atypical evolution of a calcified lipid cyst presenting spontaneously as a suspicious cluster of microcalcifications. Eur Radiol 2002;12:1100–3.

82. Bassett LW, Gold RH, Cove HC. Mammographic spectrum of traumatic fat necrosis: the fallibility of "pathognomonic" signs of carcinoma. AJR Am J Roentgenol 1978;130:119–22.

83. Liberman L, Zakowski MF, Avery S, et al. Complete percutaneous excision of infiltrating carcinoma at stereotactic breast biopsy: how can tumor size be assessed? AJR Am J Roentgenol 1999;173:1315–22.

84. Philpotts LE, Shaheen NA, Jain KS, Carter D, Lee CH. Uncommon high-risk lesions of the breast diagnosed at stereotactic core-needle biopsy: clinical importance. Radiology 2000;216:831–7.

85. Carder PJ, Liston JC. Will the spectrum of lesions prompting a "B3" breast core biopsy increase the benign biopsy rate? J Clin Pathol 2003;56:133–8.

86. Clinical Guidelines for Breast cancer screening assessment 2nd ed. Sheffield: 2005.

Content

6

PATHOLOGICAL DIAGNOSIS IN SURGICAL SPECIMENS

THOMAS DECKER, WERNER BOECKER, MONIKA RUHNKE, UTE KETTRITZ, RAINER OBENAUS,
KATY ROTERBERG, KRISZTINA ZELS, HEIKE JACOB AND GUENTER MORACK

The aim of this chapter is to highlight the importance of pathological examination of surgical specimens in very early breast cancer. With respect to pathological work-up, DCIS is a prototype of early breast cancer and, therefore, a challenge for the surgical pathologist. Firstly, identifying lesions is difficult. They are macroscopically nonpalpable, invisible and, therefore, as a rule, detected due to microcalcifications at mammography. Secondly, breast-conserving therapy (BCT) is a serious option in DCIS. However, the therapeutic decision to proceed with BCT depends on a number of pathologic features. There is no doubt that all the information submitted in the pathology report is primarily based on the correct sampling of specimens. This requires an optimal macroscopic examination and work-up of surgical specimens. Microscopic identification of the target lesion is a prerequisite for its histopathological classification. The data obtained are of decisive importance for planning further clinical management. Inadequate evaluation of surgical specimens can lead to both over- and undertreatment. Only by providing all clinically relevant information can the pathologist meet his commitments as a member of a multidisciplinary breast team.

In this chapter, we discuss different ways of examining surgical specimens, present results of our own experience and propose a rational strategy. The implications of pathological data for therapeutic decision-making are derived from the experience of 12 years of team work within a multidisciplinary breast unit.

Pathological diagnosis in surgical specimens

■ PRINCIPLES OF DISTRIBUTION OF DCIS
▒ IN THE BREAST

Knowledge of the lobar architecture of the mammary gland is a prerequisite for understanding DCIS (see Chapter 1 for details). In 1975 Wellings et al. were able to show by means of extensive submacroscopic examinations of 196 breasts with DCIS [1] that, with few exceptions, DCIS takes its origin from the terminal duct lobular unit (TDLU), starting with distension of the ductular structures and unfolding of lobules by the proliferating tumor cells. Further expansion then leads to the involvement of the extralobular ductal system. Thus, the neoplasia spreads within the pre-existing ductal lobular system. It follows that the architecture of the mammary ductal system itself is one of the key factors determining the variations in patterns of distribution observed in these tumors (Fig. 6.1) [1, 2]. The ductal-lobular system forms segments from the nipple to the periphery, which appear to be pyramid-shaped: the base lying in the periphery of the breast with its peak pointing towards the nipple [3].

Using computer-assisted three-dimensional reconstruction, Ohtake and co-workers were able to show that the various segments are of different size and usually overlapping in their parenchymal structures [4]. Therefore, these segments do not follow the geometry of the artificial system of quadrants. Furthermore, an analysis of complete galactograms of 85 breasts [5] disclosed that 37% of segments are aligned in an outer subcutaneous layer, 41% in an inner layer beneath this, and 22% are aligned centrally. This explains why segmentectomy can contain several independent segments [6].

DUCTAL-SEGMENTAL EXPANSION OF DCIS

Due to the complex architecture of breast tissue only three-dimensional analysis is able to deliver realistic DCIS extension patterns [3, 4, 6, 7].

Thus, data from two such studies have provided evidence that DCIS most frequently occurs within one segment [8, 9]. DCIS foci are only rarely found in clearly different segments.

Findings from Ohtake and co-workers who examined the intraductal growth of DCIS components in invasive carcinomas [6] also indicate that:
1. in total 81.3% of DCIS showed some type of intraductal expansion towards the nipple; and
2. that tumors obviously also spread in a retrograde fashion into the periphery of segments.

In addition, Ohtake et al. established so-called network models and determined the maximum angle of the segment of DCIS growth from the mamillary pole towards the periphery [4]. In all cases cone- or pyramid-like shapes with a broad base towards the periphery were found. Furthermore, overlap of ductal lobular systems from different segments could be detected, as well as connecting anastomoses at different levels of the ductal system.

Under these preconditions, even DCIS sizes of up to 100 mm could be explained as unicentric lesions with continuous segmental growth via connecting channels between different segments (Fig. 6.1). Although information in the literature relating to DCIS sizes (including those treated with mastectomy) is rare, these large lesions seem to account for a considerable number of cases. Holland and co-workers found, that 51% of DCIS lesions [42, 82] had a diameter of more than 50 mm [10]. This data is confirmed by our own experience: more than half of the DCIS cases in our patients (56%) (232/411) were found to be larger than 40 mm.

DISCONTINUOUS INTRADUCTAL GROWTH OF DCIS

In DCIS cases treated by breast-conserving therapy discontinuous growth may cause serious clinical problems. DCIS foci discontinuous to the main lesion may remain in the breast as residual tumors and cause local recurrence. In order to estimate the risk of such recurrence, it is essential to consider DCIS expansion patterns and the likelihood of distant foci elsewhere in the breast.

Unfortunately, due to the use of inconsistent definitions, the data in the literature concerning the incidence of multicentricity of DCIS range between 0 and 78% [11–14]. We define multicentricity as the presence of two or more separate foci in the breast more than 40 mm apart. Holland et al. detected only a single case containing two foci of completely isolated DCIS that fulfilled these criteria. In our own material consisting of 232 mastectomy specimens with DCIS, we found two cases with multicentric foci that were more than 45 mm apart. Multicentric DCIS as defined above therefore seems to be the exception. Furthermore, this conclusion is supported by data showing that local recurrence after breast-conserving therapy usually occurs within the area of previous surgery and that bilateral DCIS is extremely rare [13,15].

In another study 60 cases of DCIS were analyzed with a combination of radiologic and pathologic tech-

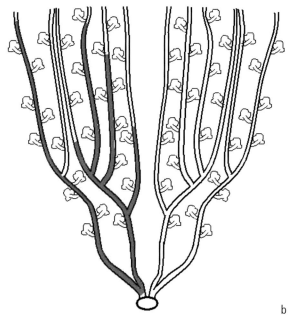

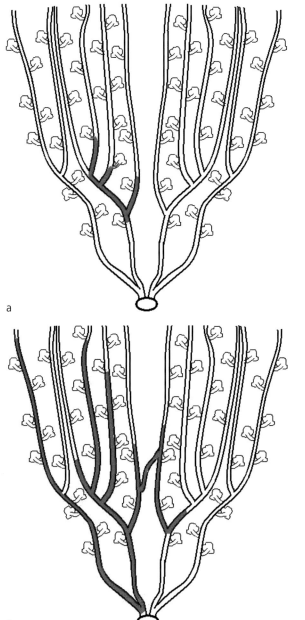

a

b

c

Fig. 6.1a–c Ductal-segmental expansion of DCIS.
6.1a Small circumscribed lesion within the center of the segment (unicentric, unisegmental).
6.1b Large DCIS involving almost all of a segment including the retromamillar region (unicentric, unisegmental).
6.1c Extended DCIS involving more than one segment as the result of intersegmental anastomoses (unicentric, multisegmental).

niques in a three-dimensional approach [7, 9]. In 50% of cases only continuous growth expansion was found, while the other half displayed discontinuities (gaps) in their intraductal growth. When the distances between discontinuous DCIS areas were measured, their length was less than 5 mm in 63%, and less than 10 mm in 83% of cases. In total, only 8% of DCIS cases showed discontinuities between DCIS foci of more than 10 mm. Furthermore, Faverly and co-workers found a correlation between the respective grade of a given

DCIS and the frequency and size of gaps between foci: while 90% of poorly-differentiated DCIS (high grade) showed no gaps at all, 70% of well-differentiated (low grade) DCIS did. In addition, the gaps were shorter in poorly-differentiated lesions, while intermediate and well-differentiated DCIS displayed larger gaps. All gaps of more than 10 mm were found in the latter group. The only case of multicentric DCIS with a distance of more than 40 mm between foci was a well-differentiated DCIS.

In summary, based on the architecture of the ductal lobular tree, the expansion of DCIS can be seen to start within the terminal ductal lobular unit (TDLU) and extend in different directions, preferentially towards the nipple. Therefore, DCIS growth occurs within one segment due to the anatomic lobar units of the mamillary gland. However, DCIS can involve several lobes or segments via intersegmental anastomoses and thus affect a larger area of breast tissue.

■ EXAMINATION OF SURGICAL SPECIMENS

GROSS PATHOLOGY AND RADIOLOGICAL FEATURES

DCIS detected by mammography very rarely displays specific macroscopic features. More than 92% of our patients with DCIS showed no clinically palpable lesions or macroscopically detectable foci. In about 80% of 573 patients included in the NSABP protocol B17 no foci were palpable [16]. The overwhelming majority of DCIS is therefore detected as a result of microcalcifications in clinically asymptomatic patients, and the pathologist must, consequently, be familiar with its radiological patterns (see Chapters 4 and 5).

DCIS WITH MACROSCOPIC FINDINGS

The small number of DCIS cases which are macroscopically detectable usually show a polycyclic tumor referred to as comedo-type DCIS in the literature (Chapter 20). These findings, however, are not specific, they can also be seen in periductal mastitis. In our material the size of such lesions varies between 7 and 57 mm. We cannot confirm the observations of those who claim a close relationship between palpability, macroscopic tumor development and size on the one hand and the possibility of breast conserving therapy on the other.

In agreement with a large number of publications, we have found tumor-forming DCIS only in lesions of high grade and in papillary DCIS. All our cases of papillary DCIS revealed additional DCIS in the adjacent tissue, usually within only slightly dilated ducts outside the intracystic tumor visible to the naked eye. These findings have led us to the conclusion that papillary lesions must be regarded as part of the segment involved by the DCIS.

DCIS WITHOUT MACROSCOPIC FINDINGS

Radiological findings are often the only clue when determining where tissue should be sampled for histological examination. In 72–98% of DCIS, microcalcifications are associated with the lesion [17–19]. However, in spite of this association, the size of a given DCIS cannot be solely determined by radiological analysis of the tissue containing these microcalcifications. Low grade DCIS may grow in ducts without forming such microcalcifications [20]. Discrepancies between the area of microcalcifications and histological size of the DCIS have been examined systematically in mastectomy specimens by Holland and co-workers [10]. In 34 cases with areas of microcalcifications of up to 30 mm in diameter on mammography, 66% of the corresponding DCIS exceeded the radiological findings by more than 1 cm, 20% by more than 2 cm and as much as 11% by more than 3 cm.

It should be borne in mind that DCIS can also be detected as incidental finding showing no microcalcifications. Goldstein and co-workers found this to be true in 17% of cases included in their DCIS series [20].

Macroscopic findings are rarely useful in the pathological examination of excision specimens with DCIS. In general, the pathologist must rely on radiologically detected microcalcifications to identify areas suspicious for DCIS. Due to obvious discrepancies in size between the area of microcalcifications and the histological lesion, the surrounding tissue must also be embedded to ensure that the entire lesion is examined.

■ INTERDISCIPLINARY PREREQUISITES

In DCIS cases (as well as in cases suspicious of DCIS) the pathologist is fundamentally confronted with three tasks: the lesion must be found and classified, the size of the lesion must be determined and, lastly, resection margins must be assessed.

In order to examine DCIS lesions appropriately, the pathologist needs the support of radiologists and surgeons.

Finding and classifying DCIS lesions. As mammographic microcalcifications are the principal and often the only indication of DCIS, the mammographic report and images, as well as the specimen radiograph are needed by the pathologist to identify the target lesion. Even in rare cases of DCIS with a macroscopically visible, tumor-forming focus specimen radiography should be utilized in order to identify possible DCIS-associated microcalcifications external to the main lesion.

Determining the size of DCIS lesions. When considering the segmental architecture of the ductal lobular system, it becomes immediately obvious that the ducts of the segment contained in a given specimen are generally oriented along virtual lines between the nipple and the periphery. The surgeon should therefore clearly mark the mamillary and peripheral resection margins in excisional specimens (Fig. 6.2)

Assessment of resection margins. The histological examination of resection margins is essential when deciding on additional treatment and determining the size of the DCIS by means of a three-dimensional reconstruction. Most importantly, an intact surgical specimen is required for an exact pathological examination. Cuts and tears in the specimen can impede reliable diagnosis, while fragmentation renders it virtually impossible.

PRACTICAL ROUTINE WITHIN AN INTER-DISCIPLINARY PROTOCOL

The following interdisciplinary procedure, specified in the Berlin-Buch practice protocol, has proven efficient in our breast center.

Immediately after removing the surgical specimen the surgeon should mark the mamillary margin of resection (the mamillary pole is relatively small). The pectoral fascia should be removed in every BCT specimen in such a way that the dorsal resection margin is formed by the fascia. The external surface of the dorsal resection margin should be marked with blue dye. The surgeon then places the excision specimen on a foil with a schematic drawing of the breast outlines (Fig 6.2), and the excision specimen is fixed with cannulas. Alternatively the surgeon can mark the surface of the mamillary, peripheral and, additionally, the ventral subcutaneous margin with sutures of different lengths to ensure proper orientation.

The radiologist then performs specimen radiography and marks the margins of the microcalcification area with several pins (Figs 6.2 and 6.3). This marking for the pathologist is done independently of the preoperative marking for the surgeon.

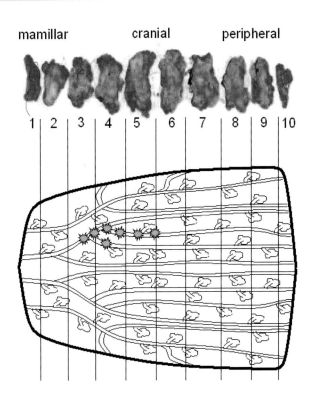

Fig. 6.3 Slicing of a segmental resection specimen containing microcalcifications. Slicing is done perpendicular to most of the ducts running between nipple and periphery. Microcalcifications invisible to the pathologist (blue stars in the scheme) have been marked by the radiologist.

The final goal of the macroscopic pathological examination is a systematic (segment-related) approach, guided by microcalcifications. This is only possible if the surfaces of the resection margins and the in-situ positioning of the operative specimen are marked by the surgeon. Furthermore, specimen radiography and marking of microcalcification by the radiologist is essential for the pathologist in the process of orientation. Therefore, detailed information from the other members of a multidisciplinary team enables targeted and efficient sampling of the specimen.

EXAMINATION OF EXCISION SPECIMENS

Examination of the excision specimen is guided by clinical mammography and specimen radiography.

MEASUREMENT OF SPECIMENS

Measurement of a given specimen's dimensions – the lengths of the mamillary-peripheral, the dorsal-ventral and the third axis – is indispensable for later recon-

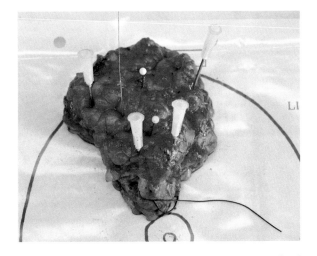

Fig. 6.2 Segmental resection for DCIS. Marked specimen fixed on a drawing by the surgeon.

struction of the size of a DCIS (see below) and should therefore be the first step in examination. Determining the weight of the specimen gives little additional information and is not helpful in pathological assessment of therapeutic excisional specimens of the breast. Weight is important only in diagnostic surgery – to minimize the size of excisions of benign lesions, the most suitable discriminatory factor is the specimen weight. Over 90% of diagnostic biopsies for nonpalpable lesions that subsequently prove benign weigh less than 30 g [21]. The vast majority of excision specimens in modern breast medicine are performed for therapeutic reasons however, and weight is no longer an important factor in segmental operations following preoperative, minimally invasive biopsies.

MARKING OF MARGINS

Marking the surface of excision tissue is essential for microscopic identification of the original resection margins. This can be done by painting the specimen's surface with marker substances that adhere to the tissue during fixation, dehydration, embedding, cutting and staining and must also be visible at microscopy. Various substances such as ink, gelatin, dyes, latex (correction fluid) or silver nitrate can be used. If marking of the surface is done by the surgeon before specimen radiography, radio-opaque substances (latex, silver nitrate) should be avoided. As a rule, all these materials adhere better to fresh than to fixed tissue. To avoid seeping of the marking substance into crevices of the surface, the specimen should not be dipped. Rather, the surface marker should be applied carefully

with a small brush or a cotton applicator. It is possible to mark different margins by using different colors for recognition on the microscopic slide.

SYSTEMATIC AND GUIDED EXAMINATION

The **systematic** pathological examination of the excision specimen has to consider the ductal-lobular extension and segmental growth of the DCIS with special emphasis on resection margins. Generally, the ducts run from the nipple to the peripheral resection margin. If the specimen is sliced perpendicularly to the mamillary-peripheral axis, it is quite obvious that most ducts will be cross-sectioned, which increases the chance of recognizing as many ducts as possible within the histological slide (Fig. 6.3). To identify non-visible DCIS detected as a result of mammographic calcifications the pathologist must be **guided**, for example, by pins marking the microcalcification area observed in the specimen radiograph. In addition, slice radiographs provide an even more precise orientation by identifying individual slices containing microcalcifications (Fig. 6.4).

SAMPLING

As illustrated, the specimen should be serially sectioned from the mamillary pole to the periphery of the segment (Fig. 6.5a). Care should be taken to slice the tissue thinly (about 4 mm). It is obvious that tissue samples with macroscopically suspicious findings and manifest microcalcifications must be examined completely. In our protocol, all macroscopically visible

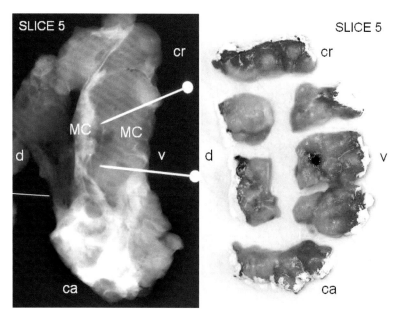

Fig. 6.4 Sampling of a slice of a segmental resection containing microcalcifications. The slice radiogram allows precise orientation. Every tissue sampled is identified by slice number (5) and the direction of the margin (MC = microcalcifications, cr = cranial, ca = caudal, d = dorsal, v = ventral).

findings as well as all areas with microcalcifications identified by slice radiography must be embedded for histological examination. Due to the discrepancy between the size of areas of microcalcification and of the histologically detected DCIS, we also embed the corresponding tissue of the neighboring slices (Fig. 6.5b). Furthermore, assessment of the resection margins is mandatory. Finally, the two first mamillary as well as the two last peripheral slices are embedded for assessment of 10 mm margins in these directions (Fig. 6.5c). Tangential slices of the nipple and peripheral margins are therefore also embedded for processing. Two cassettes for the mamillary slice and four to six cassettes for the peripheral slice are usually required. The other resection margins are contained in the slices cut perpendicular to the mamillary peripheral axis of the resection specimen. We also include the dorsal and ventral margins in the examination even when the pectoral

fascia is removed. This is indispensable for three-dimensional size determination and for quality control of the surgical techniques. Both three-dimensional reconstruction of the lesion and exact information about the direction of an involved margin require recognition of the original location of every tissue block. Since the color of the surface-marking substance is not sufficient for this purpose, we use a coding system to designate the original slice location of the excision specimen examined: the serially sectioned slices are labeled by ascending numbers from mamillary to peripheral slice. Abbreviations are used to designate the direction of the margin (ma = mamillar, p = peripheral, cra = cranial, cau = caudal, d = dorsal, v = ventral, m = medial, and l = lateral). For example, the code 39004/05-3-cau would indicate patient number 39004 from year 2005, with tissue of the third slice containing the caudal resection margin.

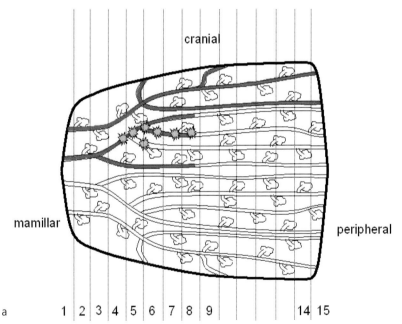

a

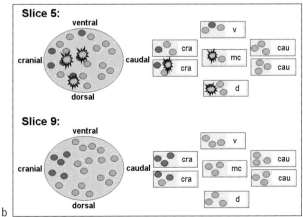

b

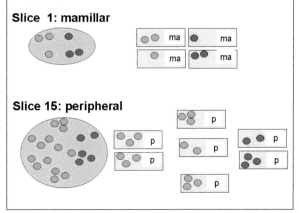

c

Fig. 6.5a−c Systematic and oriented sampling of a segmental resection specimen with microcalcifications. DCIS (red) within the ducts is invisible to the naked eye and partly even radiographically. The mamillary-peripheral axis gives information on the distribution of ducts and allows a systematic work-up. Microcalcifications (blue stars) detected by specimen or slice radiography allow oriented sampling (for details see text).

6.5a Serial sectioning: perpendicular to the mamillary-peripheral axis.

6.5b Tissue sampling: embedding of the slice(s) containing microcalcifications and neighboring slices.

6.5c Tissue sampling: embedding of the two first mamillary and the two last peripheral slices for assessment of 10 mm margins.

■ Standardized sampling enables the pathologist to identify all lesions and determine their size. Size of breast carcinoma is the most important feature for management of patients eligible for breast-conserving therapy. The results of the assessment of resection margins give highly reliable information about residual tumors in the event of re-excisions.

INTRAOPERATIVE DIAGNOSTICS

DCIS is the prototypical nonpalpable lesion of the breast. DCIS microcalcifications, which are the only evidence of DCIS in more than 90% of cases, are neither palpable nor visible to the naked eye. The surgeon depends on the support of the other team members in order to achieve optimal results, namely definitive identification of the lesion and its complete removal in a single excision.

Specimen radiography enables a quick assessment of whether microcalcifications have been successfully excised. Furthermore, assessment of the distances between areas of microcalcifications and the six re-section margins can be made. The result can then be compared to the distances preoperatively planned around the microcalcification area. We perform spec-imen radiography in two planes to control the quality of operative procedures. Theoretically, the second plane is negligible if a standardized operation is performed – requiring removal of the pectoral fascia in dorsal and the strictly subcutaneous resection in ventral direction (as described in our protocol).

Slice radiography. Macroscopic examination and sampling is carried out during the operation using fresh tissue. This allows oriented sampling. A second operation can often be avoided when radiographs of the slices are included in the decision-making process, especially in cases with suspicious or inconclusive specimen radiographs. In view of such results the extra time required is negligible.

Frozen section examination. Diagnosis and differ-ential diagnosis of DCIS should not be performed on intraoperative frozen sections. A definitive diagnosis can usually be made by means of minimal invasive biopsy techniques in more than 95% of cases (see Chapters 4 and 5) (98% of patients in our breast center).

Intraoperative frozen section examinations can only be justified in two situations. Both are exceptionally rare. In the first case an invasive tumor which was neither detected by mammography nor ultrasound may be discovered in the course of the intraoperative macroscopic examination. In this case the frozen section offers the chance to continue with axillary lymph node dissection, thereby sparing the patient

separate surgery of the axilla. However, the size of the foci must allow for 50% of the tumor to be left for paraffin histology, which, in general, only applies to tumors with a diameter of more than 10 mm. Secondly, a frozen section should be considered in an operation for centrally located DCIS with preservation of the nipple. In this case, the (disc-shaped) mamillary resec-tion margin of the excision specimen can be examined for DCIS on a frozen section. Both the pathologist and the surgeon must be aware of the risk involved. There-fore, only positive findings should be regarded as valid, whereas negative findings in frozen sections are insufficient for exclusion of involvement. This applies in particular to non-high grade DCIS. Knowing the type and grade of previously biopsied/excised DCIS is very helpful.

■ Intraoperative diagnostics in DCIS is an inter-disciplinary task for radiologists and pathologists who support the surgeon. Essentially, intraoperative diagnostics consists of quality control by means of specimen and slice radiography as well as by macro-scopic examination. Main aims are complete removal of the DCIS, including a defined margin of tissue free of microcalcifications, and the search for undetected invasive foci. Both help in avoiding further operations, such as re-excisions or secondary axillary dissections. Use of intraoperative frozen sections is not an integral part of diagnostics or therapy in DCIS and is only recommended in exceptional cases.

EXAMINATION OF RE-EXCISION SPECIMENS

Re-excisions become necessary when the examination of the primary operation specimen shows evidence of DCIS at the resection margin or within the safety margin. This may also occur when an excision for diagnostic purposes reveals malignant lesions. In principle, two re-excision variants exist: complete excision of the former operation area and directed re-excision. The resulting excision specimens show parts of the border of the older excision cavity (at the inside) as well as new resection margins (outside). Re-exci-sion specimens are more difficult to assess regarding possible residual tumor, size and definite resection margins than their primary counterparts. The pathol-ogist requires precise information on localization and markings. In **circular re-excisions** the former excision cavity is localized in a more or less central position. Apart from the subcutaneous defect (mostly ventral), such a specimen looks similar to its primary counter-part. The former operation cavity can be filled with gauze. The pathological examination is then carried out according to the protocol detailed above. After determining the size of the defect, the specimen is sliced perpendicularly to the mamillary-peripheral axis. After that, the maximum diameter of the cavity as well as the distances to the six resection margins must be measured. Since the cavity margin and the outer resection margin are included within the same tissue block and, naturally, the same histological slide, the amount of residual tumor and the distances to the resection margins can be measured. Based on systematic work-up, the findings allow spatial reconstruction, as in primary excision specimens. The number of blocks examined is equivalent to the number required for a primary excision. Two mamillary and two peripheral slices are completely embedded as well as all slices containing the cavity resulting from the primary excision and the two neighboring slices in mamillary and peripheral directions. **Directed re-excisions** are performed to clear a single resection margin of a primary specimen in only one direction. Consequently, the tissue flaps must be at least as long as the original margin-containing tumor. In such re-excisions, two surfaces are recognized: one corresponding to the former excisional cavity and another in the opposite position. Further work-up depends on orientation of the specimen and marking of the outer surface. Ideally, the specimen is marked in-situ in an appropriate fashion and positioned for transfer (Fig. 6.6). Because such specimens do not show the exact borders of the original excisional cavity, a complete work-up for the histological examination is recommended. For a tissue slice measuring 150 × 40 mm with a maximum thickness of 25 mm approximately 20 tissue cassettes will be required.

■ EXAMINATION OF MASTECTOMY SPECIMENS

Examination of mastectomy specimens in DCIS is more demanding than in invasive carcinoma. In addition to confirming the DCIS diagnosis made by minimal invasive biopsy, the size of the lesion needs to be determined and invasive growth excluded. In view of the amount of tissue to be examined, even specialized centers are unable to cope with complete work-ups as a routine procedure. Therefore, selection of tissue for the microscopic examination is essential. Naturally, the DCIS area should be examined with the help of specimen and slice radiography. We also try to examine mastectomy specimens immediately after the operation, because in specimens of this size even complete fixation does not stop autolytic processes deeper within, and this is how artifacts associated with considerable diagnostic difficulties generally arise.

Basic information. Similar to the examination of BCT specimens, macroscopic examination should draw upon imaging findings, the complete clinical data, information on size and localization, results of minimal invasive biopsy and characteristics of findings.

Marking. In addition to indicating the side, the cranial direction must be marked to enable radiopathological correlation of the localization. In simple and skin-sparing mastectomies, consideration should be given to the fact that a spindle-shaped flap of skin is not always arranged symmetrically in a horizontal plane. This can easily be solved by an arrow-shaped colored marking of the cranial direction on the surface

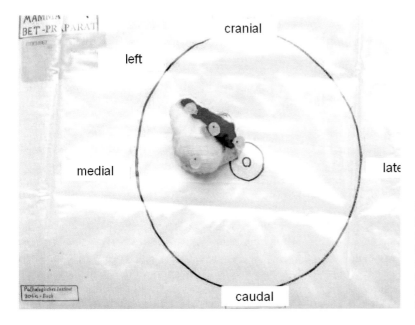

Fig. 6.6 Re-resection specimen. Directed re-excisions for clearing a single involved resection margin of a primary specimen are difficult to handle. Work-up depends on orientation of the specimen and marking of the outer surface. The figure shows an ideally marked specimen in an in-situ appropriate position.

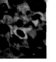

of the skin. For subcutaneous mastectomies the cranial direction must be marked by a suture.

Macroscopic description. The gross protocol should include the surgical method (simple, skin-sparing or subcutaneous mastectomy), the extension of the specimen in three dimensions (medial-lateral, cranial-caudal, ventral-dorsal) and information on abnormalities of the nipple or the covering skin. Furthermore, all focal findings – their maximum diameter as well as the localization (quadrant, central portion, axillary tail) – should be described. In secondary mastectomies, describing the cavity of the previous excision is mandatory, including the condition of the margins, the maximum diameter and the localization.

Slicing. We perform slicing perpendicular to the medial-lateral axis of the specimen (and not of the covering flap of skin, which mostly runs in a cranio-lateral to medial-caudal direction). The slices should ideally be about 5 mm. A thickness of 10 mm or more is not acceptable. All slices should be labeled and their number recorded. A special note should be made of the slice containing the mamilla. This slice gives information on the medial-lateral position of the sample: All slices with lower numbers represent the medial part of the breast, those with higher numbers the lateral one. If the other slices are separately processed by upper and lower half, it is possible to orient each individual tissue sample within the four quadrants of the breast.

Slice radiography. In the majority of cases microcalcifications visible in the slices help to localize the lesion, even if there are no macroscopic findings. Furthermore, microcalcification areas can be made visible that mammography failed to detect.

Sampling. The areas containing microcalcifications and macroscopically suspicious findings are embedded for histological examination. A block of unsuspicious fibrous glandular tissue is then routinely taken from each quadrant. Depending on breast size the retro-mamillary part of the central portion is examined in one or two blocks regardless of macroscopic findings. Finally, the nipple including the area containing the sinus lactiferi is embedded.

Reconstruction. The anatomical region of each paraffin block and histological slide may be identified by a code number (quadrants, central portion, axillary tail). It is possible to reconstruct the lesion's size by adding the number of adjacent blocks and the thickness of the individual slices.

In such a way, the size of a given DCIS can be approximately estimated. Quality control of mastectomies requires utmost precision. Lesions less than 40 mm in diameter can be distinguished safely enough from larger lesions. Furthermore, the position of the DCIS in relation to the system of quadrants and

especially its extent into the central portion can be precisely determined. Finally, microinvasion or larger invasive tumor components undetected by imaging diagnostics should be safely excluded. The data by Lagios, Holland, Ohtake and Mai and co-workers [3, 6, 12, 22] confirms that this is absolutely mandatory, as invasive foci were always found in close proximity to DCIS areas. Ohtake and Mai uncovered a close relation with the segmental architecture, the invasive tumor being mostly localized in the periphery of the involved segment [3, 6].

Examination of resection margins is not as important for mastectomy specimens as in breast-conserving therapy: the predominant part of the specimen is limited by the pectoral fascia representing the dorsal resection line. Naturally, no intraductal neoplasia can exceed this boundary. Zones with an increased risk of undiscovered invasive carcinoma near this margin will be detected by examination of mammographically suspicious areas. Nevertheless, remains of the glandular body are often found after mastectomy [23]. In modified radical mastectomies only marginal areas are at risk.

Due to the enormous size of the area to be examined even the most thorough pathological examination cannot yield definitively reliable clinical results. However, the residual risk is statistically relatively small, as shown by the low rate of local recurrence after mastectomy [24].

■ PATHOLOGICAL DATA FOR THERAPEUTIC DECISION-MAKING

During the last decade BCT has been established as the treatment of choice for both DCIS and invasive carcinoma. In comparison, however, to mastectomy with a local recurrence (LR) rate of 2–3% for both invasive and noninvasive carcinoma, breast-conserving therapy clearly shows a higher LR rate of 7–30% [25–28]. Irrespective of the modalities of adjuvant therapy the primary source for those LR after BCT is DCIS. This is confirmed by the fact that recurrent tumors occur almost without exception within the area of the previous operation. Therefore, complete excision of the lesion is generally regarded as a prerequisite for breast-conserving therapy, as reflected in the European and American guidelines [29].

In order to obtain this goal, pathologists have introduced a considerable number of safe-guards to the decision-making process of the multidisciplinary breast team. With reference to DCIS, such features include correlation with imaging (primarily microcalcifications), classification (with nuclear grading and presence or absence of comedonecroses), exclusion of invasion, size of the lesion and margin status. As a result of preoperative minimal invasive biopsy, the pathologist can contribute information on the mode of growth of different DCIS types to therapy planning. But only systematic pathological examination after complete removal of the surgical specimen will yield definitive information as a prerequisite for further treatment.

PREOPERATIVE DATA FROM MINIMAL INVASIVE BIOPSY

Minimal invasive biopsies (MIB) of the target lesion should be taken guided by the results of imaging. Because microcalcifications are the main feature of DCIS, mammography is the most commonly used guiding technique for minimal invasive biopsies. In evaluating these biopsies histologically, it is very important to note the type of calcification involved, its correlation with mammography and the grade of the DCIS.

Once correlation of microcalcification with the diagnosis of a minimally invasive biopsy has been confirmed, the **size of the microcalcification** area should be noted. This is an important feature in determining whether breast-conserving therapy should be recommended. In cases with microcalcification areas of more than 30–40 mm BCT is usually not possible (EUSOMA).

The **grade of DCIS** is another important feature for planning surgical excision: in high grade DCIS we recommend a 10 mm wide margin, in non-high grade DCIS a margin of 20 mm around the calcification area. In addition, we perform a preoperative biopsy of the central part of the breast, as this is a high-risk area for extension of DCIS outside the calcification area. A positive result is usually indicative of DCIS with poor correlation to the microcalcification area and a high risk of more extended lesions. Fifty-six percent (232/411) of our patients with DCIS larger than 40 mm underwent primary mastectomy after MIB-DCIS in the calcification area and central zone. In nine additional cases an **invasive component** was identified histologically within the mastectomy specimen. All patients undergoing mastectomy because of a DCIS larger than 40 mm were advised to undergo simultaneous sentinel lymph node biopsy, because if unexpected invasive cancers are found in these patients they are usually below 10 mm in size with a low risk of axillary metastases. A sentinel node procedure is impossible to apply after mastectomy. Furthermore, the decision whether to perform axillary dissection is influenced by the histological typing: invasive carcinomas of up to 2 mm in diameter and tubular carcinomas of up to 10 mm in diameter are not treated by axillary lymph node dissection [30].

MARGINS AND RESIDUAL TUMOR

The tumor-free margin of the surgical specimen in BCT correlates with the risk of residual tumor and the frequency of recurrence [31–35]. The concept of local recurrence developing from remaining DCIS in-situ is based on this correlation, which has been demonstrated in numerous studies. Nevertheless, opinion differs as to the optimal minimal distance, and there is no generally accepted standard for determining this parameter. Not until the 1980s when breast-conserving therapy was introduced for DCIS was special attention paid to resection margins. The NSABP B-17 protocol only stipulated that the DCIS must not be transected [16]. This requirement was certainly insufficient: patients whose DCIS had been treated by excision without radiotherapy suffered a local recurrence rate of 43% [36]. Tumor-free margins suggested by other experts were equally small: Lagios [37] und Silverstein [38] originally chose 1 mm, Solin 2 mm [39]. However, as early as 1994 Silverstein documented that a margin of 1 mm was insufficient [40], because residual tumor was found in 45% of mastectomy and re-excision specimens in these cases. Holland and co-workers were able to prove in 1985 that 1 mm wide resection margins involved a high risk in view of the large amounts of residual tumor tissue [22]. Therefore they proposed leaving a rim of normal glandular tissue between tumor and resection line as a criterion for a safer excision. Subsequent studies by Faverly and co-workers from the same working group provided an explanation for this finding: discontinuities in the intraductal neoplastic growth [9]. The most important finding relating to the debate on histological minimal distances is that gaps of more than 10 mm occur in only 8% of all DCIS cases. Theoretically, excision with a tumor-free margin of 10 mm should remove DCIS with a probability of 90%. These pathomorphological data correspond with the clinical results presented by the Van Nuys group in 1996 [41], the Nottingham group in 1997 [42] and the combined Children's Hospital and Van Nuys study in 1997 [43]. In DCIS excisions with at least 10 mm-wide, tumor-free margins the rate of local recurrence ranged from 8 to 6%, or was even as low as 5%. Correspondingly, local recurrence rates are higher in cases with shorter minimal distances to the resection margins. Nevertheless, several studies have yielded results that are in glaring contrast, among them the prospectively randomized NSABP B-17 study. This study revealed hardly any, or no correlation between the width of the histological tumor-free margins and residual tumor or the risk of recurrence [44].

Three main reasons for these data discrepancies are possible:

1. variable techniques used to examine resection margins;
2. variations in the extent of margin assessment; and
3. variable minimum requirements regarding the tumor-free margin.

VARIABLE TECHNIQUES

Technical difficulties may be the result of surgical shortcomings. Specimens sent in fragments for pathological examination, for instance, do not allow a definitive assessment of resection margins. Problems can also arise from irregular surfaces, tears or incisions, which impede objective measurement or render it virtually impossible as the resection area is barely recognizable. In such cases, marking specimens with ink or dye is also not helpful. However, failure to mark the surface may result in serious errors in microscopic diagnostics due to changes of contour and orientation of histological slides. When applying the method described by Carter [45] resection margins are prepared in the same fashion that an orange is peeled – resulting in very flat slices. Thus, obtaining a histological slide perpendicular to the resection surface is not possible. For this reason, sampling of margins should be carried out in such way that at least 10 mm of continuous tissue is achieved. By doing this, the 10 mm margin can be measured exactly. To estimate larger distances, findings in neighboring tissue blocks must usually be included. Estimation of margins larger than 10 mm by means of such reconstruction is more inaccurate, but of limited clinical relevance. The above-mentioned difficulties can be avoided by using large block techniques. However, an average of two out of six specimen margins cannot be assessed microscopically. Another source of technical difficulties is the fact that the exact diameter of the lesion along the mamillary-peripheral axis cannot be measured on slides. In this case it is impossible to measure the distances exactly: due to the thickness of large blocks any estimation would be inaccurate. There is no data in the literature defining the influence of these inconsistencies on the pathological data obtained.

VARIATIONS IN THE EXTENT OF MARGIN ASSESSMENT

Margin analysis is always an approximation. Complete embedding is the most appropriate option; the more complete the examination of the resection margins, the less inaccuracies in the data obtained. Incomplete embedding can only be considered if two conditions are met:

1. the radiopathological correlation by specimen radiography and slice radiography is appropriately used; and
2. the systematic sampling protocol is applied.

The total number of sampled blocks of tissue will increase not only with the size of the lesions (microcalcifications) but also with the size of the surgical specimen. Limiting the number of blocks in the sense of an 'absolute upper limit' inevitably leads to lesser levels of confidence in resection margins. It should be acknowledged that studies based on small numbers of blocks and slices per specimen pay little attention to resection margins for residual tumor or local recurrence [40, 44]. In a methodological study we investigated the influence of extent and type of sampling on the detection rate of intraductal tumor components in excision margins (Table 6.1). Before the procedures were standardized, we sampled the margins stochastically by taking six tissue blocks (median) per specimen. In the next phase we increased the median number of blocks from 6 to 20 per specimen. Finally we introduced the systematically oriented approach described above. Employing the three different approaches, we compared the rate of DCIS components within the 5 mm margins of 100 excision specimens of invasive pT1 tumors with macroscopic safety distances of 10 mm. While we could detect DCIS within 5 mm margins in only 2% of cases by stochastic examination of margins, this rate rose to 12% only by increasing the number of blocks. Finally, after introducing systematically oriented sampling as described above we found DCIS within the 5 mm margin in 32% of cases.

VARIABLE MINIMUM REQUIREMENTS

The high rate of local recurrence (43%) after 'complete' excision of DCIS without radiotherapy in the NSABP B17 study is clearly a result of the minimum demands (1 mm) regarding resection margins.

The updated results of the combined Children's Hospital and Van Nuys study [46] yielded the following recurrence rates after excision with tumor-free margins without radiotherapy: < 1 mm = 73%, 1–9 mm = 28% and ≥ 10 mm = 6%. Thus it seems quite obvious that minimum demands of less than

Tab. 6.1 Margin assessment: results of different approaches in pathology

Sampling method	Stochastic median 6 blocks*	Stochastic median 20 blocks*	Systematic oriented*
Number of cases with involved 5 mm margins**	2	12	32

* n = 100 cases with pT1 invasive breast cancers, see text
** margin involvement by DCIS

1 mm are too low to avoid local recurrence, while minimum demands of 10 mm seem to lower the rate of local recurrence considerably. Although there is no data on the risk of residual tumor or local recurrence associated with margins between 5 and 10 mm, it is evident that both risks will increase with free margins below the 10 mm limit. When, for example, limits of 2 mm were employed in studies to classify a sufficient width of resection margins, assessment was problematic. Even the best statistical analysis has not been able to demonstrate any significant difference between 'sufficient' (> 2 mm) or 'insufficient' (< 2 mm) resection margins. This line of reasoning, however, runs the risk of arriving at the erroneous conclusion that margins in general are irrelevant to the risk of local recurrence.

ANALYSIS OF DCIS EXCISION SPECIMENS AT THE BREAST CENTER IN BERLIN-BUCH

For reasons mentioned above, the data concerning residual tumor in re-excisions or mastectomy specimens with previous excision and insufficient resection margins vary considerably. We analyzed 299 excision specimens of patients with DCIS in the Breast Center in Berlin-Buch. These excision specimens were worked up between 1993 and 2003 according to the protocol described above (Table 6.2).

Tab. 6.2 Residual tumor after involved margins* in primary excisions in 299 DCIS patients

	Re-excision	Mastectomy (%)	Total
Residual tumor	142	67	209 (82.3%)
Tumor-free	45	0	45 (17.7%)
Total	187	67	254 (100.0%)

* DCIS within 10 mm

We compared resection margin findings with the results of re-excision or secondary mastectomy. Of the primary excision specimens, 254 of 299 showed DCIS exactly at the resection line or within the 10 mm margin. In each of these cases a second operation was carried out according to a protocol, if possible as a re-excision. In cases with an unfavorable relation of the lesion to breast size we advised patients to undergo mastectomy. In more than 85% of cases (254/299) residual DCIS could be detected in the re-excision specimen. The remaining 45 cases (15%) without

detectable residual tumor in re-excision specimens showed unusual features (Table 6.3).

The small subgroup of DCIS without residual tumor in the re-excisional specimen despite involvement of 10 mm margins of the primary excision shared three unusual features: the number of excision specimens with findings in only one of the six resection margins is much higher (85% vs. 65%), the mamillary margins were less often involved (50% vs. 78%), and, finally, the lesions with tumor-free re-excisions were all below 40 mm. In conclusion, this combination of features indicates a lower risk of residual tumor, despite involvement of 10 mm margins.

Most of the 142 DCIS cases (85%) that contained tumor within the 10 mm margins of the segmental excisions and that had residual tumor in re-excision specimens showed involvement of more than one of the margins (in several directions). The mamillary resection margin was far more often involved (87%) than all other five. All cases with an incompletely excised DCIS showed involved 5 mm margins along the mamillary resection line. Figure 6.7 shows combinations of various margin findings associated with different risks of residual tumor.

Tab. 6.3 Involved margins* with and without residual tumor at reoperation: pathological features of primary excisions

Primary excision	No residual tumor (%)	Residual tumor (%)
Only 1 of 6 margins involved	39 (86.6%)	159 (62.5%)
Involvement of mamillary margin	22 (48.8%)	191 (75.1%)
Size < 40 mm	45 (100%)	53 (20.8%)
Total	45	254

* DCIS within 10 mm

DCIS size, resection margin findings and evidence of residual tumor are closely related: the frequency of DCIS within 10 mm margins increases with the total size of the DCIS.

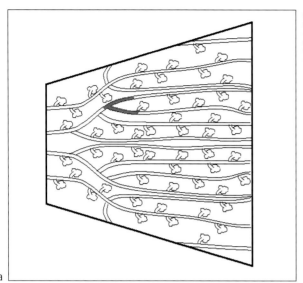

a

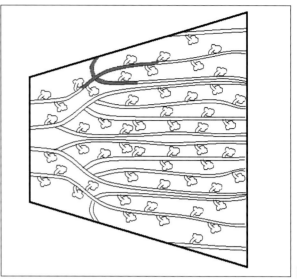

b

c

Fig. 6.7a–c Margins and residual tumor. Risk evaluation.
6.7a Low residual tumor risk. Margin > 10 mm, lesion size < 16 mm.
6.7b Intermediate residual tumor risk. Margin < 5 mm, only one margin involved, mamillary margin not involved, lesion size 16–40 mm. This combination indicates a reasonable risk of residual tumor; nevertheless there is a good chance that breast conservation by completing re-excision will be successful.

6.7c Highest residual tumor risk. Margin < 5 mm, multiple margins involved (mamillary margin included), lesion size > 40 mm. This combination indicates a very high risk of residual tumor; there is no chance of completely excising the DCIS. The patient should be advised to undergo mastectomy with reconstruction.

WIDTH OF TUMOR-FREE MARGINS

We were not able to establish any differences in the rate of residual tumors between the group with involvement of margins and the one with tumor-free margins of 1 mm or 1–5 mm. Only two cases with a minimal distance of more than 5 mm but less than 10 mm could be found: almost all cases with 5 mm wide tumor-free margins had 10 mm wide DCIS-free zones along the resection margins. This applies to all cases with complete primary excision as well as to all re-excision specimens with free resection margins.

MINIMAL FINDINGS WITHIN RESECTION MARGINS

As is characteristic of lobular cancerization in high grade DCIS [47] there may be secondary involvement of the lobular periphery by non high grade DCIS [48].

Both are the result of tumor cell growth into ductules. When localized at the resection margin, TDLUs involved by clinging type carcinoma or atypical proliferation of ductal-type may simulate flat epithelial atypia (FEA) and atypical ductal hyperplasia (ADH). In his critical review, Page pointed out how dangerous such misinterpretations can be [49]. Goldstein and co-workers analyzed the resection margins of 94 excision specimens from patients with DCIS retrospectively [48]. A significantly increased risk of recurrence was found in patients with low grade DCIS (nuclear grades 1 and 2) when a combination of DCIS and ADH was detected in resection margins. The rate of recurrence was increased in patients with high grade DCIS when DCIS and secondary lobular cancerization were detected in the margins. In line with Goldstein, we consider such minimal findings within the immediate proximity of DCIS to be direct extensions of the intraductal neoplasia. This applies to any case of secondary lobular cancerization caused by high grade DCIS. In FEA/ADH-like findings even experienced breast pathologists cannot definitely exclude surrounding non-high grade DCIS. Therefore, we consider such findings in resection margins to be an indication for re-excision. In our experience, they hardly ever occur as isolated findings along the resection line in obvious cases of DCIS: isolated findings of this kind were the sole indication for re-excision in only 7 of 152 DCIS cases. Residual DCIS was detected in six of the respective re-excision specimens. This rare situation occurred only in intermediate grade DCIS that could definitely be treated by BCT after re-excision. However, DCIS that required treatment by mastectomy due to theirsize showed clearly recognizable intraductal carcinoma within the resection margins of previous excisions.

The accuracy of histological margin assessment in DCIS increases with standardization of the pathological examination. Orientation of the specimen and marking of the margins is a precondition. Not even complete embedding (either in routine blocks or in large blocks) can allow a precise statement to be made without these preconditions being met. We consider findings of tumor tissue within a 5 mm margin along the resection line (under standardized conditions of systematic and specimen radiograph-oriented slicing) to be an indicator of residual tumor in the breast. The probability of residual tumor increases with the number of affected resection lines as well as with the involvement of the margin facing the mamilla. It is also influenced by the maximum diameter of DCIS: in cases where this is 40 mm or more, detection of tumors within the 5 mm margin with involvement of the mamillary resection margin indicates that the lesion cannot be removed completely by BCT. Under standardized examination conditions in cases with at least 5 mm wide tumor-free resection margins, we almost always achieve more than 10 mm of tissue free of DCIS.

SIZE OF DCIS AND BREAST-CONSERVING THERAPY

As DCIS is considered an obligate precursor lesion of invasive breast carcinoma, the aim of breast-conserving therapy should be complete removal of lesions. Naturally, the size of the DCIS largely determines the success of such an approach. The greater the extent of the DCIS the larger the excision must be. Many studies have explored the relationship between DCIS and specimen size, resection margin findings and recurrence risk [50–53]. Nevertheless, the available data on the influence DCIS size has on treatment

outcome is poor, mainly because of methodological problems, drawbacks in study design and the influence of patient selection.

METHODOLOGICAL PROBLEMS

The complex distribution patterns of DCIS, as determined by the glandular anatomy of the breast and the DCIS subtype, make size estimation difficult. Objective determination of size requires systematic spatial assessment of histological slices in the context of the ductal tree. Size estimations that neglect such information are fraught with error – even if the whole excision specimen is completely embedded or if large block techniques are utilized. This explains, for example, the paradox that the size of DCIS at histological examination may be smaller than the diameter of the associated area of mammographic microcalcifications. Measuring the maximum diameter on a single histological slide is only possible for lesions directly in the center of a piece of tissue and its corresponding slide. Such situations are extremely rare: most DCIS do not form visible tumors and must be 'blindly' searched for in a radiologically marked area of macroscopically unsuspicious tissue. For this reason, nonsystematic sampling does not allow a reliable estimation of the total dimension of a given DCIS. The same criticism can also be applied to the process of counting ducts containing DCIS, as the density of ducts is highly variable even within one segment. Alternatively, it has been proposed that the ratio of DCIS-containing slides to the total number of histological slides can be determined [54, 55]. This method helps to calculate the association between the rate of DCIS-involved ducts and the presence of tumor in re-excision specimens. Nevertheless, findings from differing institutions greatly vary: the percentage of DCIS-containing slides naturally depends on the total number of tissue blocks sampled as well as on the size of the surgical specimen. These methodological problems are associated with greater inaccuracies the larger the size of DCIS lesions is. In general, DCIS sizes are usually underestimated when employing such methods.

PROBLEMS IN STUDY DESIGN

As illustrated in the literature, a large number of retrospective studies have attempted to determine DCIS size from histological slides and correlate this with the effect of therapy. To the best of our knowledge, there are no reports on retrospective examinations based on a systematic work-up. Problems in the interpretation of clinical results are, therefore, most likely caused by errors in the assessment of DCIS size. Without a systematic work-up, it is impossible to assess the size of a DCIS, as the localization of tissue in the microscopic slide within the original specimen cannot be reconstructed.

The only two randomized therapy studies on DCIS ever performed, are impaired by the same problems [16, 56–58]. In about 80% of the analyzed histological findings used in the NSABP B17 study no statements on DCIS size were made [57]. A retrospective analysis could only be attempted in 40% of cases – and only on single slides taken from tissue that had not been systematically worked up [16]. In 87% of DCIS a diameter of less than 10 mm was deduced from the written protocols. The EORTC study 10853 could only provide information on DCIS size in 25% of cases under examination. This data had been partly taken from written findings and was not the result of revision of slides [59]. Despite the overall prospective design of these studies, the pathology data were obtained retrospectively and do not, therefore, allow precise estimation of the prognostic impact of pathological parameters.

THE INFLUENCE OF PATIENT SELECTION

Most data on DCIS size are derived from diagnostic or therapeutic excision specimens and not from mastectomies. Small lesions (up to 30 mm) naturally tend to prevail in this material. In the excellent retrospective analyses by Silverstein [41] DCIS with larger diameters could only be included when these patients had chosen BCT against medical recommendation. Holland and co-workers examined specimens from excisions, re-excisions and mastectomies from 59 patients with DCIS. They found only 17% were under 10 mm in diameter and 46% were larger than 30 mm. We have come to the conclusion that, in evaluating the data on DCIS size from the literature, attention must be paid to the choice of operative therapy and therefore to the extent of the operation.

BERLIN-BUCH RESULTS

Our own data on the systematic pathological and radiological examination of 299 DCIS are derived from excision as well as mastectomy specimens. About 27.2% of DCIS were smaller than 15 mm in diameter, while 16.3% were 16–40 mm and 56.4% were 40 mm or larger (Table 6.4).

Tab. 6.4 Pathological DCIS size in 411 patients*

0–15 mm	16–40 mm	> 40 mm	Total
112 (27.2%)	67 (16.3%)	232 (56.4%)	411 (100%)

* 1993–2002 Berlin-Buch Breast Center, including all DCIS patients irrespective of therapy

Complete excision of the lesion could be achieved in almost no patients with DCIS of more than 40 mm in diameter. With very few exceptions, these large DCIS showed involvement of another quadrant or of the central portion of the gland. Due to the poor anatomical definition of the central portion of the mammary gland this analysis was restricted to a retroareolar area up to 25 mm from the nipple. In cases where a lesion was mammographically detected in an overlapping area of two quadrants, only one quadrant was evaluated. Ninety-eight percent of the DCIS with diameters larger than 40 mm were also larger than 60 mm. In these cases, even in women with larger breasts, re-excisions were not successful and mastectomies had to be performed. Therefore, we consider a maximum diameter of 40 mm to be the upper limit for BCT, independent of breast size (Fig. 6.8). Such lesions have obviously outgrown their segment of origin via intersegmental anastomoses and involve large areas relative to the total size of the breast, even in cases of macromastia. Size is not only related to the total size of the breast, but equally to the number of segments involved. Due to small variations in the angle of ductal branches [6], even large breasts can show a DCIS extent of enormous volume. In the literature the relationship between DCIS size and margin status has often been emphasized [20, 41, 60]. Similar to Goldstein and co-workers, who proved a clear relationship between the degree of resection margin involvement and 'DCIS volume' [20], we found an association of positive resection margins with the size of DCIS: we were unable to excise DCIS larger than 40 mm in diameter with 10 mm tumor-free margins. Moreover, about 65% showed direct resection margin involvement and 35% contained tumor in at least five margins. In contrast, 100% of the DCIS less than 15 mm in diameter showed 10 mm wide free margins. In the remaining cases, this could only be achieved after re-excision. In the group of DCIS with diameters of 16–40 mm, the frequency of involved resection margins increased, but not to the same degree as in lesions larger than 40 mm. In this group a re-excision could not always be carried out successfully. Whenever tumor-free resection margins could be achieved by re-excision, they showed a 10 mm wide DCIS-free margin (Fig. 6.8).

Biologically, DCIS are considered to be 'early' lesions without invasion and without metastasizing potential. Nevertheless, they are not necessarily 'small' lesions – they can involve a considerable area of the glandular body. Size is the most important limiting factor for BCT, because there is a close relation between DCIS size and resection margin findings: the larger the DCIS, the greater the risk for involved resection margins. DCIS larger than 40 mm in diameter in the primary excision specimen almost

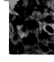

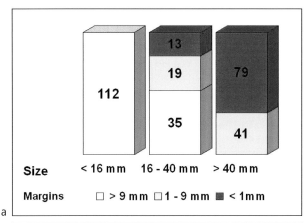

a

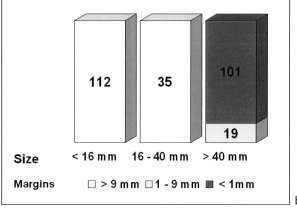

b

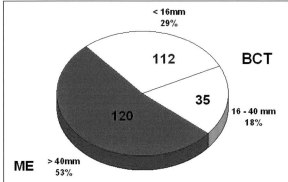

c

Fig. 6.8a–c Pathological data and therapeutic decision making in DCIS in the Berlin-Buch Breast Center (n = 299 patients, 1993–2002).

6.8a Size and margin findings in primary excisions. All patients with margins under 10 mm underwent re-excision.

6.8b Margin findings after re-excision. Whereas in all patients with lesions smaller than 40 mm free margin could be reached, this was impossible in patients with larger DCIS.

6.8c Breast conserving therapy versus mastectomy in DCIS. Therapy is decisively influenced by the final diameter of the lesion. The final decision to proceed was based on margin findings, which are surrogate markers for the definitive size of the lesion.

always show involved resection margins. Here the resection margin findings are more than just an indication for a re-excision: DCIS of more than 40 mm with involved resection margins under 5 mm always extend into the retromamillary central glandular body and/or other areas of the gland and are therefore in total much larger. Starting at 40 mm, size becomes the essential risk marker for residual tumors. The complete removal of such lesions can only be achieved by (subcutaneous or skin-sparing) mastectomy. In contrast, in our experience, small DCIS with diameters of less than 16 mm can be excised completely with 10 mm-wide free resection margins if preoperative planning is performed according to guidelines.

Finally, questions of individualized therapy within BCT are currently a topic of discussion. Which patients do not need additional radiotherapy? Which patients benefit from additional tamoxifen therapy? Trials to answer these questions must be based on prospective pathological data. In addition to histomorphological classification and biological markers, data on size and quality of the lesions is undoubtedly of importance, especially with reference to resection margins.

THE PATHOLOGIST AS A MEMBER OF A MULTIDISCIPLINARY BREAST TEAM

According to the EUSOMA guidelines, the pathologist belongs to the core team of a specialized breast unit. In this interdisciplinary setting, his task goes far beyond the histological diagnosis. His responsibilities include assessment of suspicious findings, participation in preoperative therapy planning for carcinomas, intra- and postoperative diagnostics as well as quality assurance. When assessing specimens from minimal invasive diagnostics, the pathologist must make a decision as to the validity of his findings (Chapter 5) in the context of imaging and clinical examination. Thus, he plays an essential part in the treatment of patients with a benign histology who do not undergo surgery and are instead controlled by imaging diagnostics.

In patients with malignant findings the pathologist adds essential information to preoperative planning. Before deciding whether to proceed with BCT, the correlation between DCIS and microcalcifications must be established. The size of the microcalcification area should reflect the minimal size of the DCIS. In cases with areas of microcalcifications of more than 30 mm (EUSOMA) – and certainly in those of more than 40 mm (see above) – BCT cannot be recommended.

The differentiation grade as determined by minimal invasive diagnostics is used by our team to plan macroscopic margins of the wide excision surrounding the area of microcalcifications: in high grade DCIS we plan a 10 mm margin, in non-high grade DCIS the margin is 20 mm wide (see above). In addition, our group performs a preoperative biopsy of the center of the gland, as this is a high-risk region for DCIS growth beyond a single segment. A positive result in this region suggests a very large DCIS with poor correlation to the microcalcification area. This applies to 34.7% (112/232) of patients with DCIS of more than 40 mm, who can then undergo primary mastectomy, sparing them a frustrating attempt at BCT followed by a secondary mastectomy. In some cases we are able to prove an invasive component not previously suspected at imaging diagnostics. Consequently, there is a general indication for clarification of axillary lymph node status (sentinel node biopsy or axillary lymph node dissection). In these cases histological typing is important: invasive carcinomas of up to 2 mm in diameter and tubular carcinomas of up to 10 mm are not treated by axillary lymph node dissection [30]. In addition, this therapeutic decision will be influenced by the presence of lymphatic or blood vessel invasion. In the experience of the Nottingham group, there is an increased risk of local recurrence after BCT for patients with these findings when they are younger than 50 years of age and their tumors are larger than 20 mm in diameter [61].

At present, **intraoperative diagnostics** primarily concentrates on supporting the surgeon by specimen radiography and macroscopic assessment (see above). Frozen section examination is rarely used.

When determining nuclear grade, maximal size and distances to the six resection margins the pathologist delivers the essential DCIS parameters and prerequisites for postoperative therapeutic decisions within the multidisciplinary team.

Quality assurance is also an interdisciplinary approach as it applies to all phases of treatment. Quality parameters within the preoperative phase are:
1. the time needed to obtain a histological diagnosis;
2. the rate at which patients are discussed by the interdisciplinary team;
3. the rate at which histological diagnoses are achieved with correlation to imaging diagnostics;
4. the sensitivity, specificity and positive predictive value of histological diagnosis; and
5. the false negative and false positive rate of this diagnosis (see Chapter 5).

Postoperatively, the preoperative planning data is compared with the parameters of the operative specimen, in particular the preoperative estimation of size, nuclear grade and invasion risk.

It is essential for effective quality assurance that all team members are in possession of full information regarding the case. In our experience this is best achieved by filling in a checklist.

This perioperative checklist, used by all participating physicians, documents the most important data and accompanies:
1. the patient through all clinical and imaging examinations;
2. the biopsy specimen in histological examination;
3. the physicians in the preoperative meeting;
4. the patient once more to the clinic;
5. the surgical specimen to specimen radiography and pathological examination; and finally
6. the physicians in the postoperative meeting.

By using this checklist, communication is simplified, is rendered more precise and time can be saved. In addition, all findings and images must accompany this checklist in its course throughout patient assessment and treatment.

Preoperative multidisciplinary meetings between radiologists, surgeons and pathologists are a precondition for competent decision-making leading to optimal results of therapy: All team members must agree on action to be taken. A complete interdisciplinary protocol on diagnostics and therapy is one precondition for controlling the quality of multidisciplinary team work. The other precondition is the documentation of each diagnostic and therapeutic phase for each patient. This is the only way deviations from this protocol can be noticed and analyzed. Finally, retrospective quality analysis is performed during the **postoperative meeting**.

Given complete information on clinical and imaging diagnostics based on a protocol for all participating disciplines, along with documentation and regular interdisciplinary pre- and postoperative meetings, the pathologist is able to influence the interdisciplinary breast team, thereby contributing to optimal diagnostic and therapeutic decisions. Similar to representatives of other disciplines, pathologists in the team must be known by name, must be specialized in breast diseases and must be fully replaceable by one another. The aim of this chapter has been to highlight gross pathological examination of surgical specimens in DCIS. At present, most surgical interventions in patients with DCIS are based on a histological diagnosis performed by a pathologist after minimal invasive biopsy. As a rule, therefore, operative specimens are not the result of a simple diagnostic excision but of expert oncologic surgery. It could be argued that following our proposals for dealing with specimens from every breast excision is too costly and time-consuming. From the viewpoint of the patient and her doctors, of course, the standardized pathology work-up of the specimen is justified. The comparison between the cost of standardized pathology on the one hand and unrequired adjuvant therapies in patients with DCIS or therapy due to recurrences as a result of overlooked invasive foci on the other hand has been comprehensively discussed and presented by Lagios [62, 63]. Assuming that only 10% of patients are spared radiotherapy and tamoxifen due to histologically confirmed adequate resection, Lagios estimated that unrequired therapies are 5.7 times more expensive than a (complete!) standardized tissue processing of specimens from all patients. Finally, there is a small group of patients with lesions unsuitable for minimal invasive diagnostics suspicion of malignancy is high enough to indicate diagnostic excision. If a DCIS is confirmed histologically, the pathologist is asked to provide the same parameters as for therapeutic excisions. Therefore even in diagnostic excisions for suspicious lesions, a pathological examination should be performed identical to that required for histologically proven DCIS.

Finally, early invasive cancer must be included when discussing the whole spectrum of early breast cancer. Screening mammography trials do not only show a reduction in mortality [64–66], they also provide evidence of an increasing risk of metastasis throughout the stages of tumor development after diagnosis. Moreover, it is now evident that systemic disease is not the only factor leading to death from breast cancer. Even local recurrence is an independent and important mortality factor [67, 68]. Furthermore, data exist supporting a correlation between size of recurrent tumor and five-year rates of death and of metastases [69]. This suggests that persistent locoregional residual tumor can metastasize. Therefore, the aim of therapy must be the complete removal of tumor tissue. Bearing in mind the importance of DCIS as a source of residual tumor in BCT of invasive carcinomas, the pathologist must also investigate margins of these specimens for DCIS. Taken together, we strongly recommend pathologic examination of therapeutic segmental excisions for invasive cancer in an identical fashion to that suggested in this chapter for DCIS.

REFERENCES

1. Wellings SR, Jensen HM, Marcum RG. An atlas of subgross pathology of the human breast with special reference to possible precancerous lesions. J Natl Cancer Inst 1975;55:231–73.
2. Moffat DF, Going JJ. Three dimensional anatomy of complete duct systems in human breast: pathological and developmental implications. J Clin Pathol 1996;49:48–52.
3. Mai KT, Yazdi HM, Burns BF, Perkins DG. Pattern of distribution of intraductal and infiltrating ductal carcinoma: a three-dimensional study using serial coronal giant sections of the breast. Hum Pathol 2000;31:464–74.
4. Ohtake T, Kimijima I, Fukushima T, et al. Computer-assisted complete three-dimensional reconstruction of the mammary ductal/lobular systems: implications of ductal anastomoses for breast-conserving surgery. Cancer 2001;91:2263–72.
5. Lanyi M, Lanyi. Die gesunde Brust. In: Brustkrankheiten im Mammogramm: Diagnostik und pathomorphologische Bildanalyse. Berlin, Heidelberg, New York: Springer; 2003. p.9–13.
6. Ohtake T, Abe R, Kimijima I, et al. Intraductal extension of primary invasive breast carcinoma treated by breast-conservative surgery. Computer graphic three-dimensional reconstruction of the mammary duct-lobular systems [see comments]. Cancer 1995;76:32–45.
7. Faverly DR, Holland R, Burgers L. An original stereomicroscopic analysis of the mammary glandular tree. Virchows Arch A Pathol Anat Histopathol 1992;421:115–9.
8. Holland R, Hendriks JH, Vebeek AL, Mravunac M, Schuurmans Stekhoven JH. Extent, distribution, and mammographic/histological correlations of breast ductal carcinoma in-situ. Lancet 1990;335:519–22.
9. Faverly DR, Burgers L, Bult P, Holland R. Three dimensional imaging of mammary ductal carcinoma in-situ: clinical implications. Semin Diagn Pathol 1994;11:193–8.
10. Holland R, Hendriks JH. Microcalcifications associated with ductal carcinoma in-situ: mammographic-pathologic correlation. Semin Diagn Pathol 1994;11:181–92.
11. Carter DJ. Intraductal Papillary Tumors of the Breast. A Study of 78 Cases. Cancer 1977;39:1689–92.
12. Lagios MD, Westdahl PR, Margolin FR, Rose MR. Duct carcinoma in-situ. Relationship of extent of noninvasive disease to the frequency of occult invasion, multicentricity, lymph node metastases, and short-term treatment failures. Cancer 1982;50:1309–14.
13. Rosen PP, Braun DW, Jr., Kinne DE. The clinical significance of pre-invasive breast carcinoma. Cancer 1980;46:919–25.
14. Schwartz GF, Patchefsky AS, Feig SA, Shaber GS, Schwartz AB. Clinically occult breast cancer. Multicentricity and implications for treatment. Ann Surg 1980;191:8–12.
15. Page DL, Dupont WD, Rogers LW, Landenberger M. Intraductal carcinoma of the breast: follow-up after biopsy only. Cancer 1982;49:751–8.
16. Fisher ER, Costantino J, Fisher B, et al. Pathologic findings from the National Surgical Adjuvant Breast Project (NSABP) Protocol B-17. Intraductal carcinoma (ductal carcinoma in-situ). The National Surgical Adjuvant Breast and Bowel Project Collaborating Investigators. Cancer 1995;75:1310–9.
17. Dershaw DD, Abramson A, Kinne DW. Ductal carcinoma in-situ: mammographic findings and clinical implications. Radiology 1989;170:411–5.
18. Ikeda DM, Andersson I. Ductal carcinoma in-situ: atypical mammographic appearances. Radiology 1989;172:661–6.
19. Stomper PC, Connolly JL, Meyer JE, Harris JR. Clinically occult ductal carcinoma in-situ detected with mammography: analysis of 100 cases with

radiologic-pathologic correlation. Radiology 1989;-172:235–41.
20. Goldstein NS, Kestin L, Vicini F. Intraductal carcinoma of the breast: pathologic features associated with local recurrence in patients treated with breast-conserving therapy. Am J Surg Pathol 2000;24:1058–67.
21. Perry NM. Quality assurance in the diagnosis of breast disease. EUSOMA Working Party. Eur J Cancer 2001; 37:159–72.
22. Holland R, Veling SH, Mravunac M, Hendriks JH. Histologic multifocality of Tis, T1-2 breast carcinomas. Implications for clinical trials of breast-conserving surgery. Cancer 1985;56:979–90.
23. Tewari M, Kumar K, Kumar M, Shukla HS. Residual breast tissue in the skin flaps after Patey mastectomy. Indian J Med Res 2004;119:195–7.
24. Morrow M, Strom EA, Bassett LW, et al. Standard for the management of ductal carcinoma in-situ of the breast (DCIS). CA Cancer J Clin 2002;52:256–76.
25. de Jong E, Peterse JL, van Dongen JA. Recurrence after breast ablation for ductal carcinoma in-situ. Eur J Surg Oncol 1992;18:64–6.
26. Silverstein MJ, Barth A, Poller DN, et al. Ten-year results comparing mastectomy to excision and radiation therapy for ductal carcinoma in-situ of the breast. Eur J Cancer 1995;31A:1425–7.
27. Fisher ER, Leeming R, Anderson S, Redmond C, Fisher B. Conservative management of intraductal carcinoma (DCIS) of the breast. Collaborating NSABP investigators. J Surg Oncol 1991;47:139–47.
28. Ernster VL, Barclay J, Kerlikowske K, Wilkie H, Ballard-Barbash R. Mortality among women with ductal carcinoma in-situ of the breast in the population-based surveillance, epidemiology and end results program. Arch Intern Med 2000;160:953–8.
29. Wells CA, Amendoeira I, Apostolikas N, Bellocq JP et al. Quality assurance guidelines for pathology. In: Perry N, Broeders M, de Wolf C, editors. European Guidelines for Quality Assurance in Mammography Screening. 4th ed. Office for Official Publications of the European Communities; 2005.
30. Rutgers EJ. Quality control in the locoregional treatment of breast cancer. Eur J Cancer 2001;37:447–53.
31. Silverstein MJ, Lagios MD, Groshen S, et al. The influence of margin width on local control of ductal carcinoma in-situ of the breast. N Engl J Med 1999;340: 1455–61.
32. Van Zee KJ, Liberman L, Samli B, et al. Long term follow-up of women with ductal carcinoma in-situ treated with breast-conserving surgery: the effect of age. Cancer 1999;86:1757–67.
33. Vicini FA, Kestin LL, Goldstein NS, et al. Relationship between excision volume, margin status, and tumor size with the development of local recurrence in patients with ductal carcinoma-in-situ treated with breast-conserving therapy. J Surg Oncol 2001;76:245–54.
34. Chan KC, Knox WF, Sinha G, et al. Extent of excision margin width required in breast conserving surgery for ductal carcinoma in-situ. Cancer 2001;91:9–16.
35. Douglas-Jones AG, Logan J, Morgan JM, Johnson R, Williams R. Effect of margins of excision on recurrence

after local excision of ductal carcinoma in-situ of the breast. J Clin Pathol 2002;55:581–6.
36. Fisher B, Costantino J, Redmond C, et al. Lumpectomy compared with lumpectomy and radiation therapy for the treatment of intraductal breast cancer. N Engl J Med 1993;328:1581–6.
37. Lagios MD. Duct carcinoma in-situ. Pathology and treatment. Surg Clin North Am 1990;70:853–71.
38. Silverstein MJ, Waisman JR, Gamagami P, et al. Intraductal carcinoma of the breast (208 cases). Clinical factors influencing treatment choice. Cancer 1990; 66:102–8.
39. Solin LJ, Fowble BL, Schultz DJ, Goodman RL. The significance of the pathology margins of the tumor excision on the outcome of patients treated with definitive irradiation for early stage breast cancer. Int J Radiat Oncol Biol Phys 1991;21:279–87.
40. Silverstein MJ, Gierson ED, Colburn WJ, et al. Can intraductal breast carcinoma be excised completely by local excision? Clinical and pathologic predictors. Cancer 1994;73:2985–9.
41. Silverstein MJ, Lagios MD, Craig PH, et al. A prognostic index for ductal carcinoma in-situ of the breast. Cancer 1996;77:2267–74.
42. Sibbering DM, Blamey RW. Nottingham experience. In: Silverstein MJ, editor. Carcinoma in-situ of the breast. Baltimore: Williams & Wilkins; 1997. p.271–84.
43. Lagios MD, Silverstein MJ. Ductal carcinoma in-situ. The success of breast conservation therapy: a shared experience of two single institutional nonrandomized prospective studies. Surg Oncol Clin N Am 1997;6: 385–92.
44. Fisher ER, Dignam J, Tan-Chiu E, et al. Pathologic findings from the National Surgical Adjuvant Breast Project (NSABP) eight-year update of Protocol B-17: intraductal carcinoma. Cancer 1999;86:429–38.
45. Carter D. Margins of "lumpectomy" for breast cancer. Hum Pathol 1986;17:330–2.
46. Silverstein MJ. Margin width as the sole predictor of local recurrence in patients with ductal carcinoma in-situ of the breast. In: Silverstein MJ, Recht A, Lagios MD, editors. Ductal Carcinoma in-situ of the breast. 2nd ed. Philadelphia: Lippincott, Williams and Wilkins; 2002.
47. Fechner RE. Ductal carcinoma involving the lobule of the breast. A source of confusion with lobular carcinoma in-situ. Cancer 1971;28:274–81.
48. Goldstein NS, Martinez A, Vicini F, Stromberg J. The histology of radiation therapy effect on prostate adenocarcinoma as assessed by needle biopsy after brachytherapy boost. Correlation with biochemical failure. Am J Clin Pathol 1998;110:765–75.
49. Page DL, Rogers LW, Schuyler PA, Dupont WD, Jensen RA. The natural history of ductal carcinoma in-situ of the breast. In: Silverstein MJ, Recht A, Lagios MD, editors. Ductal carcinoma in-situ of the breast. 2nd ed. Philadelphia: Lippincott Williams & Wilkins; 2002. p.17–21.
50. Fisher ER. Pathobiological considerations relating to the treatment of intraductal carcinoma (ductal carcinoma in-situ) of the breast. CA Cancer J Clin 1997;47:52–64.

51. Osteen RT. Limits of resection for ductal carcinoma in-situ. J Surg Oncol 1998;69:63–5.

52. Silverstein MJ. Ductal carcinoma in-situ of the breast. Br J Surg 1997;84:145–6.

53. Silverstein MJ. Predicting residual disease and local recurrence in patients with ductal carcinoma in-situ. J Natl Cancer Inst 1997;89:1330–1.

54. Schnitt SJ, Connolly JL. Classification of ductal carcinoma in-situ: striving for clinical relevance in the era of breast conserving therapy. Hum Pathol 1997;28:877–80.

55. Tornos C, O'Hea B. Ductal carcinoma in-situ (DCIS) of the breast: pathologic features predictive of residual disease after initial excisional biopsy. Mod Pathol 2000;13:48A.

56. Fisher ER, Costantino J. Quality assurance of pathology in clinical trials. The National Surgical Adjuvant Breast and Bowel Project experience. Cancer 1994;74: 2638–41.

57. Fisher B, Dignam J, Wolmark N, et al. Lumpectomy and radiation therapy for the treatment of intraductal breast cancer: findings from National Surgical Adjuvant Breast and Bowel Project B-17. J Clin Oncol 1998;16:441–52.

58. Julien JP, Bijker N, Fentiman IS, et al. Radiotherapy in breast-conserving treatment for ductal carcinoma in-situ: first results of the EORTC randomised phase III trial 10853. EORTC Breast Cancer Cooperative Group and EORTC Radiotherapy Group. Lancet 2000;355:528–33.

59. Bijker N, Peterse JL, Duchateau L, et al. Risk factors for recurrence and metastasis after breast-conserving therapy for ductal carcinoma-in-situ: analysis of European Organization for Research and Treatment of Cancer Trial 10853. J Clin Oncol 2001;19:2263–71.

60. Neuschatz AC, DiPetrillo T, Steinhoff M, et al. The value of breast lumpectomy margin assessment as a predictor of residual tumor burden in ductal carcinoma in-situ of the breast. Cancer 2002;94:1917–24.

61. Sibbering DM, Galea MH, Morgan DA, et al. Safe selection criteria for breast conservation without radical excision in primary operable invasive breast cancer. Eur J Cancer 1995;31A:2191–5.

62. Lagios MD. Practical pathology of ductal carcinoma in-situ: how to derive optimal data from the pathologic examination. In: Silverstein MJ, Recht A, Lagios MD, editors. Ductal carcinoma in-situ of the breast. 2nd ed. Philadelphia: Lippincott Williams & Wilkins; 2002. p.207–21.

63. Lagios MD. Pathologic procedures for mammographically detected ductal carcinoma in-situ. In: Silverstein MJ, editor. Ductal Carcinoma in-Situ of the Breast. 1st ed. Baltimore: Williams & Wilkins; 1997. p.189–93.

64. Blanks RG, Moss SM, Patnick J. Results from the UK NHS breast screening programme 1994–1999. J Med Screen 2000;7:195–8.

65. Alexander FE, Anderson TJ, Brown HK, et al. 14 years of follow-up from the Edinburgh randomised trial of breast-cancer screening. Lancet 1999;353:1903–8.

66. Nystrom L, Andersson I, Bjurstam N, et al. Long-term effects of mammography screening: updated overview of the Swedish randomised trials. Lancet 2002;359: 909–19.

67. Fortin A, Larochelle M, Laverdiere J, Lavertu S, Tremblay D. Local failure is responsible for the decrease in survival for patients with breast cancer treated with conservative surgery and postoperative radiotherapy. J Clin Oncol 1999;17:101–9.

68. Vicini FA, Kestin L, Huang R, Martinez A. Does local recurrence affect the rate of distant metastases and survival in patients with early-stage breast carcinoma treated with breast-conserving therapy? Cancer 2003; 97:910–9.

69. Voogd AC, Coebergh JW. Mortality reduction by breast-cancer screening. Lancet 2003;362:245–6.

Content

7

Basic principles of benign proliferative breast disease

Werner Boecker, Horst Buerger and Hermann Herbst

In this chapter we discuss the cellular components of benign breast lesions to provide the basis for a new and better understanding of the processes involved. **With the exception of microglandular adenosis, benign lesions contain cells expressing Ck5/14. They show differentiated bilineage characteristics comparable to normal breast epithelium. Our conclusion is that benign breast lesions can only be explained by assuming that Ck5/14+ cells and their progeny are the founding cells of these lesions.** Within this conceptual framework, the term benign proliferative breast disease (BPBD) is used to encompass and classify all benign proliferative lesions. The cellular constituents of these lesions are introduced and compared to those of breast carcinoma. **BPBD lesions can be readily distinguished from malignant epithelial lesions, which are often purely glandular in phenotype. The fundamental principles of a new understanding of the different lesions and the implications this has in distinguishing benign from malignant lesions in daily routine will be discussed.** A special paragraph is dedicated to the use of immunohistochemistry in the diagnostic context.

Basic principles of benign proliferative breast disease

■ CLASSIFICATION USED IN THIS BOOK

It is important to remember that the current system of classification for BPBD lesions – similar to a great number of nomenclature systems – consists of a mishmash of eponymous, archaic and descriptive terms. This may be attributed in some degree to the great variability of benign morphologies, to overlapping features between different categories and even to the fact that features of several categories may be found in the same lesion. In recent years the Royal College of Pathologists [1, 2], the American Society of Surgical Pathology [3, 4] and the European Breast Screening Pathology Working Group [5] have proposed almost identical classification systems for benign proliferative breast conditions. Most recent textbooks have consistently applied this terminology.

The historically sanctified term 'benign proliferative breast disease' (BPBD) has been used to define proliferative lesions without atypia, including usual ductal hyperplasia (UDH), sclerosing adenosis, papillomas and fibroadenomas [6–8]. Several studies have shown that patients with such lesions carry a slight risk of subsequently developing breast cancer in either breast 1.5–2.0 times above that of the general population when long-term follow-up is available [6–19]. They represent lesions that themselves may only occasionally progress to malignancy, with the exception of papillomas. Thus, in one study up to 30% of peripheral papillomas displayed transitions to atypical ductal proliferations [20]. We feel that, although BPBD as a diagnostic category has not been used in the most recent edition of the WHO classification of breast tumors, retaining this term is still helpful. In this book the term has therefore been adopted as a conceptual framework for proliferative lesions of epithelial type that are clearly benign and not direct precursors of invasive breast malignancies. From a cell biological viewpoint and for theoretical and practical reasons, as discussed above, we propose that tubular adenoma, nipple adenoma and benign adenomyoepithelial tumors should be included. Thus we classify BPBD lesions into eight major categories (Table 7.1).

What those lesions have in common is their glandular and myoepithelial progeny and the fact that their epithelial component is characterized by Ck5+ cells (see below). We distinguish those benign lesions from proliferations currently believed to be direct precursor lesions of invasive breast carcinoma. In our opinion, such a classification more easily communicates the clinical implications of BPBD to a predominantly clinical audience.

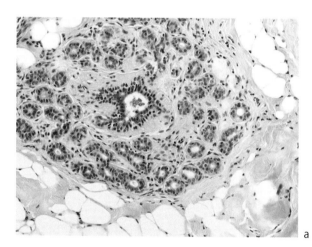

Fig. 7.1a–d Normal breast epithelium.
7.1a Normal lobule at higher magnification. Note the characteristic loose stroma against the background of collagenous tissue. Glandular and myoepithelial cells can be easily identified.

Continuation

Tab. 7.1 Benign proliferative breast disease (BPBD)

BPBD category	Features
Usual ductal hyperplasia (Chapter 8). Sclerosing adenosis and variants (Chapter 9). Radial scar/complex sclerosing lesion (Chapter 10). Papilloma and variants (Chapter 11). Tubular adenoma and variants (Chapter 12). Nipple adenoma (Chapter 13). Adenomyoepithelial tumors (Chapter 14). Fibroepithelial/phyllodes tumors (Chapter 15).	Ck5/14+ progenitor cell lesions with glandular and/or myoepithelial differentiation. Several bear a low general cancer risk. Low potential for the lesions themselves to progress to malignancy, exception: papillary lesions. No direct precursor lesions of invasive breast cancer.

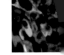

▪ CELLULAR CONSTITUENTS OF BPBD

The muddled concept of BPBD and its failure to clarify the nature of lesions can in part be attributed to the shortcomings of the current two-cell paradigm, which does not encompass the range of cell biological properties of these lesions. The use of double immunofluorescence staining for Ck5/14, Ck8/18 and the myoepithelial marker sm-actin has led to the introduction of the progenitor cell concept, opening up new insights into the cellular basis of regeneration and differentiation of normal breast epithelium (see Chapter 1). The most important finding of these immunofluorescence studies has been that Ck5 is a surrogate marker of progenitor cells and early glandular and myoepithelial cells. Thus Ck5/14+ cells give rise to glandular and myoepithelial cell lineages (Fig. 7.1).

The next logical step was to use the very tools that allowed us to recognize subtypes of cells in normal breast epithelium, to reveal the cellular components of BPBD lesions as well as their relation to each other. Interestingly, once such work was done, it became apparent that nearly all BPBD lesions share the cellular composition of normal mammary breast epithelium. This composition seems to determine the fundamental principles of the cellular evolution of these lesions [21]. With the exception of microglandular adenosis, all BPBD lesions contain Ck5/14+ cells and their glandular and/or myoepithelial progeny. This is best exemplified by comparing the cellular organization of normal breast epithelium with two classic forms of BPBD: sclerosing adenosis and UDH. In sclerosing adenosis Ck5/14+, myoepithelial and glandular progeny cells proliferate with formation of irregular tubular structures. Although the glandular-myoepithelial layering of the tubules is preserved, the

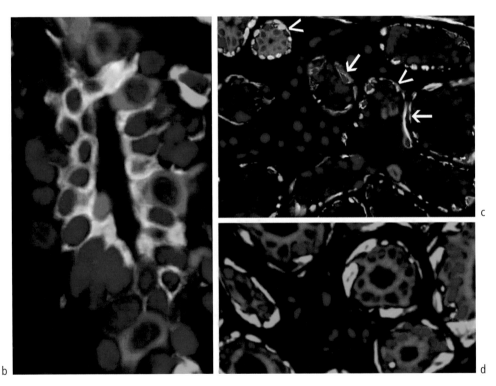

Fig. 7.1a–d Normal breast epithelium.
7.1b Double immunolabeling of a ductule for Ck5 (green signal) and Ck8/18 (red signal) displays the immunophenotypic heterogeneity of luminal epithelial cells, indicative of the presence of glandular precursor cells and their glandular progeny. Note the scarcity of differentiated glandular cells expressing Ck8/18 (red signal) in this ductule. It should be borne in mind that the Ck8/18+ cells must be regarded as transitory cells highly capable of mitotic growth.
7.1c Double immunolabeling for Ck5 (red signal) and smooth muscle actin (green signal) of ductular structures of a lobule. Intermediate myoepithelial cells express both Ck5 and sm-actin (arrows) (hybrid signal). The differentiated myoepithelial end cells show the green signal of exclusive sm-actin expression (arrow heads). Some luminal cells express Ck5 (red signal) which indicates either progenitor or early glandular precursor cells.
7.1d Double immunolabeling of ductular structures of a lobule for sm-actin (green signal) and cytokeratins 8/18 (red signal). The acinar structures display the typical architecture with luminal glandular cells expressing Ck8/18 and myoepithelial cells expressing sm-actin.

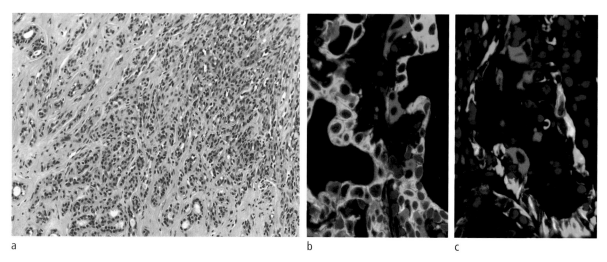

a   b   c

Fig. 7.2a–c Sclerosing adenosis.

7.2a Classic appearance of sclerosing adenosis in an H&E-stained section.

7.2b Double immunolabeling for Ck5 (red signal) and Ck8/18 (green signal) displays the same immunophenotypic heterogeneity of luminal epithelial cells as seen in normal breast epithelium (compare Fig. 7.1). Note the scarcity of Ck5+ cells (red signal) in these tubular structures. Most cells show a hybrid color indicating transitory cells that express both Ck5 and Ck8/18.

7.2c Double immunolabeling for Ck5 (red signal) and sm-actin (green signal). The myoepithelial cells display a heterogeneous staining reaction with some myoepithelial cells expressing both Ck5 and sm-actin (hybrid signal). The differentiated myoepithelial end cells show the intense green signal of exclusive sm-actin expression. Some luminal cells express Ck5 (red signal), which indicates either progenitor or early glandular precursor cells.

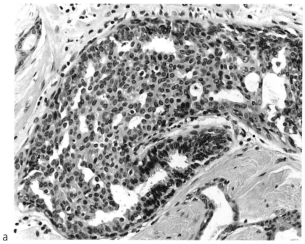

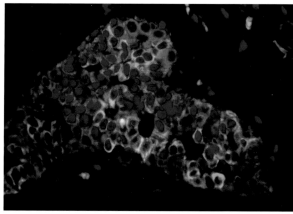

a   b

Fig. 7.3a–c Usual ductal hyperplasia.

7.3a Medium power view of a typical florid epithelial hyperplasia in an H&E-stained section.

7.3b Double immunolabeling for Ck5/6 (green signal) and Ck8/18 (red signal) highlights the heterogeneity of the glandular cell proliferation. Note the scarcity of intensely stained Ck5/6+ cells (green signal). Most cells are hybrid in color, indicating intermediate glandular cells, which express both Ck5/6 and Ck8/18. Occasionally, cells show intense red staining indicative of complete glandular differentiation. In contrast to normal breast epithelium, the regular spatial patterning and sorting are lost.

7.3c Double immunolabeling for Ck5/6 (red signal) and sm-actin (green signal). The two antibodies display a reaction pattern similar to the one seen in normal breast epithelium. The bulk of proliferating cells express Ck5. A myoepithelial differentiation of those cells is not observed.

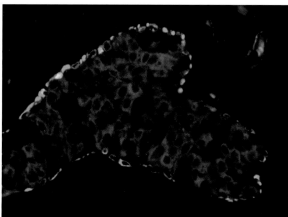

c

132

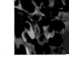

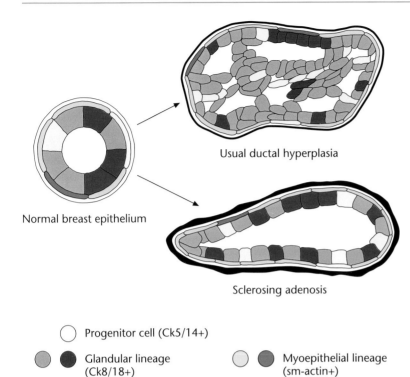

Usual ductal hyperplasia

Normal breast epithelium

Sclerosing adenosis

○ Progenitor cell (Ck5/14+)

● Glandular lineage (Ck8/18+)

○ ● Myoepithelial lineage (sm-actin+)

Fig. 7.4 Cellular epithelial components of sclerosing adenosis and usual ductal hyperplasia lesions and their architectural patterns compared to normal breast epithelium. The main features of normal breast epithelium are the symmetry of spatial patterning and the appropriate sorting of the epithelial cells. In BPBD lesions these features are lost and/or the architectural order of the glandular structures is deranged compared to the organization of normal breast epithelium.

normal architecture is lost (Figs 7.2 and 7.4). Likewise, in UDH, Ck5(14)+ cells and their glandular progeny proliferate with a loss of contact between glandular cells and myoepithelial cells. A further characteristic is the inappropriate sorting of these cells compared to normal breast epithelium (Fig. 7.3). Thus these lesions represent benign proliferative processes showing either lineage differentiation into clearly recognizable glandular cells or bilinear cell differentiation. Furthermore both lesions are characterized by the presence of Ck5/14+ cells, which we regard as precursor cells of both lineages. In contrast to the normal breast, however, the appropriate spatial patterning of the proliferating cells, and/or their histological architecture, are lost (Fig. 7.4). As will be seen in the following chapters on the various BPBD lesions, the same characteristics hold true for all other BPBD entities, although lesions may differ in their degree of glandular (Ck8/18) and/or myoepithelial lineage differentiation (sm-actin or other myoepithelial markers; Fig. 7.5).

The diversity of BPBD lesions, however, cannot be exclusively attributed to proliferation and derangement of epithelial cells. Instead it is characterized by an imbalance in the composition of epithelial cells, stromal cells and extracellular matrix constituents (Fig. 7.6). In many BPBD lesions, for example fibroadenomas and sclerosing adenosis, the stromal compartment and the extracellular matrix are major

constituents and are, therefore, likely to play a crucial role in the development of these lesions. This is clearly evident in fibroadenomas with their two components (for details see Chapter 14), but equally holds true for

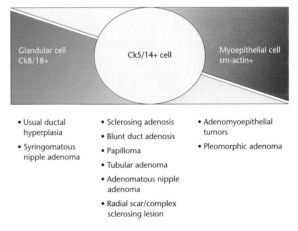

Glandular cell Ck8/18+ Ck5/14+ cell Myoepithelial cell sm-actin+

- Usual ductal hyperplasia
- Syringomatous nipple adenoma

- Sclerosing adenosis
- Blunt duct adenosis
- Papilloma
- Tubular adenoma
- Adenomatous nipple adenoma
- Radial scar/complex sclerosing lesion

- Adenomyoepithelial tumors
- Pleomorphic adenoma

Fig. 7.5 Hypothetical cellular pathogenesis of benign proliferative breast epithelium of different lesions based on data obtained in double immunofluorescence experiments using Ck5/14, Ck8/18 and a myoepithelial marker such as sm-actin. With the exception of microglandular adenosis, all entities are characterized by the presence of Ck5/14+ cells and their glandular or bilinear cell differentiation. However, the degree of glandular (Ck8/18) and/or myoepithelial lineage differentiation (sm-actin and others) may vary in these lesions.

Epithelial interactions

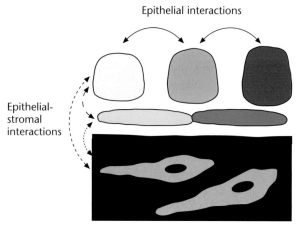

Glandular
cells

Epithelial-
stromal
interactions

Myoepithelial
cells

Basement
membrane

Stromal cells
with extracellular
matrix

Fig. 7.6 Epithelial-stromal interactions in BPBD. Many BPBD lesions must be viewed as a proliferation of epithelial structures and their mesenchymal stromal counterpart with inappropriate sorting of the epithelial and mesenchymal cell populations and violation of normal architecture. The prototypical lesion is fibroadenoma, which mimics normal lobular architecture. Many other benign lesions, however, may show a mesenchymal component. The mechanisms that regulate these processes are currently under intense investigation.

nearly all the other benign categories mentioned above (UDH being an exception). Thus papilloma, tubular adenoma, radial scar and sclerosing adenosis are – in addition to their epithelial component – principally defined by their stromal compartment. Papillomas, for example, contain typical fibrovascular stalks, whereas radial scars are characterized by their fibrous/fibroelastotic tissue. Even adenoma of the nipple may show a prominent stromal reaction. In this context it is worth reminding ourselves that, during morphogenesis of breast tissue, epithelial and mesenchymal cells proliferate, differentiate and ultimately produce the appropriate sorting of epithelial and mesenchymal compartments of the adult breast tissue.

Cross-talk between epithelium and mesenchyme seems to be an important driver of this sorting process. As a result, it may be influenced by soluble and solid phase stimuli such as cytokines, hormones, metalloproteinases and degraded matrix proteins. Although the details of this epithelial-mesenchymal interaction are still largely undisclosed, striking similarities between BPBD and developmental stages of breast tissue are currently emerging [22]. Both require cell proliferation and cell motility. Some processes may even involve epithelial invasion of the surrounding tissue and cellular differentiation of both epithelial and stromal cells. Given that both BPBD lesions and normal breast tissue share common processes of

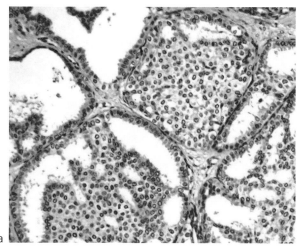

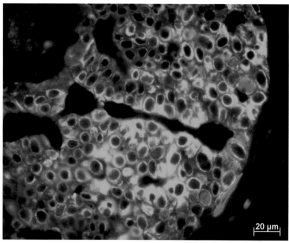

a

b

Fig. 7.7a–b Ductal carcinoma in-situ.
7.7a Higher power view of a low grade DCIS, showing a proliferation of monomorphous atypical cells with solid to cribriform pattern.
7.7b DCIS. Triple staining for Ck8/18, Ck5 and MIB1 highlights the glandular phenotype of malignant cells with Ck8/18 expression, but lack of Ck5 expression. Only one cell of the basal layer expresses Ck5. This lesion was completely surrounded by an sm-actin+ layer indicating mature myoepithelial cells.

epithelial differentiation and that both stromal cells and the extracellular matrix act as relevant modifiers of such processes, it is not surprising that the various BPBD lesions not only share distinct epithelial and mesenchymal features, but may even show over-lapping morphologies.

Usual ductal hyperplasia is not a precursor lesion of breast carcinoma. The traditional view of breast cancer development suggests a transition from normal epithelial cells via hyperplasia and atypical hyperplasia to ductal carcinoma in-situ (DCIS) and invasive breast carcinoma [23]. Of all proliferative lesions of the breast, none has been more fiercely debated and none more eloquently defended as an early step in cancer development than UDH [23, 24].

The fact that both UDH and DCIS display an intra-ductal proliferation had a large implicit impact on how the role of UDH was conceived of as one of the early lesions in cancer development. This view seemed to receive support from the epidemiological observations of Page and co-workers, according to which the risk of breast cancer increased with the degree of atypia. Thus UDH was regarded as an indicator lesion with a slightly increased general cancer risk. O'Connell et al. [25] and Lakhani et al. [26] then revealed data which indicated that at least some UDH lesions were clonal. Anecdotal evidence that synchronous UDH and invasive breast cancers share some genetic alterations [25] was interpreted as indicating a relationship between both lesions. However, it was never ruled out whether these alterations were already present in the normal breast tissue of these patients. Nevertheless, with such findings in mind, many authors endorsed the long-held view that UDH was a first step in the cascade to invasive breast carcinoma.

A number of studies published throughout the last two decades have, however, shown great differences in the cellular composition of UDH and DCIS, strongly questioning the proposed link between these two lesions [27–30]. Recent immunofluorescence, bio-chemical and molecular studies have further supported this view [21]. The main cellular trait attributed to carcinoma, as opposed to UDH and other BPBD lesions, is its almost exclusive glandular differentia-tion (Fig. 7.7) (exceptions being some high grade malignancies and certain rare specific entities such as adenosquamous carcinoma and adenoid cystic carcinoma, see next paragraph). Furthermore, the typical recurrent genetic imbalances detected by comparative genomic hybridization in noninvasive and invasive breast cancer have not been observed in UDH (Fig. 7.8). Although LOH analysis and the more refined DOP-PCR-CGH studies indicated a certain prevalence of subtle genetic changes in UDH, these aberrations were randomly distributed and not recur-rent, quite unlike those observed in ductal neoplasias

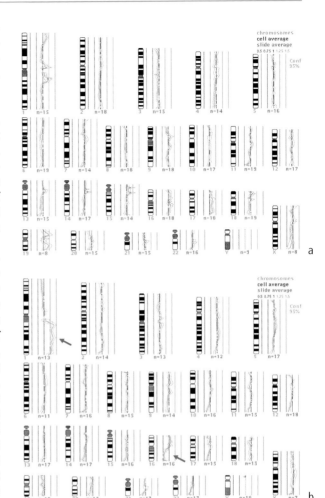

Fig. 7.8a–b CGH profiles of UDH (a) and DCIS (b). This tech-nique enables analysis of gross genetic imbalances. The CGH profiles indicate gains and losses of chromosomal material. The chromosome numbers are in green. The red curve to the right of each chromosome depicts the average ratio profile of a given tumor. Of the five lines to the right of each chromosome the black line represents a normal ratio of 1.0. Extensions of the red curve to the right reflect gains, extensions to the left, losses. The CGH study of UDH does not reveal any genetic abnormalities. This is in clear contrast to low grade DCIS which contains genetic changes, among them, typically, loss at 16q (arrows).

[25, 31, 32]. These findings suggest that some UDH lesions may be clonal and that the genetic changes associated with UDH are at least in part responsible for this type of proliferation. This, however, does not imply that UDH lesions are precursor lesions, in space or time, of ductal carcinoma. Finally, direct trans-formation of these benign lesions to invasive breast cancer has never been convincingly demonstrated.

In conclusion, apart from chance findings, there is currently no evidence that UDH is a precursor lesion of breast carcinoma.

■ CELLULAR CONSTITUENTS OF BREAST CARCINOMA

The cellular composition of BPBD lesions fundamentally differs from that of most malignant epithelial proliferations such as ADH, DCIS, lobular neoplasia and invasive breast carcinoma, whose cells usually display an entirely glandular phenotype from the onset (compare Figs 7.3 and 7.7), (for details see Chapter 17). There is evidence that this immunophenotypic difference may also be indicative of a different cellular origin. Thus, in contrast to benign lesions, breast carcinoma seems mainly to derive from Ck8/18+ transitory glandular cells of the resting breast (Fig. 7.9). Immunophenotypic characterization may be instrumental, in distinguishing benign from malignant lesions. This is achieved by application of a limited panel of antibodies with specificity for myoepithelial antigens and a set of cytokeratins such as Ck5/14 and Ck8/18.

Based on this data we propose a modified progression model (Fig. 7.10). The major difference between the old linear model and our modified progression model is that the latter does not attribute a preferential role to UDH as a precursor lesion of DCIS and invasive breast cancer. Rather, UDH and other BPBD lesions are regarded as dead ends, the cells of which rarely progress to in-situ malignancies and invasive breast carcinoma.

■ ATYPICAL PROLIFERATION (ADH/DCIS) ■ EX BPBD

As will be discussed in Chapter 17, the vast majority of ductal carcinomas arise de novo from glandular cells of the TDLUs that do not show features of any type of BPBD [33]. Nevertheless every pathologist is aware of benign lesions that clearly show a transformation to either malignant ductal or lobular-type in-situ malignancy, which may even progress to invasive carcinoma.

For benign peripheral papillary tumors, the incidence of malignant transformation of a primarily benign lesion has been reported to be as high as 30% [34–36]. The WHO characterizes these lesions by the presence of 'focal atypical epithelial proliferation with low grade nuclei' [37] (see Chapters 11 and 20). Although such malignant transformations have also been noted in other types of BPBD lesions, they are rare and represent a chance finding (for details see corresponding lesions). Thus, with the exception of papillary lesions, the risk of malignant transformation of a clearly benign lesion seems very low in each of the different categories (Table 7.2).

We therefore introduce the term atypical proliferation ex BPBD to define a process representing a malignant ductal or lobular-type transformation of a pre-existing BPBD lesion.

As discussed above, one puzzling feature of atypical ductal proliferations and invasive breast cancers is that their cells resemble the phenotype of the normal glandular cell – most of them express Ck8/18 in the absence of Ck5/14. Thus the evolution of atypical

Tab. 7.2 Epithelial malignancies ex BPBD lesions

Type of benign lesion	Type of malignancy	Frequency	Commentary
Peripheral papilloma	Atypical ductal proliferation. Atypical lobular proliferation.	10–30%. Extremely rare.	Transitions are well-documented in the literature.
Radial scar, sclerosing adenosis, fibroadenoma	Atypical ductal or lobular proliferation.	Exact incidence unknown, but probably low.	Well-documented lesions indicating a slightly increased general cancer risk, depending on size and type of proliferation.
Adenomyoepithelial tumors	Epithelial and/or myoepithelial malignancy.	Unknown.	Well-documented transition to malignancy. Malignant lesions may be epithelial, myoepithelial or both. Rarely direct transformation to malignancy.
Usual ductal hyperplasia	Atypical ductal proliferation.	Probably rare. Incidence never reported in the literature.	Precursor status of UDH unlikely. UDH is indicative of slight general cancer risk.

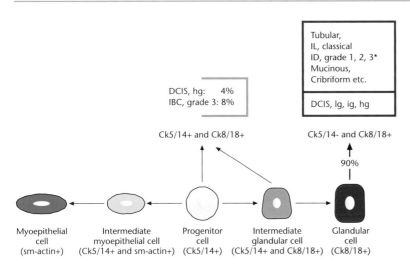

Tubular,
IL, classical
ID, grade 1, 2, 3*
Mucinous,
Cribriform etc.

DCIS, lg, ig, hg

DCIS, hg: 4%
IBC, grade 3: 8%

Ck5/14+ and Ck8/18+   Ck5/14- and Ck8/18+

90%

Myoepithelial cell (sm-actin+)   Intermediate myoepithelial cell (Ck5/14+ and sm-actin+)   Progenitor cell (Ck5/14+)   Intermediate glandular cell (Ck5/14+ and Ck8/18+)   Glandular cell (Ck8/18+)

Fig. 7.9 Hypothetical model of breast carcinoma development based on the progenitor cell concept. More than 90% of breast carcinomas and their precursors display a purely glandular phenotype and are characterized by expression of Ck8/18 and a lack of Ck5/14 expression. A small ratio of breast malignancies express or co-express Ck5/14 (see Chapter 17). There is some evidence that most breast carcinomas develop from their phenotypic glandular counterparts.

proliferation ex BPBD can be unveiled using Ck5 and Ck14 immunostaining (Fig. 7.11).

Only a small percentage of high grade DCIS and grade 3 invasive breast cancers and, possibly, some polymorphous lobular neoplasias contain tumor cells with a mixed Ck5/14+ and Ck8/18+ phenotype. According to the literature, these cases amount to 3.6% of DCIS lesions and 7.5% of invasive ductal breast carcinomas. Such cases do pose the question as to whether UDH may serve as a precursor in this type of breast carcinoma. However, as will be discussed in Chapters 17 and 20, there is currently no data to prove this hypothesis.

In summary, BPBD lesions are very common, and some of them are currently regarded as markers of increased cancer risk. At present, there is no

reasonable proof, however, that BPBD lesions per se represent obligate precursors of in-situ malignancies or even of invasive breast cancer.

DIAGNOSING BPBD

The rationale behind this book has been to use the term benign proliferative breast disease in a practical sense with inclusion of all the lesions listed in Table 7.1.

In the last century, diagnosis in breast pathology was primarily based on excisional biopsies and mastectomy specimens, careful and experienced macroscopic and light microscopic examination, and the comparison of these results with clinical data. As briefly touched upon in Chapters 4 and 5, with the spread of mammography, nonoperative diagnostic procedures such as fine needle aspiration and core biopsy have steadily gained in importance as diagnostic tools. The disadvantage of the limited tissue material has been overcome with the advent of vacuum-assisted core biopsies, which have led to high sensitivity and specificity even in problematical lesions. These techniques are currently preferred to fine needle aspiration cytology and to localization excision biopsies, as they spare women with benign lesions unnecessary surgery.

The preservation of lobular architecture, lesional symmetry and a general impression of the cellular composition of a given lesion is best seen at low power objectives. Occasionally, high power objectives may lead to the discovery of remarkable 'atypical' and worrisome nuclei in a number of benign lesions, which may therefore be misdiagnosed as malignant. On the other hand, high power objectives may be essential in recognizing the subtle atypical changes of earliest ductal in-situ neoplasia, such as clinging carcinoma and flat epithelial atypia.

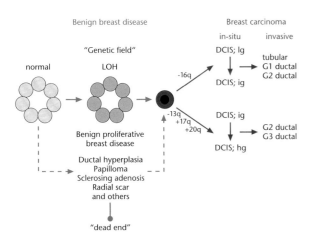

Benign breast disease   Breast carcinoma

in-situ   invasive

"Genetic field"   DCIS; lg

normal   LOH   tubular
G1 ductal
-16q   G2 ductal

DCIS; ig

Benign proliferative breast disease

-13q
+17q   DCIS; ig
+20q   G2 ductal
G3 ductal

Ductal hyperplasia
Papilloma
Sclerosing adenosis   DCIS; hg
Radial scar
and others

"dead end"

Fig. 7.10 Schematic drawing to show the two-tiered classification of proliferative breast diseases (for details see text). BPBD lesions are regarded as dead ends. The cells of these lesions – with the exception of papillary lesions – rarely progress to malignancy. In contrast, breast cancer usually derives de novo from cells of the 'normal' TDLUs.

Over a period of time, pattern recognition in combination with cytological features was used to describe the different types of BPBD. Thus the description of observed histological patterns and the regularities associated with them in terms of risk categories was regarded as the most appropriate way of characterizing clinical situations. In this system the morphologic categories were derived from H&E-stained sections.

Based on the progenitor cell concept we enhance the pattern recognition paradigm by a cell biological dimension using a small set of cellular markers, in particular Ck5/14, Ck8/18 and sm-actin. Within the framework of this concept, it is possible to correlate the composite elements of a lesion with its diagnostic category (epithelial and/or mesenchymal cells) and, implicitly, the cellular processes that have contributed to its formation. This implies that the true nature of a difficult lesion is only displayed when it is broken down into its elementary constituents. For example, the intraductal epithelial growth pattern of UDH and

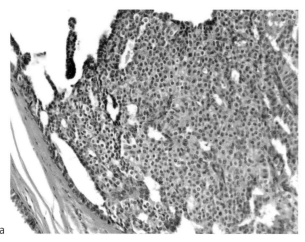 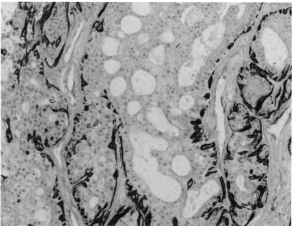

a   b

Fig. 7.11a–b Atypical ductal proliferation ex papilloma.
7.11a Medium power view of a typical papilloma with transition to low grade atypical ductal proliferation with cribriform growth pattern. This clearly indicates malignant growth.
7.11b High power view with Ck5 immunostaining highlights the Ck5– clonal proliferation of the malignant cells. The myoepithelial cells are well-preserved and their presence does not exclude malignancy (see Chapter 11).

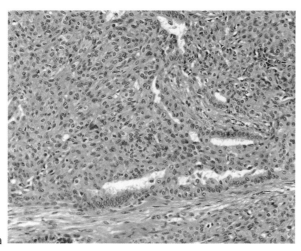 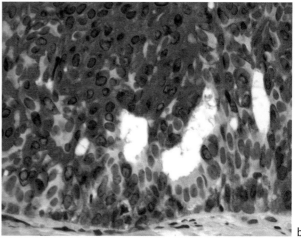

a   b

Fig. 7.12a–b Usual ductal hyperplasia.
7.12a Medium power view of typical UDH showing proliferation of heterogeneous glandular cells with variation in cytoplasmic staining, bland oval nuclei with uneven placement and peripheral slit-like lumina.
7.12b Ck5 immunostaining of the same lesion. The bulk of proliferating cells stain intensely for Ck5. A few cells are completely unstained, namely fully differentiated glandular cells which only express glandular cytokeratins 8/18 (not shown here, compare Fig. 7.3b–c).

Tab. 7.3 The most useful antibodies applicable on paraffin sections for assessment of lineage differentiation*

Cell type	First-line antibodies	Clone*	Remarks
Glandular lineage	Ck7	**OV-TL 12/30** K72.7; C68; LP5K	Expressed by cells of glandular differentiation.
	Ck8/18	**5D3** K8.8/DC10; Zym5.2	
	Ck19	**KS19.1** BA17; RCK108 A53-B/A2 26, 1533A2	
Myoepithelial	sm-actin	**1A4** α sm-actin	Very sensitive markers when applied on paraffin sections. Ck5/14 is expressed in cells in early myoepithelial differentiation.
	Calponin	CALP 26A11	
	Maspin	EAW24	
	p63	**4A4** 63PO2; Y4A3; 63PO3; 5G8; 4A4/Y4A3; 7JUL	
Progenitor cell features	Ck5/6	**D5/16B4**	Ck5/14 is expressed in progenitor cells and cells in early glandular and myoepithelial differentiation. It is lost in differentiated cells, whereas p63 is expressed in progenitor cells and in early myoepithelial cells.
	Ck14	**LL002**	
	p63	**4A4** 63PO2; Y4A3; 63PO3; 5G8; 4A4/Y4A3; 7JUL	
Squamous differentiation	Ck5/6	**D5/16B4**	Ck10 is a sensitive marker for squamous lineage that is not present in normal breast epithelium. Notice, however, that Ck5/6 is expressed in progenitor cells and their early squamous progenies.
	Ck6	**LHK 6B** LHK 6	
	Ck10	**DE-K10** DE-K13; LHP1	
Mesenchymal differentiation	Vimentin	**V9** RV202; VIM3B4	Cells of stromal origin are Ck5/14–. Note that vimentin is also expressed in progenitor cells and myoepithelial cells.

* First-line antibodies and clones we have experience with and currently use are marked in bold letters.

DCIS is the common link between both lesions. This surface similarity at H&E level was one of the strongest arguments for the traditional model of progression. The use of different cellular markers has, however, disclosed striking cellular differences in these two lesions and opened the door for new concepts. As will be discussed in the following chapters, the histological appearance of lesions is sufficient for diagnosis in most cases. In difficult cases immunophenotyping is used to identify a given lesion and to distinguish it from its benign or malignant counterparts.

Immunohistological techniques play an important role in the evaluation of proliferative breast lesions. The architecture and cellular components and even subtle features not obvious in routine pathology can be highlighted (Table 7.3). Thus immunophenotyping contributes significantly to reproducibility of diag-

noses. For benign or malignant proliferative breast lesions that are easily diagnosed on H&E sections, immunostains are not required, while they are essential for difficult and indeterminate lesions.

A large number of cytokeratin patterns have been described in normal breast epithelium and in benign and malignant proliferative breast disease [20, 27, 28, 38–50]. Cytokeratin subgroups differ in their molecular weight and isoelectric point. Specific monoclonal antibodies have been developed against many of these cytokeratins, allowing the lineage of cells to be determined. Until recently, lack of availability of antibodies with a high degree of specificity was a serious limitation. In breast pathology high molecular weight cytokeratins 5 and 14, low molecular weight cytokeratins 7/8/18/19 and squamous cell cytokeratins 6,10 and 11 [27–30, 42, 46, 51] have been shown to be extremely useful as diagnostic tools. The most important myoepithelial markers are the smooth muscle proteins sm-actin, calponin, maspin and p63 [52–62].

In general, a limited panel of antibodies including different types of cytokeratins and myoepithelial markers is usually sufficient. The antibodies that have been useful in our practice for the evaluation of proliferative breast disease are listed in Table 7.4.

BPBD lesions on the one hand and atypical ductal and lobular proliferations and their invasive counterparts on the other display a different cellular phenotypic composition. It is by now a well-established fact that almost all BPBD lesions harbor Ck5/14+ cells as their key components, whereas 90–95% of epithelial malignancies are glandular in phenotype. Furthermore, those malignancies showing Ck5/14 expression are usually high grade. These facts provide the scientific rationale behind the use of Ck5 or Ck14 immunostaining as the most reliable tool in distinguishing benign and malignant cases of diagnostically problematical proliferative lesions. Staining UDH with Ck5/14-specific antibodies reveals a characteristic Ck5/14 mosaicism, whereas the tumor cells of most breast cancers show a glandular phenotype and do not express Ck5 or Ck14 (Figs 7.11 and 7.12). Similarly, sclerosing adenosis displays Ck5/14 expression at least in some luminal and most basal cells of the tubular proliferates, whereas tubular, invasive lobular, invasive cribriform, invasive ductal, grade 1 and 2, and even most grade 3 lesions are

Ck5/14–. Thus these antigens can even be helpful in distinguishing clonal proliferative processes from different BPBD lesions. It is, however, of paramount importance that immunohistochemical findings be interpreted in the context of morphology. For example, early malignant lesions may contain Ck5/14+ residual normal cells and mimic a mosaic pattern. Furthermore, differentiated glandular cells of the resting breast or fully secretory end cells of the lactating breast do not express Ck5/14. A small number of cases defy classification. In our experience the use of broad spectrum cytokeratin antibodies such as 34βE12, which is directed against Ck1, 5, 10, 14 (and probably others), is less helpful in the context of proliferative breast lesions, since it stains both benign and malignant lesions of all grades (see Chapters 8, 9, 17 and 20).

Immunostaining must be evaluated in the context of histological findings and correlated with the cells found within the specific lesion.

As most studies have been performed on paraffin sections, the use of formalin-fixed and paraffin-embedded tissue is preferred. Furthermore, paraffin sections provide excellent cellular preservation and allow a far better distinction between normal/hyperplastic and neoplastic tissue. Molecular techniques such as comparative genomic hybridization or LOH studies are only needed if immunohistochemical and routine sections fail to provide consistent results.

Tab. 7.4 The most useful antibodies for assessing proliferative breast disease

Problem to be addressed	First-line antibodies	Remarks
Usual ductal hyperplasia vs. ductal and lobular neoplasia.	Ck5/14 and Ck8/18	Ck5/14 mosaicism in UDH as opposed to Ck5/14 negativity in most neoplasias.*
Sclerosing adenosis vs. tubular or invasive lobular carcinoma, classic type.	sm-actin, calponin, p63, maspin, Ck5/14	Positive in SA. Lack of myoepithelial cell layer in carcinomas. p63 and Ck5/14 negativity in carcinomas.
Papilloma vs. papillary carcinoma.	sm-actin, calponin, p63, maspin, Ck5/14	Myoepithelial cell layer present in papilloma, usually absent in carcinoma. Note exceptions to this rule**.
Squamous differentiation.	Ck6 and Ck10	Sensitive markers for squamous differentiation.
Adenomyoepithelial tumors vs. phyllodes tumors and spindle cell lesions.	Ck5/14, sm-actin, Ck8/18	Note that AMTs express all markers; however, tumors of mesenchymal origin are Ck5/14–. Mesenchymal parts of phyllodes tumors are also Ck5/14–.
Tubular carcinoma, other grade 1 and 2 carcinomas and most grade 3 carcinomas.	p63, sm-actin, calponin, Ck5, Ck14	Carcinomas stain negative for all these markers with few exceptions*. Note that myofibroblasts intensely stain for sm-actin.

* Grade 1 and 2 tumors are usually Ck5/14–, grade 3 tumors may be Ck5/14+.
** Some papillary DCIS may contain a well-shaped myoepithelial cell layer (see Chapter 11).

TRIPLE ASSESSMENT OF BPBD

At this juncture, it is worthwhile mentioning that, given the importance of microcalcification in the mammographic detection of precursor lesions and small breast cancers, it is mandatory for the pathologist to see the specimen radiograph before macroscopic description, specimen sectioning and obtaining blocks for histology (Chapters 5 and 6).

At imaging, benign lesions present with the whole spectrum of radiological breast abnormalities from benign lesions to suspicious tumors, ranging from asymmetric densities or architectural distortions to different types of calcifications.

In such clinical contexts malignant lesions cannot often be reliably ruled out without obtaining breast tissue, either by minimal invasive techniques such as fine needle biopsy, wide bore biopsies and/or by an open surgical diagnostic biopsy (Chapters 4 and 5). The aim of these diagnostic methods is to obtain tissue material on which a reliable morphological diagnosis can be made (see below).

THE PRINCIPLE OF RISK ASSESSMENT

Much pathological research over the last decades has been aimed at identifying lesions whose presence increases the risk of subsequent carcinoma. This has led to the identification of benign lesions that are specifically associated with a local and/or a general risk for the development of breast cancer [7]. The main pathological risk factors that have emerged during recent years are UDH, sclerosing adenosis, radial scar and benign papillary lesions. In addition to their identification per se, diagnosing these lesions is also of considerable practical value in clinical medicine as a means of identifying individuals who are at an increased risk of developing carcinoma. This topic will be addressed in more detail in Chapter 23.

REFERENCES

1. Royal College of Pathologists Working Group. Pathology Reporting in Breast Cancer Screening [abstract]. J Clin Pathol 1991;44:710–25.
2. Royal College of Pathologists Working Group and UK National Breast Screening Programme. Pathology Reporting in Breast Cancer Screening. Sheffield: NHS; 1990.
3. Hutter RV. Goodbye to "Fibrocystic Disease". N Engl J Med 1985;312:179–81.
4. Hutter RVP. Consensus meeting. Is fibrocystic disease of the breast precancerous. Arch Pathol 1986;110:171–3.
5. Perry N, Broeders M, de Wolf C, Törnberg S. European guidelines for quality assurance in mammography screening. 3rd ed. Luxembourg: Office for Official Publications of the European Communities; 2001.
6. Dupont WD, Page DL. Risk factors for breast cancer in women with proliferative breast disease. The New England Journal of Medicine 1985;312:146–51.
7. Page DL, Dupont WD, Rogers LW, Rados AM. Atypical Hyperplastic Lesions of the Female Breast. A Long-Term Follow-Up Study. Cancer 1985;55:2698–708.
8. Page DL, Rogers LW. Combined Histologic and Cytologic Criteria for the Diagnosis of Mammary Atypical Ductal Hyperplasia. Human Pathology 1992;23:1095–7.
9. Kodlin D, Winger EE, Morgenstern NL, Chen U. Chronic mastopathy and breast cancer. A follow-up study. Cancer 1977;39:2603–7.
10. Carter CL, Corle DK, Micozzi MS, Schatzkin A, Taylor PR. A prospective study of the development of breast cancer in 16,692 women with benign breast disease. Am J Epidemiol 1988;128:467–77.
11. Tavassoli FA, Norris HJ. A Comparison of the Results of Long-Term Follow-Up for Atypical Intraductal Hyperplasia and Intraductal Hyperplasia of the Breast. Cancer 1990;65:518–29.
12. Palli D, Rosselli-Del TM, Simoncini R, Bianchi S. Benign breast disease and breast cancer: a case-control study in a cohort in Italy. Int J Cancer 1991;47:703–6.
13. London SJ, Connolly JL, Schnitt SJ, Colditz GA. A prospective study of benign breast disease and the risk of breast cancer [published erratum appears in JAMA 1992 Apr 1;267(13):1780]. JAMA 1992;267:941–4.
14. Krieger N, Hiatt RA. Risk of breast cancer after benign breast diseases. Variation by histologic type, degree of atypia, age at biopsy, and length of follow-up. Am J Epidemiol 1992;135:619–31.
15. McDivitt RW, Stevens JA, Lee NC, et al. Histologic Types of Benign Breast Disease and the Risk for Breast Cancer. Cancer 1992;69:1408–14.
16. Dupont WD, Parl FF, Hartmann WH, et al. Breast cancer risk associated with proliferative breast disease and atypical hyperplasia [see comments]. Cancer 1993;71:1258–65.
17. Bodian CA, Perzin KH, Lattes R, Hoffmann P, Abernathy TG. Prognostic significance of benign proliferative breast disease. Cancer 1993;71:3896–907.
18. Marshall LM, Hunter DJ, Connolly JL, et al. Risk of breast cancer associated with atypical hyperplasia of lobular and ductal-types. Cancer Epidemiol Biomarkers Prev 1997;6:297–301.
19. Jensen RA, Page DL, Dupont WD, Rogers LW. Invasive breast cancer risk in women with sclerosing adenosis. Cancer 1989;64:1977–83.
20. Bartek J, Bartkova J, Kyprianou N, et al. Efficient immortalization of luminal epithelial cells from human mammary gland by introduction of simian virus 40 large tumor antigen with a recombinant retrovirus. Proc Natl Acad Sci U S A 1991;88:3520–4.
21. Boecker W, Moll R, Dervan P, et al. Usual ductal hyperplasia of the breast is a committed stem (progenitor) cell lesion distinct from atypical ductal hyperplasia and ductal carcinoma in-situ. J Pathol 2002;198:458–67.
22. Osin PP, Anbazhagan R, Bartkova J, Nathan B, Gusterson BA. Breast development gives insights into breast disease. Histopathol 1998;33:275–83.
23. Lakhani SR. The transition from hyperplasia to invasive carcinoma of the breast. J Pathol 1998;187:272–8.

24. Tavassoli FA. Pathology of the Breast. 2nd ed. Norwalk: Appleton and Lange; 1999.

25. O'Connell P, Pekkel V, Fuqua SA, et al. Analysis of loss of heterozygosity in 399 premalignant breast lesions at 15 genetic loci. J Natl Cancer Inst 1998;90: 697–703.

26. Lakhani SR, Collins N, Stratton MR, Sloane JP. Atypical ductal hyperplasia of the breast: clonal proliferation with loss of heterozygosity on chromosomes 16q and 17p. J Clin Pathol 1995;48:611–5.

27. Nagle RB, Bocker W, Davis JR, et al. Characterization of breast carcinomas by two monoclonal antibodies distinguishing myoepithelial from luminal epithelial cells. J Histochem Cytochem 1986;34:869–81.

28. Jarasch E-D, Nagle RB, Kaufmann M, Maurer C, Böcker WJ. Differential Diagnosis of Benign Epithelial Proliferations and Carcinomas of the Breast Using Antibodies to Cytokeratins. Hum Pathol 1988;19:276–89.

29. Böcker WJ, Bier B, Freytag G, et al. An immunohistochemical study of the breast using antibodies to basal and luminal keratins, alpha-smooth muscle actin, vimentin, collagen IV and laminin. Part I: normal breast and benign proliferative lesions. Virchows Archiv A 1992;421:315–22.

30. Böcker WJ, Bier B, Freytag G, et al. An immunohistochemical study of the breast using antibodies to basal and luminal keratins, alpha-smooth muscle actin, vimentin, collagen IV and laminin. Part II: Epitheliosis and ductal carcinoma in-situ. Virchows Archiv A 1992;421:323–30.

31. Lakhani SR, Slack DN, Hamoudi RA, Collins N, Stratton MR. Detection of Allelic Imbalance Indicates That a Proportion of Mammary Hyperplasia of Usual Type Are Clonal, Neoplastic Proliferations. Lab Invest 1996;74:129–35.

32. Jones C, Merrett S, Thomas VA, Barker TH, Lakhani SR. Comparative genomic hybridization analysis of bilateral hyperplasia of usual type of the breast. J Pathol 2003;199:152–6.

33. Azzopardi JG. Problems in Breast Pathology. 1st ed. London: W.B. Saunders; 1979.

34. Page DL, Salhany KE, Jensen RA, Dupont WD. Subsequent breast carcinoma risk after biopsy with atypia in a breast papilloma. Cancer 1996;78:258–66.

35. Ohuchi N, Abe R, Kasai M. Possible cancerous change of intraductal papillomas of the breast. A 3-D reconstruction study of 25 cases. Cancer 1984;54:605–11.

36. Raju UB, Lee MW, Zarbo RJ, Crissman JD. Papillary neoplasia of the breast: immunohistochemically defined myoepithelial cells in the diagnosis of benign and malignant papillary breast neoplasms. Mod Pathol 1989; 2:569–76.

37. MacGrogan G, Moinfar F, Raju U. Intraductal papillary neoplasms. In: Tavassoli FA, Devilee P, editors. Tumours of the Breast and Female Genital Organs. Lyon: IARC Press; 2003. p.76–80.

38. Moinfar F, Man YG, Lininger RA, Bodian C, Tavassoli FA. Use of keratin 35betaE12 as an adjunct in the diagnosis of mammary intraepithelial neoplasia-ductal-type—benign and malignant intraductal proliferations. Am J Surg Pathol 1999;23:1048–58.

39. Franke WW, Schmid E, Schiller DL, et al. Differentiation-related patterns of expression of proteins of intermediate-size filaments in tissues and cultured cells. Cold Spring Harb Symp Quant Biol 1982;46 Pt 1: 431–53.

40. Raju U, Crissman JD, Zarbo R, Gottlieb C. Epitheliosis of the Breast. An Immunohistochemical Characterization and Comparison to Malignant Intraductal Proliferations of the Breast. Am J Surg Pathol 1990;14: 939–47.

41. Moll R, Krepler R, Franke WW. Complex cytokeratin polypeptide patterns observed in certain human carcinomas. Differentiation 1983;23:256–69.

42. Moll R. Cytokeratins as markers of differentiation in the diagnosis of epithelial tumors. Subcell Biochem 1998;31205–62:–62.

43. Ramaekers FCS, van Nierkerk C, Poels L, et al. Use of monoclonal antibodies to keratin 7 in the differential diagnosis of adenocarcinoma. Am J Pathol 1990; 136:641–55.

44. Wouters FS, Markman M, de Graaf P, et al. The immunohistochemical localization of the non-specific lipid transfer protein (sterol carrier protein-2) in rat small intestine enterocytes. Biochim Biophys Acta 1995;1259: 192–6.

45. Pellegrino MB, Asch BB, Connolly JL, Asch HL. Differential expression of keratins 13 and 16 in normal epithelium, benign lesions, and ductal carcinomas of the human breast determined by the monoclonal antibody Ks8.12. Cancer Res 1988;48:5831–6.

46. Wetzels RHW, Kuijpers HJH, Lane EB, et al. Basal Cell-specific and Hyperproliferation-related Keratins in Human Breast Cancer. Am J Pathol 1991;138:751–63.

47. Savera AT, Torres FX, Linden MD, et al. Primary versus metastativ pulmonary adenocarcinoma: An immunohistochemical study using villin and cytokeratins 7 and 20. Appl Immunohistochem 1996;4:86–94.

48. Miettinen M. Keratin 20: immunohistochemical marker for gastrointestinal, urothelial, and Merkel cell carcinomas. Mod Pathol 1995;8:384–8.

49. Malzahn K, Mitze M, Thoenes M, Moll R. Biological and prognostic significance of stratified epithelial cytokeratins in infiltrating ductal breast carcinomas. Virchows Arch 1998;433:119–29.

50. Dairkee SH, Ljung BM, Smith H, Hackett A. Immunolocalization of a human basal epithelium specific keratin in benign and malignant breast disease. Breast Cancer Res Treat 1987;10:11–20.

51. Otterbach F, Bankfalvi A, Bergner S, et al. Cytokeratin 5/6 immunohistochemistry assists the differential diagnosis of atypical proliferations of the breast. Histopathol 2000;37:232–40.

52. Rudland PS. Histochemical organization and cellular composition of ductal buds in developing human breast: evidence of cytochemical intermediates between epithelial and myoepithelial cells. J Histochem Cytochem 1991;39:1471–84.

53. Bussolati G, Alfani V, Weber K, Osborn M. Immunocytochemical detection of actin on fixed and embedded tissues: its potential use in routine pathology. J Histochem Cytochem 1980;28:169–73.

54. Dairkee SH, Blayney C, Smith HS, Hackett AJ. Monoclonal antibody that defines human myoepithelium. Proc Natl Acad Sci U S A 1985;82:7409–13.

55. Ribeiro-Silva A, Zamzelli Ramalho LN, Garcia SB, Zucoloto S. Is p63 reliable in detecting microinvasion in ductal carcinoma in-situ of the breast? Pathol Oncol Res 2003;9:20–3.

56. Barbareschi M, Pecciarini L, Cangi MG, et al. p63, a p53 homologue, is a selective nuclear marker of myoepithelial cells of the human breast. Am J Surg Pathol 2001;25:1054–60.

57. Damiani S, Ludvikova M, Tomasic G, et al. Myoepithelial cells and basal lamina in poorly differentiated in-situ duct carcinoma of the breast. An immunocytochemical study. Virchows Arch 1999;434:227–34.

58. Foschini MP, Scarpellini F, Gown AM, Eusebi V. Differential Expression of Myoepithelial Markers in Salivary, Sweat and Mammary Glands. Int J Surg Pathol 2000; 8:29–37.

59. Lazard D, Sastre X, Frid MG, et al. Expression of smooth muscle-specific proteins in myoepithelium and stromal myofibroblasts of normal and malignant human breast tissue. Proc Natl Acad Sci USA 1993;90: 999–1003.

60. Moritani S, Kushima R, Sugihara H, et al. Availability of CD10 immunohistochemistry as a marker of breast myoepithelial cells on paraffin sections. Mod Pathol 2002;15:397–405.

61. Reis-Filho JS, Albergaria A, Milanezi F, Amendoeira I, Schmitt FC. Naked nuclei revisited: p63 Immunoexpression. Diagn Cytopathol 2002;27:135–8.

62. Reis-Filho JS, Schmitt FC. Taking advantage of basic research: p63 is a reliable myoepithelial and stem cell marker. Adv Anat Pathol 2002;9:280–9.

Content

8

USUAL DUCTAL HYPERPLASIA (UDH)

WERNER BOECKER AND HORST BUERGER

The term 'usual ductal hyperplasia' (UDH) is used to refer to a benign 'intraductal' epithelial proliferation within the ductal lobular system. The essential histological feature of these lesions is their cellular heterogeneity with formation of irregularly shaped secondary lumina. From the perspective of cell biology, usual ductal hyperplasia is a proliferation of Ck5/14-positive cells, intermediate cells (Ck5/14+, Ck8/18+) and differentiated glandular cells (Ck8/18+). Most lesions of usual ductal hyperplasia are microscopic in size. Sometimes usual ductal hyperplasia may, however, be associated with tumor-forming lesions such as papilloma, radial scar and adenoma of the nipple. Epidemiological studies have shown that usual ductal hyperplasia is associated with a slightly increased general breast cancer risk. Only in very rare cases do atypical ductal proliferations develop on the ground of classical florid usual ductal hyperplasia. Usual ductal hyperplasia, as such, can therefore no longer be viewed as a precursor lesion of ductal carcinoma in-situ.

Usual ductal hyperplasia (UDH)

■ DEFINITION

Synonyms: ductal hyperplasia of usual type, ordinary ductal hyperplasia, ductal hyperplasia without atypia, proliferative disease of usual or common type, intraductal hyperplasia, epitheliosis, papillomatosis, ductal intraepithelial neoplasia 1a

WHO: Usual ductal hyperplasia

Usual ductal hyperplasia is a benign, purely epithelial, intraductal proliferation characterized by great cellular heterogeneity [1–4]. The cells comprising the lesion are histologically characterized by their variability in size and shape, yet without obvious nuclear features of malignancy (Fig. 8.1). Usually the cells show a fenestrated growth pattern. Frequently located in the terminal duct-lobular unit (TDLU), the lesions can be observed anywhere in the ductal system, sometimes as a component of other benign breast lesions. Immunohistochemical studies have revealed that usual ductal hyperplasia is a lesion composed of Ck5/14+ cells, intermediate glandular (Ck5/14+; Ck8/18+) and differentiated glandular cells (Ck8/18+). Using Ck5/14 immunostaining, usual ductal hyperplasia is characterized by a typical mosaicism of Ck5/14+ cells staining at varying degrees of intensity along with occasional Ck5/14-negative cells (Fig. 8.2). The detection of Ck5/14 is absolutely crucial in differential diagnosis of UDH and Ck5/14-negative DCIS.

In Anglo-American literature, designations such as epithelial hyperplasia, usual type [4], intraductal hyperplasia [5], papillomatosis, [6–8], epitheliosis [3], and ductal intraepithelial neoplasia 1a [9] have been used to refer to, essentially, identical patterns of change. We prefer to retain the term usual ductal hyperplasia for two reasons:

1. It best signifies the special ductal pattern of benign epithelial cell increase [10].
2. It underlines the histological, cell biological and clinical differences seen in atypical ductal hyperplasia/ductal carcinoma in-situ and in lobular neoplasia [4,11–13].

Confusing and non-specific, terms such as epitheliosis and papillomatosis should be abandoned. Current evidence does not support the view that usual ductal hyperplasia represents an obligate precursor lesion to ductal carcinoma in-situ [1, 2].

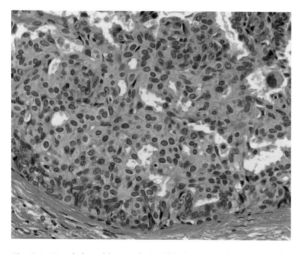

Fig. 8.1 Usual ductal hyperplasia. This is a typical example of a benign intraductal epithelial proliferation with variation of size, shape and spacing of the proliferating cells and formation of irregular lumina between the cells (fenestrated growth pattern). Note also the differences in cytoplasmic staining intensity of the proliferating cells.

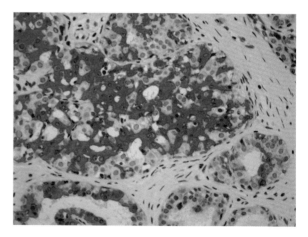

Fig. 8.2 Usual ductal hyperplasia. Cytokeratin 5 immunohistochemistry. This Ck5 staining pattern is typical for ductal hyperplasia (and is also the same staining pattern observed for Ck14). Note the uneven staining mosaicism of proliferating cells and the complete lack of staining in some cells. The presence of negatively stained cells corresponds to Ck8/18+ glandular cells which no longer express Ck5. This staining pattern contrasts with most ductal carcinomas in-situ, which only express Ck8/18 while at the same time lacking Ck5 and Ck14.

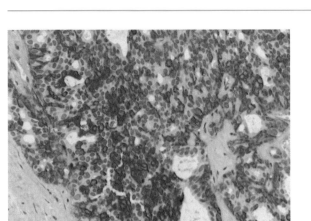

Fig. 8.11a–c Usual ductal hyperplasia.
8.11c Immunostaining for Ck5 or Ck14 reveals the typical mosaicism of the proliferating cells which is indicative of the lesion's benignity.

hard to recognize the benign nature of these lesions and clearly distinguish them from intermediate grade ductal carcinoma in-situ. Apocrine metaplasia (Fig. 8.12b) is frequently seen, while squamous metaplasia is rare. Areas of usual ductal hyperplasia may contain plenty of foam cells, a variety of other inflammatory cells and, rarely, secretory material (Fig. 8.12a and b). They are otherwise devoid of cells or secretion.

Cells in UDH lesions sometimes exhibit an appearance known as 'streaming', a characteristic arrangement of elongated cells orientated in parallel and containing fusiform nuclei – similar to cells in a leiomyoma. As the cytoplasm of these spindle cells (Fig. 8.12a) may be somewhat more eosinophilic in character, there has been speculation on a possible myoepithelial differentiation of such cells. However, sm-actin immunostaining usually fails to confirm this (see Fig. 8.5a–b). Rather, these cells tend to be intermediate glandular cells with expression of both Ck5/14 and Ck8/18.

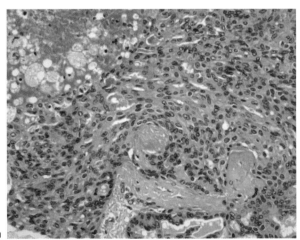

a

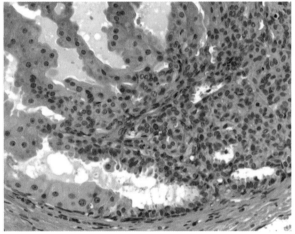

b

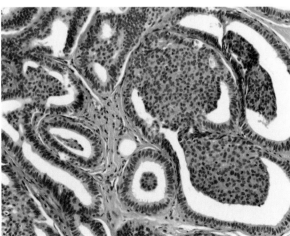

c

Fig. 8.12a–c Cellular features of usual ductal hyperplasia.
8.12a Usual ductal hyperplasia with typical spindling of cells. The long axes of nuclei are oriented in a parallel fashion to create the impression of streaming. These cells are not myoepithelial cells as they do not stain for myoepithelial markers such as sm-actin. The lumen in this case contains some secretion material, foam cells and nuclear debris.
8.12b Usual ductal hyperplasia with typical fenestrating growth pattern and focal apocrine metaplasia. The apocrine cells are characterized by their distinctly eosinophilic granular cytoplasm. The lumina contain some secretion material.
8.12c Usual ductal hyperplasia with part of the original duct lumen remaining as a crescentic space, lined by monotonous, cylindrically shaped cells with bland nuclei (cylinder cell change). The luminal proliferation shows the typical heterogeneous cellular pattern.

Pre-existing normal or cylinder cell changes may occur along the basement membrane of the peripheral spaces (Fig. 8.12). Furthermore, a minor fraction of the proliferating cells may sometimes show a more glandular maturation with negativity for Ck5/14. Such a finding should be considered in the context of the whole lesion and indicates a maturational process rather than a malignant diagnosis.

GROWTH PATTERN

Another important feature of usual ductal hyperplasia are its growth patterns. These are commonly referred to as fenestrating, micropapillary/gynecomastoid and solid.

Considering the diversity of the proliferating epithelial cells, it is only logical that the ensuing lumina between cells are irregular, varying in size and shape from angulated to slit-like spaces (Figs 8.11 and 8.12). This is one of the most characteristic structural features of usual ductal hyperplasia – referred to as 'fenestrated growth pattern' by Azzopardi – and hence a crucial feature in distinguishing usual ductal hyperplasia from the regular cribriform growth pattern of low grade DCIS. Part of the original duct lumen may remain as a crescentic space or spaces with persistent cuboidal or cylindrical cells at the edge of the duct, the central mass of epithelial cells attached to the peripheral pre-existing glandular cell lining only by cellular bridges (Fig. 8.12c). Often, focal luminal tufting and bridging of spindle-shaped epithelial cells can be observed which, in addition to the streaming pattern, are an important hallmark of usual ductal hyperplasia.

The term gynecomastoid/micropapillary epithelial hyperplasia is used to describe epithelial proliferations which bear a striking resemblance to the changes seen in gynecomastia in men. There is multilayering of the epithelium along with occasional tongue-like projections (Fig 8.13). These micropapillae are irregularly shaped fronds of epithelium, which are usually narrower and flattened at the tips. The nuclei are often more crowded, variable in size and unevenly spaced [70]. Small lesions of epithelial hyperplasia may be indistinguishable from very early lesions of intermediate grade ductal neoplasia. Immunohistochemically, the benign lesions are composed of a mixture of the same type of cells found in classical usual ductal hyperplasia. Ck5/14 immunostaining reveals a typical mosaicism and may thus help to distinguish these lesions (see differential diagnosis).

The pure solid variant is rare and can be difficult to distinguish from intermediate grade DCIS (Fig. 8.14).

However, Ck5/14 immunohistochemistry can also aid in this differential diagnosis. Combinations of solid, micropapillary and papillary architectures may be seen.

USUAL DUCTAL HYPERPLASIA ASSOCIATED WITH BENIGN TUMOR-FORMING LESIONS

It should be emphasized that extensively developed benign epithelial hyperplasia may be associated with several tumor-forming lesions. These include solid papillomas, radial scars, juvenile papillomatosis, adenomatous-type adenomas of the nipple and even occasional fibroepithelial lesions. These benign epithelial proliferations should be clearly distinguished from their malignant counterparts.

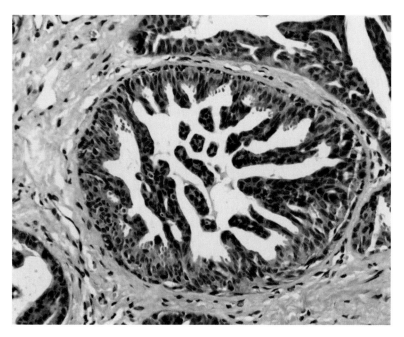

Fig. 8.13 Usual ductal hyperplasia with micropapillary architecture. This lesion displays multi-layering of cells and tongue-like micropapillary tufts. The micropapillae are irregularly shaped fronds of proliferating cells with usually smaller cells and nuclei at the tip compared to those at the base. Such cases are likely to be misdiagnosed as DCIS as they may show some nuclear irregularities. In difficult cases, Ck5/14 immunohistochemistry may be helpful, showing the typical mosaicism.

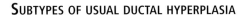

SUBTYPES OF USUAL DUCTAL HYPERPLASIA

According to the degree of intraluminal proliferation, ductal hyperplasia may be subdivided into two main subtypes:

- **Mild ductal hyperplasia:** The lower end point is defined as an increase of cells of not more than four layers above the basement membrane [10]. This category is not associated with any increased risk of later breast cancer.
- **Moderate and florid hyperplasia:** This is the characteristic lesion of usual ductal hyperplasia, as described above, and includes distension of TDLUs or ducts by proliferating epithelial cells that completely fill the distended lumina with fenestrated or solid growth patterns.

also immunostain with Ck5 and/or Ck14 antibodies. Therefore immunohistochemical staining patterns must be interpreted in the context of a proliferating cell population. The validity of the staining reaction should furthermore be ascertained by positive and negative internal controls.

A variety of other proteins, all of them involved in cell cycle progression, have been investigated. Whereas usual ductal hyperplasia is typically negative, or at best only weakly positive for p53 and e-*erb*B2 [37, 72, 73], mutations of the p53-gene or amplifications of erbB2-gene have only very rarely been described for a small minority of usual ductal hyperplasia cases [74, 75]. Varying expression patterns have also been shown for Cyclin D1 [76–78], and positive staining patterns have been described for

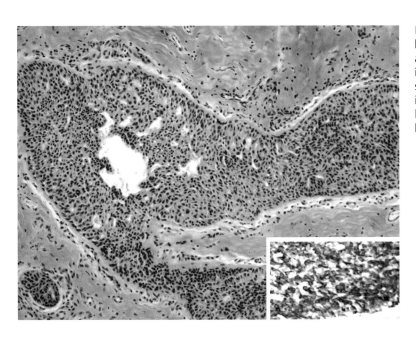

Fig. 8.14 Usual ductal hyperplasia. Small lesions of usual ductal hyperplasia which at first sight is indisdinguishable from intermediate grade ductal neoplasia. In such a case Ck5/14 immunohistochemistry is necessary to verify the nature of the lesion. (Inset) Ck5 immunohistochemistry highlights the Ck5 mosaicism.

IMMUNOHISTOCHEMISTRY

Recent immunohistochemical findings are discussed above under 'conceptual approach'. **Ck5/14 mosaicism** is regarded as a constitutive feature of usual ductal hyperplasia (Figs 8.2, 8.11, 8.14) and is in stark contrast to the clonal Ck5/14 negativity of lobular and ductal neoplasias. A number of studies have confirmed the reliability of these antibodies in the differential diagnosis of intraductal epithelial proliferations [11, 14–16, 18, 71] and have recommended them in this differential diagnostic setting. Due consideration should, however, be given to the fact that, occasionally, high grade DCIS displays a Ck5/14-positive immunophenotype. Furthermore, residual normal or hyperplastic epithelium in DCIS containing lesions may

Cyclin B, cdc2, S-100, p68, SF/c-met, PLP, MR52,000, and p63. The loss of TGF-β2 expression in usual ductal hyperplasia has been suggested as a predictive factor for the development of invasive breast cancer in the future [43], in contrast to TGF-α which showed an increasing staining intensity in malignant tumors [79]. The same could be shown for the expression of ER-α and Ki-67 [80], whereas expression of ER-β seemed to be associated with a protective effect [81].

GENETICS

Several studies have shown that loss of heterozygosity (LOH) at many different loci can be identified in usual ductal hyperplasia, varying in frequencies from

0–15% at different loci. However, although LOH is not a rare event in these lesions, the alterations do not seem to be recurrent [20, 82, 83]. Nevertheless, this data was initially interpreted as supporting the concept of a linear tumor progression, with usual ductal hyperplasia being the first step in this process [84, 82].

Recent investigations, however, which identified subtle genetic changes even in normal breast epithelium, modified this hypothesis, suggesting that such genetic alterations might be an indicator of an inherent genetic instability of breast epithelium [16]. This would also confirm epidemiological studies, according to which the general cancer risk associated with these lesions is slightly increased [33]. Nevertheless, some of the cytogenetic data is still conflicting. Whereas the largest CGH study undertaken so far failed to provide evidence for the presence of unbalanced chromosomal alterations in cases of usual ductal hyperplasia [13], other authors using the DOP-CGH method described genetic changes which were not recurrent and thus in stark contrast to the results in DCIS [85–87]. In one of these studies, however, as many as six alterations were found on average in each case of usual ductal hyperplasia adjacent to invasive breast cancer [85]. Given the figures published in this study, the results are more likely to reflect differences in morphological classification systems of intraductal epithelial proliferations used by this group, rather than any biological principle. Investigations of clonality [88, 89], morphometric parameters [90], and integrin [91] in usual ductal hyperplasia revealed heterogeneous findings.

ATYPICAL DUCTAL PROLIFERATION (ADH/DCIS) EX USUAL DUCTAL HYPERPLASIA

Atypical ductal hyperplasia ex usual ductal proliferation is a malignant transformation of a pre-existing usual ductal hyperplasia. This transformation is discussed at length by Azzopardi, who noted that 'with rare exceptions, usual ductal hyperplasia is and remains benign.' [3] Intriguingly, there are no studies on the incidence of ADH/DCIS in usual ductal hyperplasia, a fact which may indicate how exceptional such findings are in our daily practice. Nevertheless, the similarity in growth pattern between usual ductal hyperplasia and atypical ductal proliferations has resulted in a continuing overemphasis on the relationship between ADH/DCIS and usual ductal hyperplasia. In conclusion, a progression of simple epithelial hyperplasia towards DCIS may occur (ADH/DCIS ex usual ductal hyperplasia) in individual cases, but these probably represent an exception to the rule. Such information is not of purely academic interest; the view that these lesions represent precursor malignan-

cies leads pathologists to look for the early stages of cancer in usual ductal hyperplasia foci, and possibly results in over-diagnosis of simple epithelial hyperplasias.

INTERPRETATION OF CORE AND VACUUM-ASSISTED BIOPSIES

In most cases usual ductal hyperplasia is easily diagnosed in H&E sections. In cases where diagnosis is uncertain, Ck5/14 immunohistochemistry should be applied, usually resulting in correct diagnosis. This is discussed in more detail in the paragraphs on immunohistochemistry and differential diagnosis. An unequivocal diagnosis of usual ductal hyperplasia is classified as B2. It should, however, be emphasized that simple epithelial hyperplasia per se, if not part of a benign tumor forming lesion such as papilloma or radial scar, is not recognized on mammography. The appropriate management of these patients, therefore, needs to be discussed in an interdisciplinary conference.

DIFFERENTIAL DIAGNOSIS

Differential diagnosis includes all types of intraductal epithelial proliferation and lobular neoplasias. Diagnosis is not a problem in most cases of usual ductal hyperplasia cases due to the presence of a heterogeneous cell proliferation with a fenestrating growth pattern. They can be easily distinguished from low grade DCIS, with its monotonous cell growth and cribriform pattern, and from high grade DCIS, with its overtly malignant nuclear features. However, there may be a considerable overlap both in cellular features and growth patterns between usual ductal hyperplasia and some cases of intermediate grade DCIS.

Thus, the morphological similarity of the intraluminal growth pattern of usual ductal hyperplasia and atypical ductal hyperplasia/DCIS may harbor a risk of misdiagnosis, sometimes even resulting in unnecessary surgical procedures. In order to avoid such tragic errors, the pathologist should have a very good understanding of the extreme morphological variants of usual ductal hyperplasia and different subtypes of DCIS. In our experience, Ck5/14 mosaicism is a constitutive feature and the most important diagnostic element of usual ductal hyperplasia. This is in sharp contrast to low and intermediate grade, and even to most high grade DCIS, in which Ck8/18-positive clonal proliferation lacking Ck5/14 expression is the characteristic hallmark (Figs 8.15 and 8.16). If the intraductal epithelial proliferation is Ck5/14-negative, this excludes the diagnosis of usual ductal hyperplasia and implies in-situ malignancy of either lobular or

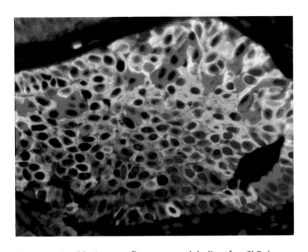

Fig. 8.15 Double immunofluorescence labeling for Ck5 (green signal) and Ck8/18 (red signal). Usual ductal hyperplasia contains the typical heterogeneous cell population as shown in Fig. 8.3. Note the staining pattern which is similar to normal glandular breast epithelium.

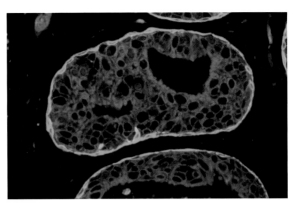

Fig. 8.16 Ductal carcinoma in-situ. The tumor cells display a differentiated glandular phenotype with expression of Ck8/18 (red signal), whereas only the myoepithelial cells express the basal cytokeratin 5. With the exception of some high grade DCIS, this is the characteristic phenotype of ductal carcinoma in-situ.

ductal-type. The only exceptions are some high grade DCIS lesions and benign apocrine proliferations, which are Ck5/14-negative by definition (see Chapter 3).

It should be emphasized that cases of lobular carcinoma in-situ, atypical ductal hyperplasia and DCIS may contain small aggregates of Ck5/14-positive residual or even hyperplastic cells which may lead to an incorrect benign diagnosis. The distinction is, however, usually quite simple, as the Ck5/14-negative clonal uniformity of the tumor cells stands out against the background of Ck5/14-positive normal cells. It is equally important to bear in mind that the neoplastic cells of some DCIS cases, particularly high nuclear grade ones, stain positively with Ck5/14 antibodies. As a result, the pathologist should be extremely careful in interpreting such findings as indicating usual ductal hyperplasia. Over a period of more than two decades, one of the authors (W. B.) has come across a mere three cases of low grade atypical ductal proliferations which homogeneously expressed Ck5/14, but not Ck8/18 (see Chapter 19).

The results of approximately 100 cases published in the literature so far confirm the practical importance of Ck5/14 immunohistochemistry in this area of breast pathology. The practical algorithm for assessment of intraductal proliferations using Ck5/14 immunohistochemistry is depicted in Fig. 8.17. The contrasting features of usual ductal hyperplasia and DCIS are listed in Table 8.2. It is worth noting that the E12β34 antibody, which is directed against cytokeratin subtypes 1/5/10/14 [34, 35], shows a positivity to usual ductal hyperplasia, but it also stains some 20–30% of atypical ductal hyperplasia and ADH/DCIS cases of all grades respectively. A related study showed that this antibody also stains lobular neoplasia tumor cells [92]. Based on this data we recommend an antibody directed solely against basal cytokeratin 5 and/ or 14 as the first-order choice for the differential diagnosis of intraductal epithelial proliferations in routine practice.

The most important applications in daily routine pathology are discussed below.

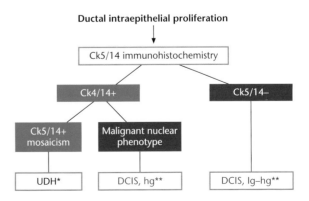

Fig. 8.17 Algorithm of intraductal epithelial proliferations.

Tab. 8.2 Contrasting features of usual ductal hyperplasia (UDH), atypical ductal hyperplasia (ADH) and ductal carcinoma in-situ (DCIS)

	UDH	ADH, classical type	DCIS
Definition	■ Intraductal proliferation of Ck5/14-positive cells and their glandular progeny	■ Intraductal proliferation of monomorphic neoplastic glandular cells that express Ck8/18 but not Ck5/14, usually confined to a TDLU	■ Intraductal proliferation of neoplastic glandular cells that usually express Ck8/18 but not Ck5/14
Cellular proliferation	■ Mixed cell population ■ Variability in cell size and shape ■ Apocrine change frequent	■ Single cell population, uniform	■ Single cell population, uniform but may be variable in cell size and shape, occasionally dimorphic pattern
Nuclei	■ Variable in size and shape ■ Crowding and overlapping ■ Parallel orientation of long axes (streaming)	■ Even nuclear size and shape	■ Even nuclear size and shape in DCIS, low grade ■ Variable in size and shape in DCIS, intermediate grade ■ Enlarged malignant nuclei in DCIS, high grade
Architecture	■ Variable, uneven spacing of cells with formation of irregular lumina (slit-like spaces, fenestrating growth pattern)	■ Regular rigid spacing of cells with rounded lumina (bridges, bars, cribriform patterns, micropapillae)	■ Regular rigid spacing of cells with rounded lumina in DCIS, low grade (bridges, bars, cribriform patterns, micropapillae) ■ May be variable and irregular in DCIS, intermediate and high grade
Myoepithelial layer	■ Present	■ Present	■ Present
Immunohisto-chemistry	■ Ck5/14-mosaicism (constitutive) Ck8/18+; Ck5/14+	■ Neoplastic cells are Ck8/18+ but Ck5/14–	■ in > 95% of DCIS cases neoplastic cells are Ck8/18+ but Ck5/14–
Comparative genomic hybridization (CGH)	■ No recurrent genetic changes	■ Recurrent genetic changes	■ Recurrent genetic changes
B classification	■ B 2 (benign)	■ B 3 (unknown potential)	■ B 5 (malignant)

USUAL DUCTAL HYPERPLASIA VS. ATYPICAL DUCTAL HYPERPLASIA/LOW GRADE DCIS

Such lesions are readily identifiable at low magnification under the microscope. Cytology and growth patterns are features used to distinguish between those lesions (Table 8.2). Monotonous vs. mixed cellular composition and fenestrated vs. cribriform growth are the most important differential diagnostic features. Atypical ductal hyperplasia/low grade DCIS is char-

acterized by its rigid and/or geometric configuration [93] and these features are virtually diagnostic of malignancy (Fig. 8.19). In contrast, usual ductal hyperplasia is composed of heterogeneous epithelial cells with a fenestrated growth pattern (Fig. 8.18). Sometimes, however, usual ductal hyperplasia may contain relatively homogeneous cell populations of solid growth pattern simulating ductal or lobular neoplasia. Mitoses are not helpful in this setting. In such difficult cases, Ck5/14 immunostaining may be helpful in

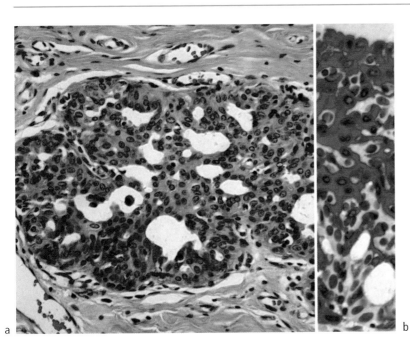

Fig. 8.18a–b Usual ductal hyperplasia vs. ductal carcinoma in-situ low grade. H&E-stained sections with a heterogeneous cell population with fenestrating growth pattern (8.18a). Ck5 immunohistochemistry reveals the typical Ck5 mosaicism (8.18b).

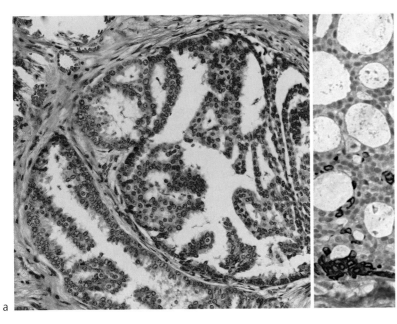

Fig. 8.19a–b DCIS. H&E-stained section displays the monotonous cell population with a cribriform growth pattern of low grade ductal carcinoma in-situ (8.19a). Ck5 characteristically is negative in these lesions (8.19b).

confirming which decision is ultimately made. Usual ductal hyperplasia lesions inherently contains a large number of Ck5/14-positive cells, whereas the neoplastic cells of solid type DCIS display a purely glandular phenotype (Ck8/18+, Ck5/14–).

Usual ductal hyperplasia vs. high grade DCIS

The cytological and nuclear details which help to distinguish usual ductal hyperplasia from high grade DCIS are an important issue in this context. Overall, malignant nuclei, high mitotic rates and abnormal mitoses are among the hallmarks of high grade DCIS and help to distinguish it from more worrisome types of usual ductal hyperplasia. In addition, this subtype of DCIS often presents with comedo-type necrosis. As some high grade DCIS neoplastic cells express Ck5/14, every positive staining reaction has to be interpreted in the context of histology.

Usual ductal hyperplasia vs. intermediate grade DCIS

The most difficult differential diagnosis may indeed be the one between solid/compact usual ductal hyperplasia and intermediate grade DCIS, (Figs 8.20– 8.22). In both cases, cytological and architectural features are of little help as variation in cell size and shape and even secondary irregular lumina may be found in both lesions. Definitive diagnosis may be even more difficult if the lesion is small or if only a limited amount of material is available (needle core biopsy). However, even for such lesions, the fundamental principles of the constituent cells, discussed above, hold true. Thus Ck5/14 immunohistochemistry is of defining significance. Ck5/14 mosaicism is indicative of usual ductal hyperplasia whereas intermediate grade DCIS shows a distinct Ck5/14-negative, Ck8/18-positive phenotype. In conventional histology such features may be virtually unrecognizable. In such a crucial situation any tool which allows analysis of the cellular constituents of a given lesion in a more objective way is most welcome.

MICROPAPILLARY EPITHELIAL HYPERPLASIA VS. MICROPAPILLARY DUCTAL CARCINOMA IN-SITU

Occasionally a purely micropapillary growth pattern may be recognized in ductal non-high grade in-situ lesions. Malignant micropapillae are usually composed of monotonous cells with low grade nuclei. The micropapillae vary greatly in size and shape, but are often long and slender in structures (Fig. 8.23). Sometimes the neoplastic cells of the micropapillae have a smaller sized or somewhat more hyperchromatic nuclei than their neoplastic counterparts at the periphery of the glands. Hyperplastic micropapillae usually contain crowded cells of different sizes and shapes with hyperchromatic nuclei (Fig. 8.24). In difficult cases, CK5/14 immunostaining is helpful.

USUAL DUCTAL HYPERPLASIA VS. SPINDLE-TYPE DCIS

The distinction between these lesions in H&E sections may be difficult and sometimes arbitrary, but it is important for patient management purposes. Although spindling of cells may sometimes be extensive in usual ductal hyperplasia, it is rarely seen throughout the entire lesion. In the event of any unusual looking spindle cell proliferation, therefore, the lesion should be examined for areas that are more diagnostic and contain features of usual ductal hyperplasia. The presence of only one type of spindle cell in a lesion should raise the suspicion of DCIS, spindle type. In our experience, Ck5/14 helps in this differential diagnostic setting as staining of DCIS, spindle-cell type, is negative, whereas usual ductal hyperplasia is positive.

USUAL DUCTAL HYPERPLASIA VS. LOBULAR NEOPLASIA

Occasional cases of usual ductal hyperplasia may show more uniform cells with bland nuclei and solid growth pattern, and a differential diagnosis should therefore include lobular neoplasia. Classical-type lobular neoplasia is Ck5/14-negative. Additional immunostains may confirm the diagnosis of lobular neoplasia by demonstration of loss of E-cadherin adhesion molecules in cells.

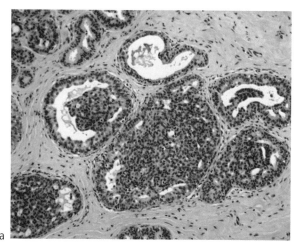

a

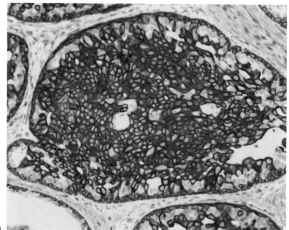

b

Fig. 8.20a–b Usual ductal hyperplasia.
8.20a This image shows a lobule with an epithelial proliferation that is more monotonous (less variability in size, shape and staining intensity) than usual. Such lesions are much more difficult to interpret than lesions such as in Figs 8.11 and 8.12. However, most pathologists would probably favor a benign diagnosis.
8.20b The benign diagnosis is confirmed by positive Ck5 staining showing a mosaic pattern.

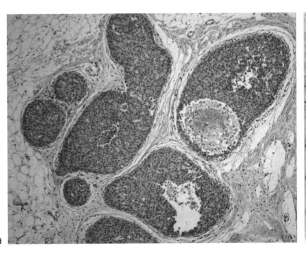

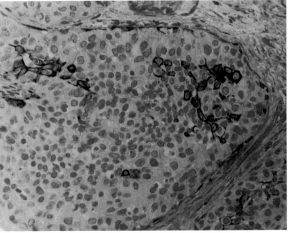

a b

Fig. 8.21a–b Ductal carcinoma in-situ, intermediate grade.
8.21a This image shows a lobule with an epithelial proliferation. The appearance of the nuclei is similar to the lesion in Fig. 8.20. Furthermore the secondary lumina are irregular similar to those in UDH. However, the comedo-type necrosis points to malignancy.
8.21b The Ck5 negativity of the tumor cells of this lesion confirms the diagnosis of a ductal carcinoma in-situ. Note that there are some residual Ck5-positive normal cells. This staining pattern should not be interpreted as Ck5 mosaicism.

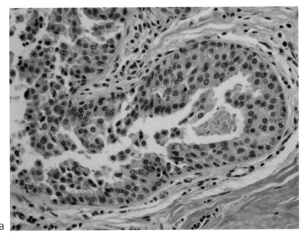

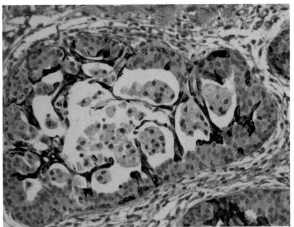

a b

Fig. 8.22a–b Ductal carcinoma in-situ, intermediate grade.
8.22a Higher magnification of an intermediate lesion with a nuclear appearance similar to Fig. 8.21a. This area is not diagnostic of malignancy, although the overall appearance suggests malignancy.
8.22b Ck5 immunostaining shows that the tumor cells are negative, whereas some residual normal cells express Ck5. This is indicative of a clonal cell proliferation.

USUAL DUCTAL HYPERPLASIA AND THEIR BENIGN COUNTERPARTS

USUAL DUCTAL HYPERPLASIA VS. ADENOMYOEPITHELIOMA

It is not uncommon for the proliferating cells of usual ductal hyperplasia to acquire a spindle cell shape possibly leading to a false diagnosis of adenomyoepithelioma. As discussed above, the cells of usual ductal hyperplasia differentiate along the glandular pathway and therefore do not express myoepithelial markers. Thus sm-actin immunohistochemistry is of great help in making a correct diagnosis (details see Chapter 14).

CK5/14-POSITIVE CLONAL INTRADUCTAL EPITHELIAL PROLIFERATIONS

Exceptionally rare cases of intraductal epithelial proliferations with a homogeneous Ck5/14 positivity may be observed. One of the authors (W.B.) with the experience of a large consultation practice has seen three

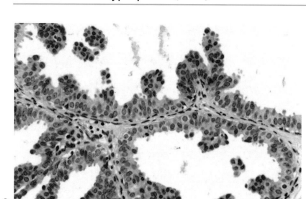
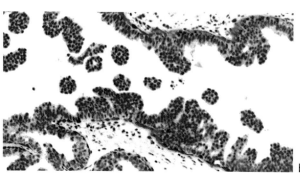

a

b

Fig. 8.23a–b Micropapillary low grade DCIS.
8.23a High power view of micropapillary growth of a low grade DCIS. Note micropapillae of variable size.
8.23b Immunostaining for Ck14 shows that expression of this high-molecular weight cytokeratin is largely absent. In contrast to the Ck5/14 mosaicism of benign micropapillary epithelial growth, this is clearly indicative of neoplastic cell growth.

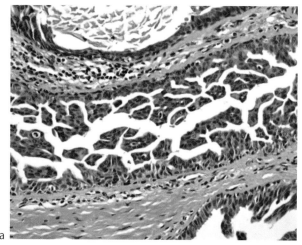
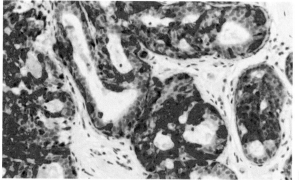

a

b

Fig. 8.24a–b Micropapillary type of benign epithelial proliferation in an adenoma of the nipple.
8.24a High power view of benign micropapillary epithelial proliferation which usually displays a broader base.
8.24b Immunostaining for Ck5 showing the classic Ck5 mosaicism of benign epithelial proliferations.

such cases. They are characterized by a monomorphic proliferation of round to oval epithelial cells and bland looking nuclei. In contrast to the Ck5/14 mosaicism of usual ductal hyperplasia, the proliferating cells of this lesion homogeneously express Ck5 and Ck14. Glandular cytokeratins such as Ck8/18 are not expressed. Their clinical significance is currently unknown. We regard these extremely rare lesions, however, as neoplastic progenitor cell lesions, probably with a very low malignant potential (compare Chapter 19).

References
1. Koerner FC. Epithelial proliferations of ductal-type. Semin Diagn Pathol 2004;21:10-7.
2. Walker RA. Are all ductal proliferations of the breast premalignant? J Path 2001;195:401-3.
3. Azzopardi JG. Problems in Breast Pathology. 1st ed. London: W.B. Saunders; 1979.
4. Page DL, Anderson TJ, Rogers LW. Epithelial hyperplasia. In: Page DL, Anderson TJ, editors. Diagnostic Histopathology of the Breast. Edinburgh: Churchill Livingstone; 1988. p.120–56.
5. Tavassoli FA, Norris HJ. A Comparison of the Results of Long-Term Follow-Up for Atypical Intraductal Hyperplasia and Intraductal Hyperplasia of the Breast. Cancer 1990;65:518-29.

6. Foote FW, Stewart FW. Comparative studies of cancerous versus non-cancerous breasts. Basic morphologic characteristics. Ann Surg 1945;121:6-53.

7. Haagensen CD. Anatomy of the Mammary Glands. In: Haagensen CD, editor. Diseases of the Breast. 3rd ed. Philadelphia: Saunders; 1986. p.1–46.

8. McDivitt RW, Holleb AI, Foote F-WJ. Prior breast disease in patients treated for papillary carcinoma. Arch Pathol 1968;85:117-24.

9. Tavassoli FA. Ductal intraepithelial neoplasia (IDH, AIDH and DCIS). Breast Cancer 2000;7:315-20.

10. Elston CW, Ellis IO. The Breast. 1st ed. Edinburgh: Harcourt Brace and Company Ltd; 1998.

11. Böcker WJ, Bier B, Freytag G, et al. An immunohistochemical study of the breast using antibodies to basal and luminal keratins, alpha-smooth muscle actin, vimentin, collagen IV and laminin. Part I: normal breast and benign proliferative lesions. Virchows Archiv A 1992; 421:315-22.

12. Böcker WJ, Bier B, Freytag G, et al. An immunohistochemical study of the breast using antibodies to basal and luminal keratins, alpha-smooth muscle actin, vimentin, collagen IV and laminin. Part II: Epitheliosis and ductal carcinoma in-situ. Virchows Archiv A 1992;421:323-30.

13. Boecker W, Moll R, Dervan P, et al. Usual ductal hyperplasia of the breast is a committed stem (progenitor) cell lesion distinct from atypical ductal hyperplasia and ductal carcinoma in-situ. J Pathol 2002;198:458-67.

14. Nagle RB, Bocker W, Davis JR, et al. Characterization of breast carcinomas by two monoclonal antibodies distinguishing myoepithelial from luminal epithelial cells. J Histochem Cytochem 1986;34:869-81.

15. Jarasch E-D, Nagle RB, Kaufmann M, Maurer C, Böcker WJ. Differential Diagnosis of Benign Epithelial Proliferations and Carcinomas of the Breast Using Antibodies to Cytokeratins. Hum Pathol 1988;19:276-89.

16. Boecker W, Moll R, Poremba C, et al. Common Adult Stem Cells in the Human Breast Give Rise to Glandular and Myoepithelial Cell Lineages: A New Cell Biological Concept. Lab Invest 2002;82:737-46.

17. Lakhani SR. The transition from hyperplasia to invasive carcinoma of the breast. J Pathol 1999;187:272-8.

18. Otterbach F, Bankfalvi A, Bergner S, et al. Cytokeratin 5/6 immunohistochemistry assists the differential diagnosis of atypical proliferations of the breast. Histopathol 2000;37:232-40.

19. Buerger H, Otterbach F, Simon R, et al. Comparative genomic hybridization of ductal carcinoma in-situ of the breast-evidence of multiple genetic pathways. J Pathol 1999;187:396-402.

20. Lakhani SR, Slack DN, Hamoudi RA, Collins N, Stratton MR. Detection of Allelic Imbalance Indicates That a Proportion of Mammary Hyperplasia of Usual Type Are Clonal, Neoplastic Proliferations. Lab Invest 1996;74:129-35.

21. Moinfar F, Man YG, Arnould L, et al. Concurrent and independent genetic alterations in the stromal and epithelial cells of mammary carcinoma: implications for tumorigenesis. Cancer Res 2000;60:2562-6.

22. O'Connell P, Pekkel V, Fuqua SA, et al. Analysis of loss of heterozygosity in 399 premalignant breast lesions at 15 genetic loci. J Natl Cancer Inst 1998;90:697-703.

23. Boecker W, Buerger H, Schmitz K, et al. Ductal epithelial proliferations of the breast: a biological continuum? Comparative genomic hybridisation and high-molecular-weight cytokeratin expression patterns. J Path 2001; 195:415-21.

24. Lakhani SR. The transition from hyperplasia to invasive carcinoma of the breast. J Pathol 1999;187:272-8.

25. Deng G, Lu Y, Zlotnikov G, Thor AD, Smith HS. Loss of heterozygosity in normal tissue adjacent to breast carcinomas. Science 1996;274:2057-9.

26. Larson PS, de las Morenas A, Cupples LA, Huang K, Rosenberg CL. Genetically abnormal clones in histologically normal breast tissue. Am J Pathol 1998; 152:1591-8.

27. Lakhani SR, Chaggar R, Davies S, et al. Genetic alterations in "normal" luminal and myoepthelial cells of the breast. J Pathol 1999;189:496-503.

28. Li Z, Moore DH, Meng ZH, et al. Increased risk of local recurrence is asociated with allelic loss in normal lobules of breast cancer patients. Cancer Res 2002; 62:1000-3.

29. Shoker BS, Jarvis C, Sibson DR, Walker C, Sloane JP. Oestrogen receptor expression in the normal and precancerous breast. J Path 1999;188:237-44.

30. Shoker BS, Jarvis C, Clarke RB, et al. Estrogen receptor-positive proliferating cells in the normal and precancerous breast. Am J Pathol 1999;155:1811-5.

31. Iqbal M, Rossoff LJ, Marzouk KA, Steinberg HN. Yellow nail syndrome: resolution of yellow nails after successful treatment of breast cancer. Chest 2000; 117:1516-8.

32. Sloane JP. Biopsy Pathology of the Breast. Vol. 24, 2nd edition ed. London: Arnold; 2001.

33. Dupont WD, Page DL. Risk factors for breast cancer in women with proliferative breast disease. The New England Journal of Medicine 1985;312:146-51.

34. Raju U, Crissman JD, Zarbo R, Gottlieb C. Epitheliosis of the Breast. An Immunohistochemical Characterization and Comparison to Malignant Intraductal Proliferations of the Breast. Am J Surg Pathol 1990;14:939-47.

35. Moinfar F, Man YG, Lininger RA, Bodian C, Tavassoli FA. Use of keratin 35betaE12 as an adjunct in the diagnosis of mammary intraepithelial neoplasia-ductal-type – benign and malignant intraductal proliferations. Am J Surg Pathol 1999;23:1048-58.

36. Schnitt SJ, Conolly JL, Tavassoli FA, et al. Interobserver Reproducibility in the Diagnosis of Ductal Proliferative Breast Lesions Using Standardized Criteria. Am J Surg Pathol 1992;16:1133-43.

37. Allred DC, O'Connell P, Fuqua SAW, Kent Osborne C. Immunohistochemical studies of early breast cancer evolution. Breast Cancer Res Treat 1994;32:13-8.

38. Dupont WD, Parl FF, Hartmann WH, et al. Breast cancer risk associated with proliferative breast disease and atypical hyperplasia [see comments]. Cancer 1993;71:1258-65.

39. Black MM, Speer FD. Nuclear structure in cancer tissues. Surg Gynaecol Obstet 1957;105:97-105.

40. Cutler SJ, Black MM, Mork T, Harvei S, Freeman C. Further observations on prognostic factors in cancer of the female breast. Cancer 1969;24:653-67.
41. Goldstein NS, Murphy T. Intraductal carcinoma associated with invasive carcinoma of the breast. A comparison of the two lesions with implications for intraductal carcinoma classification systems. Am J Clin Pathol 1996;106:312-8.
42. Deng G, Lu Y, Zlotnikov G, Thor AD, Smith HS. Loss of heterozygosity in normal tissue adjacent to breast carcinomas. Science 1996;274:2057-9.
43. Gobbi H, Dupont WD, Simpson JF, et al. Transforming growth factor-beta and breast cancer risk in women with mammary epithelial hyperplasia. J Natl Cancer Inst 1999;91:2096-101.
44. Bodian CA, Perzin KH, Lattes R, Hoffmann P. Reproducibility and validity of pathologic classifications of benign breast disease and implications for clinical applications [see comments]. Cancer 1993;71:3908-13.
45. Kodlin D, Winger EE, Morgenstern NL, Chen U. Chronic mastopathy and breast cancer. A follow-up study. Cancer 1977;39:2603-7.
46. Dupont WD, Page DL. Breast cancer risk associated with proliferative disease, age at first birth, and a family history of breast cancer. Am J Epidemiol 1987;125:769-79.
47. Krieger N, Hiatt RA. Risk of breast cancer after benign breast diseases. Variation by histologic type, degree of atypia, age at biopsy, and length of follow-up. Am J Epidemiol 1992;135:619-31.
48. Davis HH, Simons M, Davis JB, et.al. Cystic disease of the breast. relationship to carcinoma. Cancer 1964; 17:957-78.
49. Carter CL, Corle DK, Micozzi MS, Schatzkin A, Taylor PR. A prospective study of the development of breast cancer in 16,692 women with benign breast disease. Am J Epidemiol 1988;128:467-77.
50. Page DL, Dupont WD, Rogers LW, Rados AM. Atypical Hyperplastic Lesions of the Female Breast. A Long-Term Follow-Up Study. Cancer 1985;55:2698-708.
51. Ma L, Boyd NF. Atypical hyperplasia and breast cancer risk: a critique. Cancer Causes Control 1992;3:517-25.
52. Ashikari R, Huvos AG, Snyder RE, et al. A clinicopathologic study of atypical lesions of the breast further follow up. Pathol Res Pract 1980;166:481-90.
53. Black MM, Barclay TH, Cutler SJ, Hankey BF, Asire AJ. Association of atypical characteristics of benign breast lesions with subsequent risk of breast cancer. Cancer 1972;29:338-43.
54. Bodian CA, Perzin KH, Lattes R, Hoffmann P, Abernathy TG. Prognostic significance of benign proliferative breast disease. Cancer 1993;71:3896-907.
55. Donnelly P, Baker K, Carney J. Benign breast lesions and subsequent breast carcinoma in Rochester, Minnesota. Mayo Clin Proc 1975;50:650-6.
56. London SJ, Connolly JL, Schnitt SJ, Colditz GA. A prospective study of benign breast disease and the risk of breast cancer [published erratum appears in JAMA 1992 Apr 1;267(13):1780]. JAMA 1992;267:941-4.
57. McDivitt RW, Stevens JA, Lee NC, et al. Histologic Types of Benign Breast Disease and the Risk for Breast Cancer. Cancer 1992;69:1408-14.
58. Moskowitz M, Gartside P, Wirman JA, McLaughlin C. Proliferative disorders of the breast as risk factors for breast cancer in a self-selected screened population: pathologic markers. Radiology 1980;134:289-91.
59. Page DL. Cancer Risk Assessment in Benign Breast Biopsies. Hum Pathol 1986;17:871-4.
60. Page DL, Dupont WD. Anatomic markers of human premalignancy and risk of breast cancer. Cancer 1990; 66:1326-35.
61. Page DL, Dupont WD, Rogers LW. Ductal involvement by cells of atypical lobular hyperplasia in the breast: a long-term follow-up study of cancer risk. Hum Pathol 1988;19:201-7.
62. Page DL, Vander Zwaag R, Rogers LW, et al. Relation Between Component Parts of Fibrocystic Disease Complex and Breast Cancer. J Natl Cancer Inst 1978; 61:1055-60.
63. Palli D, Rosselli-Del TM, Simoncini R, Bianchi S. Benign breast disease and breast cancer: a case-control study in a cohort in Italy. Int J Cancer 1991;47:703-6.
64. Rosen PP, Holmes G, Lesser ML, Kinne DW, Beattie EJ. Juvenile papillomatosis and breast carcinoma. Cancer 1985;55:1345-52.
65. Rosen PP, Kimmel M. Juvenile papillomatosis of the breast. A follow-up study of 41 patients having biopsies before 1979 [see comments]. Am J Clin Pathol 1990; 93:599-603.
66. Marshall LM, Hunter DJ, Connolly JL, et al. Risk of breast cancer associated with atypical hyperplasia of lobular and ductal-types. Cancer Epidemiol Biomarkers Prev 1997;6:297-301.
67. Tavassoli FA. Pathology of the Breast. 2nd ed. Norwalk: Appleton and Lange; 1999.
68. Rohan TE, Hartwick W, Miller AB, Kandel RA. Immunohistochemical detection of c-erbB2 and p53 in benign breast disease and breast cancer risk. J Natl Cancer Inst 1998;90:1262-9.
69. Dehner LP. The continuing evolution of our understanding of juvenile papillomatosis of the breast [editorial; comment]. Am J Clin Pathol 1990;93:713.
70. Tham KT, Dupont WD, Page DL, Gray GF, Rogers LW. Micro-papillary hyperplasia with atypical features in female breasts, resembling gynecomastia. In: Progress in Surgical Pathology. Heidelberg: Springer; 1989. p.101–9.
71. Lacroix-Triki M, Mery E, Voigt JJ, Istier L, Rochaix P. Value of cytokeratin 5/6 immunostaining using D5/16 B4 antibody in the spectrum of proliferative intraepithelial lesions of the breast. A comparative study with 34betaE12 antibody. Virchows Arch 2003;442: 548-54.
72. Siziopikou KP, Prioleau JE, Harris JR, Schnitt SJ. bcl-2 expression in the spectrum of preinvasive breast lesions. Cancer 1996;77:499-506.
73. Umekita Y, Takasaki T, Yoshida H. Expression of p53 protein in benign epithelial hyperplasia, atypical ductal hyperplasia, non-invasive and invasive mammary carcinoma: an immunohistochemical study. Virchows Arch 1994;424:491-4.
74. Done SJ, Arneson NC, Ozcelik H, Redston M, Andrulis IL. p53 mutations in mammary ductal carcinoma in-

situ but not in epithelial hyperplasias. Cancer Res 1998;58:785-9.

75. Stark A, Hulka BS, Joens S, et al. HER-2/neu amplification in benign breast disease and the risk of subsequent breast cancer. J Clin Oncol 2000;18:267-74.

76. Alle KM, Henshall SM, Field AS, Sutherland RL. Cyclin D1 protein is overexpressed in hyperplasia and intraductal carcinoma of the breast. Clin Cancer Res 1998; 4:847-54.

77. Weinstat SD, Merino MJ, Manrow RE, et al. Overexpression of cyclin D mRNA distinguishes invasive and in-situ breast carcinomas from non-malignant lesions. Nature Medicine 1995;1:1257-60.

78. Mommers EC, van Diest PJ, Leonhart AM, Meijer CJ, Baak JP. Expression of proliferation and apoptosis-related proteins in usual ductal hyperplasia of the breast. Hum Pathol 1998;29:1539-45.

79. Parham DM, Jankowski J. Transforming growth factor alpha in epithelial proliferative diseases of the breast. J Clin Pathol 1992;45:513-6.

80. Shaaban AM, Sloane JP, West CR, Foster CS. Breast cancer risk in usual ductal hyperplasia is defined by estrogen receptor-alpha and Ki-67 expression. Am J Pathol 2002;160:597-604.

81. Roger P, Sahla ME, Makela S, et al. Decreased expression of estrogen receptor beta protein in proliferative preinvasive mammary tumors. Cancer Res 2001;61: 2537-41.

82. O'Connell P, Fischbach K, Hilsenbeck S, et al. Loss of heterozygosity at D14S62 and metastatic potential of breast cancer [see comments]. J Natl Cancer Inst 1999; 91:1391-7.

83. Kaneko M, Arihiro K, Takeshima Y, Fujii S, Inai K. Loss of heterozygosity and microsatellite instability in epithelial hyperplasia of the breast. Journal of Experimental Therapeutics and Oncology 2002;2:9-18.

84. Maitra A, Wistuba II, Washington C, et al. High-resolution chromosome 3p allelotyping of breast carcinomas and precursor lesions demonstrates frequent loss of heterozygosity and a discontinuous pattern of allele loss. Am J Pathol 2001;159:119-30.

85. Werner M, Mattis A, Aubele M, et al. 20q13.2 amplification in intraductal hyperplasia adjacent to in-situ and invasive ductal carcinoma of the breast. Virchows Arch 1999;435:469-72.

86. Gong G, DeVries S, Chew KL, et al. Genetic changes in paired atypical and usual ductal hyperplasia of the breast by comparative genomic hybridization. Clin Cancer Res 2001;7:2410-4.

87. Jones C, Merrett S, Thomas VA, Barker TH, Lakhani SR. Comparative genomic hybridization analysis of bilateral hyperplasia of usual type of the breast. J Pathol 2003; 199:152-6.

88. Noguchi S, Aihara T, Koyama H, et al. Clonal analysis of benign and malignant human breast tumors by means of polymerase chain reaction. Cancer Lett 1995;90: 57-63.

89. Diallo R, Schaefer KL, Poremba C, et al. Monoclonality in normal epithelium and in hyperplastic and neoplastic lesions of the breast. J Pathol 2001;193:27-32.

90. Mommers EC, Page DL, Dupont WD, et al. Prognostic value of morphometry in patients with normal breast tissue or usual ductal hyperplasia of the breast. Int J Cancer 2001;95:282-5.

91. Koukoulis GK, Virtanen I, Korhonen M, et al. Immunohistochemical localization of integrins in the normal, hyperplastic, and neoplastic breast. Correlations with their functions as receptors and cell adhesion molecules. Am J Pathol 1991;139:787-99.

92. Bratthauer GL, Moinfar F, Stamatakos MD, et al. Combined E-cadherin and high molecular weight cytokeratin immunoprofile differentiates lobular, ductal, and hybrid mammary intraepithelial neoplasias. Hum Pathol 2002; 33:620-7.

93. Weidner N. The Difficult Diagnosis in Surgical Pathology. Philadelphia: W.B. Saunders; 1996.

Content

SCLEROSING ADENOSIS AND OTHER FORMS OF ADENOSIS

WERNER BOECKER AND UTE KETTRITZ

This chapter will focus on the morphological and clinical features of sclerosing adenosis and its variants. In the most recent classification published by the WHO, sclerosing adenosis is described as the prototypical lesion among the different types of adenosis and their variants [1]. **The basic features of sclerosing adenosis are sprouting and branching of glandular tissue to form irregular tubular structures and associated hyaline sclerosis in a basically lobular architecture. On a cellular level, sclerosing adenosis is a lesion that consists of Ck5/14+ cells and their glandular and myoepithelial progeny cells.**

A number of variants of this prototypical lesion have been described, with lesions differing in architecture and degree of sclerosis. They may further be modified by apocrine metaplasia. One important feature shared by sclerosing adenosis and its variants is their tendency to clinically and morphologically mimic invasive carcinoma. Malignant transformation of pre-existing sclerosing adenosis to in-situ malignancies (carcinoma in-situ ex adenosis) is rare.

In contrast to sclerosing adenosis and its variants, **microglandular adenosis** is a purely glandular lesion displaying significantly premalignant potential.

Sclerosing adenosis and other forms of adenosis

■ DEFINITION

WHO: Adenosis

Sclerosing adenosis is the prototypical lesion of this group of proliferative disorders. The single lesion is characterized by a benign proliferation of distorted, irregular, tubular/trabecular, acinar structures in a round or oval lobular architecture (Fig. 9.1), which is best seen at low magnification. The epithelial structures contain a glandular and myoepithelial cell layer surrounded by a basement membrane. Varying degrees of fibrosis and hyaline sclerosis may be observed [2–6]. In immunofluorescence experiments these lesions are characterized by Ck5/14+ cells and their glandular and myoepithelial progenies. Sclerosing adenosis is a common finding in mammographically detected lesions.

Variants of this prototype are characterized by formation of prominent tubules [7] (tubular adenosis), apocrine metaplasia [8–12] (apocrine adenosis, adenomyoepithelial adenosis), by coalescence of multiple adjacent 'lobules' so that a tumor mass is formed [13] (nodular adenosis, adenosis tumor), or by the prevalence of myoepithelial cells [14, 15] (myoepithelial adenosis). The term blunt duct adenosis refers to an organoid hyperplasia and hypertrophy of lobular structures [16, 17].

Microglandular adenosis is distinct from all other types of adenosis as it usually lacks the 'normal' cellular composition observed in the latter [12, 18, 17, 19–22]. Microglandular adenosis will, however, be discussed in this chapter as these lesions have a similar clinical setting and display the same differential diagnostic spectrum. Many adenosis lesions may show an infiltrative pattern and therefore be mistaken for invasive carcinoma.

The development of in-situ malignancies ex adenosis is extremely rare [23–25].

To prevent overdiagnosis, frozen section diagnosis should be avoided.

■ CONCEPTUAL APPROACH

Sclerosing adenosis is considered to be a benign proliferative process [26–29]. Subgross preparations of sclerosing adenosis by Wellings SR et al. [28] have shown that these lesions are characterized by proliferation of disarrayed tubules and ductules in a lobular architecture. It is generally assumed that the lesions evolve from lobules. From their stereomicroscopic studies, Tanaka and Oota [27] have,

however, suggested that sclerosing adenosis can evolve from sprouting of parallel arrays of tubular ductules originating from ducts to form irregular 'bundles of noodles'. Such tubules tend to run parallel to or around the ductal system forming knots or whorls. Sometimes, the developing mass may even extend into the lumen of the duct.

Immunostaining for cytokeratins 8/18 and myoepithelial markers clearly demonstrates the glandular-myoepithelial nature of this lesion. The spatial ordering of the epithelial double layer of the prototypical tubule of sclerosing adenosis is usually preserved along with its basement membrane. Further insights into the cellular composition of these lesions were derived from double immunofluorescence experiments. The results of these experiments clearly confirm that the cellular phenotypes of the tubular structures are identical to

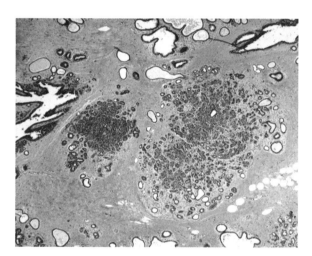

Fig. 9.1 Hematoxylin-eosin stained specimen showing two lobulocentric lesions. Microcystic change can be observed at the periphery of the lesions.

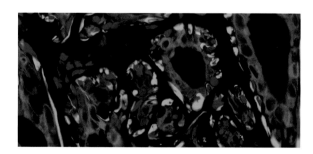

Fig. 9.2 Sclerosing adenosis. Double immunofluorescence labeling for sm-actin (green signal) and glandular Ck8/18 (red signal). The sm-actin+ myoepithelial cell lineage (green signal) outlines some of the tubular proliferations. The glands contain cells of the Ck8/18+ lineage (red signal).

10

RADIAL SCAR

WERNER BOECKER AND UTE KETTRITZ

Radiologically and morphologically, radial scar lesions have a stellate appearance. **Their histological hallmark is a central area of fibroelastotic tissue surrounded by radiating benign epithelial structures embedded in fibrous tissue.** The significance of radial scars is their striking resemblance to breast cancer, both on imaging and at pathology. **Radial scar,** according to the most recent WHO classification [1], **is a variant of sclerosing adenosis** (see Chapter 9 'Sclerosing adenosis and other forms of adenosis'). Although radial scars are obviously similar in many respects to adenosis and its variants, we feel that these lesions share important features with other benign proliferative breast disease lesions such as usual ductal hyperplasia or papillomas as these are themselves often a component part of radial scars. In addition, **radial scars possess their own unique clinical and morphological characteristics,** further strengthening the case for their inclusion in a separate chapter. Mention must also be made of the development of ductal or lobular neoplasia from these primarily benign lesions (atypical ductal or lobular proliferation ex radial scar).

Radial scar

■ DEFINITION

WHO: Complex sclerosing lesion/radial scar

Radial scar is a benign proliferative breast lesion classically characterized by a central fibroelastotic core, from which benign glandular structures embedded in a fibrous tissue radiate giving lesions their irregular stellate appearance (Fig. 10.1). The central core usually contains distorted tubular structures. The peripheral zone of glandular structures may show a number of changes such as usual ductal hyperplasia, sclerosing adenosis or papillary proliferations.

The descriptive term radial scar (German: *strahlige Narbe*) was introduced by the German pathologist H. Hamperl [2] along with the Danish pathologist F. Linell and his coworkers [3]. It is one of a multitude of names found in the literature referring to the same lesion, including non-encapsulated sclerosing lesions [4] sclerosing papillary proliferations [5], complex compound, heteromorphic lesions [6], scleroelastotic lesions [7], infiltrating epitheliosis [8], benign sclerosing ductal proliferation [9] and indurative mastopathy [10]. Anderson and Gram [11, 12] designate 'sclerotic lesions' to be those with a diameter of less than one centimeter, while 'complex sclerotic lesions' are defined as those greater than one centimeter in diameter. We prefer to use the term radial scar for all lesions independent of their size and to specify any additional features which may occur, such as usual ductal hyperplasia or atypical ductal or lobular proliferation.

Schnitt's group recently performed a study on radial scar lesions, including lesions as small as four millimeters. They reported that the number of lesions and the presence of usual ductal hyperplasia and/or atypical ductal proliferation within their architecture seem to be of value in predicting the general risk for development of breast carcinoma [13]. Furthermore the lesion has received widespread attention due to a possible association with carcinomas developing in a radial scar.

■ CONCEPTUAL APPROACH

The pathogenesis of radial scar lesions with their specific architecture and typical fibroelastotic core is still not clear. Inflammatory reactive processes to injury and ductal obliteration have been proposed as possible causes [2, 14, 15], resulting in the formation of a scar with radial distortion of the surrounding glandular structures. Chauhan et al. [16]

recently demonstrated the loss of CD34, a sialomucin expressed by normal breast fibroblasts, and the acquisition of sm-actin in radial scar fibroblasts. They suggest that the very focal change in phenotype implies the involvement of local signaling mechanisms, probably epithelial in origin.

Cell biologically, the epithelial structures of radial scar contain the same glandular and myoepithelial component cells as normal epithelium of resting breast tissue. Thus the basal cells are immunoreactive for sm-actin, calponin, p63 and Ck5/14, while the glandular cells show great variability in staining for Ck8/18 and Ck5/14. The tubular/trabecular ductules in the central elastotic/hyaline area and, in particular, the ductal hyperplasia components are immunoreactive for Ck5/14. Both the luminal and the basal cells of the tubular structures stain heavily. The outer radial glandular structures may consist of contracted TDLUs [17]. They may also contain areas characteristic of other lesions such as ductal hyperplasia, sclerosing adenosis, papilloma and blunt duct adenosis.

As with other benign proliferative breast lesions, all types of atypical epithelial proliferations may develop in the milieu of the epithelial structures of a radial scar, including flat epithelial atypia, atypical ductal hyperplasia, ductal carcinoma in-situ and lobular neoplasia [14, 18, 19]. In addition, it has been demonstrated that tubular carcinoma may arise within radial scars [17]. Although a correlation between the incidence of such atypical epithelial proliferation, the lesion size and patients' age has been shown [19], such a transition seems to occur only rarely and by chance.

■ CLINICAL FEATURES AND IMAGING

CLINICAL FEATURES

In the premammographic era the main clinical symptom associated with radial scars was that of a palpable mass [20]. In the present, however, they are mostly likely to be detected at mammography as a small, nonpalpable, spiculated mass or as a pattern of microcalcifications (Table 10.1) [21]. It is often impossible to distinguish a radial scar in such mammograms from a small invasive cancer [22–25]. In several studies the incidence of radial scar in biopsy material varied significantly (1.7–28%) [2, 23, 14, 26–28], with most lesions detected as an incidental microscopic finding of small size. Some, however, do form a palpable mass [19]. Autopsy studies by Nielsen et al. [29] on 82 unselected female autopsies have shown that radial scars are common, with an incidence of 28%, and that multicentricity and bilaterality are frequently observed (67% and 43% of cases respectively). These figures are in line with the observation that the widespread use of mammography has led to an increase in the detection of smaller lesions, which present as spiculated masses and, more rarely, as microcalcifications. Although Linell et al. [3] suggested that radial scar may be a precursor lesion of tubular carcinoma, the evidence that the lesion itself may be preneoplastic is far from conclusive [19, 30–32]. The data in the literature suggests that the incidence of malignancy in scars of less than six millimeters and in patients under 50 years of age is rare [19]. This also applies to cases detected at screening [33]. A possible general increase in breast cancer risk associated with radial scars [20, 34, 35] has also been proposed. Follow-up in the study of Jacobs et al. [36] disclosed that radial scar is an independent histologic overall risk factor with a relative risk of 1.8. Women with radial scar have a higher risk of cancer than those with no proliferative breast disease, the risk increasing with the size and number of lesions.

The prognosis is also aggravated by associated ductal hyperplasia or atypical ductal hyperplasia [37]. In conclusion, the authors recommend that patients with radial scars be regularly followed up clinically and mammographically.

In a follow-up study averaging 19.5 years, Anderson and Gram, however, found a lower than expected incidence compared to that in a control population [38]. Similar results had already been obtained by Fenoglio and Lattes [20].

IMAGING

MAMMOGRAPHY

Only 5–10% of radial scars clinically present as a lump [19]. Most radial scars are small and detected during histologic examination of breast tissue excised for other reasons. In recent years the increasingly widespread use of screening mammography has, however, led to the discovery of larger numbers of radial scar cases on imaging.

Fig. 10.1a–b Radial scar.
10.1a Submacroscopic view of a radial scar with the typical radial arrangement of the parenchymal structures.

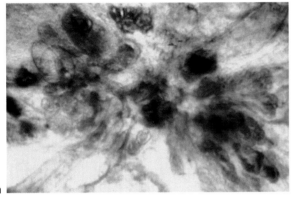
a

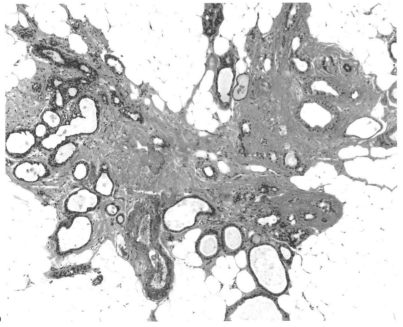
b

10.1b Histologic view of a radial scar characterized by a compact field of fibro-elastotic tissue with simple glandular structures radiating outwards from the center of the lesion. Some of the glands show apocrine change.

The classic description of the mammographic appearance of a radial scar as a 'spiculated mass' with the following characteristics was provided by Tabár and Dean [39].

1. Long slender white spicules consisting of sclerosed soft tissue, radiating from the center of the lesion ('white star').
2. The presence of radiolucent black, linear structures representing distorted fat parallel to the white spicules. The black structures may occasionally dominate the overall appearance creating a 'black star' effect.
3. The absence of a central tumor mass formation. In its place a radiolucent area can be observed.
4. A varying appearance in different projections.
5. A palpable lesion on physical examination is usually absent.

Thus the prototypical lesion is characterized by a spiculated mass with a radiolucent center in two projections but with varying appearances on two orthogonal views (Figs 10.2–10.4). A palpable abnor-

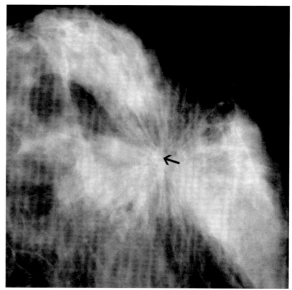

Fig. 10.3 Radial scar. Craniocaudal mammogram of a 46-year-old woman showing a stellate lesion with long radiating spicules against a small dense center (arrow). The typical radiolucent central area can be obscured in a very dense parenchymal background.

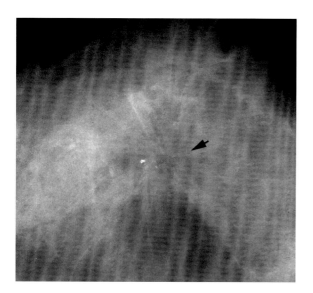

Fig. 10.2 Radial scar. Craniocaudal mammogram of a 48-year-old woman showing an area of architectural distortion with radiating spicules against a radiolucent central area (arrow). These mammographic findings are typical of radial scar, but may be indistinguishable from architectural distortion due to an invasive carcinoma. Some coarse microcalcifications with an indeterminate appearance are also present.

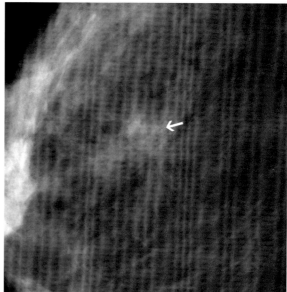

Fig. 10.4 Radial scar. Mediolateral oblique mammogram of a 45-year-old woman showing an area of architectural distortion with a stellate appearance. A dense center is present (arrow), rendering the lesion indistinguishable from carcinoma.

mality is usually absent even in cases in which the mammographic lesion involves larger areas close to the surface of the skin. Spot compression views may be helpful in gaining further insights into the internal architecture of the distorted epithelial and soft tissue structures. In dense breast tissue, stromal distortion may only be seen as barely visible convergences of a few spicules towards a central area. Although the absence of a solid central tumor mass may be a helpful mammographic feature in differentiating radial scar from carcinoma, it does not preclude malignancy. Furthermore, a dense central nidus may even be found in cases of radial scars [40, 41]. Microcalcifications may be present, and their incidence is currently increasing due to the improved quality of mammograms [42–44].

A radiolucent center is one of the typical features of radial scar on mammography. The feature is, however, not exclusive to radial scar as it may be seen in stellate malignancies such as sclerosing tubular carcinomas. Thus Ciatto et al. [45] noted a radiolucent center in 35 of 38 radial scars and in 6 of 30 impalpable stellate carcinomas. Mitnick et al. [46] observed a radiolucent center in 5 of 9 radial scars and in 14 of 73 nonpalpable stellate carcinomas. In summary, these authors emphasized that the radiological features used to differentiate between benign and malignant stellate lesions are unreliable [47]. Excision of mamographically detected radial scars is therefore mandatory.

ULTRASOUND

Radial scars can be visible on ultrasound (Fig. 10.5). Cohen et al. [48] found a lesion on ultrasound in 8 of 12 mammographically identified radial scars, while Finlay et al. [49] identified 21 radial scars by ultrasound. Sonographic features of the lesion include an irregular hypoechoic mass with ill-defined borders or, less characteristically, areas of poorly defined tissue with diminished posterior sound transmission. The posterior acoustic shadowing can be the dominant feature when no circumscribed mass is visible. However these sonographic features are similar to those of invasive carcinoma and are therefore not diagnostic [50–52].

Sonography may be used to guide core biopsy, if the lesion is more clearly seen on ultrasound than on mammography.

MAGNETIC RESONANCE MAMMOGRAPHY

Contrast-enhanced magnetic resonance mammography cannot reliably distinguish radial scar from malignant lesions. Baum et al. [53] evaluated mammographically detected spiculated lesions suggestive of radial scar by contrast-enhanced magnetic resonance mammography. In cases which had been surgically removed and which proved to be radial scars, 3 of 15 displayed criteria typical of malignancies, whereas 3 of 9 cases of invasive carcinomas lacked these features.

In conclusion, typical radiological features may be present in many radial scars, though they fail to reliably distinguish these lesions from carcinoma [54–56].

■ PATHOLOGY

MACROSCOPY

Only larger lesions can be seen with the naked eye (Fig. 10.6). Lesions have a stellate architecture with pale creamy streaks of elastosis. Usually the consistency of such a lesion is more elastic than that of an invasive cancer of similar size.

MICROSCOPY

The prototypical radial scar has a characteristic stellate appearance with peripheral sclerosed or nonsclerosed

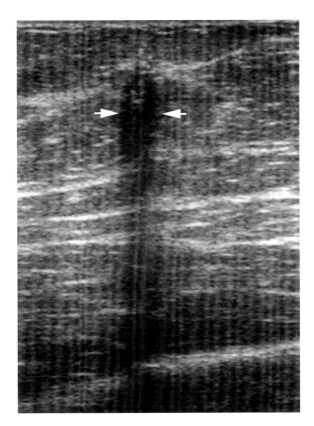

Fig. 10.5 Radial scar. Ultrasound in a 56-year-old woman demonstrates marked posterior acoustic shadowing (arrows) caused by an area of architectural distortion without a visible circumscribed mass.

10 Radial scar

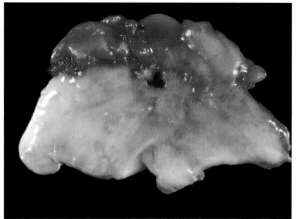

Fig. 10.6a–c Radial scars.

10.6a Cut section of an excision biopsy showing the typical aspect of a radial scar with chalky yellow streaks in a glassy irregular tumor mass about 1.5 cm in diameter. The core biopsy defect is seen in the upper field.

10.6b Radial scar showing typical elements of hyalinized (h) and elastotic tissue (e) with entrapped elongated tubules (arrows), and an adenotic proliferation in the left field.

10.6c Low power view of another radial scar with the typical stellate appearance of fibroelastic stroma with entrapment of distorted tubular structures. The radiating structures in the right field and a dilated gland in the center show a marked epithelial proliferation of usual type.

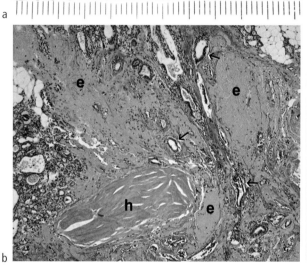

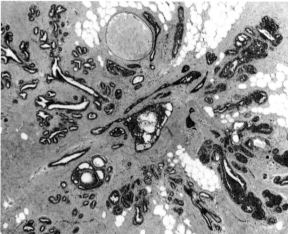

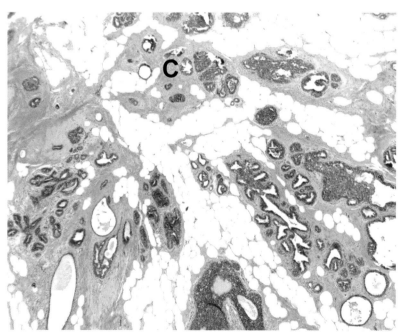

Fig. 10.7 Low power view of a radial scar. This image shows part of a spiculated mass with a central fibroelastotic area (c) and radiating arms at the periphery containing parenchymal structures with florid usual ductal hyperplasia. Note that the central area and the radiating structures are associated with larger amounts of fatty tissue causing more radiolucent black structures on mammography (so-called black star).

200

Tab. 10.1 Characteristics of radial scars

Definition	Lesions are composed of fibroelastotic tissue and benign epithelial structures in a stellate appearance.
Radiological diagnosis	Radiologically, no specific criteria exist to distinguish radial scar from carcinoma.
Epithelial composition	Epithelial structures contain the same glandular and myoepithelial component cells as normal breast epithelium. They may be associated with adenosis, usual ductal hyperplasia or papilloma.
Stromal changes	Lesions usually contain a fibroelastotic core with a radial arrangement of fibrous tissue.
Immunohistochemistry	Myoepithelial cells show staining for p63, calponin, sm-actin and Ck5/14. Glandular cells are positive for Ck8/18 and, partially, for Ck5/14. Usual ductal hyperplasia shows a typical Ck5/14 mosaicism. Note that the tubular structures in fibroelastotic areas are always Ck5/14+.
Malignancy	Lobular neoplasia/atypical ductal proliferations rarely develop in radial scars.
B-classification	B3
Differential diagnosis	Invasive carcinoma, malignancy ex radial scar.

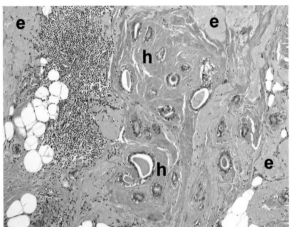
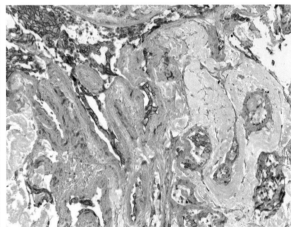

Fig. 10.8a–b Central part of a radial scar.
10.8a Higher magnification of a central area with hyaline (h) and elastotic (e) change and entrapped distorted tubular structures. In a core biopsy such a field may lead to a mistaken diagnosis of invasive carcinoma, yet careful examination usually confirms the myoepithelial cell layer. In difficult cases, immunostaining for sm-actin or Ck5/14 is helpful in distinguishing these benign lesions from tubular carcinoma.
10.8b Immunostaining for Ck14 showing intense staining of both glandular and myoepithelial cells, highlighting the immaturity of this epithelium. Such a staining pattern is indicative of a benign tubular proliferation (compare Figs 10.11–10.14). Note the intense elastosis surrounding some tubular structures.

parenchymal tissue growth radiating from a central fibroelastotic core [8, 57–60]. This central core is usually composed of dense, often hyalinized and poorly cellular fibrous tissue with areas of elastosis (Figs 10.6–10.8). Typically it also contains entrapped distorted and sometimes compressed tubular structures (Fig. 10.8) which usually lack an organoid distribution. The tubules are lined by a double layer of regularly arranged glandular/myoepithelial cells, but the myoepithelial layer may be attenuated and barely visible in H&E routine sections. The glandular cells may contain enlarged nuclei similar to those of tubular carcinoma which may cause diagnostic difficulties when found in needle biopsies.

While the peripheral zone of small radial scars may be exclusively composed of radiating tubules (Fig. 10.1b), larger ones often disclose complex parenchymal tissue around the periphery showing foci of adenosis, collagenous spherulosis, ductal hyperplasia (Fig. 10.9), papilloma, apocrine metaplasia and cysts. For this reason some experts in the field employ the term 'radial scar' for lesions smaller than 10 mm and the term 'complex sclerosing lesions' for larger ones. In our opinion applying the term

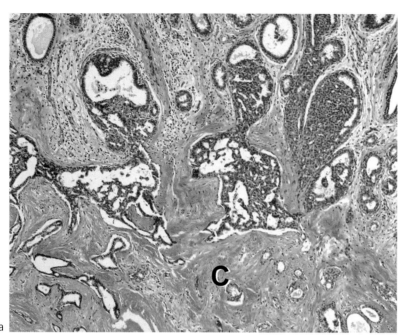

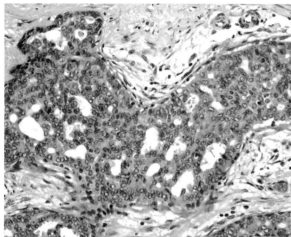

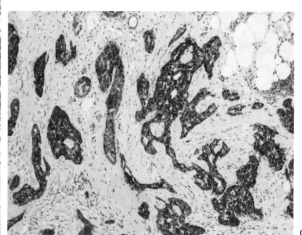

Fig. 10.9 a–c Radial scar with usual ductal hyperplasia.
10.9a Another radial scar showing a fibrous stroma with marked hyaline change around some ductular structures in the lower field, which represents the core (c) of the lesion.
10.9b High power view of the same lesion showing florid epithelial hyperplasia with a fenestrating growth pattern.
10.9c Ck14 immunostaining with a mosaic staining pattern characteristic of benign epithelial proliferations. Note the contrasting staining pattern of atypical epithelial proliferations in Fig. 10.11.

'radial scar' to both groups independent of size is justified, since the most characteristic feature is the shape of the lesion and larger lesions show the same histological features, albeit on a larger scale [61].

VARIATIONS OF RADIAL SCARS

Some radial scars contain a central area with a more cellular fibroblastic tissue without evidence of significant scarring or elastosis [62] (Fig. 10.10). Furthermore, a moderate chronic inflammatory reaction may be observed at the interface of the central fibroblastic reaction and the peripheral zone in these 'early' lesions.

IMMUNOHISTOCHEMISTRY

In radial scar, the central tubular structures immunostain intensely for Ck5 and Ck14 in almost all cases. These basal cytokeratins are found in both the glandular and myoepithelial cells (Figs 10.10 and 10.15). Furthermore, immunostains for myoepithelial markers such as p63 and sm-actin decorate the myoepithelial cells of these tubular structures [63].

Immunostaining of the radiating parenchymal tissues surrounding the central core varies according to the component cells. The parenchymal structures are usually invested by a myoepithelial layer which immunostains for myoepithelial markers and basal Ck5/14. The glandular double-layered epithelium usually contains Ck5/14+ cells but areas of Ck5/14–

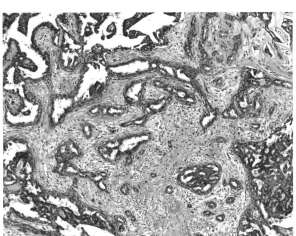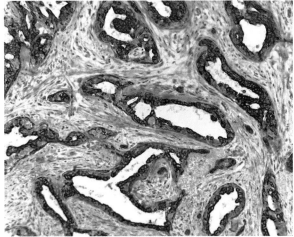

a   b

Fig. 10.10a–b Central part of a radial scar.
10.10a Radial scar with entrapped tubular structures and a moderately cellular (myo-) fibroblastic stroma. It may be very difficult to distinguish such a lesion from the tubules of a tubular carcinoma, although the presence of a myoepithelial layer usually helps. In difficult cases the use of p63 or Ck5/14 may solve this problem.
10.10b Immunostaining for Ck14. The benign epithelial structures of radial scars always express Ck5 and Ck14. Therefore cytokeratin immunohistochemistry is such a valuable tool for confirming the benign nature of a tubular lesion in difficult cases.

glandular epithelium do exist. Benign epithelial proliferations of usual ductal hyperplasia type display the characteristic Ck5/14 mosaicism pattern as described in Chapter 9 (Fig. 10.9).

In contrast, atypical epithelial proliferations such as flat epithelial atypia, atypical ductal proliferation, DCIS and lobular neoplasia do not express Ck5 and Ck14 (Chapter 22). Similarly, metaplasias derived from glandular cells such as apocrine cells are Ck5/14–, regardless of whether they are benign or malignant.

■ ATYPICAL PROLIFERATIONS OF DUCTAL OR ■ LOBULAR-TYPE EX RADIAL SCAR

Being able to distinguish the type of epithelial proliferation found in radial scar is of fundamental importance. Ductal hyperplasia shows the typical features described in detail in Chapter 8. Occasionally, atypical proliferations of lobular or ductal-type may be seen (Fig. 10.11). The criteria used to diagnose these atypical proliferations are the same as elsewhere in the breast. Characteristically, neoplastic cells prove to be Ck5/14– (see Chapters 17–20). In an analysis of 126 cases of radial scar, Sloane and Mayers [19] found 26 cases containing atypical ductal proliferations (atypical ductal hyperplasia and ductal carcinoma in-situ). They proposed a cutoff point in lesions of about 6–7 mm, below which such proliferations were very uncommon and above which they were relatively frequent. A similar relationship was seen with patient age (see also Douglas-Jones et al. [64]). Atypical

ductal proliferations were not seen in lesions removed from women under forty, were rare in the fifth decade and relatively common above this age [19]. These atypical lesions involve a variable percentage of the epithelium of the lesions, with a mean of 25–32% for the different types of atypical proliferations. Occasionally invasive breast carcinoma is found in association with radial scars [3, 65].

■ INTERPRETATION OF CORE AND ■ VACUUM-ASSISTED BIOPSIES

Current imaging techniques and criteria for radial scar cannot reliably exclude malignancy. A thorough histologic assessment of these lesions is therefore mandatory.

Image-guided percutaneous needle breast biopsy has been increasingly used as an alternative to surgical biopsy for the evaluation of indeterminate or suspicious breast lesions (see Chapter 4). It has been demonstrated that fine needle aspiration is not useful in the assessment of stellate lesions [66]. Core needle biopsy is more sensitive due to the greater amount of tissue that is sampled. Recent studies showed a high accuracy in the diagnosis of radial scar, especially when a greater number of samples were removed [67] or vacuum-assisted biopsy was used [68]. Philpotts et al. [43] reported nine radial scars which were diagnosed by core biopsy and confirmed by excisional biopsy. Brenner et al. [69] and Kirwan et al. [70] were able to show that core biopsy is probably a reliable

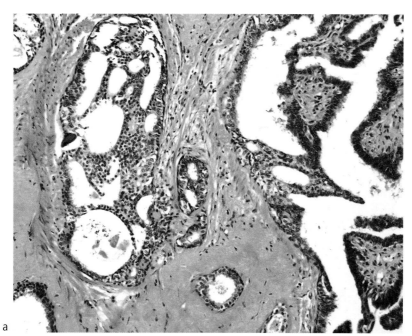

Fig. 10.11a−b Radial scar with atypical ductal proliferation.

10.11a Towards the left there is an atypical epithelial proliferation of monomorphic cells with cribriform growth pattern and a lamellar microcalcification against a background of fibroelastic tissue. A larger cystic space with mainly benign papillary structures is located at the right side.

a

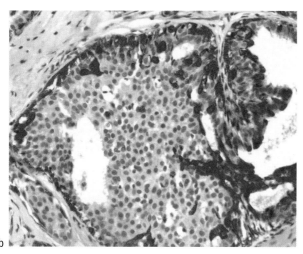

10.11b Ck14 immunostaining confirms that the atypical epithelial proliferation does not express Ck14. Note the positive reaction of myoepithelial cells and some normal epithelial cells in the periphery of the lesion.

b

method of diagnosing radial scar. They suggest that surgery may not be necessary to confirm a diagnosis when core biopsies show features of radial scar with no evidence of atypia and when mammographic findings are reconciled with histologic findings. Radiologists and pathologists must carefully review evidence garnered from histology and imaging in interdisciplinary meetings to plan further management of a given lesion. As controversy still exists concerning the increased risk of malignancies associated with a diagnosis of radial scar [71, 72], radial scars diagnosed at core biopsy require deliberate management recommendations.

The morphology of core or vacuum-assisted biopsies varies considerably depending on the size of the lesion and on whether tissue is obtained from central and/or peripheral sections of the lesion. In addition to radial scar's most predominant feature –

distinctive fibroelastotic tissue associated with double layered epithelial tubules – a number of other variable features may also be present. Those include areas of more fibrous tissue with hyalinization and a variety of benign parenchymal proliferations such as usual ductal hyperplasia, papillomas, and adenotic changes. The frequent presence of tubular structures within the fibroelastotic core closely resembles tubular carcinoma in H&E sections. Tubular carcinoma and radial scar can, however, be clearly distinguished using Ck5/14 immunostaining. If the typical features of radial scar are present, the lesion should be categorized as B3. Usually a surgical excision is recommended in this situation. When the lesion is small and extensive sampling has resulted in complete removal of the mammographic lesion, the B2 category may be appropriate, provided that histological examination confirms the diagnosis of radial scar and

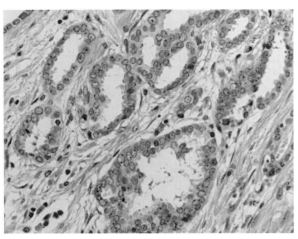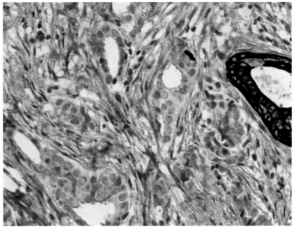

a   b

Fig. 10.12a–b Tubular carcinoma.
10.12a Tumor area with open tubular structures and a desmoplastic fibrous stroma. Note that the myofibroblasts of the desmoplastic stroma may mimic myoepithelial cells, even more so because they stain for sm-actin (see also Chapter 9).
10.12b Immunostaining for Ck14 showing no reaction within the tumor in contrast to the positive reaction of a normal duct in the right field.

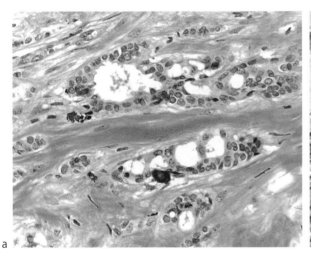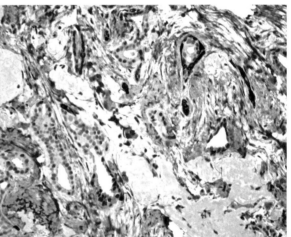

a   b

Fig. 10.13a–b Another case of tubular carcinoma.
10.13a High power view of a tubular carcinoma with slight desmoplastic stromal reaction. The tubules are lined by a monomorphous glandular epithelium.
10.13b Immunostaining for Ck5 highlights the negativity of the neoplastic tubules.

excludes atypical changes. In some cases it may be difficult to determine the specific nature of the lesion. The differential diagnosis of these indeterminate sclerosing lesions falls into four main groups that have been discussed in the corresponding chapters:
1. sclerosing adenosis (Chapter 9);
2. sclerosing papilloma (Chapter 11);
3. radial scar;
4. some types of adenomyoepithelial tumors (Chapter 14).

To determine the further clinical management in this situation, discussing the needle biopsy findings in the context of radiological and clinical findings in an interdisciplinary approach is mandatory.

DIFFERENTIAL DIAGNOSIS

The differential diagnosis of radial scar includes invasive carcinoma and in-situ malignancies ex radial scar.

Distinguishing radial scar from invasive carcinoma, in particular low grade invasive ductal and tubular carcinoma, is a common and very difficult problem. It can prove challenging even in good paraffin sections, let alone frozen sections. Diagnosing frozen sections

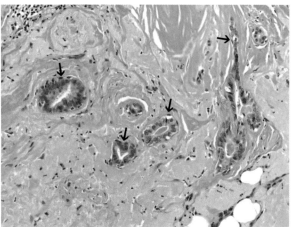
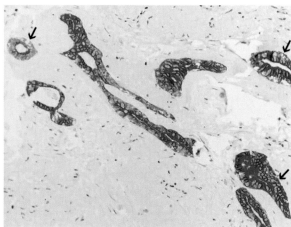

a · b

Fig. 10.14a – b Central area of radial scar.
10.14a High power view of the lesion in Fig 10.8a with hyaline-elastotic background containing tubular structures with a barely visible myoepithelial layer (arrows). The nuclear features do not allow a clear distinction from tubular carcinoma.
10.14b Ck14 immunostaining with positive reaction of both myoepithelial (arrows) and glandular cells. This is the typical staining pattern of the tubular structures of radial scars and allows a clear distinction from the Ck5/14− reaction of tubular carcinomas (see Figs 10.12 and 10.13)

from surgical biopsies of small lesions should be strictly avoided.

In biopsies containing the whole lesion, the most important feature to be identified is the underlying architecture of the lesion. The histologic hallmark of the lesion, as mentioned, is its zonal pattern of a fibroelastotic core with radiating parenchymal structures. This complex pattern is usually not found in invasive carcinoma. Moreover, invasive carcinoma is often associated with desmoplastic stromal response (Fig. 10.12). The most important feature distinguishing benign lesions from invasive carcinoma, however, is the type of cellular proliferation. The benign tubules of radial scar consist of an epithelial double layer, the myoepithelial cells of which are usually attenuated. This is in clear contrast to the open, angulated malignant tubules of tubular carcinoma with their single glandular layer and complete absence of myoepithelial cells. Taking these different features into account it is usually possible to reach a final diagnosis at the H&E level.

In cases where little material is available, such as needle biopsies, the cytoarchitectural and nuclear features may however be of little help in distinguishing benign from malignant tubules (Figs 10.13 and 10.14). Radically distorted architecture, furthermore, may rule out a conclusive decision. In this context, demonstrating the presence of myoepithelial markers or of high molecular weight cytokeratins 5/14 in immunostaining is consistently discriminatory. Furthermore, this is essential in the setting of significantly different treatment protocols. Benign tubular proliferations are Ck5/14+. The myoepithelial cells can be highlighted by markers such as p63, calponin or sm-actin. Invasive low grade ductal and tubular carcinomas are Ck5/14− and lack the myoepithelial layer.

The distinguishing features of intraductal epithelial proliferations are discussed in Chapters 8 and 11.

REFERENCES
1. Tavassoli, F.A. WHO Histological Classification of Tumours of the Breast. IARC Press, Lyon (2003).
2. Hamperl,H. Strahlige Narben und obliterierende Mastopathie. Virchows Archiv A 369, 55–68 (1975).
3. Linell,F., Ljungberg,O. & Andersson,I. Breast carcinoma. Aspects of early stages, progression and related problems. Acta Pathol Microbiol. Scand. Suppl 1–233 (1980).
4. Fisher, E.R., Palekar, A.S., Kotwal, N. & Lipana, N. A nonencapsulated sclerosing lesion of the breast. Am J Clin Pathol 71, 240–246 (1979).
5. Semb, C. Fibroadenomatosis cystica mammae. Acta Chir Scand. 10, 1–484 (1928).
6. Wellings, S.R., Jensen, H.M. & Marcum, R.G. An atlas of subgross pathology of the human breast with special reference to possible precancerous lesions. J Natl Cancer Inst 55, 231–273 (1975).
7. Eusebi, V., Grassigli, A. & Grosso, F. [Breast scleroelastotic focal lesions simulating infiltrating carcinoma]. Pathologica 68, 507–518 (1976).
8. Azzopardi, J.G. Problems in Breast Pathology. W.B. Saunders, London (1979).
9. Tremblay, G., Buell, R.H. & Seemayer, T.A. Elastosis in benign sclerosing ductal proliferations of the female breast. Am J Surg Pathol 1, 1155–1158 (1977).
10. Rickert, R.R., Kalisher, L. & Hutter, R.V.P. Indurative Mastopathy: a benign sclerosing lesion of breast with elastosis which may simulate carcinoma. Cancer 47, 561–571 (1981).

11. Andersen, J.A. & Gram, J.B. Radial scar in the female breast. A long-term follow-up study of 32 cases. Cancer 53, 2557–2560 (1984).

12. Page, D.L. & Anderson, T.J. Diagnostic histopathology of the breast. Page, D.L. & Anderson, T.J. (eds.), pp. 89–103 (Churchill Livingstone, Edinburgh,1987).

13. Jacobs, T.W., Byrne, C., Colditz, G., Connolly, J.L. & Schnitt, S.J. Radial scars in benign breast-biopsy specimens and the risk of breast cancer. N Engl J Med 340, 430–436 (1999).

14. Wellings, S.R. & Alpers, C.E. Subgross pathologic features and incidence of radial scars in the breast. Hum Pathol 15, 475–479 (1984).

15. Andersen, J.A., Carter, D. & Linell, F. A symposium on sclerosing duct lesions of the breast. Pathol Annu. 21 Pt 2, 145–179 (1986).

16. Chauhan, H. et al. There is more than one kind of myofibroblast: analysis of CD34 expression in benign, in-situ, and invasive breast lesions. J Clin Pathol 56, 271–276 (2003).

17. Linell, F. & Rank,F. Breast cancer. Schmidt,W. (ed.), pp. 18–68 (Universitetsförlaget Dialogos, Lund,1989).

18. Nielsen, M., Jensen, J. & Andersen, J.A. An autopsy study of radial scar in the female breast. Histopathol 9, 287–295 (1985).

19. Sloane, J.P. & Mayers, M.M. Carcinoma and atypical hyperplasia in radial scars and complex sclerosing lesions: importance of lesion size and patient age. Histopathol 23, 225–231 (1993).

20. Fenoglio, C. & Lattes,R. Sclerosing papillary proliferations in the female breast. A benign lesion often mistaken for carcinoma. Cancer 33, 691–700 (1974).

21. Orel, S.G., Evers, K., Yeh, I.T. & Troupin, R.H. Radial scar with microcalcifications: radiologic-pathologic correlation. Radiology 183, 479–482 (1992).

22. Adler, D.D., Helvie, M.A., Oberman, H.A., Ikeda, D.M. & Bhan, A.O. Radial sclerosing lesion of the breast: mammographic features. Radiology 176, 737–740 (1990).

23. Ciatto, S. et al. Radial scars of the breast: review of 38 consecutive mammographic diagnoses. Radiology 187, 757–760 (1993).

24. Orel, S.G., Evers, K., Yeh, I.T. & Troupin, R.H. Radial scar with microcalcifications: radiologic-pathologic correlation. Radiology 183, 479–482 (1992).

25. Vega, A. & Garijo, F. Radial scar and tubular carcinoma. Mammographic and sonographic findings. Acta Radiol. 34, 43–47 (1993).

26. Andersen, J.A. & Gram, J.B. Radial scar in the female breast. A long-term follow-up study of 32 cases. Cancer 53, 2557–2560 (1984).

27. Jacobs, T.W., Byrne, C., Colditz, G., Connolly, J.L. & Schnitt, S.J. Radial scars in benign breast-biopsy specimens and the risk of breast cancer. N Engl J Med 340, 430–436 (1999).

28. Fisher, E.R., Palekar, A.S., Kotwal, N. & Lipana, N. A nonencapsulated sclerosing lesion of the breast. Am J Clin Pathol 71, 240–246 (1979).

29. Nielsen, M., Jensen, J. & Andersen, J.A. An autopsy study of radial scar in the female breast. Histopathol 9, 287–295 (1985).

30. Bahrmann, E. Die Mastopathie als Vorläufer des Mamma-Karzinoms. Dtsch. Gesundh. Wis. 17, 1762–1765 (1962).

31. Douglas-Jones, A.G. & Pace, D.P. Pathology of R4 spiculated lesions in the breast screening programme. Histopathol 30, 214–220 (1997).

32. Anderson, T.J. & Battersby, S. Radial scars of benign and malignant breasts: comparative features and significance. J Pathol 147, 23–32 (1985).

33. Douglas-Jones, A.G. & Pace, D.P. Pathology of R4 spiculated lesions in the breast screening programme. Histopathol 30, 214–220 (1997).

34. Andersen, J.A. & Gram, J.B. Radial scar in the female breast. A long-term follow-up study of 32 cases. Cancer 53, 2557–2560 (1984).

35. Jacobs, T.W., Byrne, C., Colditz, G., Connolly, J.L. & Schnitt, S.J. Radial scars in benign breast-biopsy specimens and the risk of breast cancer. N Engl J Med 340, 430–436 (1999).

36. Jacobs, T.W., Byrne, C., Colditz, G., Connolly, J.L. & Schnitt, S.J. Radial scars in benign breast-biopsy specimens and the risk of breast cancer. N Engl J Med 340, 430–436 (1999).

37. Jacobs, T.W., Byrne, C., Colditz, G., Connolly, J.L. & Schnitt, S.J. Radial scars in benign breast-biopsy specimens and the risk of breast cancer. N Engl J Med 340, 430–436 (1999).

38. Andersen, J.A. & Gram, J.B. Radial scar in the female breast. A long-term follow-up study of 32 cases. Cancer 53, 2557–2560 (1984).

39. Tabar, L. & Dean, P.B. Basic principles of mammographic diagnosis. Diagn. Imaging Clin Med 54, 146–157 (1985).

40. Mitnick, J.S., Vazquez, M.F., Harris, M.N. & Roses, D.F. Differentiation of radial scar from scirrhous carcinoma of the breast: mammographic-pathologic correlation. Radiology 173, 697–700 (1989).

41. Ciatto,S. et al. Radial scars of the breast: review of 38 consecutive mammographic diagnoses. Radiology 187, 757–760 (1993).

42. Orel, S.G., Evers, K., Yeh, I.T. & Troupin, R.H. Radial scar with microcalcifications: radiologic-pathologic correlation. Radiology 183, 479–482 (1992).

43. Philpotts, L.E., Shaheen, N.A., Carter, D. & Lee, C.H. Comparison of rebiopsy rates after stereotactic breast core biopsy with 11-gauge vacuum suction probe vs. 14-gauge needle and automated gun. AJR Am J Roentgenol. 170 (Suppl.), 83 (abst.) (1998).

44. Patel,A. et al. Radial scars: a review of 30 cases. Eur. J Surg Oncol 23, 202–205 (1997).

45. Ciatto,S. et al. Radial scars of the breast: review of 38 consecutive mammographic diagnoses. Radiology 187, 757–760 (1993).

46. Mitnick, J.S., Vazquez, M.F., Harris, M.N. & Roses, D.F. Differentiation of radial scar from scirrhous carcinoma of the breast: mammographic-pathologic correlation. Radiology 173, 697–700 (1989).

47. Mitnick, J.S., Vazquez, M.F., Harris, M.N. & Roses, D.F. Differentiation of radial scar from scirrhous carcinoma of the breast: mammographic-pathologic correlation. Radiology 173, 697–700 (1989).

48. Cohen,M.A. & Sferlazza, S.J. Role of sonography in evaluation of radial scars of the breast. AJR Am J Roentgenol. 174, 1075–1078 (2000).

49. Finlay, M.E., Liston, J.E., Lunt, L.G. & Young, J.R. Assessment of the role of ultrasound in the differentiation of radial scars and stellate carcinomas of the breast. Clin Radiol. 49, 52–55 (1994).

50. Cohen,M.A. & Sferlazza, S.J. Role of sonography in evaluation of radial scars of the breast. AJR Am J Roentgenol. 174, 1075–1078 (2000).

51. Finlay, M.E., Liston, J.E., Lunt, L.G. & Young, J.R. Assessment of the role of ultrasound in the differentiation of radial scars and stellate carcinomas of the breast. Clin Radiol. 49, 52–55 (1994).

52. Vega,A. & Garijo, F. Radial scar and tubular carcinoma. Mammographic and sonographic findings. Acta Radiol. 34, 43–47 (1993).

53. Baum, F. et al. [The radial scar in contrast media-enhanced MR mammography]. Rofo Fortschr. Geb. Rontgenstr. Neuen Bildgeb. Verfahr. 172, 817–823 (2000).

54. King, T.A. et al. A better understanding of the term radial scar. Am J Surg 180, 428–432 (2000).

55. Frouge, C. et al. Mammographic lesions suggestive of radial scars: microscopic findings in 40 cases. Radiology 195, 623–625 (1995).

56. Vega, A. & Garijo, F. Radial scar and tubular carcinoma. Mammographic and sonographic findings. Acta Radiol. 34, 43–47 (1993).

57. Elston, C.W., Ellis, I.O. & Goulding, H. The Breast. Elston, C.W. & Ellis, I.O. (eds.), pp. 107–132 (Churchill Livingstone, Edinburgh,1998).

58. Sloane, J.P. Biopsy Pathology of the Breast. Arnold, London (2001).

59. Rosen, P.P. Rosen's Breast Pathology. Lippincott Williams & Wilkins, Philadelphia (2001).

60. Tavassoli, F.A. Pathology of the Breast. Appleton and Lange, Norwalk (1999).

61. Anderson, T.J. & Battersby, S. Radial scars of benign and malignant breasts: comparative features and significance. J Pathol 147, 23–32 (1985).

62. Anderson, T.J. & Battersby, S. Radial scars of benign and malignant breasts: comparative features and significance. J Pathol 147, 23–32 (1985).

63. Werling, R.W., Hwang, H., Yaziji, H. & Gown, A.M. Immunohistochemical distinction of invasive from noninvasive breast lesions: a comparative study of p63 versus calponin and smooth muscle myosin heavy chain. Am J Surg Pathol 27, 82–90 (2003).

64. Douglas-Jones, A.G. & Pace, D.P. Pathology of R4 spiculated lesions in the breast screening programme. Histopathol 30, 214–220 (1997).

65. Battersby, S. & Anderson, T.J. Myofibroblast activity of radial scars. J Pathol 147, 33–40 (1985).

66. Patel, A. et al. Radial scars: a review of 30 cases. Eur. J Surg Oncol 23, 202–205 (1997).

67. Kirwan, S.E., Denton, E.R., Nash, R.M., Humphreys, S. & Michell, M.J. Multiple 14G stereotactic core biopsies in the diagnosis of mammographically detected stellate lesions of the breast. Clin Radiol. 55, 763–766 (2000).

68. Brenner, R.J. et al. Percutaneous core needle biopsy of radial scars of the breast: when is excision necessary? AJR Am J Roentgenol. 179, 1179–1184 (2002).

69. Brenner, R.J. et al. Percutaneous core needle biopsy of radial scars of the breast: when is excision necessary? AJR Am J Roentgenol. 179, 1179–1184 (2002).

70. Kirwan, S.E., Denton, E.R., Nash, R.M., Humphreys, S. & Michell, M.J. Multiple 14G stereotactic core biopsies in the diagnosis of mammographically detected stellate lesions of the breast. Clin Radiol. 55, 763–766 (2000).

71. Jacobs, T.W., Byrne, C., Colditz, G., Connolly, J.L. & Schnitt, S.J. Radial scars in benign breast-biopsy specimens and the risk of breast cancer. N Engl J Med 340, 430–436 (1999).

72. King, T.A. et al. A better understanding of the term radial scar. Am J Surg 180, 428–432 (2000).

Content

11

PAPILLOMA

WERNER BOECKER AND SYLVIA HEYWANG-KOEBRUNNER

The term 'papilloma' (papillary adenoma) applies to benign proliferative epithelial breast lesions with a papillary architecture. The papillae in such lesions are constructed of arborizing fibrovascular cores, lined by glandular surface epithelium, a basal myoepithelial layer and a basement membrane. Papilloma may occur at any site in the ductal lobular system from the nipple to the terminal ductal-lobular unit (TDLU). Papillomas are subdivided into two categories: **solitary (central) papillomas** which are located in the major nipple/sub-areolar ducts or large segmental ducts and **multiple (peripheral) papillomas** in cystically dilated TDLUs. **The latter are more often associated with low grade DCIS.** The prototypical papillary lesion may be modified by further epithelial or stromal changes. **Benign papillary lesions must be distinguished from papillary-type DCIS, in-situ malignancies developing in papillomas and from invasive papillary carcinoma.**

Papilloma

■ DEFINITION

WHO: Intraductal papilloma
ICD code: 8503/0

Papilloma is a benign proliferative epithelial lesion of the ductal-lobular system with a papillary growth pattern (Fig. 11.1). The single prototypical papillary structure is characterized by fibrovascular cores with a glandular-myoepithelial surface epithelium. Papilloma of the breast may be located both in large ducts and in the ducts of the nipple (central papilloma and adenoma of the nipple) and in peripheral TDLUs (peripheral papilloma).

Prototypical papilloma can undergo modification as a result of epithelial and/or 'stromal' changes, in extreme cases even leading to a distortion of the specific papillary nature of lesions. Like the terminal duct lobular units, papilloma may serve as the site of benign epithelial proliferations. Thus, epithelial hyperplasia may accumulate on the surface of the papillary structures, and, in occasional cases, the exaggerated epithelial proliferation may lead to a solid tumor mass. In contrast, in the stroma of the papillary stalks one may observe secondary 'endophytic' inverse sprouting of the surface epithelial layer leading to an adenosis-like appearance (ductal adenoma) or sclerosis (sclerosing papilloma). In rare cases, myoepithelial cells may also be the dominant component with spilling of these elements into the surrounding stroma. Such lesions should be correctly designated as 'adeno-myoepithelioma' (see Chapter 14). Furthermore, papilloma may be modified by apocrine metaplasia. The term 'papillomatosis', previously used both for usual ductal hyperplasia and for multiple papillomas, should be abandoned.

Atypical ductal proliferation and, rarely, lobular neoplasia may develop in a primarily benign papillary adenoma (atypical ductal proliferation or lobular neoplasia ex papilloma).

Papillomas must be distinguished from their malignant counterparts. Due to difficulties that may arise in distinguishing these lesions even on paraffin sections, any attempt at frozen-section diagnosis of papillary lesions is strongly discouraged.

■ CONCEPTUAL APPROACH

The great variability of papillary lesions is clear evidence that several morphogenetic processes must ultimately determine the different morphologies of papillomas. Although the

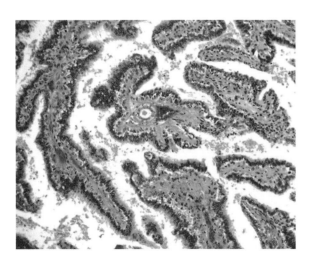

Fig. 11.1 Papilloma. Typical proliferative epithelial breast lesion with papillary arborizing fibrovascular cores in a cystically dilated duct. Note that, even at this low magnification, the glandular-myoepithelial layer can be identified.

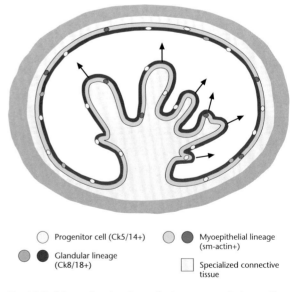

Fig. 11.2 Schematic drawing of the prototypical papillary lesion. Epithelial-myoepithelial tufts protrude into the lumen forming branching fibrovascular cores. Note that this core tissue develops from the specific periductal and perilobular stroma.

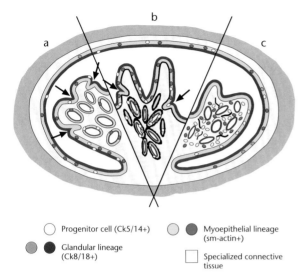

Progenitor cell (Ck5/14+)   Myoepithelial lineage (sm-actin+)

Glandular lineage (Ck8/18+)   Specialized connective tissue

Fig. 11.3 Variations of prototypical papilloma. Hypothetical mechanisms that may lead to variations of prototypical papilloma include modifications caused by 'endophytic' inverse sprouting of the surface epithelium into the specific stroma (arrows) with formation of tubular structures (ductal adenoma) (a), excess formation of basement membrane material (sclerotic papilloma) (b), or radial sprouting of 'myoepithelial' cells (adenomyoepithelial lesions) (c). Further modifications may be caused by epithelial changes such as usual ductal hyperplasia or apocrine metaplasia.

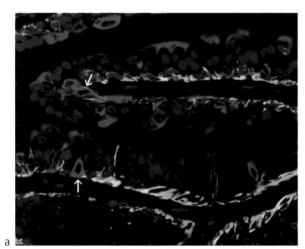

a

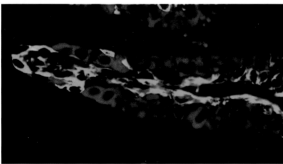

b

details of many of these changes are still poorly understood, it is nevertheless possible to outline and identify at least some of the developmental processes at work by focusing on the specific organization of the cellular and extracellular matrix components. The following key processes must be addressed in a conceptual approach:
1. the papillary structure;
2. the complex epithelial and stromal changes that may take place in the stalk of a papilloma;
3. surface epithelial changes.

The basic morphogenetic processes that can be recognized are shown schematically above (Figs 11.2 and 11.3).

THE PAPILLARY STRUCTURE

The most important feature of papilloma is its characteristic structure. Muir [1] postulated that papillary growth is primarily triggered by proliferation of the epithelium with an increase in surface area, which in turn leads to a coordinated growth of connective tissue. Typical papillary structures are the end result, which may give rise to secondary branches. It is important to emphasize that the epithelium of a papilla displays a two-lineage differentiation – identical to normal breast epithelium – with glandular and myoepithelial cells. Double immunofluorescence labeling studies have shown that the luminal epithelium is often very mature and immunostains for Ck8/18, but not for basal type cytokeratins 5/14. Ck5/14+ cells may, however, be observed at the tips or at sites where new papillae are starting to sprout. This indicates that the cells are an important morphogenetic driver of the papillary process. The basal layer contains Ck5/14+ cells, intermediary myoepithelial cells (Ck5/14+ and sm-actin+) and usually only a few differentiated myoepithelial end cells (sm-actin+) (Figs 11.2–11.4).

Fig. 11.4a–b Papilloma.
11.4a Double immunofluorescence labeling for cytokeratin 5/6 (red signal) and sm-actin (green signal). The basal layer contains cells of the myoepithelial lineage in different states of maturation with intermediate myoepithelial cells (hybrid signal) and differentiated myoepithelial cells (green signal). There are few cells in the outer layer expressing only Ck5, which is indicative of a precursor status (arrows). In this case the luminal cell layer also contains Ck5+ cells. Note that many luminal cells are Ck5–. These represent Ck8/18+ glandular cells.
11.4b Double immunofluorescence staining for Ck5/6 (green) and glandular Ck8/18 (red) demonstrates that the luminal layer contains many differentiated glandular cells (red signal) with only few Ck5/6+ progenitor cells. The basal cells express Ck5/6, which is indicative of immature myoepithelial cells.

Continuation

213

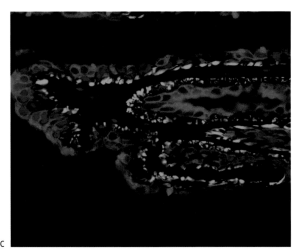

c

Fig. 11.4c Papilloma.
11.4c Double immunofluorescence labeling for Ck8/18 (red) and sm-actin (green). Note that the glandular cells comprise Ck8/18+ cells and that the basal layer contains sm-actin+ myoepithelial cells.

PAPILLARY STROMAL CHANGES

Prototypical papillae in papillomas are arborizing with delicate fibrovascular cores. However, the papillae can also be broad, with the cores containing epithelial proliferations and/or hyalinized tissue. Without doubt, such morphological change originates in the stroma of the papillary stalks, which is composed of specific lobular or periductal mantle stroma pulled into the evolving papilloma. It follows, therefore, that the morphogenetic processes associated with these changes are related to the type of the stroma as well as the properties of the epithelium. The key feature in this process seems to be a secondary endophytic inverse sprouting of the surface epithelial layer into the specific stroma of the papillary stalks (Fig. 11.5). Such inverse sprouting can form tubular structures similar to the structures seen in adenosis. They consist of an inner layer of glandular cells, an outer myoepithelial cell layer and a basement membrane. In other cases the epithelial elements may be accompanied by excessive formation of hyaline material, similar to the changes seen in sclerosing adenosis (Fig. 11.6). The hyaline tissue contains abundant collagen IV and laminin, typical components of basement membranes. There is some evidence that this type of sclerosis may be the result of the secretory activity of myoepithelial cells. Moreover, (myo-)fibroblasts may also play a role in the formation of the characteristic hyaline stroma of sclerosing papilloma. Last but not least, the process of inverse epithelial sprouting may be associated with an increase in the number of abluminal 'myoepithelial' cells radiating into the surrounding stroma of the fibrovascular cores so that features of an 'adenomyoepithelioma' may evolve (compare Chapter 14). The spectrum of changes observed in papillomas can therefore be compared to the processes taking place in adenosis/sclerosing adenosis [2].

SURFACE EPITHELIAL CHANGES LEADING TO PAPILLOMA VARIANTS

In addition to these two basic growth and differentiation processes, the surface epithelium may show other changes producing architecturally complicated patterns. Thus the specific papillary structure may be modified by apocrine metaplastic epithelium replacing or overgrowing the luminal epithelium, or by a benign proliferating epithelium similar to the one observed in usual ductal hyperplasia (see Chapter 6). Finally, focal squamous epithelial metaplasia may occur – usually associated with infarction. This metaplasia is thought to originate from Ck5/14+ progenitor cells (see Chapter 3).

The variants of papillary lesions described above are not mutually exclusive; a single tumor may fit the descriptions of all variants. The broad morphological spectrum with overlapping features of different cellular and architectural patterns results in a great diversity of papillary lesions. Thus an ability

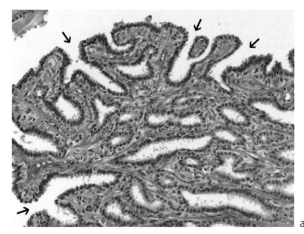

a

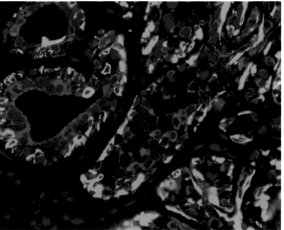

b

Fig. 11.5a–b Papilloma.
11.5a Papilloma with inverse sprouting of glandular-myoepithelial structures into the 'specific' papillary stroma (arrows).
11.5b Double immunofluorescence labeling for Ck8/18 (red) and sm-actin (green signal) showing the organized proliferation of tubular structures in a papillary stalk.

to recognize the basic architectural growth patterns, the cellular organization and the extracellular stromal components is important in making an informed diagnosis.

The relationship between papillomas and DCIS is described below.

■ CLINICAL FEATURES AND IMAGING

CLINICAL FEATURES

Papilloma encompasses a wide range of clinical symptoms and morphological findings with considerable variation in size and location of the lesions. Sandison [3] found papillomas in 3.7% of a total of more than 1,000 surgical specimens (Table 11.1).

SOLITARY (CENTRAL) PAPILLOMA

Clinically manifest central papillomas are usually located in the main ducts and may extend into segmental or even subsegmental interlobular ducts. The lesions usually measure 4–5 mm in diameter, but occasionally may be as large as 4–5 cm. Although they occur most often in the fourth and fifth decade of life, they may also be seen in adolescents and in the elderly. Central papilloma can also include the nipple area (adenoma of the nipple). In an autopsy study of 800 cases with no previous history of breast disease, Sandison [3] and his collaborators found 10 solitary papillomas, an incidence of 1.2%.

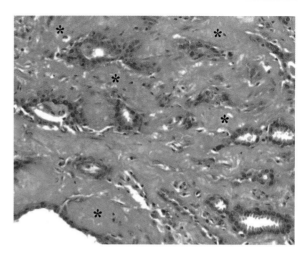

Fig. 11.6 Sclerosing papilloma. Note that the glands are surrounded by basement membrane-like hyaline material (asterisks). Immunohistochemically, these structures can be shown to contain collagen IV and laminin (not shown here).

Clinically, most central papillomas present as serous or serosanguinous nipple discharge [4]. Less often they can also present as a mammographic mass in a dilated duct [5, 6] and as microcalcifications or nodularities [5, 6]. Although controversy concerning the malignant potential of central papillomas still persists in the literature [7–13], there is no conclusive evidence that patients with a single central papilloma have an increased risk of developing breast carcinoma [14].

Tab. 11.1 Differences between solitary and multiple papillomas

	Solitary papilloma	Multiple papillomas
Mean age of patient	48 years.	40 years.
Nipple discharge	Nipple discharge usually present.	Usually no nipple discharge. Ill-defined mass or nodularity.
Site	Mainly subareolar.	Mainly in the periphery.
Bilaterality	1.5%	25%
Mammography	Usually normal, calcification rare.	Nodular, round or lobulated mass. Calcification may be present.
Ultrasound	Presence of a dilated duct and a hypoechoic or isoechoic intraductal mass.	Smooth-walled solid to cystic lesion with intraductal mass.
Ductogram	Filling defect.	–
Malignancy ex papilloma	Rare.	Up to 30% of cases.

Modified according to Azzopardi, 1978 and Chinyama, 2004

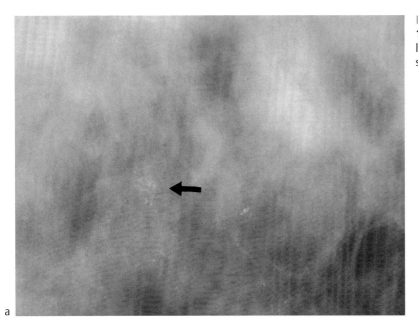

Fig. 11.7a–c Central papilloma.
11.7a Mammography showing a lobulated mass of low density with no surrounding architectural distortion.

a

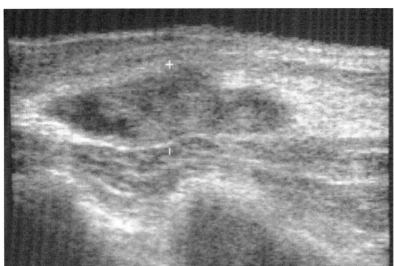

11.7b Ultrasound shows a clearly delineated smooth-walled, cystic lesion with a hypoechoic to isoechoic solid mass arising from the wall.

b

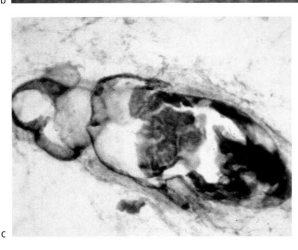

11.7c Submacroscopic slide of the lesion in 11.7b showing a cystically dilated duct with papillary projections.

c

MULTIPLE (PERIPHERAL) PAPILLOMA

Multiple (peripheral) papillomas have different clinical features due to their origin in cystically dilated TDLUs at the periphery of the ductal lobular system. The median age of patients with multiple papilloma is slightly lower than of those with central papilloma [15–17]. Patients with multiple papillomas show a certain propensity to develop in-situ malignancies. In some cases nipple discharge may be seen.

IMAGING

Small papillomas without calcification are mammographically occult. Larger lesions display a well-circumscribed nodular, rounded or lobulated mass of low density with no surrounding architectural distortion (Fig. 11.7) and/or a dilated duct. Microcalcifications may present as polymorphous, punctate or popcorn-like forms [5, 6, 18]. Sonographically, the lesions are smooth-walled, solid or cystic with hypoechoic to isoechoic solid intraductal masses, which are usually well-defined. [19]. Neither mammography nor ultrasound are able to distinguish between papilloma and carcinoma. Galactography may be helpful in identifying and localizing small central lesions prior to surgery [5] as it may show an obstruction of the duct or an irregular filling defect (Fig. 11.8). MR mammography is not a reliable method to identify papillomas (Fig. 11.9).

RELATIONSHIP OF PAPILLOMA TO CARCINOMA

Determining the frequency of recurrence or of the rate of subsequent development of carcinoma is difficult due to a lack of consistency in the published data when classifying benign, atypical and malignant papillary lesions. After local excision, the recurrence rate ranges from 10–30% [20]. Some authors found only a slightly elevated risk of subsequently developing invasive breast cancer (4–8%) [21–24, 7–9], whereas others deny such an increase [9–11, 25]. In an analysis of 368 women with papillomas, Page and coworkers found a relative risk of developing invasive breast carcinoma approaching 3.5 times that of the general population. Interestingly, the risk was higher in micropapillomas (< 3 mm) than in larger papillomas (> 3 mm). Patients with papillomas without atypia had a relative risk of 1.8. The risk increased further with the presence of epithelial atypia within the papilloma or in the surrounding breast tissue, amounting to 7.5 and 15.8 respectively [25]. The carcinomas tended to arise in the ipsilateral rather than in the contralateral breast. The importance of atypia as an additive risk factor is further supported by the work of Raju and coworkers who showed that 3 out of 12 patients with

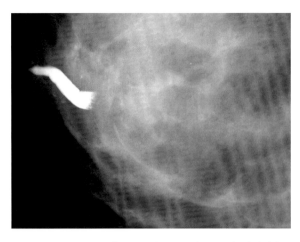

Fig. 11.8 Central papilloma. Galactography may be helpful in localizing lesions. Here a large subareolar duct has been completely obstructed.

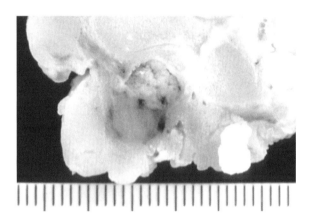

Fig. 11.9 Central papilloma. The cut surface shows a well-encapsulated, tan-pink, friable tumor about five millimeters in diameter obliterating the cystically enlarged duct.

papilloma and associated atypical ductal hyperplasia were later diagnosed at follow-up with in-situ or invasive carcinoma [26].

There is clearly a greater risk of recurrence after local excision of peripheral papillomas [27].

Furthermore, several studies revealed an increased frequency of malignancies in the lesions themselves (carcinoma ex papilloma) [28–31]. Areas of atypical ductal proliferation (usually referred to as atypical ductal hyperplasia or DCIS) in an otherwise clearly benign lesion are more common in multiple peripheral than in central solitary papillomas. To elucidate the precancerous nature of papillomas, Ohuchi et al. [31] studied 25 cases by using three-dimensional reconstruction. Of the 15 cases with multiple papillomas included in the study, 5 were associated with DCIS in which anatomic continuity existed between benign and malignant tissue. In contrast, only one of the solitary papillomas showed a transition to in-situ malignancy. Raju et al. [26] studied 97 cases of papillary lesions, 22 of which showed atypical ductal proliferations which the authors classified as ADH. The malignancy may evolve from the papilloma itself, or it may appear separately and merge with the papilloma. Ali-Fehmi et al. found 12 of 28 multiple papillomas contained atypical ductal proliferations (43%) [32]. Papotti et al. [33] studied 18 cases of combined intraductal papillomas and DCIS immunohistochemically (sm-actin and carcinoembryonic antigen [CEA]) and found transitions from benign lesions to malignancy. It is clear therefore that, regardless of the location of a tumor, the papillomas themselves and the surrounding breast tissue must be carefully screened for malignancy.

PATHOLOGY

MACROSCOPY

Central papillomas are generally solitary and have an average size of 2–3 cm, but they may also be smaller, measuring less than 5 mm. In some cases no macroscopic abnormality is seen, and it may therefore be necessary to carefully open the involved duct using a fine pair of scissors [34]. Solitary papillomas are well-circumscribed (Fig. 11.10). The tumor may obstruct the dilated duct and even lead to a cystic space (intracystic papilloma), which may contain clear fluid or blood. The tan-pink, friable tumor is usually attached to the wall of the duct by a stalk. Occasionally the tumor may show hemorrhagic infarction. The duct wall may be thickened and fibrosed.

Peripheral papillomas are usually multiple and located in cystically dilated TDLUs [20, 31, 33] (Fig. 11.11). Larger papillary lesions and multiple papillomas may form a solid tumor mass likely to be detected by palpation or mammography. Alternatively, such large lesions may present as a cystic mass with induration of tissue. In some cases this tumor mass may expand to several centimeters in diameter.

MICROSCOPY

As discussed above (see 'Conceptual approach'), the histological spectrum of individual papillomas can be very broad, and there is considerable morphologic overlap between the prototypical papilloma and its variants on the one hand and entities such as ductal adenoma and adenomyoepithelioma on the other. Papillomas may display epithelial changes such as apocrine change, squamous cell metaplasia and usual ductal hyperplasia. Furthermore, it is crucial that atypical ductal proliferations are recognized. The overall cellular, architectural and stromal features discussed below should therefore be carefully taken into consideration before making a diagnosis (Table 11.2).

CLASSIC PAPILLOMA
Papillary lesions usually present as a circumscribed solitary or aggregate lesion within a cystic duct or cystically dilated TDLU. Histologically, prototypical papillomas are composed of papillary structures, each papilla containing fibrovascular cores attached to the duct wall. Papillae may be delicate and arborizing, or, alternatively, broad. The branching fibrovascular cores are usually lined by a luminal glandular and a

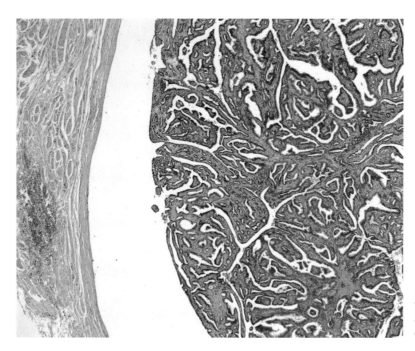

Fig. 11.10 Central papilloma with the typical papillary architecture with arborizing papillae and the fibrous capsule of the enlarged duct on the left.

Tab. 11.2 Histology of papilloma

Definition	Benign epithelial proliferation with papillary growth pattern. Glandular-myoepithelial surface epithelium (two-cell type differentiation) with 'normal' spatial symmetry of the epithelial double layer and its basement membrane.
Epithelial composition	Glandular cells with ovoid, normochromic nuclei. Apical snouts or blebbing may be present. Myoepithelial cell layer may vary from subtle to prominent.
Stromal composition	Formation of 'specific' papillary stroma.
Immunohistochemistry	Ck8/18+ glandular cells, Ck5/14+ cells and sm-actin+ myoepithelial cells. Collagen IV and laminin in basement membrane material.
Modifications	Sclerosis, infarction, hemorrhage, apocrine change and squamous cell change. Usual ductal hyperplasia may be prominent.
B-classification	B3
In-situ malignancy ex papilloma	Atypical ductal proliferation ex papilloma up to 30% in peripheral papillomas. Lobular neoplasia exceptionally rare.

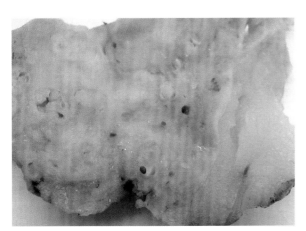

a

Fig 11.11a−b Large peripheral papilloma.
11.11a This patient refused surgical excision for several years, in which time her tumor grew to more than seven centimeters in diameter. Macroscopy reveals the tumor-forming papilloma. Note the cystically dilated ductal system occupied by solid proliferations in a fibrous stroma.

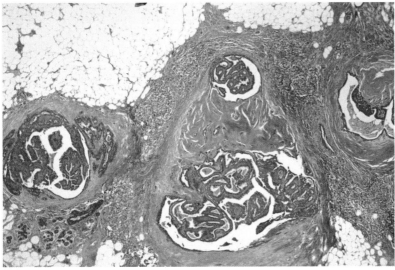

b

11.11b Another case of peripheral papilloma. Part of the lesion with three dilated TDLUs containing broad sclerosing papillary proliferations. Note the entrapped tubular structures within the papillary stalks, which themselves may cause diagnostic problems.

basal myoepithelial cell layer representative of the two different cell lineages (Fig. 11.12). The basal membrane is often inconspicuous. The surface epithelium of the basic papillary structure is a continuous layer of glandular cells, which are usually cuboidal to cylindrical in morphology. Often, the cells are uniform with bland, round to oval and normochromic nuclei. Apocrine snouts may be present at the luminal border of the glandular cells. Classic papillomas contain a continuous myoepithelial cell layer which can be highlighted by special immunostains such as sm-actin and p63 (Fig. 11.13). p63 is preferable to sm-actin, because it does not react with smooth muscle cells of small blood vessels, interfering with the localization of myoepithelial cells. The stroma in the cores consists of fibrocellular, edematous or dense hyaline tissue with small blood vessels. Usual ductal hyperplasia, apocrine metaplasia [13, 27], squamous metaplasia [35, 36], myoepithelial hyperplasia [26] and mesenchymal metaplasia of the papillary stalks have been described [37] (see below: 'Variants of papilloma'). Furthermore, the lesions may display endocrine characteristics [38–40]. All these changes contribute to the great diversity of benign papillary lesions and are discussed below.

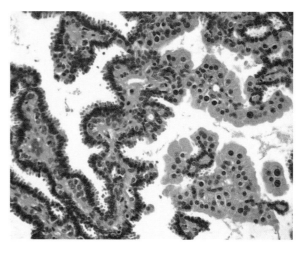

Fig. 11.12 Typical benign papillary lesion demonstrating the prototypical histological appearance of papilloma lesions: papillae containing delicate fibrovascular cores lined by a bland luminal glandular cell layer, normochromic basally located nuclei and a basal myoepithelial cell layer. Note the apocrine metaplasia on the right.

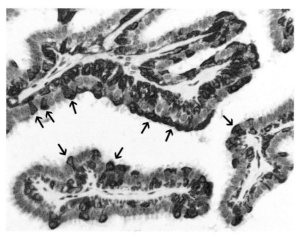

a

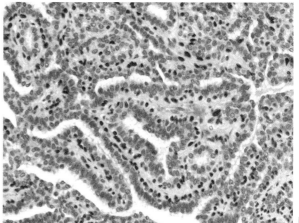

b

Fig. 11.13a–b Papilloma immunostained for Ck5/6 and p63.
11.13a Papilloma immunostained for cytokeratins 5/6. The myoepithelial cells stain intensely. The luminal cells are unevenly stained containing Ck5+ cells (arrows). Note, however, that, in many papillomas the single-layered luminal cells do not stain for Ck5/6.
11.13b Papilloma immunostained for p63, highlighting the myoepithelial cell layer.

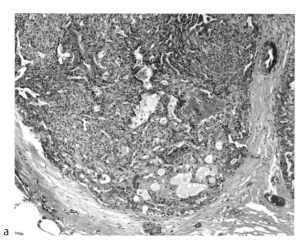

a

Fig. 11.14a An unusual case of a papilloma with associated usual ductal hyperplasia.
11.14a The solid epithelial proliferation between the hyaline papillary fronds shows a cell population with unevenly placed, normochromic nuclei and some anisonucleosis. This lesion thus would classify as tumor-forming papilloma with extensive usual ductal hyperplasia. *Continuation*

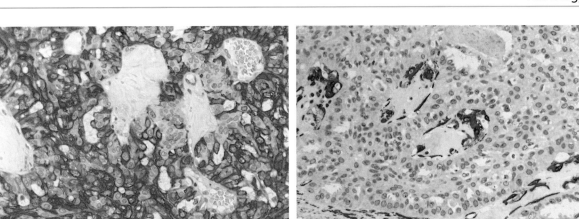

b

c

Fig. 11.14b–c An unusual case of a papilloma with associated usual ductal hyperplasia.
11.14b The same case immunostained for Ck5/6 with the typical patchwork pattern of usual ductal hyperplasia. In this area the myoepithelial cells are absent. In long-standing lesions such regression of myoepithelial cells may be found. This finding should not lead to a false diagnosis of malignancy.
11.14c Immunostaining for sm-actin which can only be identified in some basal and smooth muscle cells of small blood vessels. Note that the myoepithelial cell lining in this lesion is discontinuous. Myofibroblasts in the surrounding capsular stroma also immunostain for sm-actin.

VARIANTS OF PAPILLOMA

Epithelial and/or 'stromal' changes often lead to more complex papillomas, sometimes even to a distortion of the typical papillary structure of lesions.

PAPILLOMA WITH USUAL DUCTAL HYPERPLASIA OR METAPLASIA

Usual ductal hyperplasia or apocrine metaplasia (Fig. 11.12) are found in approximately 20–30% of cases. Less common changes include squamous, mucinous, clear cell and sebaceous gland metaplasia [19, 27, 35, 36, 41–43]. Epithelial proliferation is common in both central and peripheral papillomas [43]. When benign epithelial proliferation of usual type accumulates on the surface of the papillary structures, this may lead to a fenestrated or even solid cell mass. The papillary pattern of such cases may be completely obliterated, and the epithelial growth appears to be traversed by fibrovascular septa. The standard cytological, architectural and immunohisto-chemical criteria used to designate these epithelial proliferations as benign can be employed. Thus the lesions show immunostaining for Ck5/14 with the typical mosaicism pattern [42, 44] (Fig. 11.14a–c), (see Chapter 7). The epithelial cells also express vimentin. The histological patterns of solid papilloma should be interpreted with great caution to avoid misdiagnosing lesions as adenomyoepithelial tumors (see Chapter 14) and, more importantly, papillary-type DCIS.

PAPILLOMA WITH INFARCTION

Partial or complete infarction (Fig. 11.15a–b) of papilloma is common and may be associated with hemorrhagic debris and macrophages in the duct lumen [35, 41, 43, 45, 46]. This is often accompanied by squamous epithelial metaplasia [35], resulting in growth patterns that may lead to an incorrect diagnosis of carcinoma. It should be noted that these metaplasias originate from Ck5/14+ cells (see Chapter 3). Partial or total infarction may be the cause of serosanguinous discharge in central papillomas. In the event of complete necrosis, differentiation between benign and malignant lesions may become impossible. In such cases, the surrounding tissue should be carefully screened for signs of malignancy.

SCLEROSING PAPILLOMA

In cases of sclerosing papilloma, hyaline sclerosis of the intrinsic papillary structures with entrapment of irregular glandular myoepithelial tubules is commonly found. The glandular cells may exhibit enlarged nuclei of worrisome dimensions. As the myoepithelial cells may be inconspicuous in H&E sections, the compressed and distorted epithelial structures can simulate invasive carcinoma. As discussed in Chapter 9, the epithelial proliferations of such changes intensely stain for Ck5/14, both in the luminal and basal cell layer of the epithelial structures (Fig. 11.16a). The hyaline tissue contains collagen IV and laminin, typical

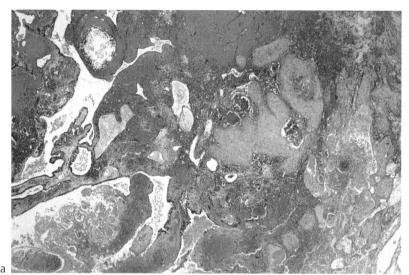

Fig. 11.15a – b Solitary papilloma showing infarction and intense squamous cell metaplasia.
11.15a Low power view with many papillary fronds showing hemorrhages and infarction and extensive squamous metaplasia.

a

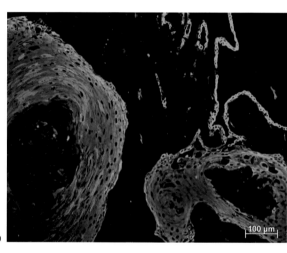

11.15b Squamous cell metaplasia in the same case as shown in 11.15a, double immunostained for Ck5/6 and Ck10. Squamous cell metaplasia is strongly positive for Ck5/6 and also expresses Ck10, indicative of squamous differentiation. Note the normal Ck5/6+ glandular epithelium in the right upper field.

b

components of basement membranes. Histologically, sclerosing papilloma often presents as a broad papillary mass with hyaline sclerosis of the papillary stalks. Occasionally, florid sclerosing adenosis may be seen around the ducts or even merging with the ductal papilloma.

PAPILLOMAS WITH REACTIVE PERIDUCTAL FIBROSIS
Periductal fibrosis (Fig. 11.16c), which is usually more cellular than the hyaline areas observed in the fibrovascular cores of sclerosing papilloma, probably originates as fibrosis secondary to focal necrosis or hemorrhage. It may also harbor distorted and irregular tubular epithelium, which may be mistaken for invasive carcinoma. Usually these tubules show a luminal and myoepithelial layer in H&E sections. Immunostaining for p63 and Ck5/14 is helpful in cases of papilloma with periductal fibrosis which are difficult to distinguish from tubular carcinoma (consistently Ck5/14–).

TUBULAR ADENOMA
Papilloma, tubular adenoma and adenomyoepithelioma seem to form a morphological continuum [6]

(Fig. 11.17). Areas with the classic morphological pattern of papilloma may merge with areas of tubular adenoma or adenomyoepithelioma. The final diagnosis rests on an identification of the overall features of the lesion (see Chapter 12).

DUCTAL ADENOMYOEPITHELIOMA
Papilloma may be associated with such an abundant proliferation of 'myoepithelial' cells that the term 'ductal adenomyoepithelioma' appears appropriate. The key feature of such lesions is that the myoepithelial cells of the papillary structures merge with the stroma of the papillary stalks. The myoepithelial cells may have a spindle, clear or epithelioid cell appearance (see Chapter 14). Immunohistochemically, the cells stain strongly for myoepithelial markers such as p63 or sm-actin and most cells coexpress Ck5 and Ck14, the latter being indicative of an overgrowth of Ck5/14+ myoepithelial progenitor cells (Ck5/14+ and sm-actin+), which differentiate to myoepithelial cells (sm-actin+).

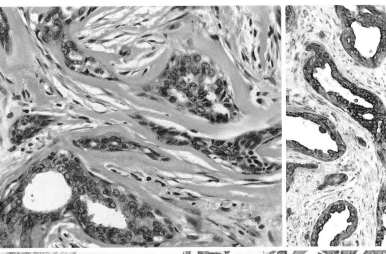

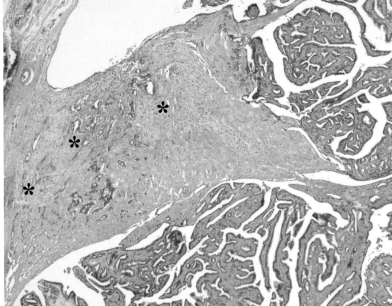

Fig. 11.16a–c Sclerosing papilloma and papilloma with periductal fibrosis.
11.16a Sclerosing papilloma with entrapment of irregular tubules. Such a lesion may be misdiagnosed as malignant. These tubules are, however, always Ck5/14+ and can thus be distinguished from Ck5/14– carcinoma.
11.16b The same case as 11.16a. Ck5 immunohistochemistry shows strong reactivity of both glandular and myoepithelial cells of the tubular structures, indicating their benign nature. In this case, p63 immunostaining revealed strong reactivity of the myoepithelial cells.

11.16c Papilloma with extensive periductal fibrosis and entrapped tubular structures in the left field (asterisks). If there is doubt as to the nature of the tubular structures immunostaining for myoepithelial markers and Ck5/14 usually helps to solve the problem.

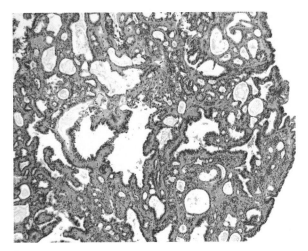

Fig. 11.17 Solitary papilloma with adenosis-like appearance. Low power view which shows a broad papilla with intense 'endophytic' inverse sprouting of the surface glandular-myoepithelial layer into the stroma of the papillary stalks, leading to the formation of irregularly sized tubular structures. The intertubular stroma is inconspicuous. If the whole lesion shows this pattern, a diagnosis of tubular adenoma may be appropriate.

JUVENILE PAPILLOMATOSIS

Juvenile papillomatosis is characterized by cysts and a combination of intraductal proliferation of UDH type, papillary lesions, and sclerosing adenosis (see Chapter 8).

IMMUNOHISTOCHEMISTRY

Papillomas have a similar immunophenotype to normal breast epithelium. The basal layer can be demonstrated using antibodies to sm-actin [26, 47], calponin, sm-myosin heavy chain, p63 or Ck5/14 (Figs 11.4 and 11.13) [48]. It is important to mention that sm-actin antibodies not only decorate the myo-epithelial cells, but also the smooth muscle cells of small vessels of the papillary stalks.

The glandular epithelium of papilloma displays Ck8/18 positivity, usually with a homogeneous expression in the luminal cells. The luminal epithelium may contain no or only few Ck5/14+ cells. However, if associated with usual ductal hyperplasia, the hyperplasic epithelium shows a typical Ck5/14 mosaicism (Figs 11.13 and 11.14). Furthermore, glandular and myoepithelial cells of the tubular structures of sclerosing papillary lesions and periductal fibrosis are usually strongly Ck5/14+. Estrogen and progesterone receptors are expressed by the luminal epithelium in a heterogeneous staining pattern.

MOLECULAR GENETICS

Papillomas appear to be clonal proliferations, as demonstrated by X-chromosomal analysis. Furthermore, chromosomal abnormalities such as loss of heterozygosity [49], microsatellite instability [50] and interstitial deletion of 3p [51] have been observed in benign papillomas.

ATYPICAL DUCTAL AND LOBULAR PROLIFERATION EX PAPILLOMA

WHO: Atypical papilloma

Several prominent physicians in breast pathology did not initially regard papilloma as premalignant due to the low prevalence of malignancy in these lesions [11, 41]. With the increase of pathological knowledge and the application of immunohistochemical markers it has become easier to appreciate the different types of intraductal epithelial lesions (see Chapter 8) and to recognize even minute lesions of atypical proliferations. The defining criteria of an atypical ductal or – extremely rare – lobular proliferation ex papilloma are:
1. recognition of residual benign papilloma;
2. identification of atypical epithelial proliferation within the benign papillary process (Fig. 11.18a–b).

To make a reliable diagnosis of malignancy in such cases, at least one or two low power fields should display convincing cytological and architectural atypicality with complex growth patterns characteristic of a DCIS. We would like to emphasize that atypical ductal proliferations ex benign papilloma often consist of cells with finely granular, eosinophilic cytoplasm, which may be misinterpreted as benign apocrine cells. Furthermore, benign papillary lesions may be found to contain the typical glandular-myoepithelial layers, but exhibit a focal appearance of clearly atypical glandular epithelium comparable to that described in the literature under the term 'flat epithelial atypia' (Figs 11.19a–b), (see Chapter 18). The neoplastic cells are usually columnar, and the nuclear/cytoplasmic ratio tends to be high with darkly staining, hyperchromatic and monomorphic nuclei. Apocrine apical blebs or truncated luminal cell margins may be present. Although, in some cases, mitoses may be found more readily in this type of epithelium, this is of no help in distinguishing it from the bland glandular epithelium of a benign papilloma. In all these lesions excluding malignancy in the adjacent breast tissue is mandatory.

As noted above, it has been shown by several authors that primarily benign peripheral papillomas are more susceptible to malignant transformation than central solitary papillomas [34, 52, 53].

INTERPRETATION OF CORE AND VACUUM-ASSISTED BIOPSIES

Because a variety of benign and malignant breast lesions may exhibit papillae and areas of sclerosis, both the architecture and the cytology of needle biopsy lesions must be carefully assessed in reaching an appropriate diagnosis. Full-blown papillary lesions are easily diagnosed in needle biopsies. In difficult cases H&E-stained sections at different levels and immunohistochemical staining may be helpful in reaching a final decision. On account of the intralesional heterogeneity of papillomas, the whole papillary lesion and the surrounding tissue must be assessed to exclude atypical ductal proliferations. As needle core and even vacuum-assisted biopsies usually do not provide sufficient material for a complete excision of the whole lesion with its surrounding normal tissue (excluding small microscopic papillomas), a surgical excision is more prudent in most cases. The majority of these lesions should, therefore, be classified as B3 (lesion of uncertain malignant potential).

The final judgment, however, on whether a small lesion has been successfully removed by extensive mammotome sampling can only be made by taking into account mammographic findings, requiring an

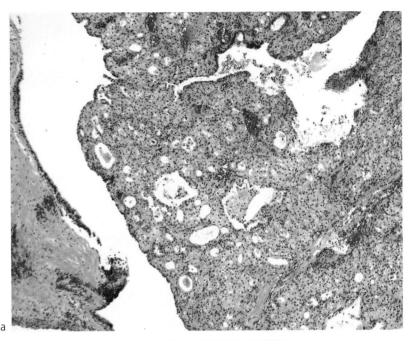

Fig. 11.18a – b Atypical ductal proliferation ex papilloma.

11.18a H&E-stained section showing solid to cribriform cell growth among some residual normal papillary epithelium with darker staining nuclei. Other areas contain typical benign papillary areas. On the left, the duct wall is composed of normal epithelium. Note that, with these lesions, it is mandatory to exclude malignancy in the adjacent breast tissue.

a

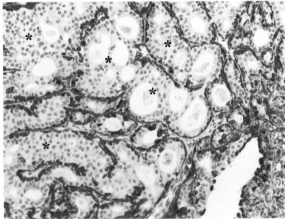

b

11.18b Immunostaining for Ck5/6 highlights the intensely stained basal myoepithelial layer. The atypical cells (asterisks) are Ck5/6– which, in this context, is indicative of neoplastic cell growth. This example demonstrates that the presence of myoepithelial cells does not always exclude malignancy.

interdisciplinary approach. In these cases a benign classification may be considered. Conversely, when a sample of a papillary lesion in a core biopsy shows atypical epithelial proliferations, a B4 designation may occasionally be more appropriate.

DIFFERENTIAL DIAGNOSIS

Surgical specimens should contain the whole papillary lesion along with a suitable amount of the surrounding normal breast tissue. A more conservative approach to treatment is justified when this normal tissue contains no evidence of atypical ductal proliferation. If, however, a lesion is identified as a papillary malignancy, appropriate therapeutic measures must be taken (see Chapters 22 and 27).

THE DIFFERENTIAL DIAGNOSTIC APPROACH

The classic histological features used to distinguish benign and malignant papillary lesions were first described by Kraus and Neubecker [11] and Azzopardi [41]. Neubecker reported that, in two series, approximately 10% of papillary lesions were erroneously misdiagnosed as malignant [11, 12]. The differential diagnoses should include papillary-type ductal carcinoma in-situ, atypical ductal proliferations (ADH/DCIS) ex papilloma and invasive papillary carcinoma. In this context, recognizing pseudoinvasion in sclerosing lesions and in reactive periductal fibrosis is particularly important. Furthermore, distinguishing papillomas with usual ductal hyperplasia from adenomyoepithelial lesions may pose a severe problem. In difficult cases of papillary lesions with an intraductal

Tab. 11.3 Contrasting features of benign papilloma and papillary type DCIS

	Papilloma	Papillary type DCIS
Epithelial cells	Glandular-myoepithelial surface epithelium. Glandular cells with bland normochromic nuclei. Apocrine change and usual ductal hyperplasia may be present.	Single cell population with nuclear hyperchromasia and striking nuclear uniformity. Stratified atypical cylindrical cells or cells with micropapillary, cribriform or solid cell growth. Basal neoplastic cells may be pagetoid in appearance (dimorphic pattern).
Myoepithelial cells	Myoepithelial layer always present.	Myoepithelial layer usually absent. Note, however, exceptions do exist.
Fibrovascular cores	Stroma is often well-developed.	Usually delicate stroma.
Surrounding tissue	Normal. May occur in combination with other types of benign proliferative breast disease.	Usually contains DCIS.
Immunostaining	Cells of basal layer immunostain for sm-actin, p63 and Ck5/14. Luminal cells may be negative for Ck5/14. Ck5/14 mosaicism in UDH.	Neoplastic cells express Ck8/18, but do not express Ck5/14.

epithelial proliferation, immunohistochemical staining may be used as an adjunct to routine evaluation by light microscopy. As papillary lesions may pose considerable difficulties, even on paraffin sections, frozensection diagnosis should be abandoned.

Examples

Papilloma vs. papillary-type ductal carcinoma in-situ

Distinguishing papilloma and papillary-type DCIS may occasionally be difficult [33]. The main distinguishing features are summarized in Table 11.3.

Important clues are:
1. the morphology of glandular cells covering the papillae;
2. the absence of a myoepithelial cell layer.

All other features represent additional clues leading to a correct diagnosis, but are relatively insignificant in problematic cases.

Glandular cell morphology

A benign epithelial proliferation should not be confused with the malignant proliferation of a papillary DCIS. The glandular cells of prototypical papillomas are cuboidal to cylindrical. They have regular round, normochromic nuclei, which are usually located basally.

A type of papillary carcinoma, likely to prove challenging at differential diagnosis, is the cylindrical cell variant of papillary carcinoma in-situ (Fig. 11.12). The cells lining this type of carcinoma are usually larger and more crowded. The cylindrical cells often show pseudostratification with nuclear hyperchromasia, high nuclear cytoplasmic ratio and nuclear uniformity. The tumor cells may show apical snouts. Careful attention to cellular details of the glandular cells is thus required for a correct diagnosis. Since papillomas often contain 'differentiated' glandular cells that lack expression of Ck5/14 and since the presence of myoepithelial cells does not, in principle, exclude malignancy, staining for p63 and Ck5/14 should be interpreted with the full histological context in mind (compare Fig. 11.19a–b).

The dimorphic pattern of papillary carcinoma (see Chapter 20) may also create problems in distinguishing it from papilloma with prominent myoepithelial cells. The basal tumor cells of such a pattern may be mistaken for myoepithelial cells. However, the coincidence of the two cell types seen in these tumors is the result of divergent glandular phenotypes, contrasting with the presence of two cell lineages as typically seen in benign papilloma (Fig. 11.20a–b). In this context, sm-actin or p63 immunostaining helps to identify the lesion as composed of only glandular cell type.

Papilloma with usual ductal hyperplasia must be distinguished from cribriform, solid and spindle cell papillary-type DCIS. In contrast to papilloma with associated usual ductal hyperplasia, cribriform, solid, and spindle cell papillary-type DCIS lesions are composed of a single cell population. The tumor cells are characterized by monotonous Ck5/14 negativity [27, 54, 55]. Usual ductal hyperplasia is characterized by a heterogeneous epithelial proliferation with great

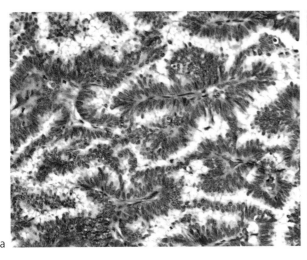
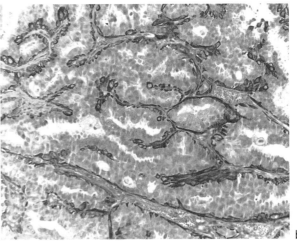

a   b

Fig. 11.19a–b Papillary type ductal carcinoma in-situ.
11.19a Papillary type DCIS. H&E-stained section with an arborizing papillary carcinoma. Note the typical appearance of malignant cylinder cell epithelium on the fine fibrovascular cores.
11.19b Papillary type DCIS from the same case as 11.19a, but immunostained for Ck5/14. Note the Ck5/14 negativity of the tumor cells and the strong reaction of the myoepithelial cell layer.

histological variability of its cellular and nuclear features and Ck5/14 mosaicism (Fig. 11.14). This is discussed in more detail in Chapter 8.

THE PRESENCE OF A MYOEPITHELIAL LAYER

Immunohistochemical staining of the myoepithelial layer may prove helpful, since it can usually be demonstrated in papillomas and is lacking in most papillary carcinomas. A rule of thumb is that papillary lesions lacking a myoepithelial lining can be interpreted as carcinomas, whereas most benign papillomas do contain a clearly recognizable myoepithelial cell layer. However, the presence of myoepithelial cells in papillary lesions does not, in principle, exclude malignancy (Figs 11.18 and 11.19) [26]. Lesions of early papillary-type DCIS, in particular, and those with focal atypical proliferation may display a well-shaped myoepithelial cell layer. In such cases, the epithelial features are most important in distinguishing papillary-type DCIS from its benign counterparts.

It is certainly true, that well-stained smooth muscle cells of small blood vessels and myofibroblasts may be difficult to distinguish from myoepithelial cells. In such cases, specific immunohistochemical myoepithelial markers such as p63 or Ck5/14 may be of more help in reaching a correct diagnosis (Fig. 11.19).

PAPILLOMA VS. ATYPICAL DUCTAL PROLIFERATION (ADH/DCIS) EX PAPILLOMA (PAPILLOMA WITH ADH/DCIS)

In some cases, a malignant transformation of a pre-existing benign papillary lesion can be demonstrated (Fig. 11.18). The same criteria discussed in the first differential diagnosis also apply to the detection of focal areas of malignant growth. Features that should be sought for are monomorphic epithelial proliferations between the papillary stalks. As atypical proliferations are nearly always negative for Ck5/14, immunostaining is instrumental in distinguishing them from benign epithelial proliferation. Myoepithelial markers are not helpful in such cases due to the presence of a myoepithelial layer [33].

SCLEROSING PAPILLOMA VS. INVASIVE CARCINOMA

Fibrosis and sclerosis with entrapped epithelial tubules are often seen within papillae and in periductal tissue of larger involved ducts. In addition, papillomas may merge with sclerosing adenosis or may be part of a radial scar. Such lesions should be interpreted with care. H&E-stained sections usually allow detection of a compressed myoepithelial cell layer around the entrapped tubules. Sometimes, findings are inconclusive, and even features such as comparatively large nuclei are insufficient evidence in reaching a conclusive diagnosis. As discussed in Chapter 9, sm-actin and Ck5/14 immunostaining play a key role in the identification of the entrapped benign epithelial structures (Figs 11.16a–b). To avoid overinterpretation

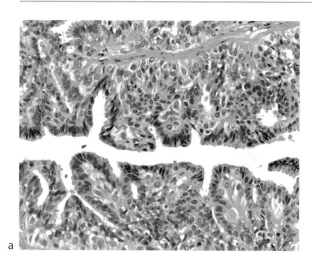

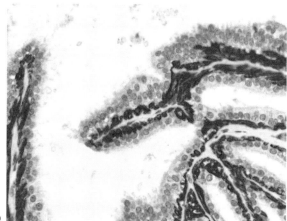

Fig. 11.20a–b Papilloma with prominent myoepithelial layer.
11.20a H&E staining showing a prominent differentiation of two different cell types. The luminal cells display features of cylindrical and basal cells with large nuclei and polygonal, vacuolated cytoplasm. As this lesion mimics the dimorphic pattern of papillary type DCIS, immunostaining for myoepithelial markers may be helpful.
11.20b Ck5 immunostaining discloses a prominent myoepithelial cell layer. Identical results were obtained with myoepithelial markers such as p63 or calponin. Based on these findings the lesion was interpreted as benign.

of malignancy in difficult cases, especially wide-bore needle biopsies, immunostaining for myoepithelial markers and/or cytokeratin 5/14 may be necessary (also see Chapter 13). The feature that distinguishes sclerosing papilloma from cancer is the detection of these antigens in the epithelial cell proliferations which, in our experience, is diagnostic for benign lesions (Fig. 11.16). In contrast, tubular carcinoma, invasive lobular and cribriform carcinoma have a glandular phenotype with expression of Ck8/18, but not of Ck5/14, and, furthermore, they lack a myoepithelial cell layer.

PAPILLOMA WITH EXTENSIVE UDH VS. ADENOMYOEPITHELIOMA

Papilloma with UDH and some adenomyoepithelial tumors may cause problems in differential diagnosis. In H&E-stained sections it may be impossible to distinguish between these lesions as they all contain a considerable amount of spindle cells. To render a diagnosis of an adenomyoepithelial tumor, the myoepithelial lineage differentiation of the proliferating cells must be demonstrated by staining for Ck5/14 and a myoepithelial marker (see Chapter 14), whereas in usual ductal hyperplasia the glandular lineage must be visualized by Ck5/14 and Ck8/18 immunohistochemistry (see Chapter 8).

PAPILLOMA WITH EXTENSIVE UDH VS. PAPILLARY DCIS WITH SQUAMOUS DIFFERENTIATION

Distinguishing between these two types of lesion is a particular pitfall as the proliferating cells of both show intense Ck5/14 reactivity. Squamous cell papillary carcinomas are exceptionally rare. The only two lesions we have ever witnessed had clearly identifiable papillary connective tissue cores covered by a high grade atypical epithelium with individually keratinizing cells. The distinguishing features are clear malignancy of squamous tumors with clearly malignant nuclei and mitoses. Furthermore, Ck10 highlights individual or groups of keratinizing cells. Squamous metaplasia in ductal hyperplasia may occur but usually displays a more organoid keratinization than those metaplastic cells of atypical lesions which show the cellular and nuclear features discussed in Chapter 8. Ck5/14 immunostains are of little help in this differential diagnostic problem.

REFERENCES

1. Muir R. The evolution of carcinoma of the mama. J Pathol Bacteriol L II 1945;2:155–72.
2. Lammie GA, Millis RR. Ductal adenoma of the breast – a review of fifteen cases. Hum Pathol 1989;20:903–8.
3. Sandison AT. A study of surgically removed specimens of breast, with special reference to sclerosing adenosis. J Clin Pathol 1958;11:101–9.
4. Sloane JP. Biopsy Pathology of the Breast. Vol. 24, 2nd edition ed. London: Arnold; 2001.
5. Woods ER, Helvie MA, Ikeda DM, et al. Solitary breast papilloma: comparison of mammographic, galactographic, and pathologic findings. Am J Roentgenol 1992;159:487–91.
6. Cardenosa G, Eklund GW. Benign papillary neoplasms of the breast: mammographic findings. Radiology 1991; 181:751–5.
7. Kilgore AR, Fleming R, Ramos MD. The incidence of cancer with nipple discharge and the risk of cancer in the presence of papillary disease of the breast. Surg Gynaecol Obstet 1953;96:649–60.

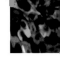
8. Moore SW, Pearce J, Ring E. Intraductal papilloma of the breast. Surg Gynaecol Obstet 1961;112:153–8.

9. Lewison EF, Lyons JJ. Relationship between benign breast disease and cancer. Arch Surg 1953;66:94–114.

10. Hendrick JW. Intraductal papilloma of the breast. Surg Gynaecol Obstet 1957;105:215–23.

11. Kraus FT, Neubecker RB. The differential diagnosis of papillary tumors of the breast. Cancer 1962;15:444–55.

12. Haagensen CD, Stout AP, Philips JS. The papillary neoplasms of the breast. Ann Surg 1951;133:18–36.

13. Azzopardi JG. Problems in Breast Pathology. 1st ed. London: W.B. Saunders; 1979.

14. Page DL, Dupont WD. Premalignant conditions and markers of elevated risk in the breast and their management. Surg Clin North Am 1990;70:831–51.

15. Murad TM, Swaid S, Pritchett P. Malignant and benign papillary lesions of the breast. Hum Pathol 1977; 8:379–90.

16. Rosen PP. Papillary duct hyperplasia of the breast in children and young adults. Cancer 1985;56:1611–7.

17. Betta PG, Merlini E, Seymandi PL. Juvenile papillomatosis of the breast in a 2 1/2 year-old female infant after exposure to an estrogen ointment. Breast Dis 1993;6:207–10.

18. Lanyi M. Diagnosis and differential diagnosis of breast calcifications. Berlin, Heidelberg, New York: Springer; 1986.

19. Jiao YF, Nakamura S, Oikawa T, Sugai T, Uesugi N. Sebaceous gland metaplasia in intraductal papilloma of the breast. Virchows Arch 2001;438:505–8.

20. Carter DJ. Intraductal Papillary Tumors of the Breast. A Study of 78 Cases. Cancer 1977;39:1689–92.

21. Rosen PP, Caicco JA. Florid papillomatosis of the nipple. A study of 51 patients, including nine with mammary carcinoma. Am J Surg Pathol 1986; 10:87–101.

22. Ciatto S, Andreoli C, Cirillo A, et al. The risk of breast cancer subsequent to histologic diagnosis of benign intraductal papilloma follow-up study of 339 cases. Tumori 1991;77:41–3.

23. Hart D. Intracystic papillomatous tumors of the breast. A study of 78 cases. Arch Surg 1927;14:793–835.

24. Buhl JS, Fischermann K, Johansen H, Petersen B. Cancer risk in intraductal papilloma and papillomatosis. Surg Gynecol Obstet 1968;127:1307–12.

25. Page DL, Salhany KE, Jensen RA, Dupont WD. Subsequent breast carcinoma risk after biopsy with atypia in a breast papilloma. Cancer 1996;78:258–66.

26. Raju U, Vertes D. Breast papillomas with atypical ductal hyperplasia: a clinicopathologic study. Hum Pathol 1996;27:1231–8.

27. Murad TM, Contesso G, Mouriesse H. Papillary tumors of large lactiferous ducts. Cancer 1981;48:122–33.

28. Wellings SR, Jensen HM, Marcum RG. An atlas of subgross pathology of the human breast with special reference to possible precancerous lesions. J Natl Cancer Inst 1975;55:231–73.

29. Tavassoli FA, Norris HJ. A Comparison of the Results of Long-Term Follow-Up for Atypical Intraductal Hyperplasia and Intraductal Hyperplasia of the Breast. Cancer 1990;65:518–29.

30. Tavassoli FA, Norris HJ. Intraductal apocrine carcinoma: a clinicopathologic study of 37 cases. Mod Pathol 1994;7:813–8.

31. Ohuchi N, Abe R, Kasai M. Possible cancerous change of intraductal papillomas of the breast. A 3-D reconstruction study of 25 cases. Cancer 1984;54:605–11.

32. Ali-Fehmi R, Carolin K, Wallis T, Visscher DW. Clinicopathologic analysis of breast lesions associated with multiple papillomas. Hum Pathol 2003;34:234–9.

33. Papotti M, Gugliotta P, Ghiringhello B, Bussolati G. Association of breast carcinoma and multiple intraductal papillomas: A histological and immunohistochemical investigation. Histopathol 1984;8:963–75.

34. Schnitt SJ, Conolly JL. Pathology of benign breast disorders. In: Harris JR, editor. Diseases of the Breast. 2004.

35. Flint A, Oberman HA. Infarction and squamous metaplasia of intraductal papilloma: a benign breast lesion that may simulate carcinoma. Human Pathology 1984;15:764–7.

36. Rosen PP. Rosen's Breast Pathology. 2nd ed. Philadelphia: Lippincott Williams & Wilkins; 2001.

37. Smith BH, Taylor HB. The occurence of bone and cartilage in mammary tumors. Am J Clin Pathol 1969; 51:610–8.

38. Maluf HM, Koerner FC. Solid papillary carcinoma of the breast. A form of intraductal carcinoma with endocrine differentiation frequently associated with mucinous carcinoma. Am J Surg Pathol 1995;19:1237–44.

39. Maluf HM, Zukerberg LR, Dickersin GR, Koerner FC. Spindle-cell argyrophilic mucin-producing carcinoma of the breast. Histological, ultrastructural, and immunohistochemical studies of two cases. Am J Surg Pathol 1991;15:677–86.

40. Tsang WY, Chan JK. Endocrine ductal carcinoma in-situ (E-DCIS) of the breast: a form of low grade DCIS with distinctive clinicopathologic and biologic characteristics. Am J Surg Pathol 1996;20:921–43.

41. Azzopardi JG. Papilloma and papillary carcinoma. In: Problems in Breast Pathology. 1st ed. Philadelphia: WB Saunders; 1979. p.150–66.

42. Raju UB, Lee MW, Zarbo RJ, Crissman JD. Papillary neoplasia of the breast: immunohistochemically defined myoepithelial cells in the diagnosis of benign and malignant papillary breast neoplasms. Mod Pathol 1989; 2:569–76.

43. Tavassoli FA. Papillary Lesions. In: Pathology of the Breast. 2nd ed. Stanford: Appleton & Lange; 1999. p.325–71.

44. Boecker W, Moll R, Dervan P, et al. Usual ductal hyperplasia of the breast is a committed stem (progenitor) cell lesion distinct from atypical ductal hyperplasia and ductal carcinoma in-situ. J Pathol 2002; 198:458–67.

45. Rosen PP. Papilloma and Related Benign Tumors. In: Rosen's Breast Pathology. 2nc ed. Philadelphia: Lippincott Williams & Wilkins; 2001. p.77–119.

46. Walker AN, Betsill WL. Infarction of intraductal papilloma associated with hyperprolactinemia. Arch Pathol Lab Med 1980;104:280.

47. Papotti M, Macri L, Bussolati G, Reubi JC. Correlative study on neuro-endocrine differentiation and presence of

somatostatin receptors in breast carcinomas. Int J Cancer 1989;43:365–9.

48. Otterbach F, Bankfalvi A, Bergner S, et al. Cytokeratin 5/6 immunohistochemistry assists the differential diagnosis of atypical proliferations of the breast. Histopathol 2000;37:232–40.

49. Lininger RA, Park WS, Man YG, et al. LOH at 16p13 is a novel chromosomal alteration detected in benign and malignant microdissected papillary neoplasms of the breast. Hum Pathol 1998;29:1113–8.

50. Kasami M, Vnencak-Jones CL, Manning S, Dupont WD, Page DL. Loss of heterozygosity and microsatellite instability in breast hyperplasia. No obligate correlation of these genetic alterations with subsequent malignancy. Am J Pathol 1997;150:1925–32.

51. Dietrich CU, Pandis N, Teixeira MR, et al. Chromosome abnormalities in benign hyperproliferative disorders of epithelial and stromal breast tissue. Int J Cancer 1995;60:49–53.

52. O'Malley FP, Page DL, Nelson EH, Dupont WD. Ductal Carcinoma In-Situ of the Breast With Apocrine Cytology. Definition of a Borderline Category. Hum Pathol 1994;25:164–8.

53. Rosner D, Lane WW, Penetrante R. Ductal carcinoma in-situ with microinvasion. A curable entity using surgery alone without need for adjuvant therapy. Cancer 1991;67:1498–503.

54. Carter D, Orr SL, Merino MJ. Intracystic papillary carcinoma of the breast. After mastectomy, radiotherapy or excisional biopsy alone. Cancer 1983;52:14–9.

55. Lefkowitz M, Lefkowitz W, Wargotz ES. Intraductal (intracystic) papillary carcinoma of the breast and its variants: a clinicopathological study of 77 cases. Hum Pathol 1994;25:802–9.

Content

12

ADENOMA OF THE BREAST AND VARIANTS

WERNER BOECKER AND UTE KETTRITZ

Adenomas of the breast are benign epithelial tumors consisting of cells with glandular (luminal) and myoepithelial (abluminal) differentiation, a basement membrane and a small amount of stroma. These tumors usually form tubular structures and are well-circumscribed. They present clinically as a slowly growing, painless mass.

Adenoma of the breast and variants

◼ DEFINITION

WHO: Adenoma
   ICD-O code: 8211/0 (tubular adenoma)
   ICD-O code: 8204/0 (lactating adenoma)
   ICD-O code: 8401/0 (apocrine adenoma)
   ICD-O code: 8503/0 (ductal adenoma)

The term 'tubular adenoma' is applied to benign epithelial tumors composed entirely of uniform, acinar or tubular structures, which are lined by a glandular/myoepithelial cell layer (Fig. 12.1). Variants are tubular, ductal and basal cell adenoma. They are solid lesions that are thought to derive from ductules of terminal duct lobular units. In 1984, Azzopardi and Salm [1] described a solid benign lesion of the breast ducts, proposing the term 'ductal adenoma'. Further studies extended these observations. Such lesions can be interpreted as variants of papillary lesions [2, 3]. A further variant is basal cell adenoma.

Adenomas are characterized by formation of tubular and/or alveolar structures with typical luminal and myoepithelial cell lining, surrounded by a basement membrane. The tubules are separated by a scant stroma [4]. Changes in the glandular epithelium may modify the appearance of adenomas, resulting in lactating, apocrine or clear cell adenomas [5, 6]. In addition, the luminal layer may show usual epithelial hyperplasia. A further type of mammary adenoma, the basal cell adenoma, is more commonly found in the salivary gland and is an exceptionally rare finding in the breast. It is characterized by anastomosing tubular to trabecular structures consisting nearly mainly of Ck5+ and Ck8/18– basal type cell proliferations. Combinations with papillomas and fibroadenomas may be found.

◼ CONCEPTUAL APPROACH

Cell biologically, the prototypical adenoma is characterized by acinar/tubular structures, which display a double epithelial layer of glandular and myoepithelial cells surrounded by a basement membrane. Data from double fluorescence experiments clearly shows that the cellular phenotypes of the tubular structures and of normal resting breast epithelium are identical. Thus the histoarchitectural symmetry of the epithelial double layer and its basement membrane is preserved. The tubular structures consist of Ck5/14+ cells, intermediate glandular cells (Ck5/14+ and Ck8/18+) and phenotypically differentiated glandular cells (Ck8/18+) in the luminal layer, as well as intermediate myoepithelial cells (Ck5/14+ and sm-actin+) and myoepithelial end cells (sm-actin+) in the outer layer (Figs 12.2

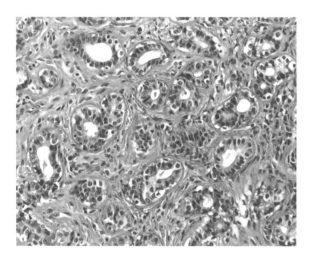

Fig. 12.1 Tubular adenoma shows tubular structures lined by a double layer of glandular and myoepithelial cells with scant fibrous tissue. This example also contains a focal inflammatory reaction with lymphocytes and plasma cells.

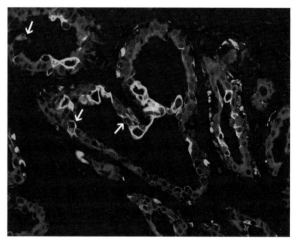

Fig. 12.2 Ductal adenoma. Double staining for Ck5 (green signal) and Ck8/18 (red signal). The glandular structures contain mainly Ck8/18+ cells. Few cells express Ck5 (green signal), indicative of progenitor cells (arrows). In the outer layer the myoepithelial cells stain weakly for Ck5 (green signal). The cell layers are organized in exactly the same way as in normal resting breast epithelium.

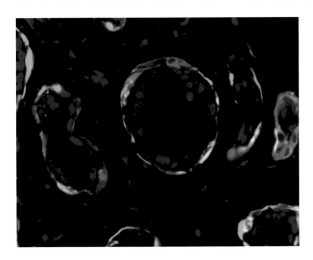

Fig. 12.3 Double staining for Ck5 (red signal) and sm-actin (green signal). Some of the myoepithelial cells express mainly Ck5 (red signal) or both Ck5 and sm-actin (hybrid signal), which is typical of cells of the myoepithelial differentiation pathway. The luminal cells in this area are not stained, indicating that they are differentiated glandular cells.

and 12.3). As described in Chapter 11, the development of ductal adenomas seems to be related to papillomas. Thus some of these lesions might develop by an inverse proliferation of tubular structures into the stroma of the papillary stalk. Lammie and Millis [3] compare the spectrum of changes seen in ductal adenomas with those observed in adenosis. It therefore seems likely that similar developmental mechanisms are at work in tubular adenomas (compare Chapter 11).

In the rare basal cell adenoma the trabecular/tubular structures consist mainly of Ck5+ basal-type cells, which are surrounded by a layer of myoepithelial cells.

■ CLINICAL FEATURES AND IMAGING

CLINICAL FEATURES

Adenomas are very rare benign epithelial tumors of the breast. They present as a circumscribed or nodular mass, which is indistinguishable from fibroadenoma on mammography and ultrasound. The size of tumors ranges from 1 to 4 cm. Similar to fibroadenomas these lesions usually occur in younger females [7]. The age of patients presenting with ductal adenoma ranges from 22 to 77 years, with a mean of 51 years [3, 1]. Adenomas may rarely be seen bilaterally [8]. Although cases of malignancy have been described in adenomas [4, 9–11], there is agreement that adenomas are not considered to be a risk factor for subsequent development of cancer [3, 4, 12].

IMAGING

MAMMOGRAPHY

Tubular adenomas in younger women present as well-circumscribed masses similar in appearance to noncalcified fibroadenomas [7, 13]. They are usually well-circumscribed, round or lobulated masses with smooth margins (Fig. 12.4). In older women, tubular adenomas may resemble malignant masses with microcalcifications. Soo et al. [13] found microcalcifications, initially considered suspicious of malignancy, in three of five tubular adenomas in older women detected by screening. The microcalcifications were dense, punctate or irregular without cast-like or branching forms and tightly grouped within a nonpalpable mass.

ULTRASOUND

On ultrasound, tubular adenomas are similar to fibroadenomas. They present as well-circumscribed, oval or lobulated, solid masses with a homogeneous hypoechoic structure and without posterior acoustic shadowing (Fig. 12.5). Sound transmission can be enhanced or equal to that of the surrounding tissue. In older, calcified adenomas, sonographic features can resemble malignant lesions as a result of ill-defined margins and posterior acoustic shadowing [13].

MAGNET RESONANCE IMAGING

Similar to fibroadenomas, tubular adenomas show enhancement in magnetic resonance imaging. Uptake

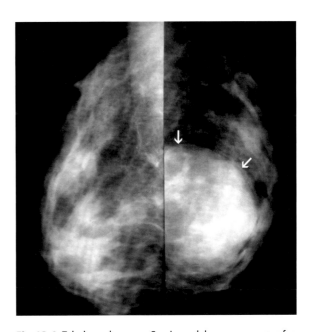

Fig. 12.4 Tubular adenoma. Craniocaudal mammogram of a 35-year-old woman with a palpable nodule, showing a round, well-defined mass (arrows) similar in appearance to that of fibroadenoma.

of contrast agent may vary. Even though a delayed type of enhancement is considered to be characteristic of adenomas [14, 15], there is a far-reaching overlap in the appearance of benign and malignant lesions. Malignancy may not be distinguishable from adenomas with strong enhancement [16].

CLASSIFICATION

The typical mammographic appearance with well-defined margins places adenomas in category 3 of the BI-RADS classification of the American College of Radiology [17]. These lesions have a very low probability of malignancy and imaging follow-up may be sufficient. If imaging findings are not typical or the lesion is increasing in size, core needle biopsy is recommended to exclude malignancy [13, 16].

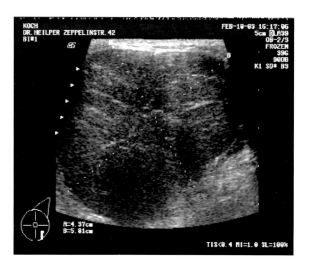

Fig. 12.5 Ultrasound shows a fairly well-circumscribed solid mass with a homogeneous hypoechoic structure.

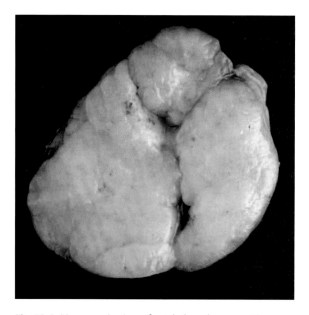

Fig. 12.6 Macroscopic view of a tubular adenoma with a gray cut surface.

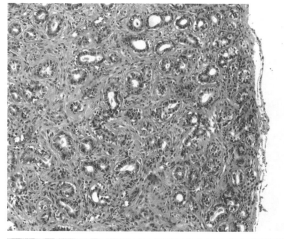

a

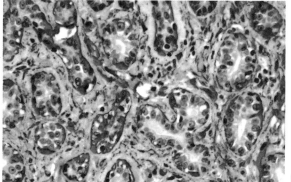

b

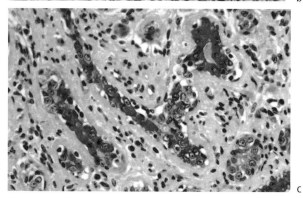

c

Fig. 12.7a–c Tubular adenoma.
12.7a Low power view showing the characteristic composition of acinar structures and scant fibrous stroma. A typical capsule is not present.
12.7b Immunostaining for collagen IV. In contrast to adenomyoepithelial tumors the tubular structures are sharply delineated from the stroma.
12.7c Immunostaining for Ck5 highlights the myoepithelial and luminal cells which in part express Ck5. The myoepithelial cells form a continuous outer layer which is heavily stained for sm-actin (not shown here).

PATHOLOGY

MACROSCOPY

Tubular adenoma presents as a circumscribed mass with a uniform gray-white to yellowish, often gritty cut surface [3] (Fig. 12.6). Ductal adenoma, which arises in the interlobular or larger ducts, is typically encapsulated, and in half of cases consists of multiple, discontinuous nodules [1]. Occasionally the lesion may be found in a cystically dilated ductal lumen.

MICROSCOPY

TUBULAR ADENOMA

The prototypical tubular adenoma is a well-demarcated lesion sometimes surrounded by a thin capsule. The histological appearance consists of narrow tubular structures with luminal glandular cells enveloped by myoepithelial cells and a basement membrane (Fig. 12.7a–c) [4]. The luminal cells are indistinguishable from the epithelium of normal lobules. The luminal layer may consist mainly of Ck8/18+ glandular cells or may be more immature with many interspersed Ck5/14+ cells (Fig. 12.7c). The myoepithelial cell layer and the myofibroblasts of the stroma stain for sm-actin. In contrast to adenomyoepitheliomas, where the myoepithelial cells submerge in the supporting stroma, the individual tubules of the adenoma are well-delineated and set apart from the scant fibrovascular stroma. In lactating adenomas, the luminal epithelium is vacuolated with some secretory material being found in the lumen [18, 19]. In apocrine adenomas typical apocrine metaplastic change is found [9, 11, 20].

DUCTAL ADENOMA

The ductal adenoma prototype consists of single or multiple adenomatous nodules. These are encapsulated with an occasionally thickened and fibrosed capsule (Fig. 12.8), which in special stains reveals the presence of fragmented elastica. The adenoma may obliterate the ductal lumen, or it may be present as a nodule in one or several broad papillary stalks connected to the walls by a fibrous basis (Fig. 12.9). The tubules are lined by inner glandular cells and an outer layer of myoepithelial cells. They may be cystically dilated or compressed. Occasionally and some form of lactating, clear cell, or apocrine change (Fig. 12.10) and usual ductal hyperplasia can be observed making the overall appearance less orderly than in tubular adenoma. The relative proportion of stroma and epithelium varies. Sometimes

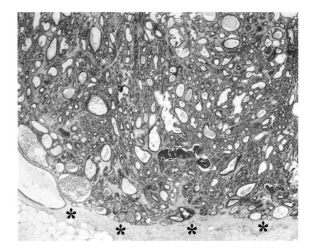

Fig. 12.8 Ductal adenoma showing more complex proliferation of ductular structures with some cystically dilated tubules. Ductal adenomas are usually well-circumscribed with a fibrous capsule (asterisks).

Tab. 12.1 Tubular adenoma

Definition	Tumor consisting of acinar or tubular glandular elements with scant fibrous tissue.
Cellular composition	Bilayer with glandular cells and myoepithelial progeny cells and a basement membrane.
Extracellular matrix	Scant fibrous tissue. May contain myofibroblasts (sm-actin+).
Immunohistochemistry	Ck5/14+, Ck8/18+, sm-actin+, collagen IV+.
Variants	Lactating, apocrine and basal-cell types.
Core biopsies/B-classification	B2
Differential diagnosis	Adenomyoepithelial tumors, solid papilloma.

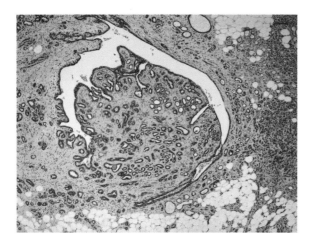

Fig. 12.9 An interlobular dilated duct showing a broad papillary stalk with glandular structures, which some experts might refer to as ductal adenoma. We tend to use the term 'papilloma' or 'sclerosing papilloma' for this lesion. This lesion is surrounded by areas of sclerosing adenosis, which are similar in appearance to the papillary structures.

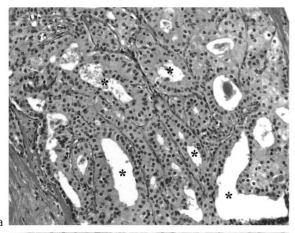

a

Fig. 12.10a – b Apocrine ductal adenoma.
12.10a The tubular structures (asterisks) are composed of apocrine and barely recognizable myoepithelial cells. Although the apocrine cells show some intraluminal proliferation, the complex growth pattern needed for a diagnosis of atypical apocrine hyperplasia is not present.

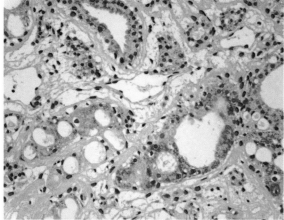

b

12.10b Immunostaining for p63 highlights the nuclear expression of this protein in myoepithelial cells. The apocrine cells show some non-specific granular staining in the cytoplasm.

BASAL CELL ADENOMA

Basal cell adenomas are very rare benign tumors composed of basaloid cells sharply delineated from the surrounding stroma by an eosinophilic hyaline sheath that is made up of basement membrane material (Fig. 12.11). The lesions may show a solid papillary structure and exhibit compact monotonous trabecular growth patterns similar to those described in basal cell adenomas of the parotid gland [21]. The broad trabecular structures are composed of distinctive,

the center of the lesion may show a fibrous hyaline scar with entrapped or distorted tubular structures. Myxoid change or chondroid metaplasia are rare [3]. Peripheral fibrosis may be considerable with entrapment of epithelial structures similar to the appearance seen in ductal papillomas, which may produce worrying pseudoinfiltrative patterns. Azzopardi and Salm also described a further type of ductal adenoma [1], which, although well-delineated and smoothly contoured, does not seem to be clearly ductal in origin.

somewhat monotonous Ck5/14+ basal-type cells. In contrast to usual ductal hyperplasia the basaloid cells can also express p63. Myoepithelial markers are confined to the outer border of the trabecular structures. The inner cells can show a glandular differentiation which is highlighted by expression of Ck8/18. Squamous cell metaplasia may also be present. Tumors may show an interposition of hyaline material among the tumor cells. Thus, these lesions must also be distinguished from adenoid cystic carcinoma. Lack of infiltration, a still recognizable organoid pattern and the presence of an obvious basement membrane around the epithelial proliferations all favor a diagnosis of basal cell adenoma.

■ IMMUNOHISTOCHEMISTRY

Immunohistochemically, classic adenoma displays the typical Ck5/14, Ck8/18 and sm-actin staining patterns well-known from the resting breast epithelium. The luminal cells express Ck8/18 as well as, to various degrees, Ck5/14. The myoepithelial layer usually contains a great number of Ck5/14+ and sm-actin+ cells. Estrogen shows a heterogeneous expression, often with only focal positivity of luminal cells.

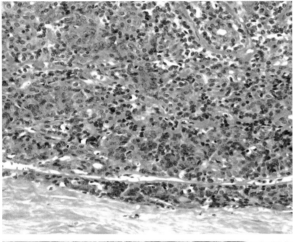

a

Fig. 12.11a−e Basal cell adenoma.
12.11a Low power view of a lesion rich in basal-type cells and poor in stroma. Broad trabecular epithelial proliferations with a fibrous capsule. In contrast to papilloma with usual ductal hyperplasia, the proliferating epithelial cells have a more monotonous basaloid appearance.
12.11b Immunostaining for Ck5/14. Note the intense staining for Ck5/14 of many epithelial cells close to the papillary stalks. The Ck5/14 mosaicism of usual ductal hyperplasia is not seen.
12.11c Immunostaining for Ck8/18. Only luminal cells show a glandular differentiation with expression of Ck8/18. The basaloid cells are negative. Transitions from basal cells to these glandular luminal cells cannot be convincingly demonstrated.
12.11d Immunostaining for collagen IV showing a papillary ground structure with fine papillary stalks.
12.11e Immunostaining for p63 shows intense staining of the smaller basaloid cells close to the papillary stromal stalks.

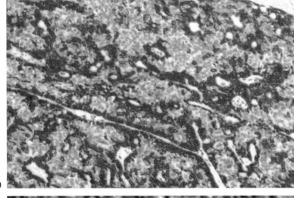

b

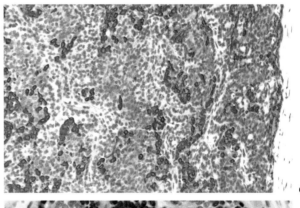

c

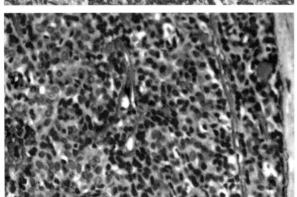

d

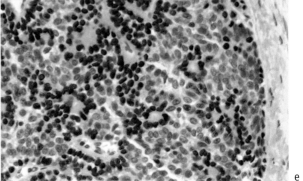

e

■ INTERPRETATION OF CORE AND VACUUM-ASSISTED NEEDLE BIOPSIES

The appropriate category for adenoma is B2.

■ DIFFERENTIAL DIAGNOSIS

Typical adenoma poses no difficulty at diagnosis. The main diagnostic challenge facing the pathologist is to distinguish adenoma from differentiated tubular adenomyoepithelioma. However, the tubular structures of adenoma have the characteristic spatial order of normal breast epithelium with a bilayer and a basement membrane, in contrast to adenomyoepithelial tumors in which the myoepithelial cells disperse ('melt') into the surrounding stroma. Differential diagnosis of basal cell adenoma must consider solid papilloma associated with extensive usual ductal hyperplasia obliterating the papillary structure. The latter shows the characteristic Ck5/14 mosaicism not seen in basal cell adenomas.

REFERENCES

1. Azzopardi JG, Salm R. Ductal adenoma of the breast: a lesion which can mimic carcinoma. J Pathol 1984; 144:15–23.
2. Gusterson BA, Middwood C, Gazet JC, et al. Ductal adenoma of the breast – a lesion exhibiting a myoepithelial/epithelial phenotype. Histopathol 1987;11:103–10.
3. Lammie GA, Millis RR. Ductal adenoma of the breast – a review of fifteen cases. Hum Pathol 1989;20:903–8.
4. Hertel BF, Zaloudek C, Kempson RI. Breast Adenomas. Cancer 1976;37:2891–905.
5. Tesluk H, Amott T, Goodnight JE. Apocrine Adenoma of the Breast. Arch Pathol Lab Med 1986;110:351–2.
6. De Potter CR, Cuvelier CA, Roels HJ. Apocrine adenoma presenting as gynaecomastia in a 14-year-old boy. Histopathol 1988;13:697–9.
7. Nishimori H, Sasaki M, Hirata K, et al. Tubular adenoma of the breast in a 73-year-old woman. Breast Cancer 2000;7:169–72.
8. Tavassoli FA. Pathology of the Breast. 2nd ed. Norwalk: Appleton and Lange; 1999.
9. Costa A. Una variante non conosciuta di adenoma puro della ghiandola mammaria: l'adenoma puro a cellule apocrine (con una classificazione degli adenomi mammari) [A little known variant of pure adenoma of the breast: pure apocrine cell adenoma (with a classification of breast adenomas)]. Arch De Vecchi Anat Patol 1974;60:393–401.
10. Hill RP, Miller FN. Adenomas of the breast. Cancer 1954;7:318–24.
11. Rosen PP. Proliferative breast "disease". An unresolved diagnostic dilemma. Cancer 1993;71:3798–807.
12. Geschickter CF. Diseases of the Breast. Diagnosis-Pathology-Treatment. 2nd ed. Philadelphia: JB Lippincott; 1945.
13. Soo MS, Dash N, Bentley R, Lee LH, Nathan G. Tubular adenomas of the breast: imaging findings with histologic correlation. AJR Am J Roentgenol 2000; 174:757–61.
14. Stack JP, Redmond OM, Codd MB, Dervan PA, Ennis JT. Breast disease: tissue characterization with Gd-DTPA enhancement profiles. Radiology 1990;174: 491–4.
15. Heywang SH, Wolf A, Pruss E, et al. MR imaging of the breast with Gd-DTPA: use and limitations. Radiology 1989;171:95–103.
16. Heywang-Köbrunner S, Schreer I. Bildgebende Mammadiagnostik. Georg Thieme Verlag; 1996.
17. American College of Radiology. Illustrated breast imaging report and data system (BI-RADS). 3rd ed. Reston, VA.: American College of Radiology; 1998.
18. James K, Bridger J, Anthony PP. Breast tumour of pregnancy ('lactating' adenoma). J Pathol 1988;156: 37–44.
19. Slavin JL, Billson VR, Ostor AG. Nodular breast lesions during pregnancy and lactation. Histopathol 1993; 22:481–5.
20. Lui M, Dahlstrom JE, Bell S, James DT. Apocrine adenoma of the breast: diagnosis on large core needle biopsy. Pathology 2001;33:149–52.
21. Cheuk W, Chan JKC. Salivary gland tumors. In: Fletcher CDM, editor. Diagnostic Histopathology of Tumors. 2nd ed. London, Edinburgh, New York: Churchill Livingstone; 2000. p.231–311.

Content

13

ADENOMA OF THE NIPPLE

WERNER BOECKER AND UTE KETTRITZ

'Adenoma of the nipple' is a clinical term applied to a variety of benign proliferative mass lesions in the nipple area. Histologically, these lesions are constituted by four major distinctive groups:
1. sclerosing lesions,
2. conventional papillomas located in a nipple duct,
3. adenomatous type lesions,
4. syringomatous adenomas.

Lesions of the first two groups are also often seen in the deeper breast parenchyma, whereby the cellular composition of lesions in both locations is identical. Sclerosing lesions and papillomas are described in detail in Chapters 9, 10 and 11. Adenomatous and syringomatous lesions are quintessential lesions of the nipple area and are described in this chapter.

Adenomatous adenoma is defined as a lesion consisting of an adenomatous proliferation of tubular structures replacing the nipple tissue. The tubules are lined by a layer of glandular cells often associated with micropapillary epithelial hyperplasia and by a layer of myoepithelial cells. **Syringomatous adenoma** is an infiltrative epithelial lesion of Ck5/14+ tubular structures with glandular and squamous cell differentiation. These lesions usually lack a myoepithelial cell layer. Syringomatous adenoma is prone to local recurrence.

Combinations of the different types of lesions may be seen. The term 'nipple adenoma' was introduced by Handley and Thackray in 1962 [1].

Adenomatous nipple adenoma

■ DEFINITION

WHO: Nipple adenoma
   ICD code: 8506/0 (nipple adenoma)
   ICD code: 8503/0 (intraductal papilloma)
   ICD code: 8506/0 (adenomatous nipple adenoma)
   ICD code: 8407/0 (syringomatous adenoma)

A number of other terms have also been used in the literature to describe the most common type of nipple adenoma. This is characterized by glandular proliferation and is often associated with micropapillary epithelial hyperplasia (Fig. 13.1). The most frequently used terms have included 'erosive adenosis' [3], 'adenomatosis' [4–11], 'papillary adenoma' [12–14] and 'papillomatosis' [15–22]. For a discussion on nomenclature see Azzopardi [2].

■ CONCEPTUAL APPROACH

The prototypical adenomatous adenoma of the nipple is regarded as a proliferation of new ductules which grow into the nipple stroma (Fig. 13.2) [1, 14, 23]. The lesion consists of ramifying tubular structures with outer myoepithelial and inner glandular cells (Fig. 13.3). These lesions are usually associated with micropapillary usual ductal hyperplasia. In Taylor and Robertson's opinion [23] the more solid components consist of a proliferation of inner epithelial cells, while others have also detected myoepithelial cells. Double fluorescence staining shows that the prototypical tubule contains Ck5+ cells with a glandular lineage restricted to the inner layer, and cells of myoepithelial lineage solely in the outer layer (Figs 13.3–13.4). The cell layers are therefore organized in exactly the same way as in normal resting breast epithelium and in the tubular structures of sclerosing adenosis. Glandular lineage proliferation is also found in cases associated with epithelial hyperplasia. This is described in Chapter 8 in the context of usual ductal hyperplasia.

■ CLINICAL FEATURES AND IMAGING

CLINICAL FEATURES

The prototypical adenomatous adenoma of the nipple is rare and mainly observed in the perimenopausal period [23], although it has been reported in women of all ages [24]. Clinically, the lesion presents as sanguineous or serous discharge [14, 23], as a nodule or plaque or – less commonly – as redness, inflamma-

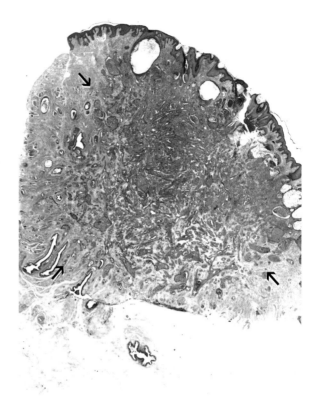

Fig. 13.1 Adenomatous adenoma. Low power view reveals a compact mass lesion composed of a complex proliferation of ductular structures. The lesion is well-circumscribed (arrows) but has no capsule. The epidermis of the nipple can be seen at the top, and some lactiferous ducts, at the bottom.

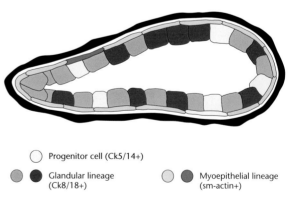

Progenitor cell (Ck5/14+)
Glandular lineage (Ck8/18+)
Myoepithelial lineage (sm-actin+)

Fig. 13.2 Schematic drawing of an adenoma of the nipple, adenomatous type. Prototypical adenomatous adenoma of the nipple is regarded as a proliferation of new ductules which grow into the nipple stroma. These consist of a glandular layer, a myoepithelial layer and a basement membrane.

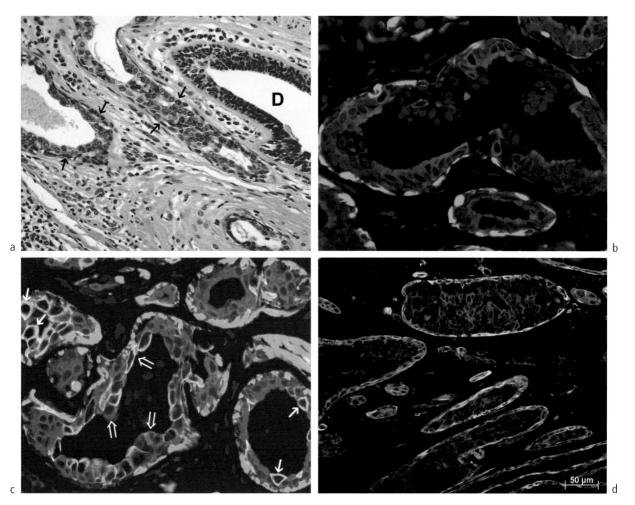

Fig. 13.3a – d Adenomatous adenoma.
13.3a Two tubular structures lined by several layers of glandular cells and clearly visible myoepithelial cells. The glandular cells of the neoplastic tubules display enlarged normochromic nuclei in contrast to the smaller hyperchromatic nuclei of the cells in an adjacent lactiferous duct (D). The myoepithelial lining and basement membrane of the tubular structures are easily recognized (arrows). The nipple stroma shows a slight edema and a lymphoplasmacytic inflammatory reaction.
13.3b Double staining for Ck8/18 (red signal) and sm-actin (green signal) shows the bilayer of this tubule.
13.3c Double staining for Ck5 (green signal) and Ck8/18 (red signal). The tubules contain a mixture of cells with progenitor cells (green signal), intermediate glandular (hybrid signal) and glandular cells (red signal). A few glandular cells express Ck5 (green signal), indicative of progenitor cells (arrows), and several coexpress Ck5 and Ck8/18 (hybrid signal), indicative of intermediate cells (double arrows). Some cells only express Ck8/18 (red signal), typical of glandular cells. Other tubules contain only Ck8/18+ glandular cells. The myoepithelial cells stain for Ck5 (green signal). The cell layers are organized in exactly the same way as seen in normal resting breast epithelium and in sclerosing adenosis.
13.3d Double staining for Ck5 (red signal) and sm-actin (green signal). Many of the basal cells express Ck5 (red signal) or both Ck5 and sm-actin (hybrid signal), which is characteristic of cells of the myoepithelial pathway. Most of the luminal cells in this neoplastic tubule express Ck5, indicating early cells of the glandular pathway.

tion and erosion/ulceration of the epidermis of the nipple [14, 20]. These symptoms may be accompanied by itching, burning or pain suggesting a clinical diagnosis of Paget's disease.

Carcinoma ex adenoma of the nipple has been described, but is equally rare [20, 25 – 27]. Synchronous invasive malignancies may occur in addition to the nipple lesion, sometimes even in the contra-

lateral breast [14, 28]. There are extremely rare reports of subsequent development of a carcinoma.

Local excision with clear margins is the therapy of choice for adenomatous nipple adenoma. This may require nipple resection [28, 29]. Local recurrence is rare [14, 20, 23] and metastases were never reported. An association with mammary carcinoma is exceedingly rare [30].

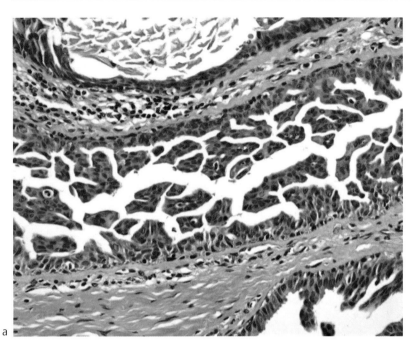

Fig. 13.4a – b Adenomatous adenoma with benign epithelial hyperplasia.

13.4a This tubule shows prominent micropapillary epithelial hyperplasia. This type of epithelial proliferation is typical of adenomatous nipple adenomas and should not be confused with an intraductal papilloma of lactiferous ducts. The nuclei show variations in size and shape. The nipple stroma displays a slight inflammatory reaction.

a

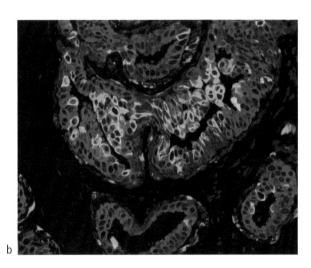

13.4b Double staining for Ck5 (green signal) and Ck8/18 (red signal). The epithelial proliferation is composed of a heterogeneous glandular cell proliferation with Ck5+ early glandular cells (green signal), Ck5+ and Ck8/18+ intermediate glandular cells (hybrid signal), and Ck8/18+ differentiated glandular cells (red signal). Myoepithelial layer weakly stained for Ck5.

b

IMAGING

MAMMOGRAPHY

Mammography only enables limited assessment of the nipple area. Due to its location, visualization of the adenoma of the nipple depends on the size of the lesion. Small adenomas may not be seen at all on mammograms [31, 32], whereas larger ones manifest as retroareolar density with or without thickening of the overlying skin. Adenomas may present as oval tumors with well-defined borders (Fig. 13.5), although irregularly shaped lesions are equally likely to occur [31, 33].

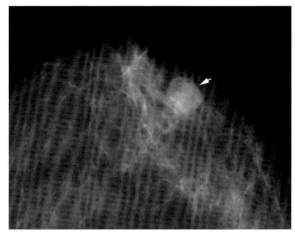

Fig. 13.5 Adenomatous adenoma. Mammography showing a round tumor with well-defined borders.

ULTRASOUND

Depending on their size, adenomas of the nipple may present as a hypoechoic mass on ultrasound (Fig. 13.6) [33], although assessment of the nipple areolar complex is limited. No specific features exist that enable a clear distinction between adenoma of the nipple and centrally located malignancies.

MAGNETIC RESONANCE IMAGING

Similar to other adenomas, there are no reliable criteria that enable a clear distinction between adenoma of the nipple and other lesions that might grow in this area.

PATHOLOGY

MACROSCOPY

Adenoma of the nipple manifests as a small nodule or mass that is usually no larger than 15 mm, sometimes

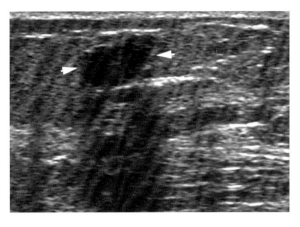

Fig. 13.6 Adenomatous nipple adenoma on ultrasound presents as a hypoechoic mass. No specific features exist which help in distinguishing adenoma of the nipple from centrally located malignancies.

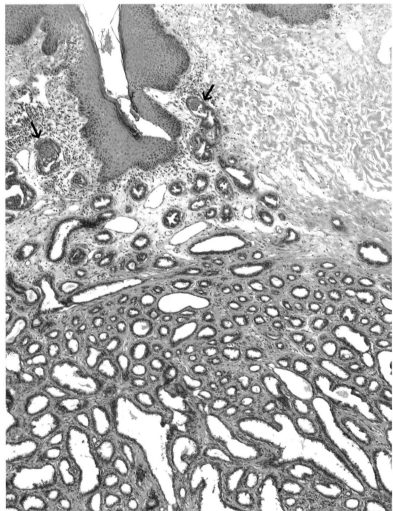

Fig. 13.7a Adenomatous adenoma with overlying epidermis of the nipple.
The tubular structures form a complex branching pattern. Note the squamous cell metaplasia in tubules close to the surface (arrows). *Continuation*

a

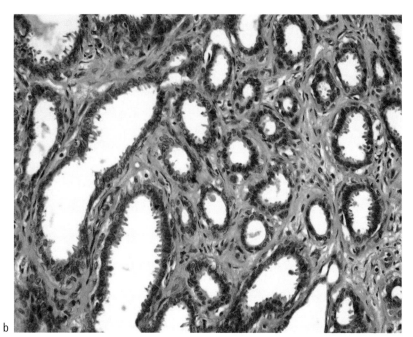

Fig. 13.7b Adenomatous adenoma with overlying epidermis of the nipple.
Higher magnification reveals the double layer of the epithelium with flattened myoepithelial cells.

b

with ill-defined borders. Whereas syringomatous lesions may show small cystic areas on the cut surface, adenomatous lesions are usually macroscopically inconspicuous.

MICROSCOPY

A low power view of adenomatous nipple adenoma displays a circumscribed mass characterized by complex tortuous and interweaving open tubules aggregating in a fibrotic nipple stroma (Fig. 13.1). The newly formed tubules are composed of a basal cell layer with myoepithelial differentiation and an inner layer with glandular differentiation (Fig. 13.7). This prototypical lesion can be modified by benign epithelial proliferations and variations in stromal reactions. Thus benign epithelial hyperplasia often coincides with these lesions [2] and is characterized by multilayering of the luminal epithelium with a typical micropapillary growth pattern (Fig. 13.8). Double layered tubular formations or usual ductal hyperplasia may predominate. As discussed more extensively in Chapters 8 and 9, the luminal cells of the bilayered tubules and the intraductal epithelial proliferation include CK5/14+ cells and their glandular progeny. Thus the cells of adenomatous adenoma stain heavily for Ck5 (Fig. 13.9). Myoepithelial cells are only seen at the periphery of the glan-

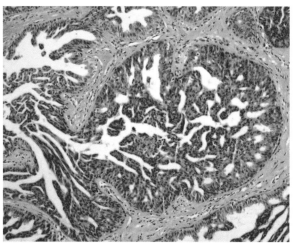

a

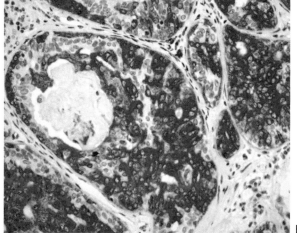

b

Fig. 13.8a–b Adenomatous adenoma with benign micropapillary and fenestrating epithelial proliferation.
13.8a Higher magnification of adenomatous adenoma of the nipple showing the epithelial growth pattern.
13.8b Immunostaining for Ck5 showing the typical Ck5 mosaicism of benign breast lesions.

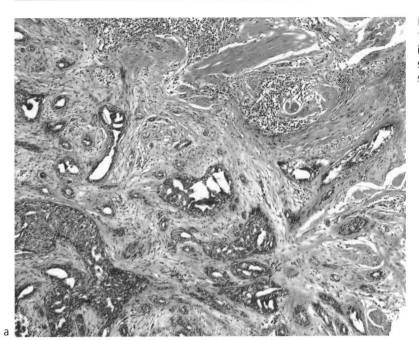

a

Fig. 13.9a–c Adenomatous adenoma.
13.9a Periphery of the adenoma with infiltrating growth pattern and prominent stromal reaction. In the right upper field smooth muscle cells of the nipple.

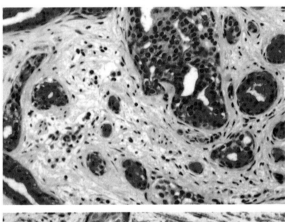

b

13.9b Immunostaining for Ck5 shows the characteristic intense reaction of both luminal and myoepithelial cells.

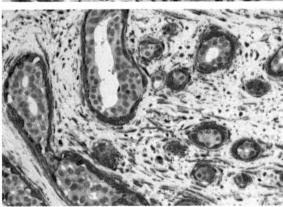

c

13.9c Immunostaining for sm-actin highlights that even the smallest epithelial islands are surrounded by strongly reacting myoepithelial cells. The stromal reaction contains a number of sm-actin+ myofibroblasts.

dular structures and are not observed as a component of intraductal epithelial proliferation. They may be highlighted by immunostaining for myoepithelial markers such as calponin, sm-actin and p63. The lesions are accompanied by various degrees of fibrous stromal reaction also containing sm-actin+ myofibroblasts (Fig. 13.9). The margins of the tumor may be ill-defined, and the lesion may even show an infiltrative pattern (Fig. 13.9). The lesion is therefore prone to be misdiagnosed as carcinoma. Squamous cell and apocrine metaplasia may occur, but the latter is rarely seen [14, 23]. The former is usually located in the superficial part of the adenoma close to the epidermis and is rarely observed in the newly formed adenomatous structures [2].

■ IMMUNOHISTOCHEMISTRY

Prototypical adenomatous adenoma contains a mosaic pattern of Ck5/14+ and Ck8/18+ cells in the luminal epithelium with sm-actin+ myoepithelial differentiation in the outer cell layer.

■ INTERPRETATION OF CORE AND VACUUM-ASSISTED BIOPSIES

Needle core biopsies are rarely performed. The most important distinction to be made is between adenoma and carcinoma. If the typical features of an adenoma of the nipple are present, the lesion should be categorized as B2.

■ DIFFERENTIAL DIAGNOSIS

See below.

Syringomatous adenoma

■ DEFINITION

ICD code: 8407/0

Syringomatous adenoma is an infiltrative epithelial lesion of Ck5/14+ tubular structures with glandular and squamous cell differentiation [15, 29, 34]. Lesions usually lack a myoepithelial cell layer. Local recurrence of syringomatous adenoma is common.

■ CONCEPTUAL APPROACH

Syringomatous nipple adenoma has a similar appearance to the syringoma of skin adnexal tumors. The tumor consists of branching tubules and solid cords of cells with glandular and squamous cell differentiation (Figs 13.10 and 13.11). The cellular origin of these lesions in the nipple is still unknown. Doctor and Sirsat [15] as well as Rosen have suggested that syringomatous nipple adenoma [35–38] may arise from sweat gland ducts. However, we are not convinced that a heterologous differentiation of a breast tumor such as syringomatous adenoma or pleomorphic adenoma of salivary gland type, necessarily indicates the development of such lesions from sweat or salivary gland tissue. Syringomatous adenomas and eccrine ducts do display some similarities (Figs 13.12 and 13.13): the prototypical tubular structures of syringomatous adenomas are solely composed of a double layer of Ck5+ cells, as seen in eccrine ducts, while a sm-actin+ myoepithelial layer is absent. However, syringomatous lesions usually contain epithelial structures that show a glandular differentiation of the luminal cells and, furthermore, display a heterologous squamous cell differentiation (Figs 13.13 and 13.14). Both of these features are absent in eccrine ducts. In addition, syringomatous tumors may also occasionally be found in the deep mammary breast tissue where eccrine glands have not been described. In view of the cellular composition of syringomatous adenoma (Ck5/14+ cells being key components) and the plasticity of these cells, there is sound evidence to support the view that syringomatous adenoma is a lesion

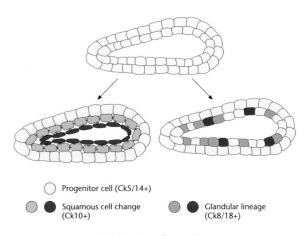

Fig. 13.10 Schematic drawing of an adenoma, syringomatous type. The prototypical syringomatous adenoma is composed of glands with a double layer of Ck5/14+ cells, lacking an sm-actin+ myoepithelial layer. The lesions usually show a glandular differentiation of the luminal cells and a heterologous squamous cell differentiation.

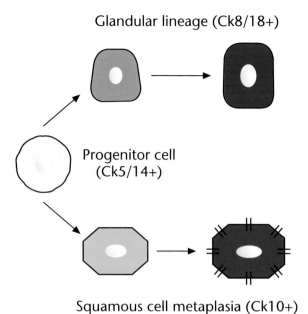

Glandular lineage (Ck8/18+)

Progenitor cell
(Ck5/14+)

Squamous cell metaplasia (Ck10+)

Fig. 13.11 Syringomatous adenoma is a lesion consisting mainly of Ck5/14+ cells that differentiate to 'normal' glandular and to heterologous squamous cells.

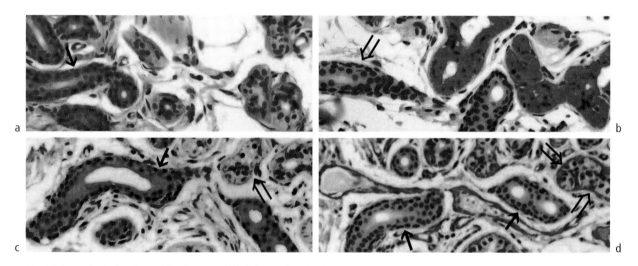

Fig. 13.12a–d Eccrine duct with adjacent acini of the eccrine gland.
13.12a H&E-stained sections show that the eccrine duct (arrow) contains a double layer of epithelium surrounded by a barely visible basement membrane.
13.12b The eccrine duct (arrow) is negative for Ck8/18, whereas the luminal cells of the acini stain heavily.
13.12c The cells of the eccrine duct are positive for Ck5, whereas the acini show a weak reaction for Ck5 in the myoepithelial cells (double arrow).
13.12d Sm-actin highlights the myoepithelial cells of acini (double arrow) and some small blood vessels, whereas the basal cells of the eccrine duct are negative. Thus the eccrine duct consists only of a bilayer of Ck5+ cells.

derived from Ck5/14+ progenitor cells of the breast epithelium that differentiate along glandular and squamous cell lines (Fig. 13.11). It should be noted that the prototypical epithelial structures and the spindle cell stroma of these lesions closely resemble early developmental stages of breast tissue. Regarding these lesions as mimicries of early embryological stages originating from Ck5/14+ cells may therefore be justified. The close proximity of squamous epithelium to the primitive budding structures in early embryological stages of the breast seems to further support this view.

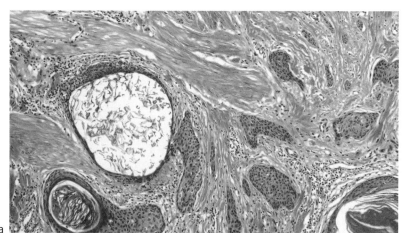

Fig. 13.13a–e Adenoma of the nipple, syringomatous type.

13.13a Prototypical syringomatous adenoma consisting of nests of comma-shaped and trabecular cords of cells with an infiltrating growth pattern. The tumor cells display glandular and squamous differentiation. Myoepithelial cells are usually not observed. In this example there was a prominent formation of keratinous cysts.

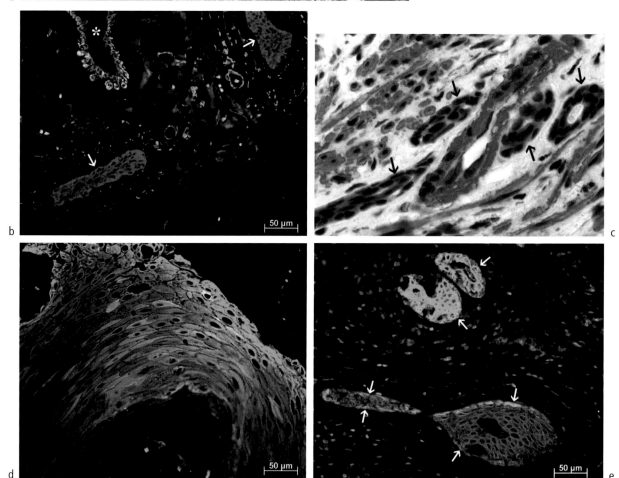

13.13b Immunostaining for sm-actin (green signal) and Ck5 (red signal) highlights the cellular composition of the epithelial structures. The prototypical syringomatous tubules (arrows) are composed of a double layer of Ck5/14+ cells which lack sm-actin+ myoepithelial cells. Sm-actin+ myofibroblasts may occasionally surround tumor cell complexes. Myoepithelial cells of a small duct (asterisk) express Ck5 and sm-actin, while myofibroblasts and smooth muscle cells only express sm-actin.

13.13c Immunostaining for sm-actin. The cells of the infiltrating syringoma (arrows) are negative because they lack a myoepithelial layer.

13.13d Double staining for Ck5 (green signal) and Ck10 (red signal). This figure highlights the evolution of squamous cells from Ck5+ progenitor cells.

13.13e Double staining for Ck8/18 (green signal) and Ck10 (red signal) shows that the epithelial cells display either the glandular differentiation or the squamous differentiation. In both epithelial structures the outer cell layer (arrows) is negative for Ck8/18 and Ck10, indicating less-differentiated cells.

In conclusion, we are convinced that there is sound evidence that syringomatous adenoma is derived from Ck5/14+ breast epithelial cells, which demonstrate both glandular and squamous cell differentiation.

CLINICAL FEATURES AND IMAGING

CLINICAL FEATURES

Clinically the lesion is characterized by a discrete mass with subtle induration of the subareolar area [34, 39].

Only a few dozen cases of syringomatous adenoma of the nipple have been described [1, 29, 34, 36, 37, 40–42]. Similar lesions are exceptionally rare in deeper breast regions [36].

Local excision with clear margins is the therapy of choice. This may require nipple resection [28, 29]. The local recurrence rate for syringomatous adenoma has been reported to be as high as 30% due to the infiltrating growth pattern of these lesions [29, 34, 41]. No patients, however, have developed metastases, nor is there any association with mammary carcinoma [30].

Syringomatous tumors of the deep breast tissue show the same cellular and architectural features. Nevertheless, some authors regard these tumors as low grade adenosquamous carcinomas [43].

IMAGING

Depending on their size, syringomatous adenomas may be visible on mammography and ultrasound (see 'Imaging' adenomatous adenoma).

PATHOLOGY

MACROSCOPY

The lesion presents as a small, ill-defined mass in the nipple stroma.

MICROSCOPY

Syringomatous adenoma contains small tubular ducts, occasionally branching in structure, which infiltrate rather than displace the nipple stroma (Figs 13.13–13.16). The tubules are angulated, comma-shaped or round, and they may show solid trabecular or open tubular structures. Mixtures of both structures may also be seen. The nipple stroma may be inconspicuous but usually shows a desmoplastic stromal reaction of collagenous tissue [34]. Prototypical syringomatous tubules are usually lined by two rows of epithelial cells which only express Ck5/14 (Fig. 13.13b). In most instances these cells are flat to cuboidal. In contrast to the tubules of adenomatous adenoma, a myoepithelial cell layer is lacking. These prototypical tubules show varying degrees of glandular and squamous cell differentiation. The former are characterized by expression of Ck8/18, the latter by compact or cystic epithelial structures with squamous differentiation (Ck10+) (Fig. 13.13e) and occasionally even luminal lamellar keratinization, which in some cases may be extensive (Fig. 13.14). A mistaken diagnosis of squamous cell carcinoma should therefore be avoided in such cases.

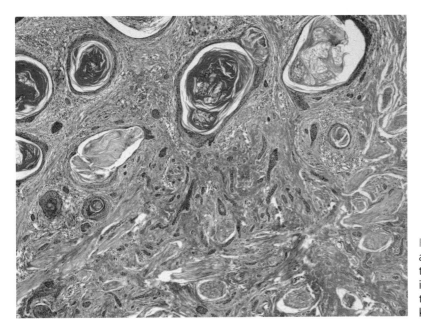

Fig. 13.14 Prototypical syringomatous adenoma consisting of small nests and trabecular cords of tumor cells with an infiltrating growth pattern. In this example there was a prominent formation of keratinous cysts.

Some tumors have only a few tubular structures distributed in the nipple stroma, and may therefore be overlooked on low power examination (Fig. 13.15). In other cases, the overall infiltrating pattern may lead to overdiagnosis of malignancy, even in paraffin sections.

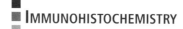

IMMUNOHISTOCHEMISTRY

The prototypical syringomatous type adenoma contains a mixture of cells expressing Ck5/14, p63, Ck8/18 (glandular differentiation) and Ck10 (squa-

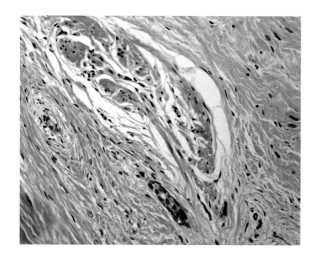

Fig. 13.15 Syringomatous nipple adenoma. This tumor displays only a few infiltrating tubular structures, which are distributed in the nipple stroma and which may easily be overlooked on low power examination. Note the absence of a stromal reaction in this case. Such a case may easily be missed due to the sparsely populated infiltrates.

Tab. 13.1 Distinguishing features of adenomatous and syringomatous nipple adenoma and tubular carcinoma

	Adenomatous type	Syringomatous type	Tubular carcinoma
Definition	Proliferation of new ductules with glandular and myoepithelial cells and a basement membrane.	Proliferation of primitive tubular and/or trabecular structures, occasionally comma-like in shape and usually with glandular and squamous cell differentiation.	Invasive breast cancer with formation of well-formed angulated tubular structures consisting of a single glandular layer only.
Architecture	Compact architecture which may be infiltrative.	Infiltrative architecture.	Infiltrative architecture.
Epithelial organization	Double layered tubular structures containing Ck5/14+ cells with glandular (Ck8/18+) and myo-epithelial (sm-actin+) differentiation. Micropapillary epithelial hyperplasia often also present.	Double layered tubular structures containing Ck5/14+ cells with glandular (Ck8/18+) or squamous cell (Ck10/11+) differentiation. Myoepithelial cells absent.	Neoplastic tubules containing Ck8/18+ uniform tumor cells. Myoepithelial cells absent.
Stroma	Varying amounts of cellular fibrous stroma, which usually contains myofibroblasts (sm-actin+).	Usually cellular fibrous stroma, containing myofibroblasts (sm-actin+).	Desmoplastic stroma, frequently with central elastosis, which usually contains myofibroblasts (sm-actin+) mimicking myoepithelial cells.
Immunohisto-chemistry (first line markers)	Ck5/14+, Ck8/18+, sm-actin+, p63+.	Ck5/14+, Ck8/18+, Ck10+ and p63+.	Ck8/18+, Ck5/14–, p63– and Ck10–.
B-classification	B2	B3	B5

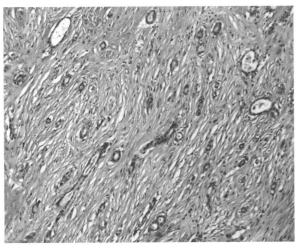 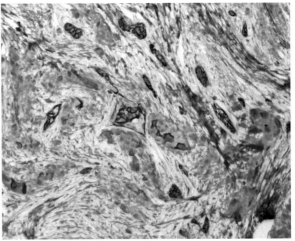

a   b

Fig. 13.16a – b Syringomatous adenoma.
13.16a In this area, tubular structures surrounded by a prominent stromal reaction may lead to an incorrect diagnosis of tubular carcinoma. A clear-cut distinction between benign and malignant lesions can be made by Ck5/6 immunohistochemistry (13.16b).
13.16b Immunostaining for Ck5/6 highlights the progenitor cell features of these lesions, clearly confirming their benign nature.

mous differentiation), but usually not sm-actin. The immunohistochemical profile of the constituent cells is only characterized by an intense reaction to Ck5/14 in prototypical tubular differentiations. Contrary to adenomatous adenoma, myoepithelial cells are usually not present.

■ INTERPRETATION OF CORE AND ■ VACUUM-ASSISTED BIOPSIES

Experience with needle core biopsies is limited. This lesion may be easily mistaken for tubular or – if squamous differentiation is pronounced – squamous cell carcinoma. Immunostaining for Ck5/14, Ck8/18, p63 and Ck10 aids in reaching a correct diagnosis. This lesion should be classified as B3.

■ DIFFERENTIAL DIAGNOSIS

GENERAL DISCUSSION

One of the greatest challenges the pathologist is faced with is differentiating nipple adenoma from tubular carcinoma. This is particularly difficult, and perhaps impossible, in frozen sections. We recommend that frozen section diagnosis is not employed in diagnosing nipple tumors. Furthermore adenomatous adenoma

must be distinguished from central papilloma of the lactiferous duct and from other sclerosing lesions.

Tubular carcinoma is easily distinguished from adenomatous adenoma since it lacks the epithelial bilayer. In difficult cases p63 and sm-actin staining may help. It should, however, be taken into consideration that the stroma may contain sm-actin+ myofibroblasts, which are likely to interfere with interpretation.

In our experience Ck5/14 immunohistochemistry should be given preference over sm-actin immunohistochemistry, because Ck5/14 allows a clear distinction between benign and malignant cases. Furthermore, syringomatous-type adenomas do not contain any myoepithelial differentiation and may thus be misdiagnosed as tubular/tubulolobular carcinoma.

Conventional papillomas of the collecting ducts resemble tumors seen at any site of the ductal lobular system. Sometimes these lesions present through the distended orifice of the involved duct as a friable or hemorrhagic papillary mass. Their histological appearance has been described in Chapter 11.

Sclerosing lesions are often similar in appearance to sclerosing adenosis, or – less frequently – to radial scars [44, 45]. The glandular structures form open or compressed tubules, which are composed of an inner luminal (Ck8/18+), an outer myoepithelial (sm-actin+) lining and a broadly thickened basement membrane, in contrast to the open tubules of adenomatous adenoma.

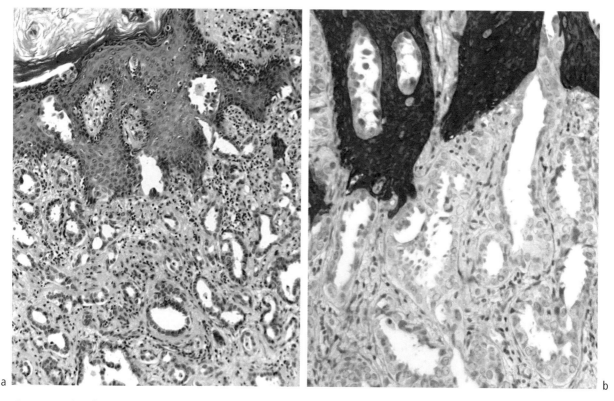

Fig. 13.17a–b Tubular carcinoma of the nipple.
13.17a Infiltration of the nipple area by open tubular structures with a moderate desmoplastic stromal reaction. The monotonous single layer of cells that comprise the tubules is helpful in arriving at a correct diagnosis. It may, however, be difficult to distinguish a lesion such as this from syringoma with only few tubular structures.
13.17b Immunostaining for Ck5/6 shows a completely negative reaction of the tubular carcinoma, in contrast to the extensive reaction of the epidermis.

Example

Adenomatous and Syringomatous Adenoma vs. Tubular Carcinoma

The distinctive feature of adenomatous lesions in H&E-stained sections is a differentiation pattern presenting two types. Syringomatous type adenoma, in contrast, is characterized by a double layer of Ck5/14+ cells with glandular and squamous cell differentiation of the luminal layer. In typical cases the diagnosis is easily made. Small or needle core biopsies may, however, contain very small clusters of cells and thus may lead to an erroneous diagnosis of breast carcinoma. The location of the lesion and its overall features are important in arriving at a correct diagnosis (Table 13.1). Immunostaining can also be employed in difficult cases.

Papilloma of the lactiferous duct vs. ductal carcinoma in-situ, papillary type (Chapters 11 and 20)

Sclerosing lesions vs. invasive carcinoma (Chapters 9 and 10)

References

1. Handley RS, Thackray AC. Adenoma of the nipple. Cancer 1962;16:187–94.
2. Azzopardi JG. Problems in Breast Pathology. 1st ed. London: W.B. Saunders; 1979.
3. Diaz NM, Palmer JO, Wick MR. Erosive adenomatosis of the nipple: histology, immunohistology, and differential diagnosis. Mod Pathol 1992;5:179–84.
4. Gros CM, LeGal Y, Bader P. L'adenomatose erosive du mamelon. Press Med 1959;67:615–6.
5. LeGal Y, Gros CM, Bader P. L'adenomatose erosive du mamelon. Ann Anat Pathol 1959;4:292–304.
6. Miller G, Bernier I. Adenomatose erosive du mamelon. Can J Surg 1965;8:261–6.
7. Lewis HM, Ovitz ML, Golitz LE. Erosive adenomatosis of the nipple. Arch Dermatol 1976;112:1427–8.
8. Moulin G, Darbon P, Balme B, Frappart L. [Erosive adenomatosis of the nipple. Report of 10 cases with immunohistochemistry]. Ann Dermatol Venereol 1990;117:537–45.
9. Shapiro L, Karpas CM. Florid papillomatosis of the nipple. First reported case in a male. Am J Clin Pathol 1965;44:155–9.
10. Smith EJ, Kron SD, Gross PR. Erosive adenomatosis of the nipple. Arch Dermatol 1970;102:330–2.

11. Smith NP, Jones EW. Erosive adenomatosis of the nipple. Clin Exp Dermatol 1977;2:79–84.
12. Brownstein MH, Phelps RG, Magnin PH. Papillary adenoma of the nipple: analysis of fifteen new cases. J Am Acad Dermatol 1985;12:707–15.
13. Montemarano AD, Sau P, James WD. Superficial papillary adenomatosis of the nipple: a case report and review of the literature. J Am Acad Dermatol 1995;33:871–5.
14. Perzin KH, Lattes R. Papillary Adenoma of the Nipple (Florid Papillomatosis, Adenoma, Adenomatosis). A Clinicopathologic Study. Cancer 1972;29:999–1009.
15. Doctor VM, Sirsat MV. Florid papillomatosis (adenoma) and other benign tumours of the nipple and Areola. Br J Cancer 1971;25:1–9.
16. Bhagvan BS, Patchefsky A, Koss LG. Florid subareolar duct papillomatosis (nipple adenoma) and mammary carcinoma: report of 3 cases. Hum Pathol 1973;4:289–95.
17. Myers JL, Mazur MT, Urist MM, Peiper SC. Florid papillomatosis of the nipple: immunohistochemical and flow cytometric analysis of two cases. Mod Pathol 1990;3:288–93.
18. Nichols FC, Dockerty MD, Judd ES. Florid papillomatosis of the nipple. Surg Gynaecol Obstet 1958;107:474–80.
19. Robert H, DeBrux J, Winaver D. La papillomatose benigne du mamelon. Presse Med 1963;71:2713–5.
20. Rosen PP, Caicco JA. Florid papillomatosis of the nipple. A study of 51 patients, including nine with mammary carcinoma. Am J Surg Pathol 1986;10:87–101.
21. Scott P, Kissin MW, Collins C, Webb AJ. Florid papillomatosis of the nipple: a clinico-pathological surgical problem. Eur J Surg Oncol 1991;17:211–3.
22. Waldo ED, Sidhu GS, Hu AW. Florid papillomatosis of male nipple after diethylstilbestrol therapy. Arch Pathol 1975;99:364–6.
23. Taylor HB, Robertson AG. Adenomas of the nipple. Cancer 1965;18:995–1002.
24. Ellis IO, Elston CW, Goulding H, Pindar SE. Miscellaneous benign lesions. In: Elston CW, Ellis IO, editors. The Breast. Edinburgh: Churchill Livingstone; 1998. p.205–30.
25. Bhagavan BS, Patchefsky A, Koss LG. Florid subareolar duct papillomatosis (nipple adenoma) and mammary carcinoma: report of three cases. Hum Pathol 1973;4:289–95.
26. Burdick C, Rinehart RM, Matsumoto T, O'Connell TJ, Heisterkamp CW. Nipple adenoma and Paget's disease in a man. Arch Surg 1965;91:835–9.
27. Gudjonsdottir A, Hägerstrand I, Östberg G. Adenoma of the nipple with carcinomatous development. Acta path microbiol scand A 1971;79:676–80.
28. Jones MW, Tavassoli FA. Coexistence of nipple duct adenoma and breast carcinoma: a clinicopathologic study of five cases and review of the literature. Mod Pathol 1995;8:633–6.
29. Rosen PP. Syringomatous adenoma of the nipple. Am J of Surg Pathol 1983;7:739–45.
30. Rosen PP. Syringomatous adenoma of the nipple. In: Rosen PP, editor. Rosen's Breast Pathology. 2nd ed. Philadelphia: Lippincott, Williams & Wilkins; 2001. p.111–4.
31. Vette J, Muller JW. Adenoma of the nipple. Diagn Imaging 1983;52:264–6.
32. Sander T, Schrocksnadel H, Heim K, Bergant A, Muller E. [Differential diagnostic and therapeutic considerations of nipple adenoma]. Geburtshilfe Frauenheilkd 1993;53:273–5.
33. Fornage BD, Faroux MJ, Pluot M, Bogomoletz W. Nipple adenoma simulating carcinoma. Misleading clinical, mammographic, sonographic, and cytologic findings. J Ultrasound Med 1991;10:55–7.
34. Jones MW, Norris HJ, Snyder RC. Infiltrating syringomatous adenoma of the nipple. A clinical and pathological study of 11 cases. Am J Surg Pathol 1989;13:197–201.
35. Rosen PP. Rosen's Breast Pathology. 2nd ed. Philadelphia: Lippincott Williams & Wilkins; 2001.
36. Suster S, Moran CA, Hurt MA. Syringomatous squamous tumors of the breast. Cancer 1991;67:2350–5.
37. Ward BE, Cooper PH, Subramony C. Syringomatous tumor of the nipple. Am J Clin Pathol 1989;92:692–6.
38. Tavassoli FA. Diseases of the nipple. In: Tavassoli FA, editor. Pathology of the Breast. 2nd ed. Stanford: Appleton & Lange; 1999. p.731–62.
39. Biernat W, Jablkowski W. Syringomatous adenoma of the nipple. Pol J Pathol 2000;51:201–2.
40. Andrac-Meyer L, Solere K, Sappa P, Garcia S, Charpin C. Syringoadenome infiltrant du mamelon: un nouveau cas. [Infiltrating syringoadenoma of the nipple: a new case]. Ann Pathol 2000;20:142–4.
41. Slaughter MS, Pomerantz RA, Murad T, Hines JR. Infiltrating syringomatous adenoma of the nipple. Surgery 1992;111:711–3.
42. Urso C. [Syringomatous breast carcinoma and correlated lesions]. Pathologica 1996;88:196–9.
43. Metaplastic carcinoma In: Tavassoli FA, Devillee P, editors. Tumours of the Breast and Female Genital Organs. Lyon: IARC Press; 2003. p.37–41.
44. Rosen PP. Adenomyoepithelioma of the breast. Hum Pathol 1987;18:1232–7.
45. Hamperl H. Strahlige Narben und obliterierende Mastopathie. Virchows Archiv A 1975;369:55–68.

Content

14

ADENOMYOEPITHELIAL TUMORS

WERNER BOECKER, DANIELA HUNGERMANN, UTE KETTRITZ AND HERMANN HERBST

Originally described by Hamperl, the entity **adenomyoepithe-lioma** encompasses a heterogeneous group of breast neoplasms. This group **comprises tumors with tubular structures and a prominent multilayered abluminal myoepithelial component at one end of the morphological spectrum or lesions with a mesenchymal appearance at the other.**

From a histogenic viewpoint, the term 'adenomyoepithelial tumors' **refers to Ck5/14+ progenitor cell lesions with glandular (Ck8/18+) and myoepithelial progeny cells (myoepithelial marker-positive).** The myoepithelial cell differentiation is usually associated with synthesis of basement membrane-like material. Diagnosis of adenomyoepithelial tumors is significantly aided by immunohistochemistry, in particular by antibodies specific for Ck5/14 and p63.

Evenly shaped glandular structures are always present in **biphasic adenomyoepithelial tumors.** However, in less differentiated lesions, the glandular cells may form a barely visible, loosely cohesive reticular component or may consist of a spindle cell component with a purely mesenchymal appearance (adenomyoepithelioma, monophasic). Expression of glandular cytokeratins such as Ck8/18 can even be found in the latter.

Most adenomyoepithelial tumors follow a benign clinical course, but some may recur and progress to malignancy. Histologically, many lesions can clearly be classified as either benign or malignant. In some lesions, however, a clear assessment of prognosis cannot be given. These lesions should be classified as 'borderline tumors'.

Purely **myoepithelial tumors** are characterized by cells that are positive for Ck5/14 and myoepithelial markers, but completely lack glandular differentiation.

The extremely rare **pleomorphic adenoma** is considered to be a variant of adenomyoepithelial tumors, characterized by mesenchymal metaplasia and formation of heterologous tissue.

Adenomyoepithelial tumors

■ DEFINITION

Synonyms: adenomyoepithelioma, malignant myoepithelioma

WHO: Benign adenomyoepithelioma; malignant (aggressive) adenomyoepithelioma, myoepithelioma

ICD-O code: 8983/0 (benign adenomyoepithelioma)

ICD-O code: 8982/3 (malignant adenomyoepithelioma)

ICD-O code: 8940/0 (pleomorphic adenoma)

In the recent WHO classification, adenomyoepithelial tumors were defined as lesions composed of a predominantly, and usually solid, proliferation of phenotypically variable myoepithelial cells around small glandular spaces [1] (Fig. 14.1). One of the lesions' defining histologic features is, therefore, a prominent myoepithelial cell proliferation. These myoepithelial cells are characterized by expression of markers such as sm-actin, calponin and p63. They are also often associated with formation of hyaline basement membrane material, which can be regarded as an important feature of this tumor, albeit currently not appreciated in the literature. The second defining cellular feature is the glandular differentiation detectable by means of morphology or immunohistochemistry. This glandular differentiation is clearly recognizable in H&E sections of better differentiated examples of adenomyoepithelial tumors. However, these tumors sometimes consist solely of cells with a mesenchymal appearance and no obvious glandular differentiation. In these cases, immunostaining for Ck8/18 and myoepithelial markers is crucial in visualizing the glandular and myoepithelial lineages of the constituent cells. We suggest that these tumors be categorized according to their appearance into biphasic (well-differentiated, tubular) and monophasic (poorly-differentiated, spindle cell type) adenomyoepithelial tumors.

Irrespective of the architectural patterns, adenomyoepithelial tumors are defined as tumors containing Ck5/14+ cells with a bilineage differentiation in which myoepithelial cells predominate.

Most malignant adenomyoepithelial tumors show a mesenchymal phenotype without obvious glandular components. In the recent literature some of these tumors have been categorized as 'metaplastic spindle cell carcinoma, fibromatosis-like' [2–5] or they have been referred to as myoepithelial carcinomas (see below).

Tumors that only contain myoepithelial cells should be referred to as **myoepitheliomas**, and their malignant counterparts as **myoepithelial carcinomas** [6–19]. This terminology is, however, not used consistently, especially with reference to myoepithelial neoplasms. We suggest that expression of Ck5/14 and

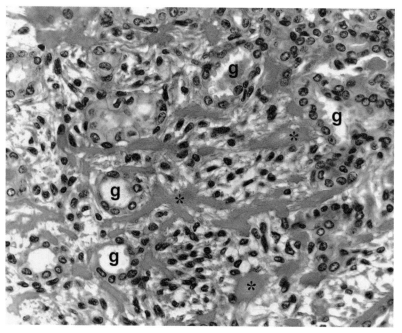

Fig. 14.1 Adenomyoepithelial tumor, differentiated. The lesion consists of glandular structures (g) and prominent myoepithelial cells with production of basement membrane material (asterisks). Note the loss of the appropriate sorting of the myoepithelial cells which shed their normal spatial order and submerge into the surrounding stroma. This is in clear contrast to the well-defined tubular structures of other benign proliferative lesions such as sclerosing adenosis, tubular adenoma and adenoma of the nipple.

sm-actin, and the absence of glandular keratins 8/18, be used as defining features in diagnosing purely myoepithelial neoplasms. In the authors' experience these tumors are exceptionally rare. In the study by Hungermann et al. [114], only 1 in 28 adenomyoepithelial tumor cases investigated displayed a purely myoepithelial lineage.

In conclusion two different types of adenomyoepithelial tumors can thus be distinguished:

1. Biphasic adenomyoepithelial tumors (differentiated, 'tubular' and 'lobular' types, according to Tavassoli et al. [1]). These are characterized by well-shaped tubular structures enveloped by mantles of myoepithelial cells, which are submerged in the surrounding stroma.

2. Monophasic adenomyoepithelial tumors (undifferentiated, 'spindle' or 'epithelioid' cell types and 'lobular' type [without tubule formation] according to Tavassoli et al. [1]). The main features of these tumors are cells with mesenchymal appearance without, or with only barely recognizable, glandular differentiation and, in many cases, intense production of hyaline basement membrane-like material.

Pleomorphic adenoma, the counterpart of the more common salivary gland tumor, is rare in the breast [11, 20–50]. Pleomorphic adenoma differs from benign adenomyoepithelial tumors by the presence of a myxoid matrix with chondroid and osseous metaplasia. In double immunofluorescence studies we have observed that, in pleomorphic adenomas, chondroid or osseous metaplasia is derived from Ck5/14+ tumor cells, hence our conclusion that adenomyoepithelial tumors and pleomorphic adenomas share the same cellular composition.

■ CONCEPTUAL APPROACH

BASIC CELLULAR ORGANIZATION

The prototypical adenomyoepithelial tumor (adenomyoepithelioma) consists of tubular structures enveloped by prominent myoepithelial cells submerged in the surrounding stroma, usually with intervening hyaline basement membrane-like material (Fig. 14.1).

Although the mechanisms underlying the pathogenesis of these rare tumors are largely unknown, it is obvious that loss of growth control and appropriate sorting of myoepithelial cells which disperse ('melt') into the surrounding stroma are important hallmarks of these lesions (Figs 14.2 and 14.3). Furthermore, these cells appear to retain some functional remnants of their normal counterparts, with an irregular production of basement membrane material [51–53]. In addition, the lesions display a glandular

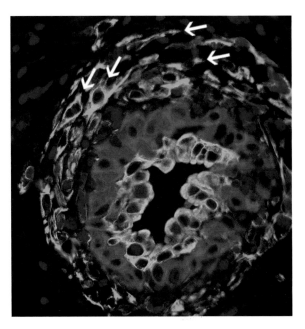

Fig. 14.2 Adenomyoepithelial tumor, differentiated. Double staining for Ck5 (green signal) and Ck8/18 (red signal) shows glandular differentiation with some undifferentiated cells in the lumen and multilayering of myoepithelial cells, which lose contact with the glandular cells (arrows).

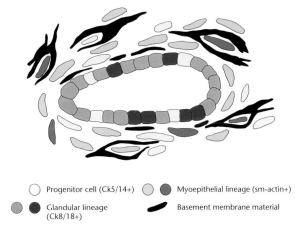

Progenitor cell (Ck5/14+)   Myoepithelial lineage (sm-actin+)
Glandular lineage (Ck8/18+)   Basement membrane material

Fig. 14.3 Schematic drawing showing the components of a differentiated adenomyoepithelial tumor (see also text).

differentiation, which is clearly evident in H&E sections in more biphasic lesions. The most important cellular constituent is a Ck5/14+ cell. Based on double fluorescence data, we assume that Ck5/14+ cells retain their potential to differentiate along both glandular and myoepithelial lineages.

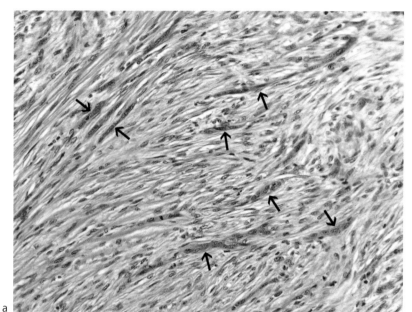

a

Fig. 14.4a–c Adenomyoepithelial tumor, poorly differentiated.
14.4a This is an example of a spindle cell lesion consisting of cells with mesenchymal appearance. Some of them are arranged in a trabecular pattern indicative of epithelial differentiation (arrows).

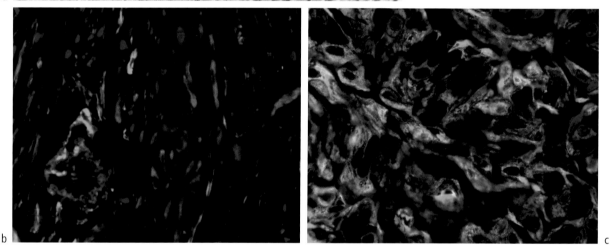

b   c

14.4b Double fluorescence staining for sm-actin (green signal) and Ck8/18 (red signal) clearly shows cells with a myoepithelial and glandular phenotype. Note the absence of hybrid colors, ruling out any transdifferentiation from one cell type to the other.
14.4c Double fluorescence staining for Ck5 (red signal) and sm-actin (green signal). This area contains immature Ck5+ progenitor cells (red signal), many intermediate myoepithelial cells co-expressing both Ck5 and sm-actin (hybrid signal), and differentiated myoepithelial cells (green signal).
Continuation

Adenomyoepithelial tumors may be more or less completely 'mesenchymal' in appearance with no, or barely recognizable, glandular differentiation in H&E-stained sections (Fig. 14.4). Using double immunofluorescence experiments we have been able to provide evidence that even these tumors display Ck5/14+ cells as a key component, as well as expressing myoepithelial or glandular markers. Another interesting finding is that many adenomyoepithelial tumors display squamous cell change (Fig. 14.5). Given the fact that the tumor contains Ck5/14+ progenitor cells as an important constituent – often the dominant cell type – and that squamous cell differentiation

evolves from Ck5+ cells (see Chapter 3), such a differentiation is not at all surprising (Fig. 14.6).

We regard myoepitheliosis as a variant of normal breast tissue, and not as a precursor lesion of adenomyoepithelial tumors (see Chapter 2). Rather, given the similarities of the more differentiated adenomyoepitheliomas and sclerosing lesions and the observation that some lesions may contain areas of typical papillary or sclerosing lesions that 'melt' into adenomyoepitheliomas, our contention is that sclerosing lesions may play a role in the development of adenomyoepitheliomas. This is in line with reports of transitions of adenosis to adenomyoepithelial tumors [54, 55]. The main

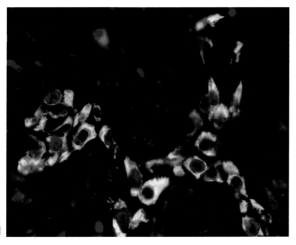

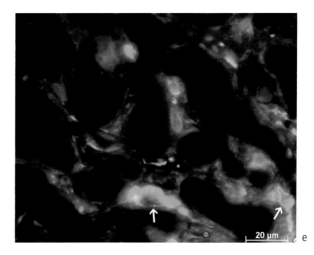

d   20 μm   e

Fig. 14.4a–e Adenomyoepithelial tumor, poorly differentiated.
14.4d Double fluorescence staining for Ck5 (red signal) and Ck8/18 (green signal). Note that the cells show a somewhat 'trabecular' appearance. This field displays a few Ck5+ progenitor cells, and many intermediate glandular cells (hybrid signal). Such a glandular differentiation is usually found in poorly differentiated adenomyoepithelial tumors and can only be detected using Ck8/18 immuno-staining.
14.4e This area shows abundant basement membrane-like material stained for collagen IV (red signal), which is regarded as a specific product of the myoepithelial cells (sm-actin+, green signal, arrows) and as a constitutive feature of most adenomyoepithelial tumors.

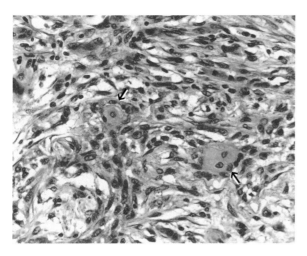

Fig. 14.5 Poorly differentiated adenomyoepithelial tumor with squamous cell differentiation. This field shows loosely cohesive epithelial cells with squamous cell metaplasia (arrows). These epithelial cells derive from Ck5/14+ progenitor cells.

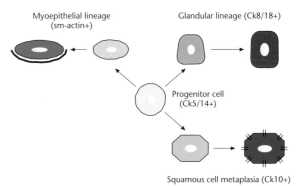

Myoepithelial lineage (sm-actin+)

Glandular lineage (Ck8/18+)

Progenitor cell (Ck5/14+)

Squamous cell metaplasia (Ck10+)

Fig. 14.6 Cellular differentiation patterns of adenomyoepithelial tumors. Ck5/14+ cells differentiate into cells of the glandular and myoepithelial cell lineage. In approximately 25% of these tumors a squamous cell differentiation can also be found.

difference between these lesions is loss of the bilayered arrangement of the glandular and myoepithelial layers in the latter lesions.

Pleomorphic adenoma is a very rare benign epithelial tumor with variable amounts of a characteristic metaplastic chondroid matrix. Based on double immunofluorescence studies, Ck5+ cells differentiate both along the glandular (Ck8/18+) and, rarely, squamous cell lineage as well as along the fibromyxoid/chondroid (vimentin-positive) lineage.

Furthermore, myoepithelial cell differentiation (sm-actin+) is also seen.

Purely myoepithelial lesions are extremely rare. They are characterized by proliferation of the Ck5/14+ progenitor cells that give rise only to the myoepithelial cell lineage. These tumors also intensely stain for other myoepithelial markers such as p63, sm-actin and calponin. Any glandular differentiation should, however, be ruled out by definition. So far, reports of malignant myoepitheliomas (myoepithelial carcinomas) have been very rare [8, 9, 15–17, 19, 56–59]. According to Tavassoli, immunoreactions for S-100 protein and actin are at least focally positive. In 27 of 28 adenomyoepithelial tumors Hungermann et al. [114] observed markers of both glandular and myoepithelial differentiation, even in tumors that appeared to be purely myoepithelial in H&E histology. In only a single case did they verify an exclusively myoepithelial composition in the absence of glandular differentiation. Some tumors that in the past were regarded as metaplastic spindle cell tumors and myoepithelial carcinomas should probably now be reevaluated, taking into account their potential to express glandular differentiation markers. According to our classification, such tumors would then be diagnosed as malignant adenomyoepithelial tumors (or adenomyoepithelial carcinomas), monophasic type.

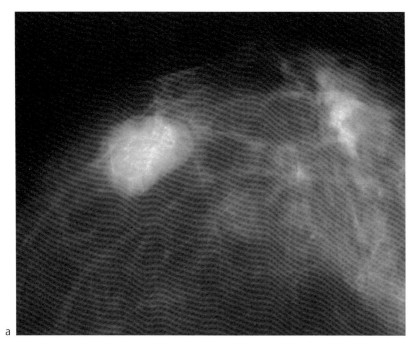

a

Fig. 14.7a–b Adenomyoepithelioma.
14.7a Craniocaudal mammogram of a 55-year-old woman showing a well-circumscribed mass.

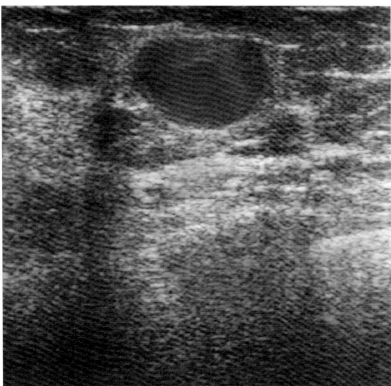

b

14.7b On ultrasound, the palpable mass presented as a well-defined hypoechoic mass. Surgery revealed adenomyoepithelioma.

Several authors reported on the **development of carcinomas arising in, or accompanied by, typical 'myoepitheliomas'** [32, 58, 60–64]. From a theoretical standpoint these malignancies may develop from one of the three differential lineages, the most commonly involved being the glandular lineage. The authors have seen cases with mainly glandular, squamous or heterologous mesenchymal differentiation. The defining feature of such tumors is Ck5/14 positivity associated with their specific lineage differentiation.

◼ CLINICAL FEATURES AND IMAGING

CLINICAL FEATURES

With approximately 200 tumors reported in the literature, adenomyoepithelial tumors are rare neoplasms of the breast [10, 14, 59, 60, 62, 64–98, 114].

According to published data, the age of patients ranges from 25 to 80 years, the majority of patients being over 50 [14]. Adenomyoepithelial tumors present as a circumscribed nodule which may be palpable [14, 58–60, 62–70, 72, 74, 77, 79–86, 88, 89, 92–95, 97, 99–105] or, if too small or located deep in the breast, as a well-circumscribed mass which can only be visualized on mammography [80, 91, 96] or ultrasound.

IMAGING

MAMMOGRAPHY

On mammography, adenomyoepithelial tumors present as round or lobulated masses, usually with fairly well-defined borders (Fig. 14.7) [65, 106]. The malignant forms can, however, present as spiculated lesions. Microcalcifications are only rarely found [14, 67, 68, 91, 105].

ULTRASOUND

Adenomyoepithelial tumors on ultrasound are usually solid, well-circumscribed masses with low echogenicity compared to the surrounding parenchyma (Fig. 14.8) [106].

PROGNOSIS AND TREATMENT

Because these tumors are extremely rare, the body of data on their prognosis is scarce. Adenomyoepithelial tumors are characterized by local recurrence rates amounting to approximately 15% of the reported cases of adenomyoepithelial tumors in the literature, and occurring from 4 months to 23 years after initial diagnosis. Recurrences were associated with incomplete removal, the presence of cellular pleomorphism,

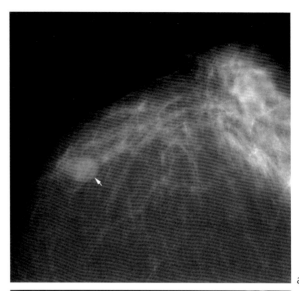
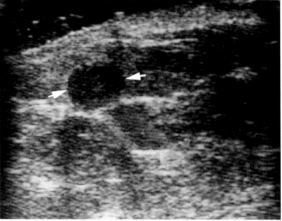

Fig. 14.8a–b Recurrence of adenomyoepithelioma.
14.8a One year later, another well-delineated mass located close to the site of the previous excision was detected on a craniocaudal mammogram.
14.8b On ultrasound, the lesion was well-circumscribed and solid (arrows). Surgery revealed a recurrence of the adenomyoepithelioma.

mitoses, necrosis, invasion into surrounding tissue or occurred as malignant tumors ex adenomyoepithelial tumors [14, 58, 59, 63, 64, 71, 80, 87, 93, 97, 100].

Bult et al. [107] regard local excision with a clear margin as the optimal choice of treatment. In tumors with features of malignancy, nodal or distant metastases have been recorded, the sites of metastases being axillary lymph nodes, lung, bones and brain, and the thyroid gland [58, 62, 64, 80, 93, 107]. Usually these are observed in adenomyoepithelial tumors, which themselves display malignant features or which are associated with other types of malignant tumors ex adenomyoepithelial tumors. Metastases retain the characteristic features of locally recurrent tumors.

Overtly malignant tumors ex adenomyoepithelial tumors should be treated in the same way as carcinoma of the breast. The distinction between myoepithelial carcinoma and metaplastic (sarcomatoid) carcinoma is primarily academic and not critical to patient management as the treatment of choice in both cases is that for carcinoma.

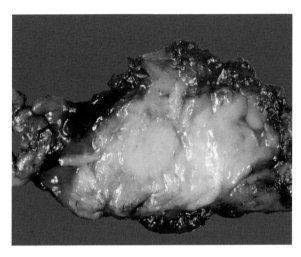

Fig. 14.9 Macroscopic appearance of a malignant adenomyoepithelial tumor. The tumor displays a glistening, white cut surface with smooth margins. In such cases only histology is capable of revealing the infiltrative pattern.

PATHOLOGY

MACROSCOPY

Adenomyoepithelial tumors present as solitary, circumscribed lesions with a smooth margin (Fig. 14.9) or with a lobulated appearance with smooth or irregular, and sometimes even spiculated borders. The cut surface glistens with a tan or yellow-tan color and tumors can contain papillary or cystic structures. They may also contain hemorrhagic or necrotic foci. The size of tumors ranges from 0.5 cm to 10 cm [10, 14, 58, 59, 62, 65–68, 70–72, 76, 77, 79–86, 88, 89, 92–105, 108]. In exceptionally rare cases, these lesions may be found as an incidental finding in excision biopsies performed for other reasons (Fig. 14.10).

MICROSCOPY

Adenomyoepithelial tumors show considerable morphological diversity with variable growth patterns and cytological differentiations ranging from those with clearly glandular structures to pure spindle cell variants. The constitutive features are invariably sm-actin+ myoepithelial cells. Furthermore, all of these tumors share a high proportion of cells that are reactive for basal cytokeratins 5 and 14 and most, even the less differentiated ones, also contain tumor cells with expression of glandular cytokeratins 8/18. Most tumors show at least foci of hyalinization, sometimes in a basal membrane-like pattern with narrow eosin red bands enmeshing groups of tumor cells, and sometimes with

Tab. 14.1 Adenomyoepithelial tumors

Definition	Tumors composed of proliferation of phenotypically variable myoepithelial cells around spaces lined by glandular epithelium. The glandular lineage may vary from well-shaped tubular structures in biphasic (differentiated) tumors to a spindle cell appearance in monophasic (undifferentiated) tumors. The disorderly formation of basement membrane material between cells is a further characteristic of such tumors.
Cellular epithelial composition	Adenomyoepithelial tumors are the result of an increased cell growth of Ck5/14+ cells and their progeny, with formation and inappropriate sorting of the cells of the myoepithelial cell lineage.
Matrix components	Highly characteristic basement-like membrane which seems to be a specific product of the myoepithelial cells.
Immunohistochemistry	Ck5/14+, p63+, sm-actin+, calponin+ and Ck8/18+.
Molecular genetics	Inconsistent genetic alterations at different chromosomal loci.
Clinical findings and radiology	Most adenomyoepithelial tumors are benign, range in size from 1–7 cm and present as a nonspecific, well-defined or asymmetric mass. Microcalcifications may be present.
Differential diagnosis	Tubular or ductal adenoma, sclerosing adenosis, papilloma, mesenchymal tumors and spindle cell metaplastic carcinomas.

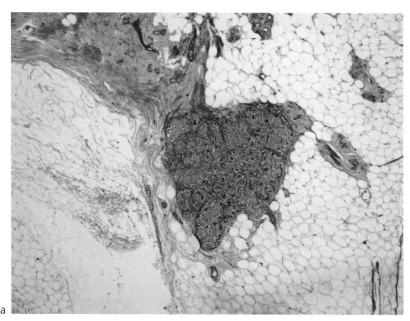

a

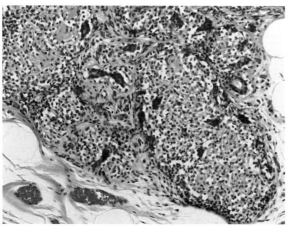

b

Incidentally found small adenomyoepithelial lesion, biphasic, differentiated.

14.10a Incidentally found adenomyoepithelial tumor, 2 mm in diameter, with a lobulated appearance.

14.10b Higher magnification highlighting the dark glandular and the clear myoepithelial cells. Even in such a small lesion, the myoepithelial cells lose contact with glandular tubules, in sharp contrast to sclerosing adenosis. The tumor shows a 'lobular' pattern in which nests or areas of tumor cells are divided by fibrous or hyaline septs of varying thickness. We do not use this feature as a criterion to distinguish a special subgroup of tumors as it is often only focally observed in adenomyoepithelial tumors.

prominent hyalinization of smaller or larger irregular areas of the tumor surrounded by or containing 'buried' myoepithelial cells.

SUBCLASSIFICATION AND VARIANTS

Tavassoli classifies adenomyoepithelial tumors into three subcategories: spindle cell, tubular and lobulated variants.

Biphasic adenomyoepithelial tumors are easy to diagnose due to the typical tubular structures and the 'melting' of the myoepithelial cells into the surrounding stroma. The monophasic types may resemble fibrous lesions, leiomyomas, fibrous histiocytomas or their malignant counterparts. Monophasic tumors may pose considerable diagnostic difficulties and may be misdiagnosed as mesenchymal tumors or spindle cell carcinomas (see differential diagnosis).

Biphasic adenomyoepithelial tumors are usually benign, well-circumscribed tumors, which may, however, be delineated with a fibrous capsule or pseudocapsule

(Fig. 14.11). The prototypical adenomyoepithelial tumor is composed of epithelial structures with abluminal proliferation of cells of the myoepithelial lineage. The epithelial structures form closed or open tubules, solid groups, loosely cohesive epithelial cells or even cystic or papillary structures. The polygonal, cubic or cylindrical epithelial cells of the tubular structures display an eosinophilic or amphophilic cytoplasm. The myoepithelial areas in these tumors are cytologically bland. Lesions may show a lobular growth pattern in which nests or areas of tumor cells are divided by fibrous septa of varying thickness (Fig. 14.10). In some cases, transitions from typical papilloma or sclerosing adenosis lesions to biphasic adenomyoepithelial tumors may be observed. Few overtly malignant biphasic adenomyoepithelial tumors have been reported. Such lesions show the architecture described above in combination with a clearly atypical cytomorphology and an invasive growth pattern.

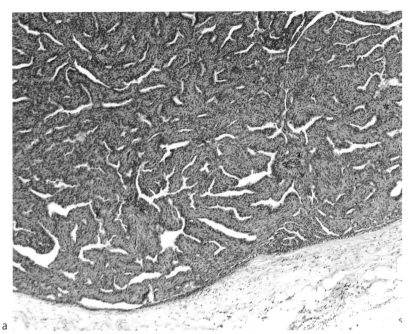

Fig. 14.11a – d Benign adenomyoepithelial tumor, biphasic type.

14.11a At low power the tumor is characteristically well-circumscribed. The tubular structures are surrounded by myoepithelial cell proliferations, which disperse ('melt') into the surrounding stroma. This is clearly distinct from the well-defined tubular structures of sclerosing adenosis and adenoma of the breast.

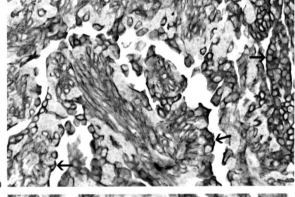

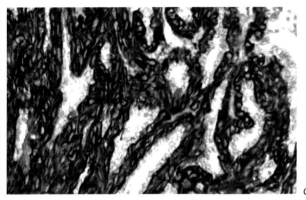

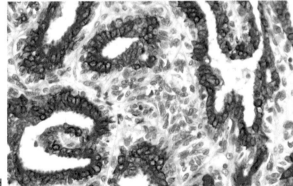

14.11b Ck5/6 immunostaining highlights the inappropriate sorting of the myoepithelial cells. The glandular cells also contain Ck5+ cells (arrows), which indicate a more immature stage.

14.11c Immunostaining for sm-actin. In contrast to 14.11b, only myoepithelial cells are stained which sets them apart from the negative reaction of the glandular cells. Similar staining results are obtained using other myoepithelial markers such as calponin and p63.

14.11d Ck8/18 immunostaining shows expression of these cytokeratins in the glandular elements.

Monophasic adenomyoepithelial tumors are characterized by their 'mesenchymal' appearance. The cells have a spindle-shaped, stellate, plasmacytoid, epithelioid or clear cell appearance. In other cases, the tumor cells may have a polygonal round to ovoid shape, containing round to oval nuclei (Fig. 14.12).

The tumor cells can be arranged in a fascicular or fibrosarcoma-like pattern, and occasionally they may show an interwoven, storiform pattern. In these monophasic adenomyoepithelial tumors the epithelial cells can form nondescript, loosely arranged aggregates of cells or sheets and trabeculae suspended in a

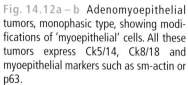

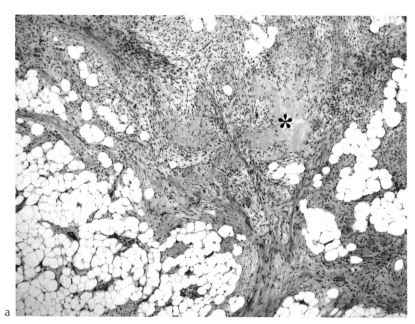

Fig. 14.12a – b Adenomyoepithelial tumors, monophasic type, showing modifications of 'myoepithelial' cells. All these tumors express Ck5/14, Ck8/18 and myoepithelial markers such as sm-actin or p63.

14.12a Malignant adenomyoepithelial tumor. This poorly-differentiated tumor is purely mesenchymal in appearance with obvious invasion. A reliable diagnosis of such a tumor can only be made using immunostaining. Immunohistochemically the tumor cells display a mixture of cells from the glandular and myoepithelial lineages. Typically irregular hyaline basement membrane deposits (asterisk) are observed which are characteristic of adenomyoepithelial tumors.

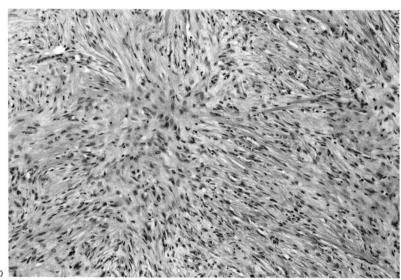

14.12b This is another case of an adenomyoepithelial tumor where storiform patterns are prominent. Immunohistochemically they display myoepithelial and glandular differentiation.

Continuation

mesenchymal background, so that their glandular or squamous differentiation is barely, or not at all, recognizable in H&E sections (Fig. 14.13). Clear cells and apocrine cells can be observed. In contrast to similar tumors of the parotid gland, tumors with solid areas and an epithelioid or plasmacytoid myoepithelial aspect are rare. Squamous cell metaplasia is often found in these tumors (25%) and is characterized by small nests of keratinizing cells, which immunoreact for Ck10. Occasionally the whole spectrum from unequivocal papilloma or sclerosing adenosis to adenomyoepithelial tumor can be seen in the same lesion.

Ck5/14+ CELLS AND THE MYOEPITHELIAL COMPONENT OF TUMORS

Ck5/14+ cells are the most important cellular component of adenomyoepithelial tumors. These cells give rise to the myoepithelial cell lineage. The key feature of adenomyoepithelial tumors is the melting growth pattern of cells of the 'myoepithelial' lineage into the surrounding stroma, often associated with formation of basement membrane-like material between the 'myoepithelial' cells.

A differentiation between Ck5/14+ cells, intermediate myoepithelial cells (Ck5/14+ and sm-actin+) and

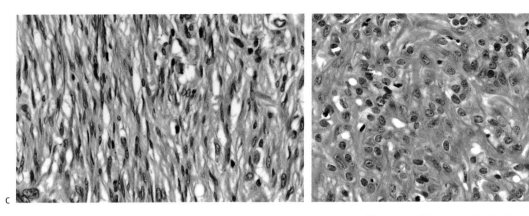

c ... d

Fig. 14.12a–d Adenomyoepithelial tumors, monophasic type, showing modifications of 'myoepithelial' cells. All these tumors express Ck 5/14, Ck 8/18 and myoepithelial markers such as sm-actin or p63.
14.12c In this example slender spindle cells with a fibrosarcoma-like appearance form the dominant cell component. Again, both cell lineages were detected immunohistochemically.
14.12d In this case nondescript epithelioid cells are seen.

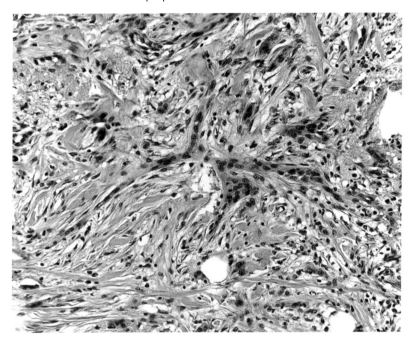

Fig. 14.13 Loosely arranged reticulated aggregates of cells or sheets and trabeculae are suspended in a 'mesenchymal' background so that the glandular or squamous differentiation is barely recognizable.

myoepithelial end cells (sm-actin+) is only possible with the help of double staining for these markers. A constitutive feature of most adenomyoepithelial tumors is the deposition of **basement membrane-like hyaline material**. This may be widespread or limited with a disorderly patchy distribution of eosinophilic material (Fig. 14.14). Laminin or collagen IV immunostaining highlights the nature of the basal membrane. Fibrillary or homogeneous hyaline material can be interspersed among the 'myoepithelial' cells and may be barely visible in H&E sections. The hyaline material seems to be particularly abundant in adenomyoepithelial tumors of the monophasic type where the material may coalesce or form greater central hyaline areas. The more cellular tumor areas are usually localized in the periphery, with more

differentiated myoepithelial cells which readily stain for sm-actin. It should be emphasized that the presence of hyaline material may be a valuable hint to correct diagnosis.

CK5/14+ CELLS AND THE EPITHELIAL COMPONENT OF TUMORS

The epithelial structures usually contain both glandular precursor (Ck5/14+ and Ck8/18+) and terminally differentiated glandular cells (Ck8/18+). In 25% of adenomyoepithelial tumors squamous cell metaplasia is observed (own data).

CRITERIA OF MALIGNANCY

More than 80% of all adenomyoepithelial tumors take a benign course [14, 15, 59, 80, 107, 109]. The criteria

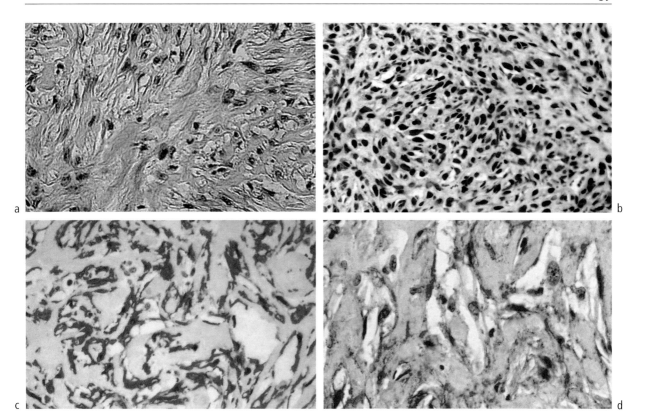

Fig. 14.14a–d Deposition of basement membrane-like hyaline material.

14.14a This can appear as fibrillary or homogeneous hyaline material interspersed among the 'myoepithelial' cells. In some cases it is barely visible in H&E sections. The hyaline material seems to be particularly abundant in adenomyoepithelial tumors of the monophasic type where the material may coalesce or form greater central hyaline areas (see 14.12a).

14.14b P63 immunostain shows extensive staining of nearly all tumor cells.

14.14c Ck5/6 immunostain highlights the progenitor cell character of this lesion. The same cells intensely stain for sm-actin.

14.14d Collagen IV immunostain highlights the basal membrane character of the hyaline material, probably produced by the myo-epithelial cells.

of malignancy are still not well-established [107]. Bland cytology, lack of mitosis and encapsulation are generally acknowledged features of benign tumors (Figs 14.1, 14.10 and 14.11).

Of the adenomyoepithelial tumors reported in the literature, 25 of the 125 cases were regarded as potentially malignant because of features shown by the adenomyoepithelial tumor itself. Number of mitoses, cellular pleomorphism, coagulative necrosis, high cellularity, and invasion (Fig. 14.12a) are all features, currently regarded as indicative of a more malignant course. Malignancy ex adenomyoepithelial tumor may occur both in the epithelial or myoepithelial component [58, 60, 62–64, 69, 71, 72, 80, 85, 87, 93, 97, 98, 100]. For benign adenomyoepithelial tumors a range of 0–13 mitoses per HPF has been reported in the literature. However lesions diagnosed as malignant may display even less than 3 mitoses per 10 HPF.

Based on molecular studies we believe that the Ki67 index of adenomyoepithelial tumors may be a reliable diagnostic tool for assessing prognosis. In lesions with a Ki67 index exceeding 10%, a tendency towards accumulation of genetic alterations and cellular pleomorphism could be demonstrated. Nevertheless, in routine diagnosis, assessment of prognosis is still difficult and rests mainly on conventional histology. Infiltrative growth patterns seem to be a 'physiological' feature of a myoepithelial phenotype rather than a clear indicator of malignancy, and may thus be seen in otherwise benign lesions with low proliferative activity. Therefore, infiltrative growth patterns must be considered in the context of other malignant features rather than being regarded as a sole indicator of malignancy.

Carcinoma ex adenomyoepithelial tumor is a malignant transformation of a pre-existing classic benign adenomyoepithelial tumor. The reported incidence is low. The malignant components may be those of a well-circumscribed in-situ malignancy or even show overtly invasive growth (Fig. 14.15). The malignant components are commonly classifiable as invasive ductal carcinoma (no specific type, Ck8/18+ with or without coexpression of Ck5/14), myoepithelial carcinoma (Ck5/14+, sm-actin+), squamous cell carcinoma (Ck5/14+, Ck10+) and variants or, more rarely, as adenoid cystic carcinoma (Ck5/14+, Ck8/18+, sm-actin+), osteosarcoma (Ck5/14+, vimentin+) and leiomyosarcoma (sm-actin+, Ck5/14+) [58–60, 62, 63, 71, 93, 100, 110].

A practical approach to assessment of the malignant potential of adenomyoepithelial tumors is shown below (Fig. 14.16). In order to be considered benign, adenomyoepithelial tumors must fulfill the following criteria: benign cytomorphology, Ki67 proliferation index not exceeding 15%, and absence of invasive features. Malignancy is diagnosed when the following criteria are met: Ki67 labeling index exceeding 15%, malignant cytomorphology, and an invasive growth pattern. Cases that do not fit into either group are regarded as borderline tumors.

■ IMMUNOHISTOCHEMISTRY

Immunostaining helps to identify Ck5/14+ cells and their glandular (Ck5/14+, Ck8/18+) and/or myoepithelial progeny (Ck5/14+, sm-actin+), depending on their degree of differentiation [10, 14, 58–60, 62–72, 74–76, 78–89, 92–105, 111].

We believe that the demonstration of Ck5/14+ cells in putative adenomyoepithelial tumors is the most important distinguishing feature in the differential diagnostic spectrum (below). Furthermore, in order to be categorized as an adenomyoepithelial tumor, a tumor should display reactivity for all three markers mentioned above. A further reliable immunostain for myoepithelial differentiation in adenomyoepithelial tumors is p63. Reactivity for S-100 protein or glial fibrillary acid protein (GFAP) is inconsistent and

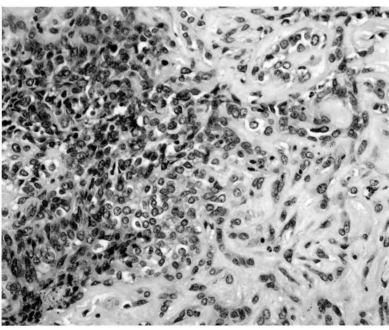

a

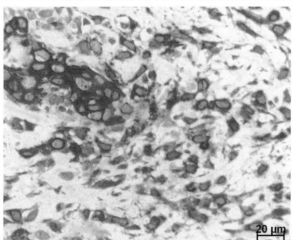

b   20 µm

Fig. 14.15a–b Invasive ductal carcinoma, grade 3, in an adenomyoepithelial tumor, monophasic type.
14.15a H&E-staining showing malignant epithelial cells in the left field. In the right field an area of adenomyoepithelial tumor, monophasic type.

14.15b Ck5 immunostaining highlights the progenitor cell character of the lesion.

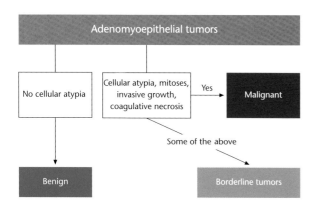

Fig. 14.16 Practical approach to the assessment of adeno-myoepithelial tumors (for details see text).

should not be used as a diagnostic tool in this context. As these tumors react for vimentin, the antibody is not useful in distinguishing adenomyoepithelial tumors from mesenchymally derived tumors. Antibodies directed against estrogen and progesterone receptors may show a patchy reactivity in the glandular component of biphasic benign lesions, whereas in undifferentiated lesions no reactivity has been observed.

MOLECULAR GENETICS

As a result of the small overall number of adenomyoepithelial tumors described in the literature, the cytogenetic data currently available is limited and inconsistent. In a series of ten malignant myoepitheliomas, Jones et al. [112] found a low incidence of chromosomal copy number alterations in purely myoepithelial carcinomas as the most striking result (mean of 2.1, compared to 8.6 in unselected ductal carcinomas). The most common alterations were loss of the 16q and 17p loci. In the series of Hungermann et al. [114] a larger number of alterations was found in malignant adenomyoepithelial tumors (mean of 6.7), the most common alteration being a loss of 17p. As no other recurrent alterations were found, the changes seem to be epiphenomena in tumor progression rather than causative genetic alterations.

INTERPRETATION OF CORE AND VACUUM-ASSISTED BIOPSIES

If there are elements of clearly identifiable differentiated adenomyoepithelial tumor, lesions should be classified as B3 (lesion with uncertain potential), and a surgical excision is recommended. Although spindle cell lesions are encountered infrequently, their presence emphasizes the importance of using a range of several antibodies to distinguish undifferentiated adenomyoepithelial tumors from other spindle cell lesions. However, as Ck5/14 may be expressed heterogeneously in core biopsies, a negative Ck5/14 reaction may not lead to a conclusive diagnosis. In these cases, wide excision with a clear margin is recommended, and the eventual therapeutic management of the patient depends on the final diagnosis of the resection specimen. Whenever possible, malignant spindle cell lesions should also be classified by use

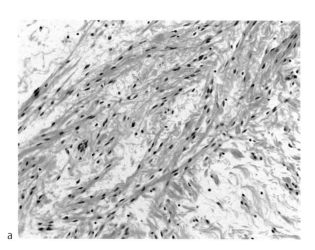
a

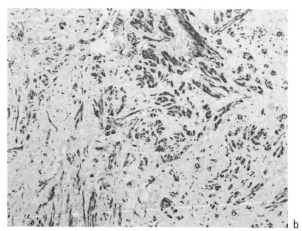
b

Fig. 14.17a–b Myofibroblastoma.
14.17a Lower magnification of a typical lesion showing cellular fibroblastic/myofibroblastic proliferations of plump bipolar spindle cells, separated by bands of collagen.
14.17b Immunostaining for sm-actin highlights the smooth muscle cell differentiation of the tumor. The tumor was completely negative for cytokeratins 5 or 14.

Tab. 14.2 Distinguishing features of spindle cell tumors of the breast

Marker	Monophasic adenomyo-epithelial tumor	Myoepithelial tumor	Metaplastic carcinoma	Phyllodes tumor, stromal tumor	Squamous cell tumor
Ck5/14	++(+)	++	+(+)	–*	+++
Ck8/18	+(+)	–	++	–*	–
Sm-actin/calponin	+(+)	+(+)	–	– to +	–
Vimentin	+(+)	++	+(+)	++	– to (+)**
Ck10	+(+)	–	+(+)**	–	+(+)

* Negative immunostaining of the stromal component, the epithelial components express both types of cytokeratins.
** Vimentin may be expressed in more immature cells, whereas squamous cells lack this intermediate filament.

of immunohistochemistry. In needle biopsies these lesions are classified as B3 to B5 according to their recognizable malignant potential.

■ DIFFERENTIAL DIAGNOSIS

GENERAL DISCUSSION

In the series of Tavassoli, 9 of 27 patients had a mastectomy as a result of an initial diagnosis of malignant tumor [1]. Adenomyoepithelial lesions therefore may be easily mistaken for a malignant tumor. Hypercellular, spindle cell adenomyoepithelial tumors must be distinguished from other spindle cell tumors of the breast (Table 14.2), and differentiated adenomyoepithelial tumors from several benign lesions.

Adenomyoepithelial tumors can be confused with tubular adenoma, adenoma of the nipple, a variety of spindle cell lesions, pleomorphic adenoma and adenoid cystic carcinoma. The latter two also show an admixture of epithelial and myoepithelial cells [21, 44, 47, 47, 81, 113].

EXAMPLES

DIFFERENTIATED ADENOMYOEPITHELIAL TUMOR VS. TUBULAR ADENOMA, SCLEROSING PAPILLOMA AND ADENOMATOUS ADENOMA OF THE NIPPLE

In differentiated adenomyoepithelial tumors the glandular cells form tubular structures with a prominent, multilayered myoepithelial component, which shows a characteristic streaming, centrifugal growth pattern that lacks sharp demarcation. This feature is clearly distinct from the tubules of tubular adenoma, sclerosing papilloma and adenoma of the nipple. Tubules in these lesions are lined by an inner and outer layer surrounded by a basement membrane, and the

individual tubules of the adenoma are well-delineated from the scant fibrovascular stroma. Mixtures and transitions of these lesions may be seen.

UNDIFFERENTIATED ADENOMYOEPITHELIAL TUMOR VS. SPINDLE CELL TUMOR

Undifferentiated adenomyoepithelial tumors are usually characterized by spindle and epithelioid cells similar to metaplastic carcinoma, malignant phyllodes tumor, leiomyosarcoma, myofibroblastoma or fibrohistiocytic tumors. As glandular differentiation is usually not observed in all these lesions, they cannot be distinguished on the grounds of H&E staining. The Ck5/14+ cell is an essential feature of adenomyoepithelial tumors, whereas the stromal component of phyllodes tumors and primary mesenchymal tumors of the breast derives from mesenchymal cells and is therefore, in contrast, Ck5/14– (Fig. 14.17). Thus Ck5/14 immunohistochemistry clearly helps to distinguish between these neoplastic lesions. The distinguishing features in relation to metaplastic carcinomas are summarized above (Table 14.2).

PLEOMORPHIC ADENOMA

This rare tumor has a biphasic appearance resulting from an intimate admixture of epithelial and stromal cells [30, 31, 33, 43–45]. Based on double fluorescence studies we interpret these tumors as a variant of adenomyoepithelial tumors and thus as a tumor derived from Ck5/14+ progenitor cells with a metaplastic stromal component (Fig. 14.18a–c). The epithelial cells display a glandular phenotype (Ck8/18+) admixed with Ck5/14+ cells. The epithelial component consists of tubules, ribbons or small solid or reticulated nests. Foci of squamous metaplasia (Ck10+) may be observed (Fig. 14.18a). The basal cells (Ck5/14+) surrounding the glandular cells merge into a fibromyxoid stroma (vimentin+) with chondroid or

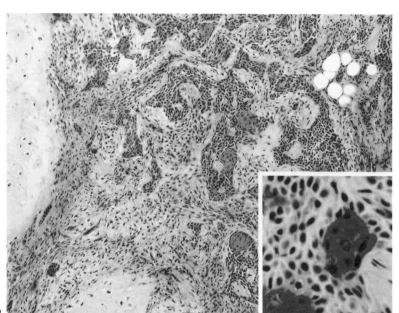

Fig. 14.18a–c Pleomorphic adenoma of the breast.

14.18a Low power view of an H&E section. Note the characteristic regional variation of cellularity, cell arrangement and extracellular matrix. A chondroid matrix is seen in the right and lower fields. The loosely adhesive epithelial structures display clearly visible squamous Ck10+ differentiation (inset). The basal cells merge with the chondroid matrix.

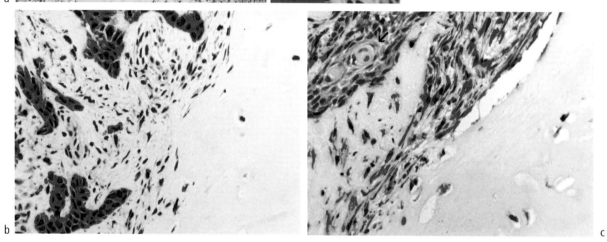

a

b

c

14.18b Ck5 immunostaining highlights precursor cells, which show transitions to vimentin-positive mesenchymal cells (compare 14.18c).

14.18c Immunostaining for vimentin showing an increase in the expression of this filament in cells with mesenchymal appearance and in those within the chondroid matrix. Note that the Ck5+ cells of the epithelial components of the tumor (compare 14.18b) lose their vimentin expression as squamous cell differentiation progresses (arrow).

lipomatous metaplasia. The myoepithelial differentiation in these rare tumors may be very minute. The stroma contains alcian blue and variably PAS+ mucosubstances produced by stromal cells.

REFERENCES

1. Tavassoli FA, Soares J. Myoepithelial lesions. In: Tavassoli FA, Devilee P, editors. Tumours of the Breast and Female Genital Organs. Lyon: IARC Press; 2003. p.86–8.
2. Brogi E. Benign and malignant spindle cell lesions of the breast. Semin Diagn Pathol 2004;21:57–64.
3. Gobbi H, Simpson JF, Borowsky A, Jensen RA, Page DL. Metaplastic breast tumors with a dominant fibro-matosis-like phenotype have a high risk of local recurrence. Cancer 1999;85:2170–82.
4. Sneige N, Yaziji H, Mandavilli SR, et al. Low grade (fibromatosis-like) spindle cell carcinoma of the breast. Am J Surg Pathol 2001;25:1009–16.
5. Kurian KM, Al Nafussi A. Sarcomatoid/metaplastic carcinoma of the breast: a clinicopathological study of 12 cases. Histopathol 2002;40:58–64.
6. Bigotti G, Di-Giorgio CG. Myoepithelioma of the breast: histologic, immunologic, and electromicroscopic appearance. J Surg Oncol 1986;32:58–64.
7. Brasseur P, Hustin J, Collard M. [Breast tumor with myoepithelial cells. Apropos of a case report]. J Belge Radiol 1990;73:197–200.

8. Cartagena N, Cabello IB, Willis I, Poppiti R. Clear cell myoepithelial neoplasm of the breast. Hum Pathol 1988;19:1239–43.

9. Enghardt MH, Hale JH. An epithelial and spindle cell breast tumour of myoepithelial origin. An immunohistochemical and ultrastructural study. Virchows Arch A Pathol Anat Histopathol 1989;416:177–84.

10. Erlandson RA. Benign adenomyoepithelioma of the breast. Ultrastruct Pathol 1989;13:307–14.

11. Kermarec J, Plouvier S, Duplay H, Daniel R. [Myoepithelial cell breast tumor. Ultrastructural study]. Arch Anat Pathol Paris 1973;21:225–31.

12. Kuwabara H, Uda H. Clear cell mammary malignant myoepithelioma with abundant glycogens. J Clin Pathol 1997;50:700–2.

13. Rode L, Nesland JM, Johannessen JV. A spindle cell breast lesion in a 54-year-old woman. Ultrastruct Pathol 1986;10:421–5.

14. Rosen PP. Adenomyoepithelioma of the breast. Hum Pathol 1987;18:1232–7.

15. Schurch W, Potvin C, Seemayer TA. Malignant myoepithelioma (myoepithelial carcinoma) of the breast: an ultrastructural and immunocytochemical study. Ultrastruct Pathol 1985;8:1–11.

16. Soares J, Tomasic G, Bucciarelli E, Eusebi V. Intralobular growth of myoepithelial cell carcinoma of the breast. Virchows Arch 1994;425:205–10.

17. Tamai M. Intraductal growth of malignant mammary myoepithelioma. Am J Surg Pathol 1992;16:1116–25.

18. Tamai M, Nomura K, Hiyama H. Aspiration cytology of malignant intraductal myoepithelioma of the breast. A case report. Acta Cytol 1994;38:435–40.

19. Thorner PS, Kahn HJ, Baumal R, Lee K, Moffatt W. Malignant myoepithelioma of the breast. An immunohistochemical study by light and electron microscopy. Cancer 1986;57:745–50.

20. Agnantis NJ, Maounis N, Priovolou-Papaevangelou M, Baltatzis I. Pleomorphic adenoma of the human female breast. Pathol Res Pract 1992;188:235–40.

21. Ballance WA, Ro JY, el Naggar AK, et al. Pleomorphic adenoma (benign mixed tumor) of the breast. An immunohistochemical, flow cytometric, and ultrastructural study and review of the literature. Am J Clin Pathol 1990;93:795–801.

22. Chen KT. Pleomorphic adenoma of the breast. Am J Clin Pathol 1990;93:792–4.

23. Cuadros CL, Ryan SS, Miller RE. Benign mixed tumor (pleomorphic adenoma) of the breast: ultrastructural study and review of the literature. J Surg Oncol 1987;36:58–63.

24. D'Allianes F, Hiely J. Tumeurs a tissus héterotopiques du sein. Ann d'Anat Pathol 1928;5:361–74.

25. Diaz NM, McDivitt R, Wick MR. Pleomorphic Adenoma of the Breast: A Clinicopathologic and Immunohistochemical Study of 10 Cases. Hum Pathol 1991;22:1206–14.

26. Gioia T, Biachi AE. Tumor mixto de la glándula mamaria en el hombre. Semen Medica 1930;2:1193–8.

27. Jakimowicz JJ, Gratama S. Three cases of rare tumors of the mammary gland. Arch Chir Neerl 1977;29:203–8.

28. Kanter MH, Sedeghi M. Pleomorphic adenoma of the breast: cytology of fine-needle aspiration and its differential diagnosis. Diagn Cytopathol 1993;9:555–8.

29. Lecene P. Les tumeurs mixtes du sein. Rev Chir 1906;33:434–49.

30. Makek M, von Hochstetter AR. Pleomorphic adenoma of the human breast. J Surg Oncol 1980;14:281–6.

31. McClure J, Smith PS, Jamieson GG. 'Mixed' salivary type adenoma of the human female breast. Arch Pathol Lab Med 1982;106:615–9.

32. Medina A, Uehlinger K. [Pleomorphic adenoma of the breast]. Helv Chir Acta 1980;47:205–8.

33. Moran CA, Suster S, Carter D. Benign mixed tumors (pleomorphic adenomas) of the breast. Am J Surg Pathol 1990;14:913–21.

34. Morris JA, Kelly JF. Multiple bilateral breast adenomata in identical adolescent Negro twins. Histopathol 1982;6:539–47.

35. Muller S, Vigneswaran N, Gansler T, et al. c-erbB2 oncoprotein expression and amplification in pleomorphic adenoma and carcinoma ex pleomorphic adenoma: relationship to prognosis. Mod Pathol 1994;7:628–32.

36. Nabert C, Kermanach G, Saout J. [Modified stroma epithelioma or mixed breast tumor: a case]. J Sci Med Lille 1968;86:507–10.

37. Nadal P. Tumeur mixte du sein a formations malpighiennes. Bull Mem Soc Ana Paris 1910;616–22.

38. Narita T, Matsuda K. Pleomorphic adenoma of the breast: case report and review of the literature. Pathol Int 1995;45:441–7.

39. Nevado M, Lopez JI, Dominguez MP, Ballestin C, Garcia H. Pleomorphic adenoma of the breast. Case report. APMIS 1991;99:866–8.

40. Paikova LV. [Mixed tumors of the breast]. Arkh Patol 1972;34:59–61.

41. Petrelli M. Pleomorphic adenomas of the breast. N Y State J Med 1986;86:232–3.

42. Rottino A, Wilson K. Osseous, cartilaginous, and mixed tumors of the human breast. A review of the literature. Arch Surg 1945;50:184–93.

43. Segen JC, Foo M, Richer S. Pleomorphic adenoma of the breast with positive estrogen receptors. N Y State J Med 1986;86:265–6.

44. Sheth MT, Hathway D, Petrelli M. Pleomorphic adenoma ("mixed" tumor) of human female breast mimicking carcinoma clinico-radiologically. Cancer 1978;41:659–65.

45. Soreide JA, Anda O, Eriksen L, Holter J, Kjellevold KH. Pleomorphic adenoma of the human breast with local recurrence. Cancer 1988;61:997–1001.

46. Stead RH, Qizilbash AH, Kontozoglou T, Daya AD, Riddell RH. An immunohistochemical study of pleomorphic adenomas of the salivary gland: glial fibrillary acidic protein-like immunoreactivity identifies a major myoepithelial component. Hum Pathol 1988;19:32–40.

47. van der Walt JD, Rohlova B. Pleomorphic adenoma of the human breast. A report of a benign tumour closely mimicking a carcinoma clinically. Clin Oncol 1982;8:361–5.

48. Willen R, Uvelius B, Cameron R. Pleomorphic adenoma in the breast of a human female. Aspiration biopsy

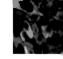

findings and receptor determinations. Case report. Acta Chir Scand 1986;152:709–13.

49. Williams RW, Leach WB. Mixed tumor of female breast of unusual duration and size. South Med J 1975;68: 97–100.

50. Zafrani B, Bourquelot R, Chleq C, Mazabraud A. [Mixed tumor of the breast (pleomorphic adenoma)]. Ann Pathol 1985;5:213–5.

51. Fu HL, Moss J, Shore I, Slade MJ, Coombes RC. Ultrastructural localization of laminin and type IV collagen in normal human breast. Ultrastruct Pathol 2002;26:77–80.

52. Gudjonsson T, Ronnov-Jessen L, Villadsen R, et al. Normal and tumor-derived myoepithelial cells differ in their ability to interact with luminal breast epithelial cells for polarity and basement membrane deposition. J Cell Sci 2002;115:39–50.

53. Slade MJ, Coope RC, Gomm JJ, Coombes RC. The human mammary gland basement membrane is integral to the polarity of luminal epithelial cells. Exp Cell Res 1999;247:267–78.

54. Tsuda H, Mukai K, Fukutomi T, Hirohashi S. Malignant progression of adenomyoepithelial adenosis of the breast. Pathol Int 1994;44:475–9.

55. Fechner RE. Lobular carcinoma in-situ in sclerosing adenosis. A potential source of confusion with invasive carcinoma. Am J Surg Pathol 1981;5:233–9.

56. Erlandson RA, Rosen PP. Infiltrating myoepithelioma of the breast. Am J Surg Pathol 1982;6:785–93.

57. Ermilova VD, Perevoshchikov AG, Anurova OA, Chipysheva TA, Gel'shtein VI. [A rare breast tumor of pluripotential cells]. Arkh Patol 1995;57:77–81.

58. Michal M, Baumruk L, Burger J, Manhalova M. Adenomyoepithelioma of the breast with undifferentiated carcinoma component. Histopathol 1994;24:274–6.

59. Tavassoli FA. Myoepithelial Lesions of the Breast. Myoepitheliosis, Adenomyoepithelioma, and Myoepithelial Carcinoma. Am J Surg Pathol 1991;15:554–68.

60. Chen PC, Chen CK, Nicastri AD, Wait RB. Myoepithelial carcinoma of the breast with distant metastasis and accompanied by adenomyoepitheliomas. Histopathol 1994;24:543–8.

61. Foschini MP, Eusebi V. Carcinomas of the breast showing myoepithelial cell differentiation. A review of the literature. Virchows Arch 1998;432:303–10.

62. Foschini MP, Pizzicannella G, Peterse JL, Eusebi V. Adenomyoepithelioma of the breast associated with low grade adenosquamous and sarcomatoid carcinomas. Virchows Arch 1995;427:243–50.

63. Rasbridge SA, Millis RR. Adenomyoepithelioma of the breast with malignant features. Virchows Arch 1998; 432:123–30.

64. Trojani M, Guiu M, Trouette H, De M, I, Cocquet M. Malignant adenomyoepithelioma of the breast. An immunohistochemical, cytophotometric, and ultrastructural study of a case with lung metastases [see comments]. Am J Clin Pathol 1992;98:598–602.

65. Accurso A, Donofrio V, Insabato L, Mosella G. Adenomyoepithelioma of the breast. A case report. Tumori 1990;76:606–10.

66. Birdsong GG, Bishara HM, Costa MJ. Adenomyoepithelioma of the breast: report of a case initially examined by fine-needle aspiration. Diagn Cytopathol 1993;9: 547–50.

67. Choi JS, Bae JY, Jung WH. Adenomyoepithelioma of the breast—its diagnostic problems and histogenesis. Yonsei Med J 1996;37:284–9.

68. Decorsiere JB, Thibaut I, Bouissou H. [Adeno-myoepithelial proliferation in the breast]. Ann Pathol 1988;8:311–6.

69. Decorsiere JB, Bouissou H, Becue J. Problèmes posés par l' adénomyoépitheliome du sein. Gynecologie 1985; 36:221–7.

70. Diomande MI, Ehouman A, Boni SA, Bialy C. [Thoughts apropos of a case of adenomyoepithelioma of the breast]. Arch Anat Cytol Pathol 1994;42:328–9.

71. Van-Dorpe J, De-Pauw A, Moerman P. Adenoid cystic carcinoma arising in an adenomyoepithelioma of the breast [see comments]. Virchows Arch 1998;432: 119–22.

72. Eusebi V, Casadel GP, Bussolati G, Azzopardi JG. Adenomyoepithelioma of the breast with distinctive type of apocrine adenosis. Histopathol 1987;11:305–15.

73. Greenberg M. Diagnostic pitfalls in the cytological interpretation of breast cancer. Pathology 1996;28:113–21.

74. Gupta RK, Dowle CS. Immunocytochemical study in a case of adenomyoepithelioma of the breast [letter]. Diagn Cytopathol 1998;18:468–70.

75. Hamperl H. The myothelia (myoepithelial cells). Normal state; regressive changes; hyperplasia; tumors. Curr Top Pathol 1970;53.

76. Hock YL, Chan SY. Adenomyoepithelioma of the breast. A case report correlating cytologic and histologic features. Acta Cytol 1994;38:953–6.

77. Jabi M, Dardick I, Cardigos N. Adenomyoepithelioma of the breast. Arch Pathol Lab Med 1988;112:73–6.

78. Kiaer H, Nielsen B, Paulsen S, et al. Adenomyoepithelial adenosis and low grade malignant adenomyoepithelioma of the breast. Virchows Arch A Pathol Anat Histopathol 1984;405:55–67.

79. Laforga JB, Aranda FI, Sevilla F. Adenomyoepithelioma of the breast: report of two cases with prominent cystic changes and intranuclear inclusions. Diagn Cytopathol 1998;19:55–8.

80. Loose JH, Patchefsky AS, Hollander IJ, et al. Adenomyoepithelioma of the breast. A spectrum of biologic behavior. Am J Surg Pathol 1992;16:868–76.

81. McCluggage WG, McManus DI, Caughley LM. Fine needle aspiration (FNA) cytology of adenoid cystic carcinoma and adenomyoepithelioma of breast: two lesions rich in myoepithelial cells. Cytopathology 1997;8:31–9.

82. Meunier B, Leveque J, Le-Prise E, Tas P, Grall JY. [Breast adenomyoepithelioma. A case report and review of the literature]. J Gynecol Obstet Biol Reprod Paris 1995;24:158–61.

83. Niemann TH, Benda JA, Cohen MB. Adenomyoepithelioma of the breast: fine-needle aspiration biopsy and histologic findings. Diagn Cytopathol 1995;12:245–50.

84. Nilsson B, Wee A, Rauff A, Raju GC. Adenomyoepithelioma of the breast. Report of a case with fine needle aspiration cytology and histologic, immunohistochemical and ultrastructural correlation. Acta Cytol 1994;38:431–4.

85. Nomura K, Fukunaga M, Uchida K, Aizawa S. Adeno-myoepithelioma of the breast with exaggerated proliferation of epithelial cells: report of a case. Pathol Int 1996;46:1011–4.

86. Parks RW, Clarke MA, Cranley B. Adenomyoepithelioma of the breast. Int J Clin Pract 1997;51:414–5.

87. Pauwels C, De-Potter C. Adenomyoepithelioma of the breast with features of malignancy. Histopathol 1994; 24:94–6.

88. Plaza JA, Lopez JI, Garcia S, De-Miguel C. Adenomyoepithelioma of the breast. Report of two cases. Arch Anat Cytol Pathol 1993;41:99–101.

89. Pogacnik A, Golouh R, Flezar M. Adenomyoepithelioma of the breast diagnosed by fine needle aspiration (FNA) biopsy; a case report. Cytopathology 1997;8:45–52.

90. Rasbridge SA, Millis RR. Carcinoma in-situ involving sclerosing adenosis: a mimic of invasive breast carcinoma [see comments]. Histopathol 1995;27:269–73.

91. Rubin E, Dempsey PJ, Listinsky CM, Crowe RD, Page DL. Adenomyoepithelioma of the breast: a case report. Breast Dis 1995;8:103–9.

92. Saez A, Serrano T, Aspeitia D, Condom E, Moreno A. Adenomyoepithelioma of the breast. A report of two cases [see comments]. Arch Pathol Lab Med 1992;116:36–8.

93. Simpson RHW, Cope N, Skálová A, Michal M. Malignant Adenomyoepithelioma of the Breast With Mixed Osteogenic, Spindle Cell, and Carcinomatous Differentiation. Am J Surg Pathol 1998;22:631–6.

94. Valente PT, Stuckey JH. Fine-needle aspiration cytology of mammary adenomyoepithelioma: report of a case with intranuclear cytoplasmic inclusions. Diagn Cytopathol 1994;10:165–8.

95. Vielh P, Thiery JP, Validire P, Annick-de MM, Woto G. Adenomyoepithelioma of the breast: fine-needle sampling with histologic, immunohistologic, and electron microscopic analysis. Diagn Cytopathol 1993;9: 188–93.

96. Weidner N, Levine JD. Spindle-cell adenomyoepithelioma of the breast. A microscopic, ultrastructural, and immunocytochemical study. Cancer 1988;62:1561–7.

97. Young RH, Clement PB. Adenomyoepithelioma of the breast. A report of three cases and review of the literature. Am J Clin Pathol 1988;89:308–14.

98. Zarbo RJ, Oberman HA. Cellular adenomyoepithelioma of the breast. Am J Surg Pathol 1983;7:863–70.

99. Berna JD, Arcas I, Ballester A, Bas A. Adenomyoepithelioma of the breast in a male [letter]. AJR Am J Roentgenol 1997;169:917–8.

100. Cameron HM, Hamperl H, Warambo W. Leiomyosarcoma of the breast originating from myothelium (myoepithelium). J Pathol 1974;114:89–92.

101. Koyama M, Kurotaki H, Yagihashi N, et al. Immunohistochemical assessment of proliferative activity in mammary adenomyoepithelioma. Histopathol 1997; 31:134–9.

102. Lukin LJ, Weinstein SR. Test and teach. Number eighty two. Diagnosis: Adenomyoepithlioma of the breast. Pathology 1997;29:41,88–31.

103. Tamura G, Monma N, Suzuki Y, Satodate R, Abe H. Adenomyoepithelioma (myoepithelioma) of the breast in a male. Hum Pathol 1993;24:678–81.

104. Tamura S, Enjoji M, Toyoshima S, Terasaka R. Adenomyoepithelioma of the breast. A case report with an immunohistochemical study. Acta Pathol Jpn 1988; 38:659–65.

105. Torlakovic E, Ames ED, Manivel JC, Stanley MW. Benign and malignant neoplasms of myoepithelial cells: cytologic findings. Diagn Cytopathol 1993;9: 655–60.

106. Aydin O, Cinel L, Egilmez R, Ocal K, Ozer C. Adenomyoepithelioma of the breast. Diagn Cytopathol 2001; 25:194–6.

107. Bult P, Verwiel JM, Wobbes T, et al. Malignant adenomyoepithelioma of the breast with metastasis in the thyroid gland 12 years after excision of the primary tumor. Case report and review of the literature. Virchows Arch 2000;436:158–66.

108. Kiaer HW, Nielsen B, Paulsen S, et al. Adenomyoepithelial adenosis and low grade malignant adenomyoepithelioma of the breast. Virchows Archiv A 1984;405:55–67.

109. Lakhani SR, O'Hare MJ, Monaghan P, Winehouse J, Gazet JC. Malignant myoepithelioma (myoepithelial carcinoma) of the breast: a detailed cytokeratin study. J Clin Pathol 1995;48:164–7.

110. Van-Hoeven KH, Drudis T, Cranor ML, Erlandson RA, Rosen PP. Low grade adenosquamous carcinoma of the breast. A clinocopathologic study of 32 cases with ultrastructural analysis. Am J Surg Pathol 1993;17:248–58.

111. Rubin E, Dempsey PJ, Pile NS, et al. Needle-localization biopsy of the breast: impact of a selective core needle biopsy program on yield. Radiology 1995; 195:627–31.

112. Jones C, Foschini MP, Chaggar R, et al. Comparative genomic hybridization analysis of myoepithelial carcinoma of the breast. Lab Invest 2000;80:831–6.

113. Ro JY, Silva EG, Gallager HS. Adenoid cystic carcinoma of the breast. Hum Pathol 1987;18:1276–81.

114. Hungermann D, Buerger H, Oehlschlegel C, Herbst H, Boecker W. Adenomyoepithelial tumours and myoepithelial carcinomas of the breast – a spectrum of monophasic and biphasic tumours dominated by immature myoepithelial cells. BMC Cancer 2005; 5:92.

Content

15

FIBROEPITHELIAL TUMORS

PAUL J. VAN DIEST, ARNO KUIJPER, RUEDIGER SCHULZ-WENDTLAND, WERNER BOECKER AND ELSKEN VAN DER WALL

These tumors represent a heterogeneous group of lesions that contain both mesenchymal (stromal) and epithelial components. According to morphology and clinical practice they are classified into fibroadenomas, phyllodes tumors, hamartomas, sclerosing lobular hyperplasia and fibroadenomatoid hyperplasias.

Fibroadenoma

■ DEFINITION

Synonyms: adenofibroma
WHO: Fibroadenoma
ICD-O code: 9010/0

The term 'adenofibroma', chiefly denoting lesions in other organs [1], has also been used for lesions of the breast. The consensus is now, however, to only use the term 'fibroadenoma' for breast lesions.

Fibroadenoma is a well-demarcated benign fibro-epithelial tumor with a relative balance between stromal and epithelial components. It contains elongated ducts surrounded by stroma. Fibroadenoma arises from the epithelium and stroma of the terminal duct lobular unit.

■ CONCEPTUAL APPROACH

Fibroadenoma is to be placed within the spectrum of fibroepithelial breast lesions as it is composed of both a stromal and an epithelial component, arising from the epithelium and stroma of the terminal duct lobular unit. Thus the epithelial structures contain Ck5/14+ progenitor cells with their glandular and myoepithelial progeny (Fig. 15.1), whereas the stromal component shows vimentin positivity.

It has been suggested that fibroadenomas arise within sclerosing lobular hyperplasia, which is present in the surrounding breast tissue of about 50% of fibroadenomas [2]. One can indeed imagine that some fibroadenomas arise as localized foci of accelerated proliferation against a background of sclerosing lobular hyperplasia. It is also known that fibroadenoma may arise from the continuous expansion of only one lobule. However, this is probably rare, as only a single case of fibroadenoma with monoclonal stroma has been described [3]. In our study, normal/hyperplastic epithelium and stroma microdissected from fibroadenomas were polyclonal in all cases using the HUMARA assay [4]. As the lobular unit is the monoclonal 'patch' of the human breast, meaning that all cells in one lobule derive from one progenitor cell [5], we conclude that most fibroadenomas probably derive from several lobules. Fibroadenomas may develop usual ductal hyperplasia [6, 7], carcinoma in-situ (CIS) – either ductal (DCIS) or lobular (LCIS) – [4, 8], and even invasive carcinoma [9–11]. Likewise, the stromal component may expand polyclonally to form benign phyllodes tumor [4], or there may be clonal expansion of phylloid areas within fibroadenomas to (benign, borderline or malignant) phyllodes tumor [3, 4, 11, 12]. Furthermore, the epithelial and/or the stromal compound of the tumor may show various forms of epithelial or mesenchymal metaplasia (see Chapter 3). Last, there may also be expansion of both epithelial and stromal compartments of fibroadenomas to form phyllodes tumors with clonal epithelial and stromal compartments [4].

Although progression of fibroadenoma to phyllodes tumor is most likely rare [4], such an event clearly demonstrates

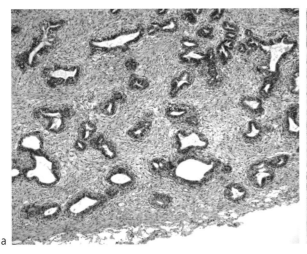
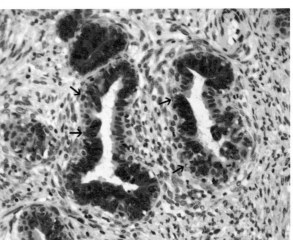

a b

Fig. 15.1a–b Pericanalicular fibroadenoma.
15.1a This type of lesion is characterized by two-layered ducts and moderately cellular stromal growth around ducts, allowing them to retain their usual shaped periductal stroma.
15.1b Immunostaining for Ck14, showing a positive reaction of myoepithelial cells (arrows) and of some luminal cells. Note the lack of staining in the periductal stroma, contrasting with the pattern of tubular adenomyoepithelial lesions.

that fibroadenomas and phyllodes tumors, in particular, are not clearly separate entities, but form a morphological and molecular genetic spectrum. This conceptual approach is illustrated below (Fig. 15.2).

The fact that fibroadenoma is a biphasic tumor makes the epithelial-stromal interactions of special interest. Mitotic figures in the stroma of fibroadenomas are located preferentially in the proximity of the epithelium, suggesting stromal stimuli are produced by the epithelial cells [13]. Indeed, both acidic fibroblast growth factor (aFGF) and one of its receptors (FGFR4) have been detected in the epithelium of fibroadenomas, whereas the stroma was strongly positive for FGFR4 but only weakly positive for aFGF [14]. These findings suggest that stromal proliferation is controlled by a paracrine loop in which aFGF is mainly produced by the epithelium and FGFR4 by the stromal compartment itself. A comparable mechanism was found for epidermal growth factor (EGF) and its receptor (EGFR) [15]. Furthermore, by assessing stromal expression of PDGF and PDGFR, Feakins et al. found evidence of autocrine stimulation of stromal growth in fibroadenomas [16].

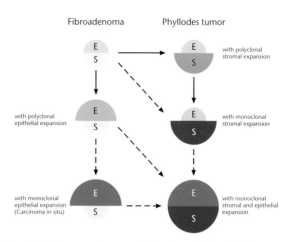

Fig. 15.2 Conceptual proposal for the relationships between fibroadenoma and phyllodes tumor by (selective) progression of epithelial (E) and stromal components (S) of these biphasic tumors (adapted from reference 145, with permission).

CLINICAL FEATURES AND IMAGING

CLINICAL FEATURES

Fibroadenoma is the most common 'benign' breast tumor. The age distribution ranges from the early teens to over 70 years, with a mean age of about 30 years [17]. Less than 5% of women with a fibroadenoma are postmenopausal. Clinically, it usually presents as a palpable well-demarcated, firm, mobile tumor, which shows a tendency to slightly enlarge at the end of the menstrual cycle and during pregnancy. However, with the advent of mammographic screening, it is likely that more and more nonpalpable fibroadenomas will be detected. The left breast is slightly more often affected than the right, and the preferred site within the breast is the upper outer quadrant [17]. In about 15% of patients, multiple fibroadenomas occur synchronously and metachronously in the same or opposite breast. Recurrences usually develop in the same quadrant as the first fibroadenoma, after a mean interval of about four years (36% of cases) [17]. The familial syndrome in which myxoid fibroadenomas are associated with cutaneous and cardiac myxomas and endocrine overactivity is known as Carney's syndrome [18]. A few cases occurring in ectopic breast tissue in the axilla have been described [19].

About 90% of fibroadenomas are smaller than 4 cm [17]. Occasionally, they grow to huge sizes to involve most, or the entire, breast, especially during adolescence. Juvenile fibroadenoma may develop as solitary or multiple tumors shortly after puberty [20–22], affecting one or both breasts.

Studies evaluating risk factors for development of fibroadenomas have been rare. Occasionally racial [23] or familial predisposition may play a role [24–26]. Use of oral contraceptives [27, 28], high Quetelet index and a large number of full-term pregnancies [29] have been shown to reduce fibroadenoma risk, but exogenous estrogen replacement therapy may increase risk [27], although not all studies agree on this [29].

Fibroadenomas also occur in the male breast, although rarely. We ourselves have described one case of fibroadenoma in a male-female transsexual [30].

IMAGING

At **mammography**, fibroadenomas are rounded and well demarcated and vary in size. Multiple fibroadenomas of different size can exist in the same breast or even bilaterally (Fig. 15.3). Due to their expansive growth, they push away the surrounding fat, which may cause a (partial) halo [31]. It is not possible to mammographically differentiate fibroadenomas from cysts, except in case of calcifications in aging fibroadenomas [32, 33]. These calcifications are large and regular and therefore differ from calcifications in adenosis and microcalcifications in cancers [34] (Fig. 15.4). Calcifications in fibroadenomas increase in size and number with the degree of degeneration. No correlation between the size of the fibroadenoma and the degenerative calcifications exists (Fig. 15.5). Hyalinized fibroadenomas can be hard to differentiate from cirrhous cancers when surrounded by tissue retractions [35, 36].

Sonography of fibroadenomas shows the typical signs of a benign lesion. The borders are sharp and

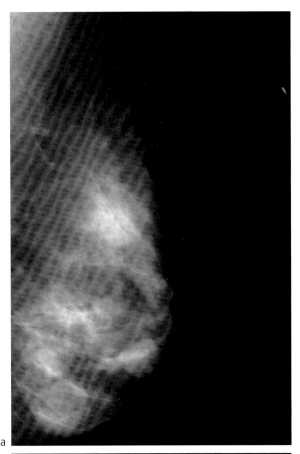

a

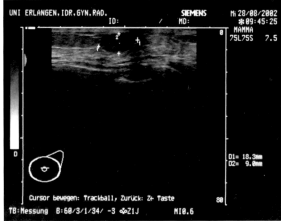

b

smooth, the inner structure is moderately to strongly and homogeneously 'echogenic', there is usually no change in echogenicity beyond the lesion, and the surrounding tissues are not affected. When the epithelial component is dominant, fibroadenomas may appear 'echo-poor', whereas, when the surrounding breast is fatty, they are moderately 'echo-rich'. Histological composition and calcifications may alter the echogenicity beyond the lesion. When the epithelial component is dominant, echogenicity is unchanged or increased, whereby a dominant fibrous composition and calcifications may lead to decrease in echogenicity ('shadow'). There is often a limited shadow at both edges of lesions. The surrounding tissue is pushed away, but no deformation of architecture is evident [37–39]. The sonographic presentation may resemble that of cysts. Cysts, however, have no inner structure and are more easily deformed.

On **magnetic resonance imaging (MRI)**, fibrotic (older) fibroadenomas show low signal intensity on T2-weighted images and little contrast enhancement with gadolinium. This is also the case in mucinous

Fig. 15.3a–b Fibroadenoma.
15.3a Mammography of fibroadenoma with multiple well demarcated, rounded mass lesions.
15.3b Ultrasound of a fibroadenoma with hypoechoic oval and well circumscribed mass. Posterior acoustic enhancement may be seen.

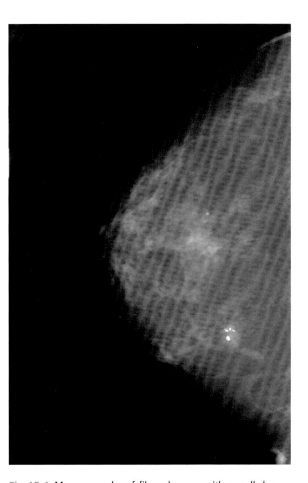

Fig. 15.4 Mammography of fibroadenoma with a well demarcated, rounded lesion containing popcorn-like calcifications.

cancers, which, however, show high signal intensity on T2-weighted images. Young, edematous, myxoid and cellular fibroadenomas, however, show intermediate to strong signal intensity and more contrast enhancement on T2-weighted images, usually with slow, but occasionally rapid, uptake [40–44].

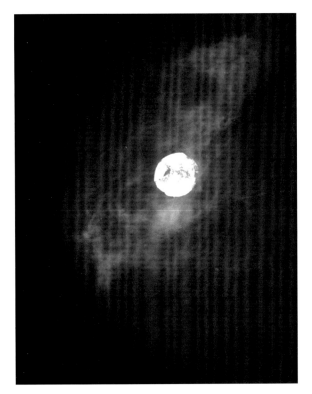

Fig. 15.5 Calcified fibroadenoma with vanished shadow, leaving only the calcifications.

PROGNOSIS AND TREATMENT

Fibroadenomas can occasionally progress in both epithelial and stromal directions [4] to malignant tumors. However, as fibroadenomas have a tendency to be self-limiting or even to regress (even giant fibroadenomas [1, 45, 46]), removal of all lesions is probably not necessary [47–49]. Continuous growth, complaints, positive family history and an age of more than 35 years, however, are indications for surgery [6]. Besides, many women prefer excision, even if fine needle aspiration or core biopsies indicate a benign lesion [47].

Most solitary fibroadenomas can well be treated by local excision. It is preferable to include some of the surrounding normal breast to allow assessment of proliferative changes adjacent to the fibroadenoma, and this helps to avoid re-excision when the tumor turns out to be a phyllodes tumor or contains carci-

noma in-situ. Adolescent fibroadenomas represent an exception to this rule; they should be excised while preserving as much breast tissue as possible, because even leaving a minimal amount of residual normal tissue may still lead to normal breast development [1].

Several epidemiological studies have shown that the risk of developing invasive breast cancer is increased in women with a history of fibroadenoma. The reported relative risks vary from 1.6 to 2.6 [50–54]. Features that further increase this risk to 3 are presence of cysts, sclerosing adenosis, calcifications, or apocrine metaplasia within the fibroadenoma ('complex fibroadenoma'), proliferative changes in the surrounding breast tissue, and a family history of breast carcinoma (relative risk of 3.7) [52, 53, 55] Interestingly, atypical (ductal or lobular) hyperplasia within fibroadenomas does not seem to indicate a further increased relative risk [56].

◼ PATHOLOGY

MACROSCOPY

Fibroadenoma usually presents with a smooth, bosselated contour. The cut surface shows a well-demarcated, firm, white to gray tumor surrounded by a fibrous pseudocapsule (Fig. 15.6). Some tumors appear to be composed of several nodules divided by septae. Cysts of varying sizes may be present.

MICROSCOPY

The typical fibroadenoma has well-defined borders and is composed of elongated ducts lined with two layers of epithelium, surrounded by a more or less cellular, fibrous stroma (Fig. 15.7). Fibroadenoma can display a large variety of histological changes otherwise seen in the nonfibroadenomatous breast. An overview of histological changes found within fibroadenomas is shown in Table 15.1.

Several studies have characterized the stromal cells of fibroadenomas as fibroblasts [57–59]. The stroma of fibroadenomas may display an intracanalicular (60%), pericanalicular (20%) or mixed (20%) growth pattern (Figs 15.1 and 15.7) [6]. In intracanalicular growth patterns, the stroma pushes into the epithelial structures from one side, forcing the ducts into slit-like, elongated, half-moon or circular shaped structures. A pericanalicular growth results from stroma growing concentrically around the ducts, allowing them to maintain their usual shape. Few, if any, mitotic figures are found in the stromal compartment.

The stroma can be sparsely cellular, myxoid or hyalinized, or moderately cellular with a modest

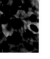

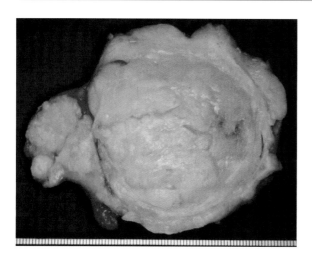

Fig. 15.6 Fibroadenoma with a smooth, bosselated contour. The cut surface shows a well demarcated, firm, white to gray vaguely multinodular tumor surrounded by a fibrous pseudocapsule.

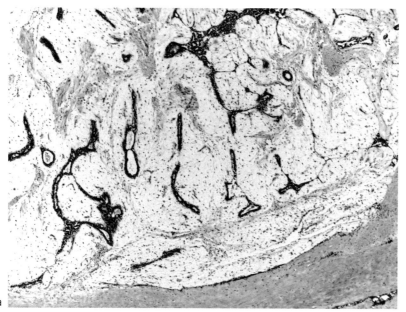

Fig 15.7a−b Fibroadenoma of intra-canalicular type.

15.7a This typical fibroadenoma has well defined borders and is composed of elongated ducts lined with two layers of epithelium, surrounded by a more or less cellular fibrous stroma with a pushing growth pattern into the epithelial strands, forcing the ducts into slit-like, elongated, half-moon shaped structures.

a

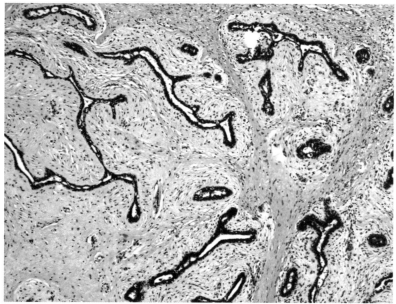

15.7b Another case of intracanalicular type with more fibrosed stroma.

b

degree of pleomorphism. Myxoid fibroadenomas are especially associated with Carney's syndrome [18]. Sometimes stromal giant cells are found, which are characterized by multiple hyperchromatic or vesicular nuclei, often arranged in a semicircular or florette pattern. They can get quite numerous, up to ten per high power field (HPF) [60–63]. Because of their disturbing morphology, detection of giant cells can cause doubt about the benign nature of lesions, especially when found in fine needle aspirates [64]. However, these cells do not influence the clinical course of lesions. Several rare forms of stromal differentiation are found in fibroadenomas. Although sometimes hard to detect, smooth muscle differentiation is present in a few percent of fibroadenomas (Fig. 15.8a–b) [6, 65, 66]. Chondroid and osseous metaplasia are seen even more seldom [67]. The latter is found almost exclusively in fibroadenomas of post-menopausal women. As these are changes of the differentiation state of fibroblasts, they are regarded as a form of mesenchymal metaplasia (sm-actin+/vimentin+). They must be distinguished from similar mesenchymal conversions of Ck5/14+ progenitor cells that occur in adenomyoepithelial tumors (see Chapter 14). Pseudoangiomatous stromal change is a rare finding (4% of fibroadenomas) [6]. Sometimes, phylloid lesions can be found in an otherwise 'normal' fibroadenoma, showing hypercellular stroma and increased numbers of mitotic figures [4, 11, 68, 69].

Tab. 15.1 Histological changes found within fibroadenomas

	No. of cases	Percent
Proliferative epithelial changes		
Mild ductal hyperplasia	46	11.6
Moderate ductal hyperplasia	106	26.8
Florid ductal hyperplasia	21	5.3
Atypical ductal hyperplasia	1	0.3
Atypical lobular hyperplasia	0	0
Lobular carcinoma in-situ	3	0.8
Ductal carcinoma in-situ	5	1.3
Invasive carcinoma	0	0
Epithelial changes		
Apocrine metaplasia	111	28.0
Cysts	20	5.1
Sclerosing adenosis	49	12.4
Calcifications	15	3.8
Microglandular adenosis	1	0.3
Papilloma	7	1.8
Pseudolactational changes	2	0.5
Squamous metaplasia	1	0.3
Stromal changes		
Pseudoangiomatous changes	15	3.8
Smooth muscle	11	2.8
Other		
Foci of tubular adenoma	2	0.5
Focal phyllodes tumor	3	0.8

Frequency of histopathological changes in 396 cases of fibroadenoma (adapted from [147], with permission, © 2001 American Society for Clinical Pathology).

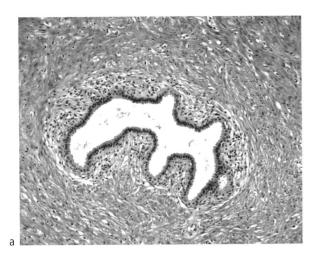

a

Fig. 15.8a–b Smooth muscle metaplasia in fibroadenoma.

Continuation

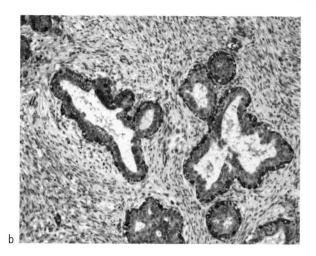

b

Fig. 15.8a−b Smooth muscle metaplasia in fibroadenoma.
15.8b Although sometimes hard to detect, smooth muscle in fibroadenomas is characterized by bundles of spindle shaped cells. This example shows leiomyomatous periductal differentiation. Note the original stromal component in the vicinity of the duct. The smooth muscle differentiation can be highlighted by sm-actin immunohistochemistry.

Recently, a clonality analysis of three fibroadenomas recurring as phyllodes tumors provided evidence for a relation between both of these lesions [70].

The epithelial component of the tumor can display a broad range of changes (Table 15.1). These include different types of benign proliferation and metaplastic changes (Fig. 15.9) described in previous chapters. A fibroadenoma should harbor at least one of these changes to be classified as complex (Fig. 15.10). Dupont et al. classified 23% of fibroadenomas as complex [53]. A recent study, however, classified nearly twice as many fibroadenomas as complex [6], possibly attributable to more extensive sampling. The most frequently found feature is apocrine metaplasia (28%) followed by sclerosing adenosis (12%) [6]. Indeed, when Azzopardi found apocrine metaplasia in 14% of fibroadenomas and sclerosing adenosis in 6% he remarked that 'more extensive sampling would reveal its presence even more' [10]. Calcifications and cysts are both found in a few percent of fibroadenomas (Figs 15.11 and 15.12). Furthermore, foci of tubular or even secretory adenoma are exceptions (Fig. 15.13) [71].

Complex changes are usually not associated with epithelial proliferative disease in the adjacent tissue [6]. Therefore, the raised relative risk associated with these changes remains unexplained. Papilloma, microglandular adenosis, pseudolactational changes and squamous metaplasia are rarely seen [6, 72]. Infarction can be found in approximately 0.5% of fibroadenomas (Fig. 15.14) [24]. Clinically, a sudden onset of pain is suggestive of infarction [73], which may occur after fine needle aspiration biopsy [74].

Using Page's criteria for diagnosing epithelial proliferative disease [75], usual ductal hyperplasia is frequently seen in breast fibroadenomas [6]. After excluding mild ductal hyperplasia, ductal hyperplasia of at least moderate grade can be found in approximately 30% of fibroadenomas (Fig. 15.15). It occurs at all ages. Although finding hyperplasia in

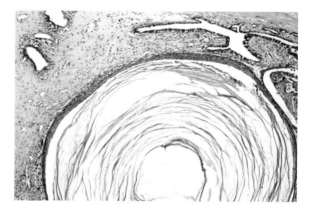

Fig. 15.9 Squamous metaplasia is rarely seen in fibroadenomas.

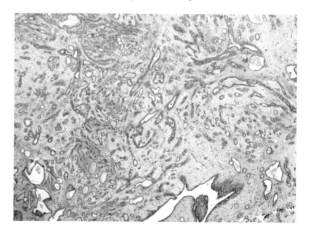

Fig. 15.10 Fibroadenoma with typical area of sclerosing adenosis.

otherwise normal breast tissue is associated with a relative risk of 2−4, the implication of ductal hyperplasia within a fibroadenoma is unknown, but it can be assumed to engender a similar risk. It is, however, not correlated with proliferative disease in the tissue adjacent to the fibroadenoma [56]. Although once thought otherwise [76], hyperplastic changes within fibroadenoma are not associated with oral contraceptive use [23, 77]. Cutting ducts tangentially represents a particular pitfall when investigating hyperplastic changes. It can lead to pseudo-multilayering of the epithelium, recognizable by the presence of dispersed myoepithelial cells. Another particular problem associated with diagnosing hyperplasia in fibroadenomas is the detachment and curling up of the epithelium into ducts, leading to widened ducts filled with epithelial strands (Fig. 15.16) [6, 11].

The study of Carter et al. [56] showed that ADH or ALH is observed at a frequency of 0.81% within fibroadenomas. It does not seem to further increase the breast cancer risk.

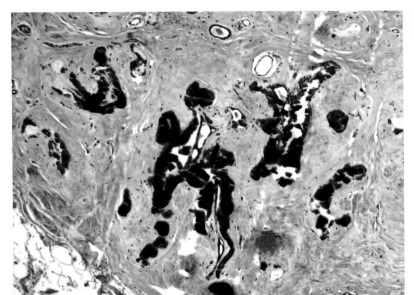

Fig. 15.11 Large irregular stromal calcifications in a fibroadenoma.

Tab. 15.2 Fibroadenoma vs. phyllodes tumor

	Fibroadenoma	Phyllodes tumor
Definition	Usually benign fibroepithelial tumor composed of proliferating glandular and stromal elements that are in balance.	Tumor composed of proliferating glandular and cellular stromal elements. Overgrowth of the stromal compartment with atypia ranging from benign to frankly malignant.
Epithelial composition	Epithelial structures with glandular and myoepithelial differentiation, with intra-canalicular or pericanalicular variants.	Epithelial structures with glandular and myoepithelial differentiation.
Epithelial modification	Modifications: ductal hyperplasia, sclerosing adenosis and several types of metaplasia possible. DCIS or LCIS rare. Infiltrating carcinoma very rare.	Modifications: usual ductal hyperplasia common. Epithelial metaplasias except squamous metaplasia are rare. LCIS rare, DCIS extremely rare. Infiltrating carcinoma exceedingly rare (lobular > ductal).
Stromal composition	Fibrous (myxoid or hyalinized stroma) and myofibroblastic differentiation. Smooth muscle metaplasia is rare.	Cellular stroma with atypia and mitoses. Clonal overgrowth of stromal elements. Stromal cellularity, atypicality and mitotic activity important for grading. Mesenchymal metaplasias may be observed, but are rare.
Immunohisto-chemistry	Glandular cells are Ck5/14+, Ck8/18+ and progesterone receptor+. Stromal cells are vimentin+. Expression of sm-actin is usually negative or weak.	Glandular cells are Ck5/14+ and Ck8/18+. Stromal cells are vimentin+, and sm-actin expression is usually negative or weak, whereby p53 is often observed in borderline and malignant tumors.
Molecular genetics	Copy number alterations on many chromosomes. Most cases are polyclonal. Genes regulating proliferations and apoptosis seem to play a role.	Complex and varying chromosomal changes, usually with losses of chromosomal material at different loci. The stromal component is usually found to be clonal.

Frequencies of CIS within fibroadenoma mentioned in the literature vary between 0.1–2.0% [6, 78–80]. Ductal carcinoma in-situ (Fig. 15.17) is found about as frequently as LCIS (Fig. 15.18) [81]. CIS in a fibroadenoma is found on average in women two decades older than the mean age of all women with fibroadenomas [6, 81]. It seems likely, therefore, that removal of fibroadenomas in women above the age of 35–40 years will reveal most fibroadenomas with CIS [6, 79]. In 38–50% of fibroadenomas with CIS the proliferation can also be found in the adjacent tissue [6, 79, 82]. Therefore, if CIS is detected in a fibro-

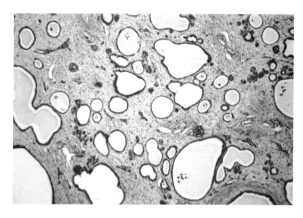

Fig. 15.12 Fibroadenoma showing cystically dilated ducts lined by a bilayer and surrounded by fibrous stroma.

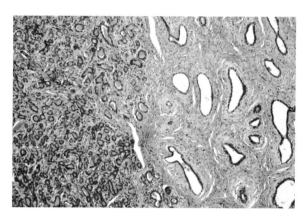

Fig. 15.13 A focus of tubular adenoma in the left field developed in this pericanalicular fibroadenoma (right field).

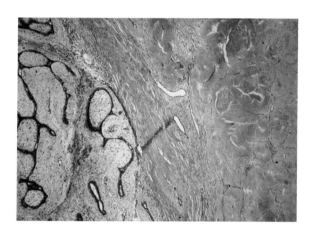

Fig. 15.14 A large (older) infarcted part of a fibroadenoma in the right field, characterized by loss of tissue architecture, absence of vital epithelial structures and hyalinized stroma. Note the intracanalicular adenoma in the left field.

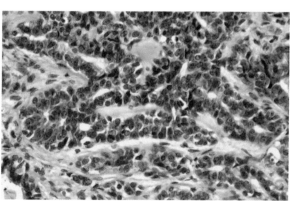

a

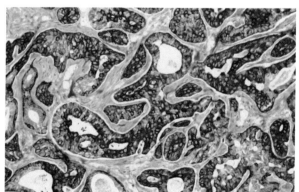

b

Fig. 15.15a–b Benign epithelial hyperplasia.
15.15a Epithelial cells filling and distending ducts reveal florid ductal hyperplasia in a fibroadenoma. In this example a micropapillary epithelial proliferation is seen.
15.15b Ck5/14 immunostaining highlights the typical mosaicism found in benign epithelial hyperplasia.

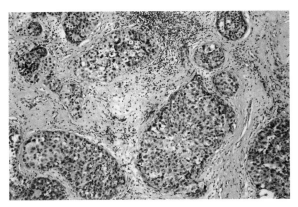

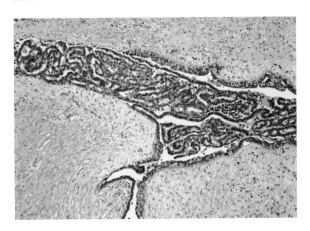

Fig 15.16 Fibroadenoma with detachment and curling of the epithelium. This pattern can be regularly observed in fibro-adenomas.

Fig. 15.17 High grade DCIS in a fibroadenoma. Even at this lower magnification the proliferation of epithelial cells with large overtly malignant nuclei is evident.

adenoma, the surrounding tissue should be explored as well. Invasive cancers arising within fibroadenoma are rare, are of ductal [83] or lobular [84] types, and should be treated as invasive carcinomas in the otherwise normal breast [79, 82].

Some consider 'juvenile fibroadenomas' to be a separate subtype, which occurs in teenage girls and is characterized by rapid growth, causing deformation of the breast. However, such lesions are not exclusively found in this age group [45, 46]. There are no features that histologically distinguish juvenile from usual fibroadenoma, although the former more frequently have a cellular stroma and contain epithelial hyperplasia [1, 46]. Few arguments therefore exist, which support the use of the term 'juvenile fibroadenoma' [45].

Cytology

Aspirates from fibroadenomas usually contain a mixture of epithelial and mesenchymal elements (Fig. 15.19). In a cytological study Bottles et al. [85] found that abundant bipolar stromal cells (usually seen as bare nuclei), 'antler horn clusters' (irregular flat stretches) and 'honeycomb sheets' (fenestrated sheets of epithelium composed of uniform polygonal cells) are the most important features that indicate a fibroadenoma. Nevertheless, when typical stroma is absent, a positive predictive value of 92% is reached by combining the presence of 'multilayered' fragments of epithelium against a background of bare nuclei [86]. Another paper found that typical stroma is present in 57%, antler horn clusters in 90% and honeycomb sheets in 81% of cytologically diagnosed fibroadenomas, somewhat reducing the clinical value of the features mentioned earlier [87]. It was determined that sensitivity and specificity of a cytologic diagnosis of fibroadenoma are 87% and 94%, respectively [88].

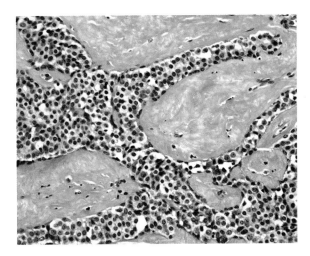

Fig. 15.18 Lobular carcinoma in-situ in a sclerosed fibroadenoma. Note the proliferation of monomorphic somewhat discohesive cells with round, hyperchromatic nuclei characteristic of lobular neoplasia.

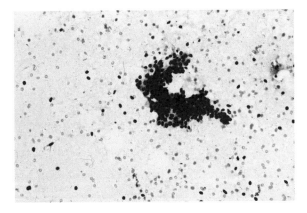

Fig. 15.19 Typical cytology of fibroadenoma with a large sheet of epithelial cells surrounded by bipolar naked nuclei (MGG staining, original magnification ×200).

Up to 50% of aspirates from fibroadenomas contain foam cells and apocrine cells [85]. Prominent nucleoli are seen in the epithelium of at least 80% and pleomorphic nuclei in 25% of fibroadenomas [85]. Failure to appreciate the cytologic variability that may be found in fine needle aspiration specimens from fibroadenomas can therefore easily lead to a false suspicion or diagnosis of carcinoma [89]. Special problems are presented by fibroadenomas harboring malignancy [90] and in pregnant women, where cytological variability is more conspicuous, epithelial cohesion is decreased and aspirates show more loose atypical cells. Occasionally, the aspirate of a breast carcinoma may mimic the cytologic appearance of fibroadenoma [88, 89, 91].

IMMUNOHISTOCHEMISTRY

The epithelial cell layers are usually Ck5/14+ and Ck8/18/19+. They normally express GCDFP-15 and the luminal sides show mucin immunostaining. The myoepithelial layer is Ck5/14+ and sm-actin+, and the stromal component shows the expected vimentin and focal sm-actin expression, but not Ck5/14.

Most fibroadenomas express the progesterone receptor, whereas the estrogen receptor is expressed in a minority of tumors [92–94]. The estrogen receptor is mainly confined to the epithelial component, whereas the progesterone receptor is located in both the epithelial and stromal compartments [92, 95, 96]. It seems that the levels of the sex hormone receptors in fibroadenoma tissue vary during the menstrual cycle [97]. In addition, it was found that levels of estrogen and sulfatase enzyme are higher in fibroadenoma than in normal breast tissue [98]. CD34 and bcl-2 staining is also more abundant in the stroma of fibroadenoma than in the normal breast [99]. In fibroadenomas p53 staining is of wild type (weak in few cells) [100].

Some authors distinguish a so-called cellular variant of fibroadenoma. This is a variant of usual fibroadenoma, which possesses a stromal cellularity of over 125 cells per high power field. Stromal cellularity was found to be correlated with bFGF and FGFR expression [101]. Based on expression patterns of several growth factors the authors have placed this variant between phyllodes tumor and usual fibroadenoma. No clonality studies have been performed to obtain further evidence for this.

Immunohistochemical evaluation of the Ki67 index can discriminate between most fibroadenomas and phyllodes tumors. The distinction between fibroadenoma with high Ki67 index and benign phyllodes tumor remains problematic [69].

Recently, frequent overexpression of insulin-like growth factor II (IGF-II) was found in the stromal component of fibroadenomas. In addition, stromal overexpression of IGF-I was related to nuclear beta-catenin accumulation. These results suggest a role for IGFs in the pathogenesis of fibroadenomas [102].

Expression of hypoxia-inducible factor 1α (HIF-1α) in fibroadenomas appeared to be rare in contrast to phyllodes tumors [103]. Although microvessel count does not seem to differ between fibroadenomas and phyllodes tumors, the distance between epithelium and nearest microvessel was smaller in fibroadenomas [103].

MOLECULAR GENETICS

In cytogenetic studies of fibroadenomas 10% to 40% of tumors seem to display clonal chromosomal aberrations [105–112]. Most authors could not assign a specific abnormality to fibroadenomas; no preferential involvement of a chromosomal region or specific breakpoint, for instance, has been recorded. A recent study, however, found that the majority of fibroadenomas (84%) are characterized by 6q alterations [113]. Since a similar high frequency of 6q alterations is found in premalignant lesions and carcinomas of the breast, the authors conclude that changes in genes located on 6q are among the earliest events in the pathogenesis of cancer. A shortcoming of most cytogenetic studies is that they do not make clear in which compartment the aberrant clone is located. By a combined immunohistochemical/cytogenetic tecnique Fletcher et al. were able to assign the clonal aberrations found in fibroadenomas to the mesenchymal compartment [109]. Dietrich et al., however, did find chromosomal abnormalities in cultures of fibroadenomas enriched for epithelial cells, which were not found, however, in cultures enriched for fibroblasts [111].

Clonality in fibroadenomas has also been studied using a different approach. Taking advantage of polymorphic repeats in X chromosome-linked genes and random inactivation of these genes by methylation, it was found that both the stromal and epithelial cells represent polyclonal cell populations [3, 12, 114, 115]. This even holds true for complex fibroadenomas [3]. Monoclonality, however, was observed in the stroma of a few simple and complex fibroadenomas. [70]. In our own study, microdissected stroma of fibroadenomas was polyclonal in all fibroadenomas, but phylloid areas in three fibroadenomas were found to be monoclonal [4].

The aberrant clones detected in cytogenetic studies are usually small and mostly balanced, which could explain why an early study by means of comparative genomic hybridization (CGH) was unable to detect any genomic imbalances in fibroadenomas [116]. This was confirmed in our own study using array CGH where 3 cases were analyzed [117]. However, a recent study did find several DNA copy number changes in fibroadenomas [118]. Gains of 5p14 (43%) and 5q34-qter (26%) were seen most frequently. A small study found copy number alterations on many chromosomes in three out of a total of eight fibroadenomas, with gains both of 8q and 5q as the most frequent changes [119]. As no microdissection was performed in these studies, it is unclear whether these cytogenetic alterations were present in stroma or epithelium.

Molecular studies found microsatellite instability (MSI) in 8% and loss of heterozygosity (LOH) in 10% of fibroadenomas, respectively [120]. Others, however, did not detect MIN, LOH or p53 gene mutations in fibroadenomas by Southern analysis [121] or by PCR-based techniques [122]. In addition, MSI, LOH or p53 mutations were not found in fibroadenomas that developed in the same breast as invasive breast cancer [123].

So far, one study has detected low levels of telomerase activity in 9 of the 20 fibroadenomas studied [124].

The reduced apoptosis to mitosis ratio in fibroadenomas compared to normal breast tissue [125] suggests that genes regulating proliferation and apoptosis may play a role in the development of these lesions.

■ INTERPRETATION OF CORE AND VACUUM-ASSISTED BIOPSIES

In general, fibroadenomas can be readily diagnosed within core biopsies. However, differentiating fibroadenoma from phyllodes tumor can, at times, be difficult [104]. In such cases the B2 category is appropriate.

■ DIFFERENTIAL DIAGNOSIS

The differential diagnosis comprises hamartoma, tubular adenoma, sclerosing lobular hyperplasia, and, in particular, phyllodes tumor.

Hamartomas show a normal lobular arrangement, and lack elongated ducts and cellular/edematous/myxoid stroma. Furthermore, fibrocystic changes and epithelial hyperplasia are rare. Sclerosing lobular hyperplasia is less well demarcated than fibroadenoma, shows vaguer and often enlarged lobular architecture, and the stromal component is more sclerotic. Tubular adenoma contains tubular/acinar structures with scant stromal tissue and is thus easily distinguished from fibroadenoma. Phyllodes tumor and fibroadenoma of intracanalicular type may be difficult to discriminate. Compared to fibroadenoma, phyllodes tumors show overgrowth of the stromal compartment with increased cellularity, especially in the periductal stromal areas. Mitotic activity is low in the stroma of fibroadenomas, and may be substantial in phyllodes tumors. The epithelial clefts are usually more elongated in phyllodes tumors, although phyllodes tumors of pericanalicular type do occur. A particular problem is presented by fibroadenomas with focal areas with phylloidal features [6, 11, 68]. Marked atypia and sarcomatous differentiation are features of phyllodes tumors.

Phyllodes tumor

■ DEFINITION

Synonyms: cystosarcoma, cystosarcoma phylloides, periductal stromal tumor

   WHO: Phyllodes tumor
   ICD-O code: 1020/1 (phyllodes tumor, NOS)
   ICD-O code: 9020/0 (phyllodes tumor, benign)
   ICD-O code: 9020/1 (phyllodes tumor, borderline)
   ICD-O code: 9020/3 (phyllodes tumor, malignant)

The term 'phyllodes tumor' was introduced by Johannes Müller in 1838 to describe tumors that were characterized by a leaf-like growth pattern (Greek: *phyllos* = leaf).

The terms 'cystosarcoma phyllodes' or 'cystosarcoma phylloides' are still used by some [11], but the term phyllodes tumor is to be preferred. To designate lesions that are often benign as 'sarcoma' is confusing for clinicians (especially 'benign [cysto]sarcoma'), and these tumors are clearly not always cystic. A term that is generically even more accurate is 'periductal stromal tumor', as it better emphasizes the putative origin from periductal stroma, and it better applies to those phyllodes tumors that do not show the typical leaf-like growth pattern. This term is yet, however, less popular.

Phyllodes tumors are mixed epithelial-mesenchymal lesions, often with a foliated structure, a double layered benign epithelial component and an overgrowth of the stromal component. The latter shows increased cellularity and proliferative activity, or even a sarcomatous appearance.

■ CONCEPTUAL APPROACH

Phyllodes tumors are thought to derive from the perilobular-periductal stroma [11]. Within the spectrum of fibroepithelial breast tumors, phyllodes tumors are to be placed at the far end of stromal progression. Phyllodes tumors may derive from clonal expansion of the stromal part of (very rarely) hamartomas [126] or fibroadenomas [4]. In fact, one could easily imagine a phyllodes tumor of intracanalicular type developing from expansion of the stroma of an intracanalicular fibroadenoma and a phyllodes tumor of pericanalicular type developing from expansion of the stroma of a pericanalicular fibroadenoma. Co-existent fibroadenomas are found in nearly 40% of phyllodes tumors [127], and phylloid areas with increased cellularity and mitotic activity [11, 69], which are clonal in HUMARA analysis, have been described [4]. We have also seen a lesion half composed of a fibroadenoma and half of phyllodes tumor (Fig. 15.20). Nevertheless, clonal expansion of a fibroadenoma to a phyllodes tumor is probably rare. Benign

phyllodes tumors may have a polyclonal stroma, indicating that they may not be truly neoplastic [4]. However, borderline and malignant phyllodes tumors do have a clonal stroma, which fits well with their neoplastic morphology and their clinical nature.

Although the stroma of phyllodes tumors is the dominant component, the epithelial component may be proliferative, showing usual ductal or lobular hyperplasia or even (lobular > ductal) carcinoma in-situ [128] and, very rarely, invasive cancer. Expression of EGFR, c-erbB3 and c-erbB4 proteins has been detected in neoplastic mesenchymal cells. In the study of Feakins et al. [16] neoplastic stromal cell positivity for PDGFR was found in almost 50% of phyllodes tumors and for PDGF in 24%, and was associated with prominent nuclear pleomorphism and stromal overgrowth. Co-positivity for stromal PDGF and PDGFR was found in 15% of phyllodes tumors, and for epithelial PDGF and stromal PDGFR in 43%, indicating the importance of autocrine and paracrine loops [16]. A similar phenomenon has been described for bFGF and FGFR [101]. Sawyer et al. found a positive relation between epithelial Wnt5a expression and

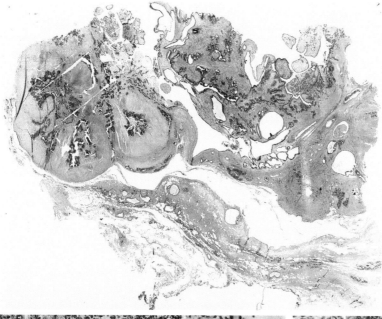

a

Fig. 15.20a−c Fibroepithelial tumor containing both areas of a fibroadenoma and phyllodes tumor.

15.20a Overview showing two close but seemingly separate nodules. In the left field the tumor shows the configuration of a pericanalicular fibroadenoma with fibrous tissue, in the right field the typical leaf-like architecture of a phyllodes tumor is seen.

15.20b Detail of the area of fibroadenoma, showing epithelium with ductal carcinoma in-situ, intermediate grade, and surrounding fibrous stroma of low cellularity.

15.20c Detail of the area of phyllodes tumor, containing highly cellular stroma with moderate atypia and occasional mitoses (indicative of borderline malignancy).

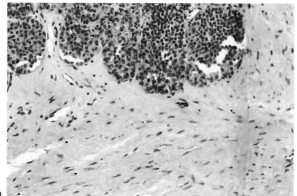

b

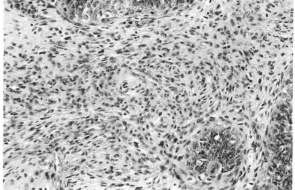

c

stromal nuclear beta-catenin accumulation in benign phyllodes tumors. Their results suggested that, in early stages of tumor development, stromal proliferation is under epithelial control [129]. In later stages, initiated by unknown mutations, stromal growth becomes autonomous. These studies suggest that the role of the epithelial component in phyllodes tumor development might be more than merely passive.

The combined expression of CD34 and bcl-2 suggests that fibroadenomas, phyllodes tumors and pseudoangiomatous hyperplasia may arise from long-lived bcl-2-positive mesenchymal cells in the breast in a manner similar to that proposed for solitary fibrous tumors [99].

CLINICAL FEATURES AND IMAGING

CLINICAL FEATURES

These tumors are rare. A population-based study conducted in the USA revealed an annual age-adjusted incidence of 2.1 per million women [130]. Patients present at a wide age range [131–135]. The mean age at diagnosis is about 45 years, approximately 15 years older than that of fibroadenoma patients [11]. Most tumors occur in 45- to 49-year-old women [130], but they can present during adolescence [133, 137–143], which may be malignant [138–140, 144], and rarely even before the age of 10 [145]. Some rare cases of phyllodes tumors in ectopic breast tissue in the vulva [146, 147] or the axilla [148] have been described.

Patients present with a well-demarcated, firm, palpable tumor, clinically indistinguishable from fibroadenoma [131]. Size varies as does growth rate, rapid growth more often indicating a malignant phyllodes tumor, especially when occurring in a previously stable pre-existing tumor. Some cases of multifocal phyllodes tumors in a single breast [127, 149] or both breasts [127, 132, 144, 150–153] have been described, as well as a few cases in men [63, 154–156]. Large tumors may invade the skin or extend into the chest wall [84, 144, 157]. One case that presented with bloody nipple discharge caused by spontaneous infarction of the tumor has been described [143].

Risk factors including ethnicity: Asian and Latino patients present at younger age than non-Latina whites, and foreign-born Latino women had a three- to fourfold higher phyllodes tumor risk than Latino women born in the United States [130]. Fibroadenoma is probably also a risk factor. Co-existent fibroadenomas are found in about 40% of phyllodes tumor cases [127], which may actually progress from fibroadenomas [4].

IMAGING

On **mammography**, phyllodes tumors present as a single, round, well-demarcated nodule (Fig. 15.21) or a conglomerate of multiple nodules, which may become very large. There are no spiculae or micro-calcifications. Degenerative changes with larger calcifications similar to those in older fibroadenomas are very rare. Larger tumors may stretch the skin and cause venous congestion. Phyllodes tumors are more easily discernible in older breasts. The dense parenchyma in younger females may obscure the well-demarcated nature of the lesion making it difficult to discriminate phyllodes tumor from breast adenocarcinomas [35, 36] (Fig. 15.22).

Sonographically, phyllodes tumor presents as an 'echo-poor' lesion in which different parts may be cystic or solid with indistinct margins [37–39].

On **MRI**, phyllodes tumors show rapid and strong uptake of gadolinium, which precludes certain discrimination from cellular fibroadenomas or well demarcated adenocarcinomas. Inhomogeneous areas or cystic areas as seen with sonography may be present [40–44].

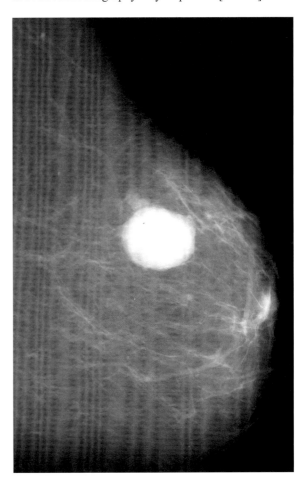

Fig. 15.21 Mammography of phyllodes tumor with well demarcated lesion with halo sign.

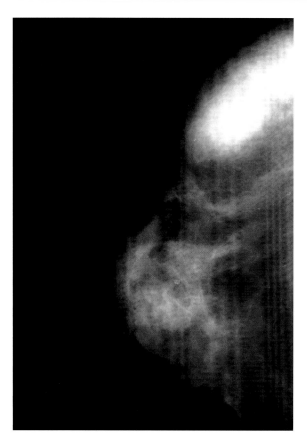

Fig. 15.22 Mammography of malignant phyllodes tumor with well demarcated lesion with spiculated margin.

TREATMENT AND PROGNOSIS

Grading of phyllodes tumors (see below) is done on the basis of their morphology which is correlated with clinical behavior. Benign phyllodes tumors do not metastasize and the probability of local recurrence is low if completely excised [11]. In a series of 51 benign phyllodes tumors, 14 (27%) recurred locally, 6 of them within a year, with the remaining recurring within 3–17 years. Borderline phyllodes tumors have a low probability (< 5%) of metastasis, and are likely (> 25%) to recur locally unless widely excised [11]. In a series of 22 borderline phyllodes tumors, 7 (32%) recurred locally, 4 of them within a year, the others taking up to 15 years. Several patients had multiple local recurrences [127]. About 25% of malignant phyllodes tumors develop metastases, and they are also prone to local recurrence [11].

The few benign or borderline phyllodes tumors that have metastasized almost always developed local recurrences with higher grade features prior to occurrence of systemic lesions [11].

Metastases usually occur at distant sites and only rarely (less than 1%) in the axillary lymph nodes [132, 149, 158, 159]. Metastases seem to be more frequent in cases with chondrosarcoma or osteosarcoma features [160–163] and are more infrequent in cases of liposarcomatous stromal metaplasia [164–167]. The most common sites of metastases are the lungs, bone, and heart [168–171]. The central nervous system has also been described [172–174].

Therapy comprises complete excision [175–179], with removal of a clear margin of about 1 cm [68]. Mastectomy is only indicated in case of large tumors that cannot be removed by local excision with acceptable cosmetic results. Following wide local excision, 8% (17/212), 29% (20/68), and 36% (16/45) of benign, borderline, and malignant phyllodes tumors recurred in the breast [180]. Routine axillary dissection is usually not indicated [181]. Little is known about the therapy of distant metastases. Phyllodes tumors initially did not seem to be responsive to chemotherapy or radiotherapy [182]. Other authors, however, have described prolonged remission or palliation with chemotherapy alone or in combination with radiotherapy [183, 184]. A recent investigation failed to detect drug resistance proteins Pgp and MRP in malignant phyllodes tumor xenografts in vivo. In addition, the xenografts were sensitive to vincristine, doxorubicin and cyclophosphamide [185]. These results suggest that at least some benefit can be expected from chemotherapy in disseminated disease.

The five-year overall survival rate of patients with phyllodes tumors is about 90% [127], and that of malignant phyllodes tumors, about 65% [11, 135, 136, 144, 186]. Most deaths due to metastatic disease occur within five years of diagnosis [143, 186, 187], and are seen in patients with high grade malignant tumors [182, 183]. The mitotic rate seems to be particularly important. In one series [127], all phyllodes tumors that developed metastases (8 of 100) had at least 15 mitoses per 50 HPF in the primary tumor or recurrence, but these numbers vary between different series [132, 188]. Similarly, Ki67 staining has prognostic value [189, 190]. Other indicators of recurrence include p53 accumulation [188, 189], S-phase characteristics [189, 191, 192], CEA [193], stromal PDGFR positivity and epithelial PDGF/stromal PDGFR co-positivity [16]. Stromal overgrowth has been reported to predict distant failure [194]. DNA ploidy does not seem to be predictive of recurrence [127, 155, 191, 192, 195, 196]. We recently found that stromal overexpression of HIF-1α, p53, cyclin A, Ki67 and pRb, tumor grade, tumor size and number of stromal cell cycle aberrations were all predictive of disease free survival [104, 197]. However, stromal p53 overexpression and number of cell cycle aberrations were the only independent prognostic parameters.

■ PATHOLOGY

MACROSCOPY

Phyllodes tumors, even if microscopically invasive, are grossly well-circumscribed, but not genuinely encapsulated. They can present as a single lesion but may be multinodular. The cut surface shows a more or less demarcated, firm gray to tan tumor, with a leaf-like appearance due to elongated circular clefts, whose rounded fragments seem to drop off when cutting (Fig. 15.23). There may be gelatinous or hemorrhagic areas due to degeneration, necrosis, and infarction, especially in malignant phyllodes tumors.

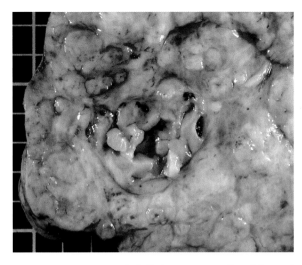

Fig. 15.23 Macroscopy of phyllodes tumor: a multinodular, well demarcated lesion with gross leaf-like structures.

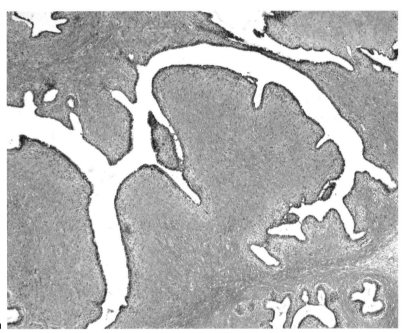

a

Fig. 15.24a−d Benign phyllodes tumor (intracanalicular type).
15.24a Leaf-like pattern with flat epithelium and moderate stromal over-growth pushing into the epithelium.

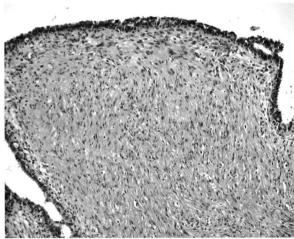

b

15.24b Detail of the stromal component with moderate cellularity, mild atypia and absent mitotic figures. *Continuation*

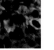

MICROSCOPY

The classical pattern consists of a fibroepithelial tumor resembling intracanalicular fibroadenoma, with half-moon to circular shaped elongated clefts lined by a thin layer of epithelium. The clefts are surrounded by a dominant hypercellular stroma (Fig. 15.24a). There are however many variants, and phyllodes tumors of pericanalicular type resembling their fibroadenoma counterpart certainly exist. Co-existent fibroadenomas are found in about 40% of cases [127].

The stroma of prototypical benign phyllodes tumors often shows condensation in the periductal areas, where mitotic activity is usually found. The stromal cellularity may, however, be more homogeneous. Myxoid stromal changes are a common finding, whereas pseudoangiomatous stroma hyperplasia (PASH) is found in a small number of phyllodes tumors. Rare changes include lipomatous, leiomyomatous, cartilaginous and osseous stromal metaplasias [126, 164], as well as intracytoplasmic inclusion bodies resembling those found in infantile digital fibromatosis [198]. Stromal mitotic activity, degree of stromal cellularity and atypia vary, and these features are important for grading (see below). In malignant phyllodes tumors, the stromal compartment often resembles that of fibrosarcoma (Fig. 5.24b), but there may be heterologous sarcomatous differentiation such as liposarcoma, chondrosarcoma [127, 160, 200] or osteosarcoma [127, 128, 161–163, 199–202].

The epithelial component in phyllodes tumor is usually sparse and is composed solely of elongated ducts, with few lobular structures. The ductal spaces may be dilated. Classically, the epithelium is composed of an attenuated layer of glandular epithelium, which is usually surrounded by myoepithelium (Fig. 15.24b–c). Apocrine metaplasia is rare [203]. Usual ductal hyperplasia may be seen [126], and atypical ductal hyperplasia [4, 127], lobular [204, 205] and ductal carcinoma in-situ and even invasive carcinoma [79, 93, 127, 204–211] may rarely be present [127]. We have seen a pericanalicular-type phyllodes tumor with extensive lobular carcinoma in-situ and focal invasive lobular carcinoma (Fig. 5.28). Myoepithelial hyperplasia is not uncommon [11].

Ductal structures may be found in locally recurrent phyllodes tumors in the breast or chest wall. Metastatic deposits, however, demonstrate the stromal component [187], which is usually fibrosarcoma-like and may also contain heterologous stromal metaplasia independent of the differentiation in the primary lesion [127, 161–165, 199, 200].

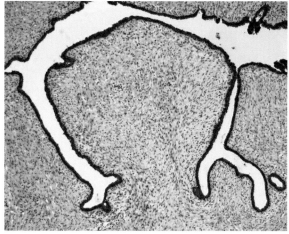

c

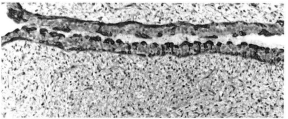

d

Fig. 15.24a–d Benign phyllodes tumor (intracanalicular type). **15.24c** Ck5/6 immunostain highlighting the immature nature of the epithelium with expression of Ck5/6 in nearly all glandular and myoepithelial cells. Note that the characteristic mosaic pattern of the glandular epithelium is frequently observed, characteristic of benign epithelial proliferation. **15.24d** Ck5/6 immunostain of another case, highlighting the myoepithelial cell layer. Most cells of the slightly hyperplastic epithelium are Ck5/6–.

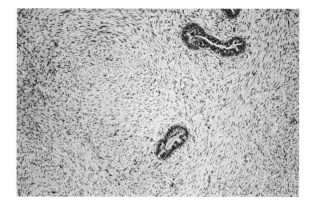

Fig. 15.25 Benign phyllodes tumor (pericanalicular type). Stromal growth with moderate overgrowth surrounding round to oval inconspicuous glandular elements.

GRADING OF PHYLLODES TUMORS

Several systems for grading of phyllodes tumors exist [10, 132, 188, 212]. Most authors use a three-tiered system and distinguish between benign, borderline and malignant cases, whereas some omit the intermediate category. Grading is based mainly on stromal cellularity, stromal overgrowth, atypia of stromal cells, mitotic activity and the microscopic character of the tumor border, but slightly different thresholds have been defined. Since intratumor heterogeneity is a characteristic of phyllodes tumors, grading should be performed on excisional biopsies to avoid undergrading due to sampling error. An automated texture analysis system of tissue architecture has been developed, resulting in good discrimination between benign, borderline and malignant cases [213].

Benign phyllodes tumor is characterized by less than 4 stromal mitoses per 10 HPF (corresponding to 1.6–2 mm^{-2}), and modest cellular overgrowth with little pleomorphism (Fig. 15.25) [188]. The stromal expansion is, in general, uniformly distributed. The tumor is usually well-circumscribed, but infiltrating margins may be present, sometimes forming secondary peripheral fibroepithelial nodules. Benign phyllodes tumors comprise approximately 64% of all phyllodes tumors [68]. Borderline phyllodes tumors more often have an invasive border, between 5–9 mitoses per 10 HPF and moderate cellularity, resembling fibromatosis or low grade fibrosarcoma [188]. Epithelial hyperplasia is more often found than in benign phyllodes tumors [127], and microvessel density is also increased compared to benign phyllodes tumors [214]. Malignant phyllodes tumors (Figs 15.26 and 15.27) comprise about 28% of all phyllodes tumors [68], show marked stromal overgrowth with 10 or more mitoses per 10 HPF, and an invasive tumor border [188]. Nuclear atypicality is often marked in the stroma (Fig. 15.26). The most common stromal pattern is that of fibrosarcoma, but heterologous mesenchymal metaplasia may be present [164, 188, 201]. Since heterologous elements and necrosis are found only in tumors that are clearly malignant by other criteria, they are not decisive for diagnostics [211]. Epithelial hyperplasia is often found [127]. Malignant phyllodes tumors comprise approximately 28% of all phyllodes tumors [68].

Pietruszka and Barnes regard mitotic activity as the most important single variable [188]. Gradation according to Moffat's criteria is less rigid [212]; only the combination of all features will assign a certain grade to a tumor. Benign tumors are characterized by less than 10% of margins showing infiltration, low to moderate stromal cellularity, atypia and overgrowth. There are fewer than 10 mitotic figures per 10 HPF. Malignant tumors show infiltration at 50% or more of

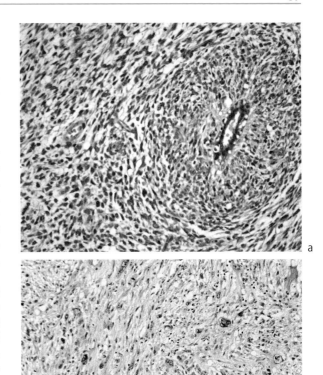

Fig. 15.26a–b Malignant phyllodes tumor.
15.26a Phyllodes tumor with hypercellular stroma containing oval to spindle-shaped cells with elongated atypical nuclei and mitotic figures.
15.26b Another case of malignant phyllodes tumor with bizarre nuclei, abundant mitotic figures and strong atypia and pleomorphism.

the margin, moderate or high stromal cellularity, pleomorphism and overgrowth, with at least one of these features classified as high. There are more than 10 mitoses per 10 HPF. Borderline tumors show some, but not all, features of tumors of malignant grade.

Ki67 expression parallels traditional grading of phyllodes tumors [69, 189, 190, 197, 215–217].

CYTOLOGY

The cytologic appearance of phyllodes tumors is much like that of fibroadenomas (Fig. 15.29). The following features are, however, more frequent in aspirates from phyllodes tumors: stromal cells with cytoplasm rather than naked bipolar nuclei [218], individual long spindle nuclei [219, 220], hypercellular stromal fragments [219–223], and large stromal fragments [224]. The aspirate from a malignant phyllodes tumor is likely to contain cellular stromal fragments composed of atypical cells and mitotic figures [11, 224], and rarely liposarcomatous elements [226]. Fine needle aspiration cytology is, however, not reliable in diag-

nosing phyllodes tumors [181, 219, 227, 228]. Cystic degeneration may make diagnosis more difficult [229]. In contrast to fibroadenomas, large, folded epithelial clusters also seem to be characteristic for phyllodes tumors [220, 230].

■ IMMUNOHISTOCHEMISTRY

The epithelial cell layers show Ck5/14 and Ck8/18/19 positivity, and CEA immunoreactivity is present in most phyllodes tumors [193]. The expression of ER and PR in the epithelial cells of phyllodes tumors has been shown to be increased compared to that in normal breast epithelium [190, 231]. Furthermore, an inverse relation between epithelial PR and ER expression and degree of malignancy has been found [232]. Stromal expression of PR and ER, on the other hand, was rarely seen. PR seems to be expressed more frequently in phyllodes tumors than ER [94, 232]. Expression of the androgen receptor seems to be low [232], although others have come to the opposite conclusion [94].

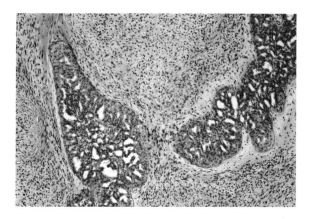

Fig. 15.27 Malignant phyllodes tumor with a ductal carcinoma in-situ demonstrating a typical cribriform growth pattern (H&E).

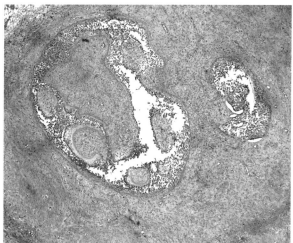

a

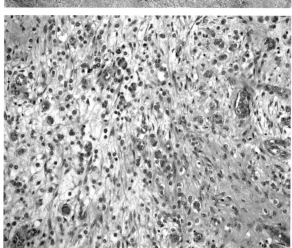

c

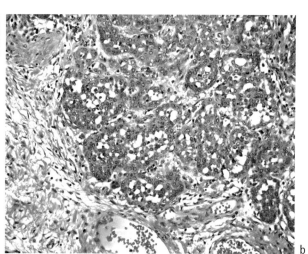

b

Fig. 15.28a–c Intracanalicular type phyllodes tumor with LCIS and invasive lobular cancer.
15.28a Low resolution showing intracanalicular growth pattern with cellular periductal stroma and an extensive dyscohesive epithelial proliferation in the ducts.
15.28b High resolution showing extensive monotonous dyscohesive intralobular proliferation to be classified as LCIS.

15.28c High resolution showing invasive lobular carcinoma with infiltrating loose epithelial cells with intracytoplasmic vacuoles.

There is also a marked production of endothelin-1 in the epithelium of phyllodes tumors [233], probably involved in a paracrine stimulation of stromal cell proliferation. Indeed, stromal mitoses tend to be more frequent close to the epithelium than in more distant stroma [13]. The myoepithelial layer is sm-actin+ and Ck5/14+ (Fig. 15.24c–d). The basic immunoreaction of the stroma is a positivity to the vimentin antibody. Depending on the metaplasias present, additional markers are expressed, such as sm-actin in myoid differentiation [234–236]. In contrast to malignant adenomyoepithelial tumors, phyllodes tumors are Ck5/14–, which may thus help in diagnosing difficult cases.

Furthermore, excess perivascular deposition of, in particular, collagen IV has been observed in the stroma of malignant phyllodes tumors [237]. Tenascin is also more diffusely present in the stroma of phyllodes tumors than in the normal breast and fibroadenomas [238].

Ki67 expression parallels traditional grading of phyllodes tumors [69, 189, 190, 197, 215, 216, 239, 240] and has prognostic value [189, 190].

Accumulation of p53 [241] is more often observed in borderline and malignant tumors [100, 101, 190, 215, 216, 240–245], is associated with increased proliferation [215, 240, 241] and had prognostic value in some studies [189, 190], but not in all [197, 240, 241]. We have recently studied expression and prognostic value of various cell cycle proteins in phyllodes tumors [197]. Our results show that, in the stromal component, increased cell cycle deregulation is associated with higher tumor grades. Cell cycle aberrations are, however, not found in the epithelial compartment.

HIF-1α is frequently expressed in the stroma of phyllodes tumors and seems to be functional in view of the co-expression of CA lX, one of its downstream targets. Stromal HIF-1α, correlates with grade, microvessel count and proliferation. Interestingly, epithelial HIF-1α and CA lX expression were often found in the morphologically normal epithelium of phyllodes tumors [103].

CD34 [99, 246] and bcl-2 [99] staining in the stroma is more conspicuous than in the normal breast and tends to be decreased adjacent to the epithelium compared to the normal breast. As CD34 is absent in spindle cell carcinomas, CD34 may help in distinguishing these types of carcinomas in difficult cases from malignant phyllodes tumors [99]. CD34 positivity was reported to be more frequent in benign than malignant phyllodes tumors [247]. In contrast, c-kit (CD117) and sm-actin are more frequent in the stroma of malignant phyllodes tumors [247]. Sawyer et al., likewise, found stromal c-kit and c-myc expression more frequently in malignant phyllodes tumors [248].

In the work of Saywer et al. on the Wnt-APC-beta-catenin pathway in phyllodes tumors, it became clear that epithelial Wnt5a expression and stromal IGF-I expression cause stromal nuclear beta-catenin accumulation in the early stages of phyllodes tumor development [102, 129]. In malignant tumors these mechanisms are lost, and the stromal component proliferates autonomously. Similar to fibroadenomas, IGF-II overexpression is frequently seen in phyllodes tumors [248].

Although microvessel count does not seem to differ between fibroadenomas and phyllodes tumors, the distance between the epithelium and the nearest microvessel was smaller in fibroadenomas [103].

It seems that there is a positive relation between numbers of microvessels and tumor grade [101, 214], reflecting adjustment to increased metabolic demands. Not much is known about the angiogenic mechanisms by which phyllodes tumors accomplish this. PDGF [16], FGF and VEGF [101] are expressed in phyllodes tumors, but their relation to microvasculature has not been evaluated. We recently studied hypoxia-inducible factor 1 (HIF-1), which has a pivotal role in the adaptive response to hypoxia [103]. Stromal HIF-1α expression was positively correlated with grade, proliferation, p53 accumulation, and the number of microvessels, and was also predictive of clinical behavior. No relation to necrosis was found, indicating that HIF-1 activation pathways in the stroma are hypoxia-independent. Although no statistically significant relation was found between grade and stromal VEGF expression, stromal VEGF expression was related to microvessel counts.

MOLECULAR GENETICS

Mutation of p53 has been demonstrated in one case in which progression from a benign to a malignant phenotype occurred [215]. In another study no allelic loss of 3p was found [216]. However, yet another found that 10/42 phyllodes tumors show allelic imbalances on one or more markers on 3p, and 14/46 on chromosome 1. Five tumors demonstrated changes in both the epithelium and stroma, eight showed changes which were only detectable in the stroma and eight displayed only epithelial changes. Three tumors exhibited low-level microsatellite instability in the epithelium but not in the stroma [249]. The authors raise the possibility that, in some phyllodes tumors, the epithelium may be neoplastic.

Initial reports assessing clonality based on X chromosome inactivation revealed the epithelial component of phyllodes tumors to be polyclonal, while the stromal component was found to be monoclonal [12, 70]. Our own study largely confirmed this,

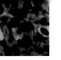

but showed that the stroma of (benign) phyllodes tumors can sometimes be polyclonal, and that the epithelium can be monoclonal [4]. Although the HUMARA technique has some inherent pitfalls, for instance those associated with 'patch size' [4], this suggests that both the stromal and epithelial components may indeed be (potentially) neoplastic.

Cytogenetic studies have uncovered complex and varying karyotypic changes in benign and malignant phyllodes tumors [110, 250–253]. Gain of 1q and structural changes of 10q emerged as frequent chromosomal changes in one study [254].

Mutations in the juxtamembrane region of the c-kit (CD117) proto-oncogene have been found in two malignant phyllodes tumors [247]. Mutation of p53 has also been occasionally found [243]. There is yet little information on telomerase activity of phyllodes tumors [255].

In a study applying comparative genomic hybridization [256], phyllodes tumors showed no evidence of genomic amplification, but frequent changes were gain of 1q (7/18) and loss of 3p (6/18), followed by gain of 7q (4/18) and loss of 6q (4/18) and 3q (3/18). Gain of 1q material was significantly associated with histologically defined stromal overgrowth. All cases with gain of 1q, without 1p gain, had a clinical history of recurrence, and 1q gain might therefore be an indicator of local aggressiveness, requiring more radical treatment. A recent study confirmed that gain of 1q is frequently found, but failed to relate it to clinical behavior or tumor grade [257]. Our own study using array CGH on frozen material of 11 phyllodes tumors revealed recurrent losses at 10q21.1–q22.2, 10q26.1–q26.3, 11q11.2, 11q13.1–q13.2, 13q14.2, 15q21.3–q22, 16q21–q24, 16p12–p13.2, 17p13 (encompassing p53), 17q, 19q13.31-qter and 19p13.12-pter. Copy number gain was frequently seen at 8q24 (harboring c-myc) and 20p12.2–p12.3 [117].

INTERPRETATION OF CORE AND VACUUM-ASSISTED BIOPSIES

Some phyllodes tumors can be readily diagnosed on core biopsies due to marked cellularity, atypia and mitotic activity of the stromal component. However, distinguishing phyllodes tumor from fibroadenoma on a core biopsy can, at times, be difficult [104]. If a biopsy contains purely stromal fragments, there may also be problems in the differential diagnosis from sarcomatoid carcinoma (cytokeratin positive) or myofibroblastoma/solitary fibrous tumor (CD34 positive).

Fibroepithelial lesions supporting phyllodes tumor should be classified as B3. In malignant lesions B4 or B5 are more appropriate. In practice, the distinction from other spindle cell lesions may be difficult or even impossible. Careful clinical assessment, however, will usually enable a suitable management of the patient.

DIFFERENTIAL DIAGNOSIS

The main differential diagnosis is that with fibroadenoma and with adenomyoepithelial tumors. Compared to fibroadenoma, phyllodes tumors show overgrowth of the stromal compartment, which shows increased cellularity, especially in the periductal stromal areas. Mitotic activity is low in the stroma of fibroadenomas and may be substantial in phyllodes tumors. The epithelial clefts are more elongated in phyllodes tumors. A particular problem is presented by fibroadenomas with focal phylloidal features [6, 11, 68]. Marked atypia and sarcomatous differentiation are features of phyllodes tumors. In cases with few epithelial elements, it may be difficult to discriminate phyllodes tumors from fibromatosis and from primary sarcoma of the breast. Fibromatosis displays bland infiltrative spindle cells with no, or very few, mitoses, while primary sarcomas lack the typical epithelial clefts. Another difficult differential diagnosis is that of poorly differentiated adenomyoepithelial tumors and metaplastic carcinomas. The latter, however, usually contain Ck5/14 and Ck8/18/19 positivity in both the epithelial and sarcomatous areas, in contrast to the stromal cells of phyllodes tumors, which lack cytokeratins. The differential diagnosis with adenomyoepithelial tumors has been discussed in more detail in Chapter 14.

Sclerosing lobular hyperplasia

DEFINITION

Sclerosing lobular hyperplasia is sometimes also called fibroadenomatoid mastopathy [11]. The former term is to be preferred as it more accurately reflects the histology of such lesions.

Sclerosing lobular hyperplasias are benign, proliferative, usually reasonably well demarcated tumors, histologically characterized by enlarged lobules with an increased number of acini and variable interlobular fibrosis.

CONCEPTUAL APPROACH

Sclerosing lobular hyperplasia is to be placed within the spectrum of fibroepithelial breast lesions as it is composed of both a stromal and an epithelial component. It can be viewed as a separate entity as it lacks the more tumorous demarcation and strict relationship between stroma and epithelium of a fibroadenoma, the more tumorous demarcation and normal lobular architecture of a hamartoma, and the clonal stromal overgrowth of a phyllodes tumor. Sclerosing lobular hyperplasia is present in the surrounding breast tissue of about 50% of fibroadenomas (with a ratio of sclerosing lobular hyperplasia to fibroadenoma of 9.3), suggesting that fibroadenoma may arise from sclerosing lobular hyperplasia, or that the same or related factors contribute to the pathogenesis of both lesions [2].

CLINICAL FEATURES AND IMAGING

CLINICAL FEATURES

This benign proliferative tumor presents between the ages of 14 and 41 [2] as a localized palpable tumor up to 5 cm in diameter, usually in the upper outer quadrant of the breast. The clinical features are unspecific, and most patients are suspected of having fibroadenoma or fibrocystic disease. There are no evident risk factors.

IMAGING

In a series of 15 patients with sclerosing lobular hyperplasia, mammography showed a well-defined mass in 8 patients (53%). Microcalcifications were present in one patient. Mammograms in two women showed asymmetric increased density compared with the opposite breast, and in five cases, the mammographic findings were interpreted as normal.

Sonography showed a solid, well-defined mass with either homogeneous or mixed echoes in 10 out of 14 patients (71%). Acoustic enhancement only occurred in one case. In the other four women, sonograms were normal. Characteristic imaging findings, suitable for discriminating sclerosing lobular hyperplasia from other well circumscribed breast masses [258], were not among them.

TREATMENT AND PROGNOSIS

Although probably not strictly indicated, most lesions will be excised, with diagnosis being made postoperatively. There are no adequate follow-up studies documenting the frequency of recurrence, but it has been suggested that these lesions may recur as fibroadenomas [11].

PATHOLOGY

MACROSCOPY

The cut surface shows nodular, tan tissue with a granular appearance, usually lacking the sharp demarcation and whiteness of a fibroadenoma.

MICROSCOPY

The lobules are enlarged and composed of an increased number of acini. The intralobular stroma is collagenized and contains variable interlobular stromal sclerosis (Fig. 15.29). Individual lobules and/or groups of lobules may have the appearance of miniature fibroadenomas. Lesions may resemble tubular adenomas due to the prominent acinar component, but the packing of acinar structures is less tight than in tubular adenomas.

Acini demonstrate normal breast architecture with distinct single layers of epithelial and myoepithelial cells. Secretory activity is minimal or absent. Sclerosing lobular hyperplasia is found in breast tissue surrounding about 50% of fibroadenomas [2], and the presence of a fibroadenoma may cause the accompanying component of sclerosing lobular hyperplasia to be overlooked.

CYTOLOGY

There are no published studies on cytology of sclerosing lobular hyperplasia, and we have ourselves little experience in the field. It may be assumed that the cytological presentation is somewhere in between that of normal breast and fibroadenoma.

IMMUNOHISTOCHEMISTRY

No immunohistochemical studies have been performed on sclerosing lobular hyperplasia.

MOLECULAR GENETICS

No molecular or cytogenetic studies have been performed on sclerosing lobular hyperplasia.

INTERPRETATION OF CORE AND VACUUM-ASSISTED BIOPSIES

No studies have been performed. Diagnosis on core biopsy is expected to be difficult.

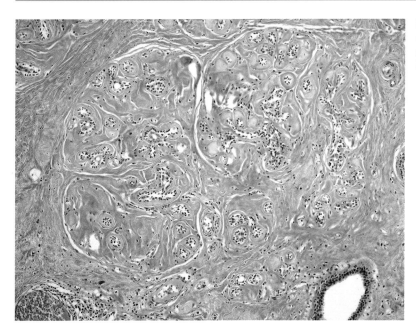

Fig. 15.29 Sclerosing lobular hyperplasia: enlarged lobules with increased number of acini and increased collagenized intralobular stroma.

■ DIFFERENTIAL DIAGNOSIS

The differential diagnosis comprises fibroadenoma, hamartoma, tubular adenoma and sclerosing adenosis. In our own series [6], 7% of tumors that were originally classified as fibroadenoma were, on revision, diagnosed as sclerosing lobular hyperplasia. Fibroadenomas are more clearly demarcated than sclerosing lobular hyperplasia and have a more regular distribution of epithelial and stromal components. The epithelial component of fibroadenomas is often hyperplastic or may show apocrine metaplasia, elongated ducts and intracanalicular growth patterns. The stroma is more often edematous or myxoid and cellular and may show some mitotic activity. It lacks the (admittedly sometimes vague and often enlarged) lobular architecture of sclerosing lobular hyperplasia. Hamartomas are also more clearly demarcated than sclerosing lobular hyperplasia, lack the enlarged lobular architecture of sclerosing lobular hyperplasia (instead showing normal lobular structures) and may contain a fatty or myxoid component. Tubular adenomas are also more clearly demarcated than sclerosing lobular hyperplasia and show a tight packing of acinar structures, no or few ductal structures and little intervening stroma. However, these lesions basically form a spectrum. Fibroadenomas may be surrounded by areas of sclerosing lobular hyperplasia and contain areas of tubular adenoma. Areas within sclerosing lobular hyperplasia may resemble tubular adenoma.

Hamartoma

■ DEFINITION

Synonyms: choristoma, mastoma
   WHO: Mammary hamartoma
   The terms choristoma [259] and mastoma are used by some, but the preferred term is hamartoma [11, 68].
   Hamartoma is a breast mass clinically and macroscopically presenting as a tumor, but microscopically composed of almost normal breast parenchyma with a distinct lobular arrangement. A conspicuous lipomatous stromal component sometimes exists.

■ CONCEPTUAL APPROACH

Although the architecture of hamartoma is much like the normal breast ('breast in breast'), it is probably not a developmental abnormality: most cases present at middle age and an association with Cowden's syndrome exists. Hamartoma is, instead, a true neoplasm, albeit with a very low tendency of epithelial or stromal progression. Little is, however, known about the pathogenesis of mammary hamartomas. The myoid component has been suggested to arise in a milieu of myoepithelial hyperplasia [260].

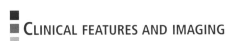

CLINICAL FEATURES AND IMAGING

CLINICAL FEATURES

Hamartomas of the breast are rare. In one large series, hamartomas accounted for 1.2% of benign lesions and 4.8% of benign breast tumors [261]. Hamartoma most often presents in premenopausal women, and an association with pregnancy has been observed [262, 263]. Growth rate is variable as is size, but lesions may be as large as 17 cm [11]. Hamartomas usually present as a painless, well-demarcated, palpable mass, but may not be palpable in macromastic women. A few cases arising in ectopic mammary tissue in the inguinal region have been described [264, 265].

Most hamartomas occur sporadically, but they are seen in high frequency in Cowden's (multiple hamartoma) syndrome. This is an autosomal dominant disorder, caused by mutation in the PTEN gene, associated with benign skin tumors, breast hamartomas and an increased risk of breast cancer [266].

IMAGING

Mammography shows a well-defined round to oval mass of homogeneous density with various amounts of fat, which may be surrounded by a narrow lucent zone [267]. Calcifications do not occur. The surrounding normal parenchyma is pushed away without architectural changes [35, 36].

The ultrasonographic appearance of mammary hamartoma is reported to be variable and nonspecific [263, 268–270]. Lesions are usually smooth and well demarcated, with or without a small 'shadow' at the edges and inside an 'echo poor' aspect with fatty islands [37–39].

Few MRI data are available [40, 42–44, 271].

TREATMENT AND PROGNOSIS

Hamartomas of the breast are almost always benign. Malignant transformation is very rare [272–275]. They can therefore be effectively treated by local excision, usually resulting in complete removal of the tumor without risk of recurrence [263, 269]. Rare cases with carcinoma in-situ or invasive cancer within the hamartoma should receive standard treatment.

PATHOLOGY

MACROSCOPY

The cut surface shows a soft, well-demarcated, sometimes lobulated mass surrounded by a thin fibrous pseudocapsule, composed of a mixed pattern of fat and fibrous breast parenchyma. If the fatty component is extensive, the lesion may macroscopically resemble a lipoma. Plate-like foci of cartilage foci have occasionally been noted [276, 277].

MICROSCOPY

Hamartoma tissue basically consists of breast parenchyma with normal lobular architecture, although the lobular arrangement may be irregular. On higher magnification, the lesion therefore loses its tumorous impression when the surrounding pseudocapsule of compressed breast tissue is no longer within the field of vision. Fibrocystic changes are common but hyperplastic epithelium is rare in most series [261, 267, 278]. One series however reported ductal hyperplasia in 27% of lesions [279], with 12% of patients having co-existent fibroadenomas. Only a few cases with carcinomas in-situ [272, 273, 275] and invasive cancer [272–274] arising from hamartomas have been described.

The stromal component may show varying proportions of mature fat cells, leading to designation as an adenolipoma [280, 281], and one case with brown fat has been described [282]. Further, there may be sharply defined islands of hyaline cartilage [277] and smooth muscle [259, 283–286], which may be cellular and show some mitotic figures [287] and epitheloid features [288]. Glandular elements were completely absent in two lesions [289, 290]. Areas of pseudo-angiomatous stromal hyperplasia are not uncommon [278, 291]. Encasement of adipocytes by hyaline collagen, or spider nevus vascular abnormalities in the hyaline interlobular connective tissue were also found to be characteristic of hamartomas [299].

CYTOLOGY

The cytology of hamartoma is non-specific and few data exists [292]. According to our own unpublished experience, the cytological presentation very much resembles that of fibroadenoma (see above), but the epithelial sheets may not be as large as in fibroadenoma. Many naked myoepithelial nuclei are present against the background. One case has been described that was cytologically diagnosed as fibrocystic change [293].

IMMUNOHISTOCHEMISTRY

The immunohistochemical pattern resembles that of the normal breast tissue [277, 294, 295]. One case with CD34 positivity has been reported [277, 278, 293, 296, 297]. Positive staining for c-erB2 and p53 is not seen in hamartomas [295].

MOLECULAR GENETICS

In view of its association with Cowden's syndrome, mutations in the PTEN gene most likely play a role in the pathogenesis of hamartomas in patients with Cowden's syndrome. It is unclear whether the PTEN gene also plays a role in sporadic hamartomas. A first hamartoma case with involvement of 6p21 and rearrangement of the HMGIY gene has been described that awaits confirmation in a larger series [298]. One case of hamartoma of the breast that was cytogenetically analyzed revealed a 12q12–15 aberration. FISH analysis showed the chromosome 12 translocation breakpoint is located within the 'multiple aberration region' (MAR). MAR is known to be a major cluster region of chromosome 12 breakpoints of benign solid tumors such as uterine leiomyoma, lipoma and pleomorphic salivary gland adenomas, suggesting that the same gene involved in hamartoma of the breast is also involved in these three benign solid tumors [105].

INTERPRETATION OF CORE AND VACUUM-ASSISTED BIOPSIES

Core biopsies from hamartomas will, in general, show histologically normal breast tissue. Diagnosis may therefore be missed. However, when it has been confirmed (sonographically for instance) that the lesion has been hit, the presence of normal breast tissue may lead to a correct diagnosis. The presence of the margin of the lesion, myoid elements or of many fat cells may also be of help.

DIFFERENTIAL DIAGNOSIS

The differential diagnosis comprises fibroadenoma and sclerosing lobular hyperplasia. Fibroadenomas lack the normal lobular arrangement of hamartomas, and have more cellular and edematous/myxoid stroma. In contrast to fibroadenomas, hamartomas do not usually show epithelial hyperplasia and fibrocystic changes. Sclerosing lobular hyperplasia is less well demarcated than hamartoma, shows vaguer and often enlarged lobular architecture and the stromal component is more sclerotic.

REFERENCES

1. Pike AM, Oberman HA (1985) Juvenile (cellular) fibroadenomas: a clinicopathologic study. Am J Surg Pathol 9:730–736
2. Kovi J, Chu H B, Leffall Jr L (1984) Sclerosing lobular hyperplasia manifesting as a palpable mass of the breast in young black women. Hum Pathol 15:336–340
3. Kasami M, Vnencak-Jones CL, Manning S, Dupont WD, Jensen RA, Page DL (1998) Monoclonality in fibroadenomas with complex histology and phyllodal features. Breast Cancer Res Treat 50:185–191
4. Kuijper A, Buerger H, Simon R, Schaefer KL, Croonen A, Boecker W, van der Wall E, van Diest PJ (2002) Analysis of progression of fibroepithelial tumors of the breast by PCR based clonality assay. J Pathol197:575–581
5. Diallo R, Schaefer KL, Poremba C, Shivazi N, Willmann V, Buerger H, Dockhorn- Dworniczak B, Boecker W (2001) Monoclonality in normal epithelium and in hyperplastic and neoplastic lesions of the breast. J Pathol 193: 27–32
6. Kuijper A, Mommers EC, van der Wall E, van Diest PJ (2001) Histopathology of fibroadenoma of the breast. Am J Clin Pathol 115:736–742
7. Magda JL, Minger BA, Rimm DL (1998) Polymerase chain reaction-based detection of clonality as a non-morphologic diagnostic tool for fine-needle aspiration of the breast. Cancer (Cancer Cytopathol) 84:262–267
8. Noguchi S, Aihara T, Koyama H, Motomura K, Inaji H, Imaoka S (1995) Clonal analysis of benign and malignant human breast tumors by means of polymerase chain reaction. Cancer Lett 90:57–63
9. Persaud V, Talerman A, Jordan R (1968) Pure adenoma of the breast. Arch Pathol 86:481–483
10. Azzopardi JG (1979) Sarcoma of the breast. In: Bennington JL (ed) Problems in breast pathology. WB Saunders Co., Philadelphia, pp 346–355
11. Rosen PP (1997) Rosen's breast pathology. Lippincott-Raven, Philadelphia
12. Noguchi S, Motomura K, Inaji H, Imaoka S, Koyama H (1993) Clonal analysis of fibroadenoma and phyllodes tumor of the breast. Cancer Res 53:4071–4074
13. Sawhney N, Garrahan N, Douglas-Jones AG, Williams ED (1992) Epithelial-stromal interactions in tumors: a morphological study of fibroepithelial tumors of the breast. Cancer 70:2115–2120
14. La Rosa S, Sessa F, Colombo L, Tibiletti MG, Furlan D, Capella C (2001) Expression of acidic fibroblast growth factor (aFGF) and fibroblast growth factor receptor 4 (FGFR4) in breast fibroadenomas. J Clin Pathol 54:37–41
15. Zelada-Hedman M, Werer G, Collins P, Backdahl M, Perez I, Franco S, Jimenez J, Cruz J, Torroella M, Nordenskjold M, Skoog L, Lindblom A (1994) High expression of the EGFR in fibroadenomas compared to breast carcinomas. Anticancer Res 14:1679–1688
16. Feakins RM, Wells CA, Young KA, Sheaff MT (2000) Platelet-derived growth factor expression in phyllodes tumors and fibroadenomas of the breast. Hum Pathol 31:1214–1222
17. Foster ME, Garrahan N, Williams S (1988) Fibroadenoma of the breast: a clinical and pathological study. J R Coll Surg Edinb 33:16–19
18. Carney JA, Toorkey BC (1991) Myxoid fibroadenoma and allied conditions (myxomatosis) of the breast. A heritable disorder with special associations including cardiac and cutaneous myxomas. Am J Surg Pathol 15:713–721
19. Aughsteen AA, Almasad JK, Al-Mutaseb MH, Al-Mutaseb MH (2000) Fibroadenoma of the supernumerary breast of the axilla. Saudi Med J 21:587–589

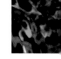

20. Block GE, Zlatnik PA (1969). Giant fibroadenomata of the breast in a prepubertal girl. Arch Surg 80:155–159

21. Farrow JH, Ashikari H (1969) Breast lesions in young girls. Surg Clin North Am 49:261–269

22. Oberman HA (1979) Breast lesions in the adolescent female. Pathol Annu 14:175–201

23. Oberman HA (1971) Hormonal contraceptives and fibroadenomas of the breast. N Engl J Med 284:984

24. Haagensen CD (1986) Diseases of the breast (3rd edition). WB Saunders Co., Philadelphia

25. Morris JA, Kelly JF (1982) Multiple bilateral breast adenomata in identical adolescent negro twins. Histopathology 6:539–547

26. Kuijper A, Preisler-Adams SS, Rahusen FD, Gille JJP, van der Wall E, van Diest PJ (2002) Multiple fibro-adenomas harbouring carcinoma in-situ in a woman with a family history of breast/ovarian cancer J Clin Pathol 55:795–797

27. Canny PF, Berkowitz GS, Kelsey JL, LiVolsi VA (1988) Fibroadenoma and the use of exogenous hormones. Am J Epidemiol 127:454–461

28. Li Volsi V, Stadel BV, Kelsey JL, Holford TR (1979) Fibroadenoma in oral contraceptive users. A histo-pathologic evaluation of epithelial atypia. Cancer 44:1778–1781

29. Yu H, Rohan TE, Cook MG, Howe GR, Miller AB (1992) Risk factors for fibroadenoma: a case-control study in Australia. Am J Epidemiol 135:247–258

30. Kanhai RC, Hage JJ, Bloemena E, Van Diest PJ, Karim RB (1999) Mammary fibroadenoma in a male-to-female transsexual. Histopathol 35:183–185

31. Sickles EA. Nonpalpable, circumscribed, noncalcified solid breast masses: likelihood of malignancy based on lesion size and age of patient (1994) Radiology 192:439–432

32. Travade A, Isnard A, Gimbergues H (1995) Imagerie de la pathologie mammaire. Masson, Paris

33. Lanyi M. Diagnostik und Differentialdiagnostik der Mammaverkalkungen (2002) Springer Verlag, Berlin

34. Cole-Beuglet C, Soriano RZ, Kurtz AB, Goldberg AB. Fibroadenoma of the breast: Sonomammography correlated with pathology in 122 patients. Am J Roentgenol 1983;140:369–375

35. Barth V (1994) Mammographie: Intensivkurs für Fort-geschrittene. Enke, Stuttgart

36. Tabár C, Dean PB (2002) Lehratlas der Mammographie. Thieme Verlag, Stuttgart

37. Madjar H (1989) Kursbuch Mammasonographie. Thieme Verlag, Stuttgart

38. Stavros AT, Thickman D, Rapp CL et al (1995) Solid breast nodules: use of sonography to distinguish between benign and malignant lesions. Radiology 196:123–134

39. Sohn C, Blohmer JU (1996) Mammasonographie. Thieme Verlag, Stuttgart

40. Heywang-Köbrunner SH, Beck R (1996) Contrast-enhanced MRI of the breast. Springer Verlag, Heidel-berg, New York

41. Heywang-Köbrunner SH, Hilbertz T (1997) The breast. In: Magnetic resonance imaging of the body. Lipping-cott-Raven Presss, New York

42. Heywang-Köbrunner SH, Schreer I (2003) Bildgebende Mammadiagnostik. Thieme Verlag, Stuttgart

43. Brinck U, Fischer U, Korabiowska M, et al (1997) The variability of fibroadenoma in contrast-enhanced dynamic MR mammogaphy. Am J Radiol 168:1331–1334.

44. Hochman MG, Orel SG, Powell CM, et al (1997) Fibroadenomas: MR imaging appearances with radio-logic-histopathologic correlation. Radiology 204:123–129

45. Fekete P, Petrek J, Majmudar B, Someren A, Sandberg W (1987) Fibroadenomas with stromal cellularity. A clinicopathologic study of 21 patients. Arch Pathol Lab Med 111:427–432

46. Mies C, Rosen PP (1987) Juvenile fibroadenoma with atypical epithelial hyperplasia. Am J Surg Pathol 11:184–190

47. Cant PJ, Madden MV, Close PM, Learmonth GM, Hacking EA, Dent DM (1987) Case for conservative management of selected fibroadenomas of the breast. Br J Surg 74:857–859

48. Wilkinson S, Anderson TJ, Rifkin E, Chetty U, Forrest APM (1989) Fibroadenoma of the breast: a follow-up of conservative management. Br J Surg 76:390–391

49. Cant PJ, Madden MV, Coleman MG, Dent DM (1995) Non-operative management of breast masses diagnosed as fibroadenoma. Br J Surg 82:792–794

50. Levi F, Randimbison L, Te V-C, LaVecchia C (1994) Incidence of breast cancer in women with fibroadenoma. Int J Cancer 57:681–683

51. Carter CL, Corle DK, Micozzi MS, Schatzkin A, Taylor PR (1988) A prospective study of the development of breast cancer in 16,692 women with benign breast disease. Am J Epidemiol 128:467–477

52. McDivitt RW, Stephens JA, Lee NC, Wingo PA, Robin GL, Gersell D, members of the Cancer and Steroid Hormone Group (1992) Histologic types of benign breast disease and the risk of breast cancer. Cancer 69:1408–1414

53. Dupont WD, Page DL, Parl FF, Vnencak-Jones CL, Plummer Jr WD, Rados MS, Schuyler PA (1994) Long-term risk of breast cancer in women with fibro-adenoma. N Engl J Med 331:10–15

54. Krieger N, Hiatt RA (1992) Risk of breast cancer after benign breast diseases, variation by histologic type, degree of atypia, age at biopsy, and length of follow-up. Am J Epidemiol 136:619–631

55. Hutchinson WB, Thomas DB, Hamlin WB, Roth GJ, Peterson AV, Williams B (1980) Risk of breast cancer in women with benign breast disease. J Natl Cancer Inst 65:13–20

56. Carter BA, Page DL, Schuyler P, Parl FF, Simpson JF, Jensen RA, Dupont WD (2001) No elevation in long-term breast carcinoma risk for women with fibroadenomas that contain atypical hyperplasia. Cancer 92:30–36

57. Ohtani H, Sasano N (1984) Stromal cells of the fibroade-noma of the human breast. An immunohistochemical and ultrastructural study. Virchows Arch [A] 404:7–16

58. Yeh I-T, Francis DJ, Orenstein JM, Silverberg SG (1985) Ultrastructure of cystosarcoma phyllodes and fibro-adenoma. A comparative study. Am J Clin Pathol 84:131–136

59. Reddick RL, Shin TK, Sawhney D, Siegal GP (1987) Stromal proliferations of the breast: an ultrastructural and immunohistochemical evaluation of cystosarcoma phyllodes, juvenile fibroadenoma, and fibroadenoma. Hum Pathol 18:45–49

60. Powell CM, Cranor ML, Rosen PP (1994) Multinucleated stromal giant cells in mammary fibroepithelial neoplasms. A study of 11 patients. Arch Pathol Lab Med 118:912–916

61. Sovani VK, Adegboyega PA (2000) Pathologic quiz case: right breast mass with atypical features. Pathologic diagnosis: fibroadenoma with atypical stromal giant cells. Arch Pathol Lab Med 124:1721–1722

62. Berean K, Tron VA, Churg A, Clement PB (1986) Mammary fibroadenoma with multinucleated stromal giant cells. Am J Surg Pathol 10:823–827

63. Nielsen VT, Andreasen C (1987) Phyllodes tumour of the male breast. Histopathology 11:761–765

64. Lanjewar DN, Raghuwanshi SR, Mathur SR, Gudi MA, Bhosale AS (1999) Fine needle aspiration diagnosis of a breast fibroadenoma with multinucleated stromal giant cells. Acta Cytol 43:530–532

65. Shimizu T, Ebihara Y, Serizawa H, Toyada M, Hirota T (1996) Histopathological study of stroma smooth muscle cells in fibroadenoma of the breast. Pathol Int 46:442–449

66. Goodman ZD, Taxy JB (1981) Fibroadenomas of the breast with prominent smooth muscle. Am J Surg Pathol 5:99–101

67. Spagnolo DV, Shilkin KB (1983) Breast neoplasms containing bone and cartilage. Virchows Arch [A] 400:287–295

68. Elston CW, Ellis IO (1998) Systemic pathology: the breast (3rd edition). Churchill Livingstone, Edinburgh

69. Umekita Y, Yoshida H (1999) Immunohistochemical study of MIB1 expression in phyllodes tumor and fibroadenoma. Pathol Int 49:807–810

70. Noguchi S, Yokouchi H, Aihara T, Motomura K, Inaji H, Imaoka S, Koyama H (1995) Progression of fibroadenoma to phyllodes tumor demonstrated by clonal analysis. Cancer 76:1779–1785

71. O'Hara MF, Page DL (1985) Adenomas of the breast and ectopic breast under lactational influences. Hum Pathol 16:707–712

72. Salm R (1957) Epidermoid metaplasia in mammary fibro-adenoma with formation of keratin cysts. J Pathol Bacteriol 74:221–223

73. Newman J, Kahn LB (1973) Infarction of fibroadenoma of the breast. Br J Surg 60:738–740

74. McCutcheon JM, Lipa M (1993) Infarction of a fibroadenoma of breast following fine needle aspiration. Cytopathology 4:247–250

75. Page DL, Anderson TJ (1987) Diagnostic histopathology of the breast. Churchill Livingstone, Edinburgh

76. Goldenberg VE, Wiegenstein L, Mottet NK (1968) Florid breast fibroadenomas in patients taking hormonal oral contraceptives. Am J Clin Pathol 49:52–59

77. Fechner RE (1970) Fibroadenomas in patients receiving oral contraceptives: a clinical and pathologic study. Am J Clin Pathol 53:857–864

78. Buzanowski-Konakry K, Harrison Jr EG, Payne WS (1975) Lobular carcinoma arising in fibroadenoma of the breast. Cancer 35:450–456

79. Ozello L, Gump FE (1985) The management of patients with carcinoma in fibroadenomatous tumors of the breast. Surg Gynecol Obstet 160:99–103

80. Deschenes L, Jacob S, Fabia J, Christen A (1985) Beware of breast fibroadenomas in middle-aged women. Can J Surg 28:372–374

81. Diaz NM, Palmer JO, McDivitt RW (1991) Carcinoma arising within fibroadenomas of the breast: a clinico-pathologic study of 105 patients. Am J Clin Pathol 95:614–622

82. Pick PW, Iossifides IA (1984) Occurrence of breast carcinoma within a fibroadenoma. Arch Pathol Lab Med 108:590–594

83. Umemura S, Tsutsumi Y, Tokuda Y, Kubota M, Tajima T, Osamura RY (1994) Epithelial Proliferative lesions and carcinomas in fibroadenomas of the breast. Breast Cancer 1:131–137

84. Gebrim LH, Bernardes Junior JR, Nazario AC, Kemp C, Lima GR (2000) Malignant phyllodes tumor in the right breast and invasive lobular carcinoma within fibroadenoma in the other: case report. Sao Paulo Med J 118:46–48

85. Bottles K, Chan JS, Holly EA, Chiu S-H, Miller TR (1988) Cytologic criteria for fibroadenoma. A step-wise logistic regression analysis. Am J Clin Pathol 89:707–713

86. Malberger E, Yerushalmi R, Tamir A, Keren R (1997) Diagnosis of fibroadenoma in breast fine needle aspirates devoid of typical stroma. Acta Cytol 41:1483–88

87. Dejmek A, Lindholm K (1991) Frequency of cytologic features in fine needle aspirates from histologically and cytologically diagnosed fibroadenomas. Acta Cytol 35:695–699

88. Lopez-Ferrer P, Jimenez-Heffernan JA, Vicandi B, Ortega L, Viguer JM (1999) Fine needle aspiration cytology of breast fibroadenoma. A cytohistologic correlation study of 405 cases. Acta Cytol 43:579–586

89. Benoit JL, Kara R, McGregor SE, Duggan MA (1992) Fibroadenoma of the breast: diagnostic pitfalls of fine-needle aspiration. Diagn Cytopathol 8:643–648

90. Gupta RK, Dowle C (1992) Fine needle aspiration of breast carcinoma in a fibroadenoma. Cytopathology 3:49–53

91. Rogers LA, Lee KR (1992) Breast carcinoma simulating fibroadenoma or fibrocystic disease by fine needle aspiration. A study of 16 cases. Am J Clin Pathol 98:155–160

92. Rao BR, Meyer JS, Fry CG (1981) Most cystosarcoma phyllodes and fibroadenomas have progesterone receptor but lack estrogen receptor: stromal localization of progesterone receptor. Cancer 47:2016–2021

93. Rosen PP, Urban JA (1975) Coexistent mammary carcinoma and cystosarcoma phyllodes. Breast 1:9–15

94. Umekita Y, Yoshida H (1998) Immunohistochemical study of hormone receptor and hormone-regulated protein expression in phyllodes tumour: comparison with fibroadenoma. Virchows Arch 433:311–314

95. Mechtersheimer G, Kruger KH, Born IA, Moller P (1990) Antigenic profile of mammary fibroadenoma and cystosarcoma phyllodes. A study using antibodies to estrogen and progesterone receptors and to a panel of cell surface molecules. Pathol Res Pract 186:427–438

96. Giani C, D'Amore E, Delarue JC, Mouriesse H, May-Levin F, Sancho-Garnier H, Breccia M, Contesso G (1986) Estrogen and progesterone receptors in benign breast tumors and lesions: relationship with histological and cytological features. Int J Cancer 37:7–10

97. Kuttenn F, Fournier S, Durand JC, Mauvais-Jarvis P (1980) Estradiol and progesterone receptors in human breast fibroadenomas. J Clin Endocrinol Metab 52: 1225–1229

98. Pasqualini JR, Cortes-Prieto J, Chetrite G, Talbi M, Ruiz A (1997) Concentrations of estrone, estradiol and their sulfates and evaluation of sulfatase and aromatase activities in patients with breast fibroadenoma. Int J Cancer 70:639–643

99. Moore T, Lee AH (2001) Expression of CD34 and bcl-2 in phyllodes tumours, fibroadenomas and spindle cell lesions of the breast. Histopathology 38:62–67

100. Millar EK, Beretov J, Marr P, Sarris M, Clarke RA, Kearsley JH, Lee CS (1999) Malignant phyllodes tumours of the breast display increased stromal p53 protein expression. Histopathology 34: 491–496

101. Hasebe T, Imoto S, Sasaki S, Tsubono Y, Mukai K (1999) Proliferative activity and tumor angiogenesis is closely correlated to stromal cellularity of fibro-adenoma: proposal fibroadenoma, cellular variant. Pathol Int 49:435–443

102. Sawyer EJ, Hanby AM, Poulsom R, Jeffery R, Gillett CE, Ellis IO, Ellis P, Tomlinson IPM (2003) β-catenin abnormalities and associated insulin-like growth factor overexpression are important in phyllodes tumours and fibroadenomas of the breast. J Pathol 200:627–632

103. Kuijper A, van de Groep P, van der Wall E, van Diest PJ (2004) Role and prognostic relevance of HIF-1α and its downstream targets in fibroepithelial tumours of the breast., submitted

104. Komenaka IK, El-Tamer M, Pile-Spellman E, Hibshoosh H (2003) Core needle biopsy as a diagnostic tool to differentiate phyllodes tumor from fibro-adenoma. Arch Surg 138:987–990.

105. Rohen C, Caselitz J, Stern C, Wanschura S, Schoen-makers EF, Van de Ven WJ, Bartnitzke S, Bullerdiek J (1995) A hamartoma of the breast with an aberration of 12q mapped to the MAR region by fluorescence in-situ hybridization. Cancer Genet Cytogenet 84:82–84

106. Ozisik YY, Meloni AM, Stephenson CF, Peier A, Moore GE, Sandberg AA (1994) Chromosome abnormalities in breast fibroadenomas. Cancer Genet Cytogenet 1994;77:125–128

107. Petersson C, Pandis N, Risou H, Mertens F, Dietrich CU, Adeyinke A, Idvall I, Bondeson L, Georgiou G, Ingvar C, Heim S, Mitelman F (1997) Karyotypic abnormalities in fibroadenomas of the breast. Int J Cancer 70:282–286

108. Calabrese G, Di Virgilio C, Cianchetti E, Guanciali Franchi P, Stuppia L, Parutti G, Bianchi PG, Palka G (1991) Chromosome abnormalities in breast fibro-adenomas. Genes Chrom Cancer 3:202–204

109. Fletcher JA, Pinkus GS, Weidner N, Morton CC (1991) Lineage-restricted clonality in biphasic solid tumors. Am J Pathol 138:1199–1207

110. Dietrich CU, Pandis N, Bardi G, Teixeira MR, Soukhikh T, Petersson C, Andersen JA, Heim S (1994) Karyotypic changes in phyllodes tumors of the breast. Cancer Genet Cytogenet 76:200–206

111. Dietrich CU, Pandis N, Teixeira MR, Bardi G, Gerdes AM, Andersen JA, Heim S (1995) Chromosome ab-normalities in benign hyperproliferative disorders of epi-thelial and stromal breast tissue. Int J Cancer 60:49–53

112. Dietrich CU, Pandis N, Rizou H, Petersson C, Bardi G, Qvist H, Apostolikas N, Bohler PJ, Andersen JA, Idvall I, Mitelman F, Heim S (1997) Cytogenetic findings in phyllodes tumors of the breast: karyotypic complexity differentiates between malignant and benign tumors. Hum Pathol 28:1379–1382

113. Tibiletti MG, Sessa F, Bernasconi B, Cerutti R, Broggi B, Furlan D, Acquati F, Bianchi M, Russo A, Capella C, Taramelli R (2000) A large 6q deletion is a common cytogenetic alteration in fibroadenomas, pre-malignant lesions, and carcinomas of the breast. Clin Cancer Res 6:1422–1431

114. Kobayashi S, Iwase H, Kuzushima T, Iwata H, Toyama T, Hara Y, Omoto Y, Ando Y,Nakamura T (1999) Consecutively occurring multiple fibroadenomas of the breast distinguished from phyllodes tumors by clonality analysis of stromal tissue. Breast Cancer 6:201–206

115. Noguchi S, Aihara T, Motomura K, Inaji H, Imaoka S, Koyama H, Tanaka H (1995) Demonstration of polyclonal origin of giant fibroadenoma of the breast. Virchows Arch 427:343–347

116. Ried T, Just KE, Holtgreve-Grez H, du Manoir S, Speicher MR, Schrock E, Latham C, Blegen H, Zetter-berg A, Cremer T, Auer G (1995) Comparative genomic hybridization of formalin-fixed, paraffin-embedded breast tumors reveals different patterns of chromo-somal gains and losses in fibroadenomas and diploid and aneuploid carcinomas. Cancer Res 55:5415–5423

117. Kuijper A, Snijders AM, Berns E, Kuenen-Bouwmeester V, Albertson DG, Van der Wall E, Van Diest PJ. Genomic profiling by array comparative genomic hybridization reveals lack of DNA copy number changes in fibroadenomas but frequent alterations in phyllodes tumours including 17p13 losses containing TP53. Submitted for publication.

118. Ojopi EP, Rogatto SR, Caldeira JR, Barbieri-Neto J, Squire JA (2001) Comparative genomic hybridization detects novel amplifications in fibroadenomas of the breast. Genes Chrom Cancer 30:25–31

119. Amiel A, Kaufman Z, Goldstein E, Bar-Sade Bruchim R, kidron D, Gaber E, Fejgin MD (2003) Application of comparative genomic hybridization in search for genetic aberrations in fibroadenomas of the breast. Cancer Genet Cytogenet 142:145–148

120. McCulloch RK, Sellner LN, Papadimitrou JM, Turbett GR (1998) The incidence of microsatellite instability and loss of heterozygosity in fibroadenoma of the breast. Breast Cancer Res Treat 49:165–169

121. Lizard-Nacol S, Lidereau R, Collin F, Arnal M, Hahnel L, Roignot P, Cuisenier J, Guerrin J (1995) Benign breast disease: absence of genetic alterations at several loci implicated in breast cancer malignancy. Cancer Res 55:4416–4419

122. Franco N, Picard SF, Mege F, Arnould L, Lizard-Nacol S (2001) Absence of genetic abnormalities in fibroadenomas of the breast determined at p53 gene mutations and microsatellite alterations. Cancer Res 61:7955–7958

123. Franco N, Arnould L, Mege F, Picard SF, Arveux P, Lizard-Nacol S (2003) Comparative analysis of molecular alterations in fibroadenomas associated or not with breast cancer. Arch Surg 138:291–295

124. Hiyama E, Gollahon L, Kataoka T, Kuroi K, Yokoyama T, Gazdar AF, Hiyama K, Piatyszek MA, Shay JW (1996) Telomerase activity in human breast tumors. J Natl Cancer Inst 88:116–122

125. Allan DJ, Howell A, Roberts SA, Williams GT, Watson RJ, Coyne JD, Clarke RB, Laidlaws IJ, Potten CS (1992) Reduction in apoptosis relative to mitosis in histologically normal epithelium accompanies fibrocystic change and carcinoma of the premenopausal human breast. J Pathol 167:25 – 32

126. Rosen PP, Romain K, Liberman L (1994) Mammary cystosarcoma with adipose differentiation (lipophyllodes tumor) arising in a lipomatous hamartoma. Arch Pathol Lab Med 118:91–94

127. Grimes MM (1992) Cystosarcoma phyllodes of the breast: histologic features, flow cytometric analysis, and clinical correlations. Mod Pathol 5:232–239

128. Nishimura R, Hasebe T, Imoto S, Mukai K (1998) Malignant phyllodes tumour with a noninvasive ductal carcinoma component. Virchows Arch 432:89–93

129. Sawyer EJ, Hanby AM, Rowan AJ, Gillett CE, Thomas RE, Poulsom R, Lakhani SR, Ellis IO, Ellis P, Tomlinson IPM (2002) The Wnt-pathway, epithelial-stromal interactions, and malignant progression in phyllodes tumours. J Pathol 196:437–444

130. Bernstein L, Deapen D, Koss RK (1993) The descriptive epidemiology of malignant cystosarcoma phyllodes tumors of the breast. Cancer 71:3020–3024

131. Cohn-Cedermark G, Rutqvist LE, Rosendahl I, Silverswärd C (1991) Prognostic factors in cystosarcoma phyllodes. A clinicopathologic study of 77 patients. Cancer 68:2017–2022

132. Norris HJ, Taylor HB (1967) Relationship of histologic features to behavior of cystosarcoma phyllodes: Analysis of ninety-four cases. Cancer 20:2090–2099

133. Andersson A, Bergdahl L (1978) Cystosarcoma in young women. Arch Surg 1978;113:742–744

134. Hart WR, Bauer RC, Oberman HA (1978) Cystosarcoma phyllodes. A clinicopathologic study of twenty-six hypercellular periductal stromal tumors of the breast. Am J Clin Pathol 70:211–216

135. Murad TM, Hines JR, Beal J, Bauer K (1988) Histopathological and clinical correlations of cystosarcoma phyllodes. Arch Pathol Lab Med 112:752–756

136. Reinfuss M, Mitus J, Smolak K, Stelmach A (1993) Malignant phyllodes tumours of the breast. A clinical and pathological analysis of 55 cases. Eur J Cancer 29A:1252–1256

137. Adachi V, Matsushima T, Kido A, Shimono R, Adachi E, Matsukurna A, Mori M, Sugimachi K (1993) Phyllodes tumor in adolescents. Report of two cases and review of the literature. Breast Dis 6:285–293

138. Briggs RM, Walters M, Rosenthal D (1983) Cystosarcoma phylloides in adolescent female patients. Am J Surg 146:712–714

139. Hoover HC, Trestioreanu A, Ketcham AS (1975) Metastatic cystosarcoma phylloides in an adolescent girl: an unusually malignant tumor. Ann Surg 181:279–282

140. Rajan PB, Cranor ML, Rosen PP (1998) Cystosarcoma phyllodes in adolescent girls and young women: a study of 45 patients. Am J Surg Pathol 22:64–69

141. Roisman I, Barak V, Okon E, Manny J, Durst AL (1991) Benign cystosarcoma phyllodes of breast in an adolescent female. Breast Dis 4:299–305

142. Senocak ME, Gögüs S, Hiçsönmez A, Büyükpamukçu N (1989) Cystosarcoma phylloides in an adolescent female. Z Kinderchir 44:253–254

143. Tagaya N, Kodaira H, Kogure H, Shimizu K (1999) A Case of Phyllodes Tumor with Bloody Nipple Discharge in Juvenile Patient. Breast Cancer 6:207–210

144. Contarini 0, Urdaneta LF, Hagan W, Stephenson Jr SE (1982) Cystosarcoma phylloides of the breast: a new therapeutic proposal. Am Surg 48:157–166

145. Sasa M, Morimoto T, Ii K, Tsuzuki H, Kamamura Y, Komaki K, Uyama T, Monden Y (1995) A malignant phyllodes tumor of the breast in a 6-year old girl. Breast Cancer 30;2:71–75

146. Chulia MT, Paya A, Niveiro M, Ceballos S, Aranda FI (2001) Phyllodes tumor in ectopic breast tissue of the vulva. Int J Surg Pathol 9:81–83

147. Tresserra F, Grases PJ, Izquierdo M, Cararach M, Fernandez-Cid A (1998) Fibroadenoma phyllodes arising in vulvar supernumerary breast tissue: report of two cases. Int J Gynecol Pathol 17:171–173

148. Saleh HA, Klein LH (1990) Cystosarcoma phyllodes arising synchronously in right breast and bilateral axillary ectopic breast tissue. Arch Pathol Lab Med 114:624–626

149. Minkowitz S, Zeichner M, Di Maio V, Nicastri AD (1968) Cystosarcoma phyllodes: a unique case with multiple unilateral lesions and ipsilateral axillary metastasis. J Pathol Bacteriol 96: 514–517

150. Bader E, Isaacson C (1961) Bilateral malignant cystosarcoma phyllodes. Br J Surg 48:519–521

151. Mrad K, Driss M, Maalej M, Romdhane KB (2000) Bilateral cystosarcoma phyllodes of the breast: a case report of malignant form with contralateral benign form. Ann Diagn Pathol 4:370–372

152. Notley RG, Griffiths HJL (1965) Bilateral malignant cystosarcoma phyllodes. Br J Surg 52:360–362

153. Reich T, Solomon C (1958) Bilateral cystosarcoma phyllodes, malignant variant, with 14-year follow-up. Ann Surg 147:39–43

154. Kahan Z, Toszegi AM, Szarvas F, Gaizer G, Baradnay G, Ormos J (1997) Recurrent phyllodes tumor in a man. Pathol Res Pract 193:653–658

155. Keelan PA, Myers JL, Wold LE, Katzmann JA, Gibney DJ (1992) Phyllodes tumor: clinicopathologic review of 60 patients and flow cytometric analysis in 30 patients. Hum Pathol 23:1048–1054

156. Reingold IM, Ascher GS (1970) Cystosarcoma phyllodes in a man with gynecomastia. Am J Clin Pathol 53:852–856

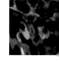

157. Browder W, McQuitty Jr JT, McDonald JC (1978) Malignant cystosarcoma phylloides. Treatment and prognosis. Am J Surg 136:239–241

158. Harada S, Fujiwara H, Hisatsugu T, Sugihara H (1987) Malignant cystosarcoma phyllodes with lymph nodes metastasis. A case report. Jpn J Surg 17:174–177

159. Treves N, Sunderland DA (1951) Cystosarcoma phyllodes of the breast: a malignant and a benign tumor. A clinicopathological study of seventy-seven cases. Cancer 4:1286–1332

160. Gisser SD, Toker C (1975). Chondroblastic sarcoma of the breast. Mt Sinai J Med 42:232–235

161. Anani PA, Baumann RP (1972) Osteosarcoma of the breast. Virchows Arch [A] 357:213–218

162. Jernstrom P, Lindberg L, Meland ON (1963) Osteogenic sarcoma of the mammary gland. Am J Clin Pathol 40:521–526

163. Rottino A, Howley CP (1945) Osteoid sarcoma of the breast: a complication of fibroadenoma. Arch Pathol 40:44–50

164. Powell CM, Rosen PP (1994) Adipose differentiation in cystosarcoma phyllodes. A study of 14 cases. Am J Surg Pathol 18:720–727

165. Jackson AY (1962) Metastasising liposarcoma of the breast arising in a fibroadenoma. J Pathol Bacteriol 83:582–584

166. Oberman HA (1965) Cystosarcoma phyllodes. A clinicopathologic study of hypercellular periductal stromal neoplasms of breast. Cancer 18:697–710

167. Qizilbash AH (1976) Cystosarcoma phyllodes with liposarcomatous stroma. Am J Clin Pathol 65:321–327

168. Kessinger A, Foley JF, Lemon HM, Miller DM (1972) Metastatic cystosarcoma phyllodes: a case report and review of the literature. J Surg Oncol 4:131–136

169. Fleisher AG, Tyers FO, Hu D, Webber EM, Essery C (1990) Dumbbell metastatic cystosarcoma phyllodes of the heart and lung. Ann Thorac Surg 49:309–311

170. Tenzer JA, Rypins RD, Jakowatz JG (1988) Malignant cystosarcoma phyllodes metastatic to the maxilla. J Oral Maxillofac Surg 46:80–82

171. Abemayor E, Nast CC, Kessler DJ (1988) Cystosarcoma phyllodes metastatic to the mandible. J Surg Oncol 39:235–240

172. Grimes MM, Lattes R, Jaretzki III A (1985) Cystosarcoma phyllodes. Report of an unusual case, with death due to intraneural extension to the central nervous system. Cancer 56:1691–1695

173. Hlavin ML, Karninski HJ, Cohen M, Abdul-Karim F, Ganz E (1993) Central nervous system complications of cystosarcoma phyllodes. Cancer 72:126–130

174. Rhodes RH, Frankel KA, Davis RL, Tatter D (1978) Metastatic cystosarcoma phyllodes. A report of 2 cases presenting with neurological symptoms. Cancer 41:1179–1187

175. Bartoli C, Zurrida S, Veronesi P, Bono A, Chiesa F, Cosmacini P, Clemente C (1990) Small sized phyllodes tumor of the breast. Eur J Surg Oncol 16:215–219

176. Hart J, Layfield LJ, Trumbull WE, Brayton D, Barker WF, Giuliano AE (1988) Practical aspects in the diagnosis and management of cystosarcoma phyllodes. Arch Surg 123:1079–1083

177. McGregor GI, Knowling MA, Este FA (1994) Sarcoma and cystosarcoma phyllodes tumors of the breast – a retrospective review of 58 cases. Am J Surg 167: 477–480

178. Salvadori B, Cusumano F, Del Bo R, Delledonne V, Grassi M, Rovini D, Saccozzi R, Andreoloa S, Clemente C (1989) Surgical treatment of phyllodes tumors of the breast. Cancer 63:2532–2536

179. Kapiris I, Nasiri N, A'Hern R, Healy V, Gui GP (2001) Outcome and predictive factors of local recurrence and distant metastases following primary surgical treatment of high grade malignant phyllodes tumours of the breast. Eur J Surg Oncol 27:723–730

180. Barth RJ Jr (1999) Histologic features predict local recurrence after breast conserving therapy of phyllodes tumors. Breast Cancer Res Treat 57:291–295

181. Ciatto S, Bonardi R, Cataliotti L, Cardona G, members of the Coordinating Center and Writing Committee of FONCAM (1992) Phyllodes turner of the breast: a multicenter series of 59 cases. Eur J Surg Oncol 18: 545–549

182. Lindquist KD, van Heerden JA, Weiland LH, Martin Jr JK (1982) Recurrent and metastatic cystosarcoma phyllodes. Am J Surg 144:341–343

183. Hawkins RE, Schofield JB, Fisher C, Wiltshaw E, McKinna JA (1992) The clinical and histologic criteria that predict metastases from cystosarcoma phyllodes. Cancer 69:141–147

184. Burton GY, Hart LL, Leight GS, Idlehart JD, McCarthy Jr KS, Cox EB (1989) Cystosarcoma phyllodes. Effective therapy with cisplatin and etoposide chemotherapy. Cancer 63:2088–2092

185. Ueyama Y, Abe Y, Ohnishi Y, Sawa N, Hatanaka H, Handa A, Tokuda Y, Yamazaki H, Kijima H, Tamaoki N, Nakamura M (2000) In vivo chemosensitivity of human malignant cystosarcoma phyllodes xenografts. Oncol Rep 7:257–260

186. West TL, Weiland LH, Clagett OT (1971) Cystosarcoma phyllodes. Ann Surg 173:520–528

187. Lester J, Stout AP (1954) Cystosarcoma phyllodes. Cancer 7:335–353

188. Pietruszka M, Barnes L (1978) Cystosarcoma phyllodes. A clinicopathologic analysis of 42 cases. Cancer 41:1974–1983

189. Niezabitowski A, Lackowska B, Rys J, Kruczak A, Kowalska T, Mitus J, Reinfuss M, Markiewicz D (2001) Prognostic evaluation of proliferative activity and DNA content in the phyllodes tumor of the breast: immunohistochemical and flow cytometric study of 118 cases. Breast Cancer Res Treat 65:77–85

190. Suo Z, Nesland JM (2000) Phyllodes tumor of the breast: EGFR family expression and relation to clinicopathological features. Ultrastruct Pathol 24:371–381

191. Palko MJ, Wang SE, Shackney SE, Cottington EM, Levitt SB, Hartsock RJ (1990) Flow cytometric S fraction as a predictor of clinical outcome in cystosarcoma phyllodes. Arch Pathol Lab Med 114:949–952

192. Samaratunga H, Clarke B, Owen L, Bryson G, Swanson C. (2001) Phyllodes tumors of the breast: correlation of nucleolar organizer regions with histopathological malignancy grading, flow cytometric

DNA analysis and clinical outcome. Pathol Int 51: 866–873.

193. Alberti O, Brentani MM, Goes JCS, Lemos LB, Torloni H (1986) Carcinoembryonic antigen. A possible predictor of recurrence on cystosarcoma phyllodes. Cancer 57:1042–1045

194. Chaney AW, Pollack A, McNeese MD, Zagars GK, Pisters PW, Pollock RE, Hunt KK (2000) Primary treatment of cystosarcoma phyllodes of the breast. Cancer 89:1502–1511

195. Layfield LJ, Hart J, Neuwirth H, Bohman R, Trumbull WE, Giuliano AE (1989) Relation between DNA ploidy and the clinical behavior of phyllodes tumors. Cancer 64:1486–1489

196. Tomita S, Deguchi S, Kusano T, Muto Y, Tamaki N, Nagamine Y (1994) Flow cytometric analysis to assess the malignant potential of phyllodes tumor. Breast Cancer 1:139–131

197. Kuijper A, de Vos RAI, Lagendijk JJ, van der Wall E, van Diest PJ (2003) Progressive deregulation of the cell cycle with higher tumor grade in the stroma of breast phyllodes tumors. Am J Clin Pathol, in press.

198. Hiraoka N, Mukai M, Hosoda Y, Hata J-I (1994) Phyllodes tumor of the breast containing the intracytoplasmic inclusion bodies identical with infantile digital fibromatosis. Am J Surg Pathol 18:506–511

199. Barnes L, Pietruszka M (1978) Rhabdomyosarcoma arising within a breast and its mimic. An immunohistochemical and cystosarcoma phyllodes. Am J Surg Pathol 2:423–429

200. Lubin J, Rywlin AM (1972) Cystosarcoma phyllodes metastasizing as a mixed mesenchymal sarcoma. South Med J 65:636–637

201. Graadt van Roggen JF, Zonderland HM, Welvaart K, Peterse JL, Hogendoorn PC (1998) Local recurrence of a phyllodes tumour of the breast presenting with widespread differentiation to a telangiectatic osteosarcoma. J Clin Pathol 51:706–708

202. Matsuo K K, Fukutomi T, Tsuda H, Hasegawa T, Akashi-Tanaka S, Nanasawa T (2001) A case of malignant phyllodes tumor of the breast with osteosarcomatous features. Breast Cancer 8:79–83

203. Salisbury JR, Singh LN (1986) Apocrine metaplasia in phyllodes tumours of the breast. Histopathology 10:1211–1215

204. Knudsen PJ Ostergaard J (1987) Cystosarcoma phyllodes with lobular and ductal carcinoma in-situ. Arch Pathol Lab Med 111:873–875

205. Padmanabhan V, Dahlstrom JE, Chong GC, Bennett G (1997) Phyllodes tumor with lobular carcinoma in-situ and liposarcomatous stroma. Pathology 29:224–226

206. Grove A, Deibjerg Kristensen L (1986) Intraductal carcinoma within a phyllodes tumor of the breast: a case report. Tumori 72: 187–190

207. Gittleman MA, Horstmann JP (1983) Cystosarcoma phyllodes with concurrent infiltrating ductal carcinoma. Breast 9:15–17

208. De Rosa G, Ferrara G, Goglia P, Ghicas C, Zeppa P (1989) In-situ and microinvasive carcinoma with squamoid differentiation arising in a phyllodes tumor: report of a case. Tumori 75:514–517

209. Klausner JM, Lelcuk S, Ilia B, Inbar M, Hammer B, Skornik Y, Rozin RR (1983) Breast carcinoma originating in cystosarcoma phyllodes. Clin Oncol 9:71–74

210. Leon AS-Y, Meredith DJ (1980) Tubular carcinoma developing within a recurring cystosarcoma phyllodes of the breast. Cancer 46:1863–1867

211. Yasumura T, Matsui S, Hamajima T, Nagashima K, Yamagishi H, Aikawa I, Oka T, Nakae T, Shimada N (1988) Infiltrating ductal carcinoma developing within cystosarcoma phyllodes-a case report. Jpn J Surg 18:326–329

212. Moffat C, Pinder S, Dixon A, Blamey R, Ellis I (1995) Phyllodes tumours of the breast: a clinicopathologic review of thirty-two cases. Histopathology 27:205–218

213. Gilles F, Gentile A, Le Doussal V, Bertrand F, Kahn E (1994) Grading of cystosarcoma phyllodes by texture analysis of tissue architecture. Anal Quant Cytol Histol 16:95–100

214. Tse GM, Ma TK, Chan KF, Law BK, Chen MH, Li KH, Chan EC, Mak MK (2001) Increased microvessel density in malignant and borderline mammary phyllodes tumours. Histopathology 38:567–570

215. Gatalica Z, Finkelstein S, Lucio E, Tawfik O, Palazzo J, Hightower B, Eyzaguirre E (2001) p53 protein expression and gene mutation in phyllodes tumors of the breast. Pathol Res Pract 197:183–187

216. Kleer CG, Giordano TJ, Braun T, Oberman HA (2001) Pathologic, immunohistochemical, and molecular features of benign and malignant phyllodes tumors of the breast. Mod Pathol 14:185–190

217. Erhan Y, Zekioglu O, Ersoy O, Tugan D, Aydede H, Sakarya A, Kapkac M, Ozdemir N, Ozbal O, Erhan Y (2002) p53 and Ki-67 expression as prognostic factors in cystosarcoma phyllodes. Breast J 8:38–44

218. Shimizu K, Masawa N, Yamada T, Okamoto K, Kanda K (1994) Cytologic evaluation of phyllodes tumors as compared to fibroadenomas of the breast. Acta Cytol 38:891–897

219. Krishnamurthy S, Ashfaq R, Shin HJ, Sneige N (2000) Distinction of phyllodes tumor from fibroadenoma: a reappraisal of an old problem. Cancer 90:342–349

220. Jayaram G, Sthaneshwar P (2002) Fine-needle aspiration cytology of phyllodes tumors. Diagn Cytopathol 26:222–227

221. Mottot C, Pouliquen X, Bastien H, Cava E, Cayot F, Marsan C (1978) Fibroadenomes et tumeurs phyllodes: approche cytopathologique. Ann Anal Pathol 23:233–240

222. Simi U, Moretti D, Iacconi P, Arganini M, Roncella M, Miccoli P, Giacomini G (1988) Fine needle aspiration cytopathology of phyllodes tumor. Differential diagnosis with fibroadenoma. Acta Cytol 32:63–66

223. Scoyler RA, McKenzie PR, Achmed D, Lee CS (2001) Can phyllodes tumours of the breast be distinguished from fibroadenomas using fine needle aspiration cytology? Pathology 33:437–443

224. Veneti S, Manek S (2001) Benign phyllodes tumour vs fibroadenoma: FNA cytological differentiation. Cytopathology 12:321–328

225. Bhattarai S, Kapila K, Verma K (2000) Phyllodes tumor of the breast. A cytohistologic study of 80 cases. Acta Cytol 44:790–796

226. Vera-Alvarez J, Marigil-Gomez M, Abascal-Agorreta M, Garcia-Prats MD, Lopez-Lopez JI, Perez-Ruiz J (2002) Malignant phyllodes tumor with pleomorphic liposarcomatous stroma diagnosed by fine needle aspiration cytology: a case report. Acta Cytol 46:50–56

227. McDivitt RW, Urban JA, Farrow JH (1967) Cystosarcoma phyllodes. Johns Hopkins Med J 120:33–45

228. Dusenbery D, Frable WL (1992) Fine needle aspiration cytology of phyllodes tumor. Potential diagnostic pitfalls. Acta Cytol 36:215–221

229. Shet T, Rege J (2000) Cystic degeneration in phyllodes tumor. A source of error in cytologicinterpretation. Acta Cytol 44:163–168

230. Shimizu K, Korematsu M (2002) Phyllodes tumor of the breast. A cytomorphologic approach based on evaluation of epithelial cluster architecture. Acta Cytol 46:332–336

231. Shoker BS, Jarvis C, Clarke RB, Anderson E, Munro C, Davies MP, Sibson DR, Sloane JP (2000) Abnormal regulation of the oestrogen receptor in benign breast lesions. J Clin Pathol 53:778–783

232. Tse GMK, Lee CS, Kung FYL, Scolyer RA, Law BKB, Lau T, Putti TC (2002) Hormonal receptors expression in epithelial cells of mammary phyllodes tumors correlates with pathologic grade of the tumor. Am J Clin Pathol 118:522–526

233. Yamashita J-I, Ogawa M, Egami H, Matsuo S, Kiyohara H, Inada K, Yamashita S-I, Fujita S (1992) Abundant expression of immunoreactive endothelin 1 in mammary phyllodes tumor: possible paracrine role of endothelin 1 in the growth of stromal cells in phyllodes tumor. Cancer Res 52:4046–4049

234. Aranda FI, Laforga JB, Lopez JL (1994) Phyllodes tumor of the breast. An immunohistochemical study of 28 cases with special attention to the role of myofibroblasts. Pathol Res Pract 190:474–481

235. Auger M, Hanna W, Kahn HJ (1989) Cystosarcoma phylloides of the breast and its mimics. An immunohistochemical and ultrastructural study. Arch Pathol Lab Med 113:1231–1235

236. Kuroda N, Sugimoto T, Ueda S, Takahashi T, Moriki T, Sonobe H, Miyazaki E, Hayashi Y, Toi M, Hiroi M, Enzan H (2001) Malignant phyllodes tumor of the breast with expression of osteonectin and vinculin. Pathol Int 51:277–282

237. Kim WH, Kim CW, Noh D-Y, Kim YI (1992) Differential pattern of perivascular type IV collagen deposits in phyllodes tumors of the breast. J Korean Med Sci 7:360–363

238. McCune B, Kopp J (1994) Tenascin distribution in phyllodes tumor is distinctly different than in fibroadenoma of the breast. Lab Invest 70:18A

239. Kocova L, Skalova A, Fakan F, Rousarova M (1998) Phyllodes tumour of the breast: immunohistochemical study of 37 tumours using MIB1 antibody. Pathol Res Pract 194:97–104

240. Shpitz B, Bomstein Y, Sternberg A, Klein E, Tiomkin V, Kaufman A, Groisman G, Bernheim J (2002) Immunoreactivity of p53, Ki-67, and c-erbB2 in phyllodes tumors of the breast in correlation with clinical and morphologic features. J Surg Oncol 79:86–92

241. Feakins RM, Mulcahy HE, Nickols CD, Wells CA (1999) p53 expression in phyllodes tumours is associated with histological features of malignancy but does not predict outcome. Histopathology 35:162–169

242. Kim CJ, Kim WH (1993) Patterns of p53 expression in phyllodes tumors of the breast – an immunohistochemical study. J Korean Med Sci 8:325–328

243. Kuenen-Boumeester V, Henzen-Logmans SC, Timmermans MM, van Staveren IL, van Geel A, Peterse HJ, Bonnema J, Berns EM (1999) Altered expression of p53 and its regulated proteins in phyllodes tumours of the breast. J Pathol 189:169–175

244. Witte F, Honig A, Mirecka J, Schauer A (1999) Cystosarcoma phyllodes of the breast: prognostic significance of proliferation and apoptosis associated genes. Anticancer Res 19:3355–3359.

245. Tse GMK, Putti TC, Kung FYL, Scolyer RA, Law BKB, Lau T, Lee CS (2002) Increased p53 protein expression in malignant mammary phyllodes tumours. Mod Pathol 15:734–740

246. Silverman JS, Tamsen A (1996) Mammary fibroadenoma and some phyllodes tumour stroma are composed of CD34+ fibroblasts and factor XIIIa+ dendrophages. Histopathology 29:411–419

247. Chen CM, Chen CJ, Chang CL, Shyu JS, Hsieh HF, Harn HJ (2000) CD34, CD117, and actin expression in phyllodes tumor of the breast. J Surg Res 94:84–91

248. Sawyer EJ, Poulsom R, Hunt FT, Jeffery R, Elia G, Ellis IO, Ellis P, Tomlinson IPM, Hanby AM (2003) Malignant phyllodes tumours show stromal overexpression of c-myc and c-kit. J Pathol 200:59–64

249. Sawyer EJ, Hanby AM, Ellis P, Lakhani SR, Ellis IO, Boyle S, Tomlinson IP (2000) Molecular analysis of phyllodes tumors reveals distinct changes in the epithelial and stromal components. Am J Pathol 156:1093–1098

250. Birdsall SH, MacLennan KA, Gusterson BA (1992) t(6;12)(q23;q13) and t(10;16)(q22;p11) in a phyllodes tumor of breast. Cancer Genet Cytogenet 60:74–77

251. Ladesich J, Damjanov I, Persons D, Jewell W, Arthur T, Rogana J, Davoren B (2002) Complex karyotype in a low grade phyllodes tumor of the breast. Cancer Genet Cytogenet 132:149–51

252. Leuschner E, Meyer-Bolte K, Caselitz J, Bartnitzke S, Bullerdiek J (1994) Fibroadenoma of the breast showing a translocation (6;14), a ring chromosome and two markers involving parts of chromosome 11. Cancer Genet Cytogenet 76:145–147

253. Woolley PV, Gollin SM, Riskalla W, Finkelstein S, Stefanik DF, Riskalla L, Swaney WP, Weisenthal L, McKenna RJ Jr (2000) Cytogenetics, immunostaining for fibroblast growth factors, p53 sequencing, and clinical features of two cases of cystosarcoma phyllodes. Mol Diagn 5:179–190

254. Polito P, Cin PD, Pauwels P, Christiaens M, Van den Berghe I, Moerman P, Vrints L, Van den Berghe H (1998) An important subgroup of phyllodes tumors of the breast is characterized by rearrangements of chromosomes 1q and 10q. Oncol Rep 5:1099–1102

255. Mokbel K, Ghilchik M, Parris CN, Newbold RF (1999) Telomerase activity in phyllodes tumours. Eur J Surg Oncol 25:352–355

256. Lu YJ, Birdsall S, Osin P, Gusterson B, Shipley J (1997) Phyllodes tumors of the breast analyzed by comparative genomic hybridization and association of increased 1q copy number with stromal overgrowth and recurrence. Genes Chromosomes Cancer 20:275–281

257. Jee KJ, Gong G, Hyun Ahn S, Mi Park J, Knuutila S (2003) Gain in 1q is a common abnormality in phyllodes tumours of the breast. Anal Cell Pathol 25:89–93

258. Poulton TB, de Paredes ES, Baldwin M (1995) Sclerosing lobular hyperplasia of the breast: imaging features in 15 cases. AJR Am J Roentgenol 165:291–294

259. Metcalf JS, Ellis B (1985) Choristoma of the breast. Hum Pathol 16:739–740

260. Daroca PJ Jr, Reed RJ, Love GL, Kraus SD (1985) Myoid hamartomas of the breast. Hum Pathol 16:212–219

261. Charpin C, Mathoulin MP, Andrac L, Barberis J, Boulat J, Sarradour B, Bonnier P, Piana L (1994) Reappraisal of breast hamartomas. A morphological study of 41 cases. Pathol Res Pract 190:362–371

262. Hogeman K-E, Ostberg G (1968) Three cases of postlactational breast tumour of a peculiar type. Acta Pathol Microbiol Scand 73:169–176

263. Linell F, Ostberg G, Soderstrom J, Andersson 1, Hildell J, Ljungqvist U (1979) Breast hamartomas. An important entity in mammary pathology. Virchows Arch [A] 383:253–264

264. Dworak O, Reck T, Greskotter KR, Kockerling F (1994) Hamartoma of an ectopic breast arising in the inguinal region. Histopathology 24:169–171

265. Reck T, Dworak O, Thaler KH, Kockerling F (1995) Hamartoma of aberrant breast tissue in the inguinal region. Chirurg 66:923–926

266. Schrager CA, Schneider D, Gruener AC, Tsou HC, Peacocke M (1998) Clinical and pathological features of breast disease in Cowden's syndrome: an underrecognized syndrome with an increased risk of breast cancer. Hum Pathol 29:47–53

267. Daya D, Trus T, D'Souza TJ, Minuk T, Yemen B (1995) Hamartoma of the breast an underrecognized breast lesion. A clinicopathologic and radiographic study of 25 cases. Am J Clin Pathol 103:685–689

268. Adler DD, Jeffries DO, Helvie MA (1990) Sonographic features of breast hamartomas. J Ultrasound Med 9:85–90

269. Hessler C, Schnyder P, Ozzello L (1978) Hamartoma of the breast: Diagnostic observation of 16 cases. Radiology 126:95–98

270. Black J, Metcalf C, Wylie EJ (1996) Ultrasonography of breast hamartomas. Australas Radiol 40:412–415

271. Kievit HC, Sikkenk AC, Thelissen GR, Merchant TE (1993) Magnetic resonance image appearance of hamartoma of the breast. Magn Reson Imaging 11:293–298

272. Coyne J, Hobbs FM, Boggis C, Harland R (1992) Lobular carcinoma in a mammary hamartoma. J Clin Pathol 45:936–937

273. Mester J, Simmons RM, Vazquez MF, Rosenblatt R (2000) In-situ and infiltrating ductal carcinoma arising in a breast hamartoma. AJR Am J Roentgenol 175:64–66

274. Anani PA, Hessler C (1996) Breast hamartoma with invasive ductal carcinoma. Report of two cases and review of the literature. Pathol Res Pract 192:1187–1194

275. Tse GMK, Law BKB, Ma TKF, Chan ABW, Pang LM, Chu WCW, Cheung HS (2002) Ductal carcinoma in-situ arising in mammary hamartoma. J Clin Pathol 55:541–542

276. Kaplan L, Walts AE (1977) Benign chondrolipomatous tumor of the human female breast. Arch Pathol Lab Med 101:149–151

277. Hayashi H, Ito T, Matsushita K, Kitamura H, Kanisawa M (1996) Mammary hamartoma: immunohistochemical study of two adenolipomas and one variant with cartilage, smooth muscle and myoepithelial proliferation. Pathol Int 46:60–65

278. Fisher C, Hanby AM, Robinson L, Millis RR (1992) Mammary hamartoma – a review of 35 cases. Histopathology 20:99–106

279. Wahner-Roedler DL, Sebo TJ, Gisvold JJ (2001) Hamartomas of the breast: clinical, radiologic, and pathologic manifestations. Breast J 7:101–105

280. Borochovitz D (1982) Adenolipoma of the breast: A variant of adenofibroma. Breast 8:32–33

281. Jackson FI, Lalani Z, Swallow J (1988) Adenolipoma of the breast. J Can Assn Radiol 39:288–289

282. Garijo MF, Torio B, Val-Bernal JF (1997) Mammary hamartoma with brown adipose tissue. Gen Diagn Pathol 1997;143:243–246

283. Benisch B, Peison B, Sarno J (1976) Benign mesenchymoma of the breast. Mt Sinai J Med 43:530–533

284. Davies JD, Riddell RH (1973) Muscular hamartoma of the breast. J Pathol 111:209–211

285. Bussolati G, Ghiringhello B, Papotti M (1984) Subaureolar muscular hamartoma of the breast. Appl Pathol 2:94–95

286. Hunkatroon M, Lin F (1984) Muscular hamartoma of the breast. An electron microscopic study. Virchows Arch (A) Pathol Anat 403:307–312

287. Khunamornpong S, Chaiwun B, Wongsiriamnuay S (1997) Muscular hamartoma of the breast: a rare breast lesion containing smooth muscle. J Med Assoc Thai 80:675–679

288. Garfein CF, Aulicino MR, Leytin A, Drossman S, Hermann G, Bleiweiss IJ (1997) Epithelioid cells in myoid hamartoma of the breast: a potential diagnostic pitfall for core biopsies. Arch Pathol Lab Med 121:354–355

289. Marsh WL Jr, Lucas JG, Olsen J (1989) Chondrolipoma of the breast. Arch Pathol Lab Med 113:369–371

290. Peison B, Benisch B, Tonzola A (1994) Case report: benign chondrolipoma of the female breast. N J Med 91:401–402

291. Rege JD, Shet TM, Pathak VM, Zurale DU (1997) Mammary hamartomas—a report of 15 cases. Indian J Pathol Microbiol 40:543–548

292. Gogas J, Markopoulos C, Gogas H, Skandalakis P, Kontzoglou K, Stavridou A (1994). Hamartomas of the breast. Am Surg 60:447–450

293. Chhieng DC, Cangiarella JF, Waisman J, Fernandez G, Cohen JM (1999) Fine-needle aspiration cytology of spindle cell lesions of the breast. Cancer 87: 359–371

294. Chiacchio R, Panico L, D'Antonio A, Delrio P, Bifano D, Avallone M, Pettinato G (1999) Mammary hamartomas: an immunohistochemical study of ten cases. Pathol Res Pract 195:231–236

295. Herbert M, Sandbank J, Liokumovich P, Yanai O, Pappo I, Karni T, Segal M (2002) Breast hamartomas: clinicopathological and immunohistochemical studies of 24 cases. Histopathology 41:30–34

296. Magro G, Bisceglia M (1998) Muscular hamartoma of the breast. Case report and review of the literature. Pathol Res Pract 194:349–355

297. Anderson C, Ricci A Jr, Pedersen CA, Cartun RW (1991) Immunocytochemical analysis of estrogen and progesterone receptors in benign stromal lesions of the breast. Evidence for hormonal etiology in pseudoangiomatous hyperplasia of mammary stroma. Am J Surg Pathol 15:145–149

298. Dal Cin P, Wanschura S, Christiaens MR, Van den Berghe I, Moerman P, Polito P, Kazmierczak B, Bullerdiek J, Van den Berghe H (1997) Hamartoma of the breast with involvement of 6p21 and rearrangement of HMGIY. Genes Chromosomes Cancer 20:90–92

299. Davies JD, Kulka J, Mumford AD, Armstrong JS, Wells CA (1994) Hamartomas of the breast: six novel diagnostic features in three-dimensional thick sections. Histopathology 24:161–168

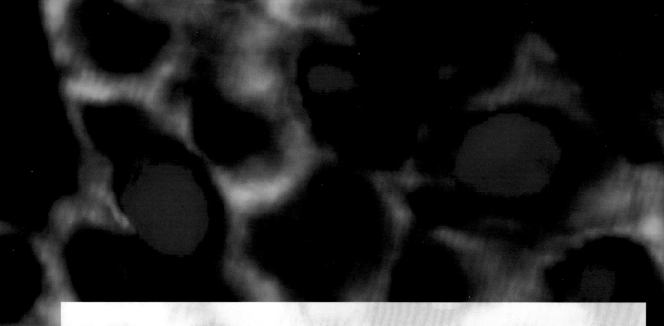

Content

16

INFLAMMATORY CONDITIONS OF THE BREAST

RAJENDRA S. RAMPAUL, SARAH E. PINDER, JOHN F. ROBERTSON AND IAN O. ELLIS

Accurate diagnosis of benign inflammatory conditions of the breast is particularly prudent. Some of these lesions can be secondary to a local insult, while others may reflect a local manifestation of systemic disease. In a small group the etiology may remain unknown. These lesions are important not only in terms of **local symptoms and discomfort** but also because many **may exhibit clinical features of malignancy.**

Duct ectasia

■ DEFINITION

A number of terms have been proposed for this condition, including 'varicocele tumor of the breast' [1–4], reflecting its clinical and various morphological features. The term 'duct ectasia' was introduced in 1951 by Haagensen [5] and is now the one most widely employed. It is a distinctive lesion involving the major, predominantly subareolar ducts. Recurrent periareolar abscesses and fistulae are related to duct ectasia in many cases. However, there appear to be at least two separate pathogenic mechanisms for this entity.

■ CONCEPTUAL APPROACH

Both the pathogenesis and the etiology of this condition remain unknown. Traditionally it was thought that duct dilatation was the primary event, with periductal inflammation following leakage of duct contents [3, 5]. More recently, periductal inflammation, which is seen more commonly in younger women, has come to be considered the initial event, followed by destruction of elastic tissue and eventually duct ectasia and periductal fibrosis (Fig. 16.1) [12–14].

It has recently been proposed that smoking may be a precipitating causal factor [15]. Pregnancy and lactation have also been cited as potential etiological factors, possibly due to mechanical damage to the major ducts. However the disease can occur in nulliparous women [16] and has been described in males [17–19] and in children [19]. Furthermore, in a study of 108 patients with duct ectasia, Dixon et al. found no differences in parity or breast feeding in these patients when compared with age-matched controls, suggesting that neither is an important etiological factor [14].

The rare reports of its occurrence in children [19] argue against Haagenesen suggestion of age-related involutional changes as an etiological factor. [20]. On the other hand, milder forms of this condition are asymptomatic, and autopsy studies indicate they are common, occurring in 25% of clinically normal breasts [21], leading to the suggestion that such cases form part of the spectrum of aberrations of normal development and involution (ANDI) [6].

Other proposed etiological factors include hyperprolactinemia [22, 23] and congenital inverted nipples [7].

The role of bacterial infection in the pathogenesis of duct ectasia remains unresolved. A variety of bacteria, including anaerobes, have been isolated from nonlactational abscesses and fistulae [24, 25], but other studies have been unable to demonstrate bacterial infection in uncomplicated or early lesions of duct ectasia [26, 27], suggesting infection is a secondary and possibly exacerbating factor.

■ CLINICAL FEATURES

The condition of duct ectasia is often asymptomatic in its mild form and may form part of the spectrum of aberrant involution (ANDI) [6]. Clinically evident disease is most common in peri- or postmenopausal women. The earliest symptom is spontaneous, intermittent nipple discharge that is usually clear, yellow, green or brown. The discharge gives a positive test for blood in about 50% of cases and a palpable lump in about 25% of presenting women. Local pain is also common and tends to be greater in young women, whereas nipple inversion or retraction is often described at a later age. Episodic acute inflammatory changes may occur and usually subside without treatment within a week or two. With disease progression, fibrotic shortening and thickening of the duct wall occurs and may result in nipple retraction [4, 7].

Such acute inflammatory episodes may result in the formation of periareolar abscesses and fistulae or sinuses [8]. Some of these features, particularly nipple retraction associated with an underlying mass, may be mistaken clinically for carcinoma and, although

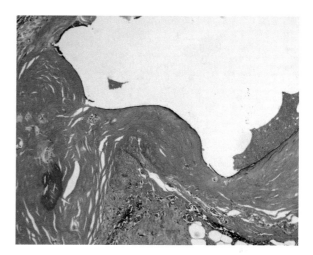

Fig. 16.1 Duct ectasia. Dilated retroareolar duct with a thick laminated layer of hyaline tissue and focal calcification obtained from a patient with long-standing disease. There is only a slight nodular inflammatory reaction of lymphocytes in the periductal tissue. The lumen contains a small amount of thick eosinophilic secretion. The epithelium is attenuated. Apocrine change and epithelial proliferation are typically absent in duct ectasia.

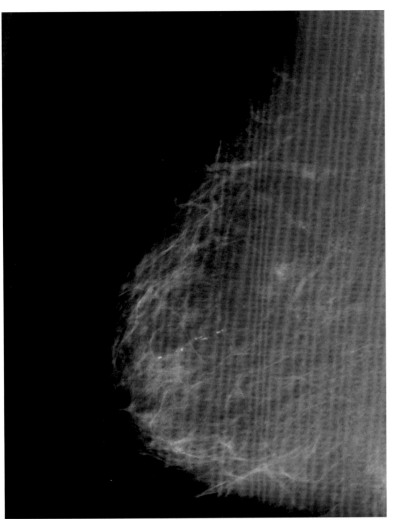

Fig. 16.2 Mammography. Rod-like calcifications along a single duct. This would be an uncommon presentation in DCIS. Clinically the patient showed spontaneous yellow discharge and a slight induration of periareolar tissue.

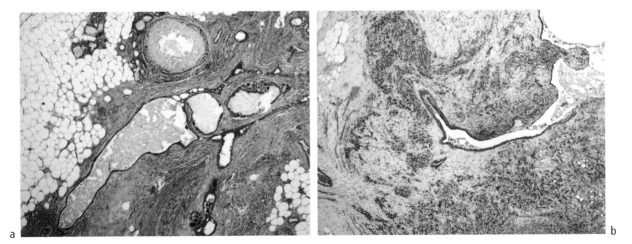

a   b

Fig. 16.3a–b Duct ectasia.
16.3a Dilation of subareolar ducts that contain stasis material with intense periductal lymphocytic inflammatory reaction and increasing fibrosis. Plasma cells are usually a minor component of the infiltrate. Focally, a granulomatous reaction with histiocytes and foreign-body giant cells can be seen (see also 16.4). The dilated duct in the upper field contains numerous foamy macrophages.
16.3b Immunohistochemistry for CD68 highlights the intense infiltration of macrophages (red).

characteristic mammographic appearances of dilated subareolar ducts and annular or tubular calcifications may be described, these may be misinterpreted or absent [9] (Fig. 16.2).

There is little evidence that antibiotics can provide long-term benefit. Symptomatic disease may require excision of the affected segment. Duct ectasia is not associated with any increased cancer risk. However, its more frequent occurrence in older women, the age group who are more likely to present with a carcinoma, together with the observation that breasts with duct ectasia tend to be more radiolucent, thereby aiding the mammographic detection of carcinoma, has led to the false impression of a relationship between the two diseases [28].

■ PATHOLOGY

MACROSCOPY

At operation the more obviously dilated ducts can be easily identified through a circumareolar incision and are best removed in a segmental excision as the disease affects the larger, predominantly subareolar ducts, although more peripheral ducts may be affected. It is usually confined to a segment containing palpable dilated ducts filled with pultaceous material and may therefore resemble comedo-type ductal carcinoma in-situ.

MICROSCOPY

Characteristically, the dilated ducts contain amorphous debris, often foamy macrophages and, occasionally,

crystalline structures. Epithelium lining the ducts, which may contain interspersed inflammatory cells and foamy macrophages, may appear ragged in the earlier stages before eventually becoming attenuated. The duct wall and periductal stroma also contain an often dense inflammatory cell infiltrate including prominent plasma cells and foamy macrophages (Fig. 16.3), the latter frequently containing brown ceroid pigment [10]. The infiltrate may be intense and granulomatous with foreign-body type giant cells (Fig. 16.4).

Alternatively, the plasma cell infiltrate may be sufficiently dense to merit the term 'plasma cell mastitis', which has also been applied to the condition [11]. As the disease progresses, fibrosis and reparative changes replace the inflammatory reaction and periductal fibrosis becomes prominent (Fig. 16.5). Azzopardi has also drawn attention to the formation of eccentric fibrous cushions that may bulge into the duct

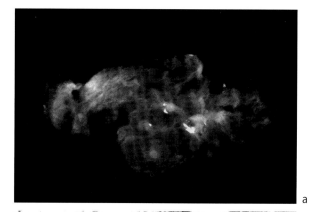

a

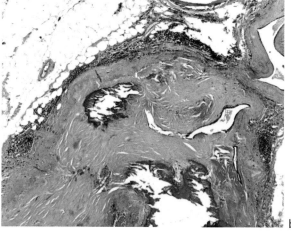

b

Fig. 16.5a–b Duct ectasia in a patient with long-standing bloody discharge associated with an underlying palpable mass.
16.5a Specimen radiography of a retroareolar specimen. The radiograph shows multiple, irregularly dilated tubular structures with coarse, polymorphous calcifications.
16.5b Specimen showing extensive hyalinization and calcification with nodular inflammatory lymphocytic infiltrates.

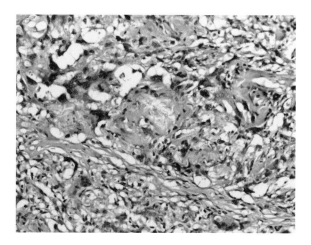

Fig. 16.4 Duct ectasia showing periductal granulomas. The granulomas contain histiocytes and foreign-body giant cells as well as foamy macrophages, which can be highlighted by their reactivity for CD68 and MAC-387.

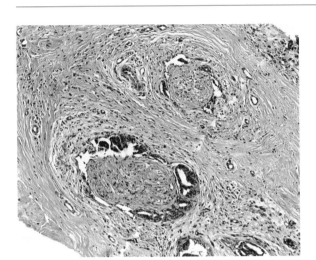

Fig. 16.6 In this case of duct ectasia the original lumina are delineated by epithelial cells and completely filled with fibrous tissue, also referred to as 'mastitis obliterans'.

lumen instead of the more usual concentric periductal fibrosis [4]. Occasionally, fibrous obliteration of the ducts may occur, leaving irregular masses of fibrous and elastic tissue with varying amounts of inflamma-

tion (Fig. 16.6) [12]. This appearance has led some authors to apply the term 'mastitis obliterans' [2]. Regenerating epithelium can produce a garland effect of epithelially-lined tubules, surrounding the fibrous tissue (Fig. 16.6) and occupying the original lumen, or, more commonly, can produce recanalization of the fibrous plug. Intraluminal mural and periductal calcification may occur.

■ DIFFERENTIAL DIAGNOSIS

As the condition is so distinctive it rarely ever presents as a diagnostic dilemma, thus differential diagnoses are few. Despite this, however, it has previously been included as part of the spectrum of fibrocystic change. Histologically, ectatic ducts are distinguished from cysts by their usually central location, linear configuration, inspissated luminal contents and presence of elastic tissue in the wall. Cysts, on the other hand, are usually round or oval, have empty lumens or contain homogeneous pale material, lack elastic tissue in their wall and often show apocrine metaplasia (see Chapter 2).

Acute mastitis

■ PUERPERAL MASTITIS

Puerperal mastitis occurs within two to three weeks at the start of lactation and is the result of infection via the mammary duct system. Cracks in the skin of the nipple or stasis of milk in lactating women may allow direct or retrograde ductal spread of bacteria (commonly *Staphylococcus aureus* or *Streptococcus pyogenes*) and thus development of localized acute inflammation of the breast. Haagensen has suggested that these skin cracks are the result of a change to an alkaline pH and that the problem may be alleviated by a slightly acidic topical application [29]. Minor inflammation often resolves itself, but occasionally, abscess formation may supervene and may require surgical drainage. Attention to the clinical setting should prevent confusion with other diseases presenting as an abscess-like lesion, such as duct ectasia and 'inflammatory carcinoma'.

■ BREAST ABSCESSES

Breast abscesses commonly associated with *Staphylococcus aureus* infection can also occur in neonates and often present in the second or third week of life [30]. The pathogenesis of these abscesses is not clear; physiological breast enlargement and breast manipulation to express colostrum, commonly regarded as etiological factors, were not identified as such in Rudoy and Nelson's review of 39 cases [30], although they admit that their records were incomplete in many cases. These abscesses are usually treated by antibiotics and surgical drainage.

■ SUB- AND PERIAREOLAR ABSCESSES

Sub- and periareolar abscesses are most common in women of reproductive age (Fig. 16.7), are found in

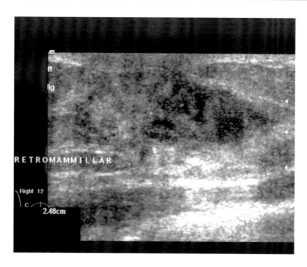

Fig. 16.7 Lactating 31-year-old woman with a focal painful retroareolar mass in the outer upper quadrant. Sonography shows a complex hypoechoic mass with increased dorsal echogenicity.

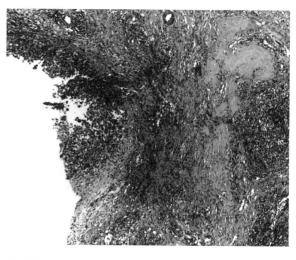

Fig. 16.8 Low power view of an abscess in a premenopausal woman associated with duct ectasia. The abscess is lined by granulation tissue with abundant neutrophil leucocytes and macrophages. Note the adjacent hyalinosis and lymphocytic infiltrates in the right field.

postmenopausal women and have also been described in men [31]. Such abscesses, most commonly associated with duct ectasia, are now much more common than those occurring in the puerperium. In a retrospective review of women presenting with breast abscesses over a ten-year period (1976–1985) Scholefield et al. found only 8.5% of all abscesses occurred in the puerperium, with only 3% occurring in women who were lactating at the time of presentation [32]. Symptoms may persist for several years, and multiple recurrences are common [31]. The disease may be bilateral and is often associated with congenital or acquired nipple retraction [24, 31]. Fistula formation between ducts and skin is common. Histologically, abscesses may be located deep in the parenchyma or in the periareolar region. Microscopically, they are

surrounded by inflamed and eventually fibrosed tissue (Fig. 16.8). They may be associated with squamous metaplasia of the lactiferous ducts and plugging by keratin debris. These cases appear to form a distinct subgroup in which the squamous metaplasia is probably congenital and associated with an inverted nipple in many cases [31]. Another large subgroup appears to be associated with duct ectasia, which is strongly implicated in the disease's pathogenesis [8, 32–34]. In contrast to abscesses occurring during lactation, a wide variety of bacteria have been isolated from the suppurative lesions, including *Staphylococcus*, *Streptococcus*, *Proteus* and *Bacteroides*; they are often mixed infections, which are predominantly anaerobic [24, 25, 32, 35]. Treatment is by drainage and surgical excision of the affected area.

Granulomatous inflammations of infective etiology

■ TUBERCULOSIS

Mammary tuberculosis is rare in Western countries but continues to be reported [36–38] and has been described as a presenting manifestation of AIDS [39]. Infection is believed to follow either hematogenous spread from an active or occult focus elsewhere or

retrograde lymphatic spread from involved axillary lymph nodes. Over a third of the 28 cases reported by Gottschalk and co-workers occurred in pregnant or lactating women [36]. Lesions may present as a mass or as recurrent infection with ulceration and sinus formation, which may be mistaken clinically for carcinoma. Indeed rarely, but not surprisingly, the two conditions may coexist [40].

Histologically, typical caseating granulomas (Fig. 16.9) are seen which destroy breast parenchyma. The axillary lymph nodes often also contain granulomas, although caseous lymphadenitis is rare and the presence of necrotizing granulomas in axillary or intramammary lymph nodes is generally due to a nontuberculous, extramammary cause such as cat-scratch disease [41, 42]. Ideally, both histological identification of acid, alcohol-fast bacilli and isolation of the organism are required for diagnosis. However, in only 2 of the 28 cases in the series studied by Gottschalk et al. were the bacilli seen and diagnostic criteria vary. Symmers [43] emphasizes the need for isolation of the organism to confirm the diagnosis as a number of other infections (e. g., syphilis and cryptococcus), infestations (e. g., hydatid cyst and cysticercosis) and iatrogenic causes (e. g., paraffin injection) may result in similar features, whereas other authors are less stringent in their requirements and place more reliance on histological features, even in the absence of identification of acid alcohol-fast bacilli in the sections [38].

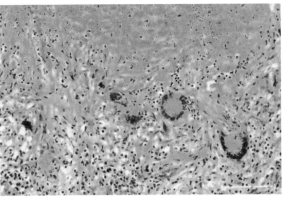

Fig. 16.9 A characteristic tuberculous granuloma, which illustrates the central caseation surrounded by epitheliod macrophages and multinucleated giant cells (Langhans giant cells) and lymphocytes at the periphery of the granuloma. Whenever a diagnosis of tuberculosis is considered, special stains for acid-fast organisms need to be performed.

FUNGAL AND OTHER INFECTIONS

Fungal infections of the breast are rare and reported cases include cryptococcosis [44, 45], histoplasmosis [45, 46] blastomycosis [47] and coccidioidomycosis [48]. They may be asymptomatic and detected mammographically or present as a mass, cyst or abscess. Many cause necrotizing granulomatous inflammation resembling tuberculous mastitis. Actinomyces infection is also very rare and usually spreads into the breast from a deep-seated infection of the lung or chest wall. Its manifestations are similar to those in other parts of the body [41, 49]. Other rare infections reported in the breast include syphilis, which results in an ulcerating gummatous mastitis [50, 51] and filiariasis [52]. Twenty cases of parasitic, mycotic and other rare infections from the files of the American Armed Forces Institute of Pathology and interpreted over a 40 year period, have been reviewed by Tavassoli [53]. They include filiarasis, which was the most common (12 cases), leprosy, histoplasmosis, syphilis, cat-scratch disease, molluscum contagiosum and schistosomiasis.

UNUSUAL INFECTIONS

Unusual infections have also been reported in association with prosthetic implants. Symmers reported a case of infection by a species of *Rhizopus* following implantation of a prosthesis [41], and more recently a case of *Mycobacterium fortuitum* infection presenting as recurrent abscesses one month after augmentation mammoplasty has been reported [54].

Continued recognition of such rare infections in the breast requires a high level of suspicion, supplemented by special stains for fungi and other micro-organisms where necessary.

Eosinophilic mastitis

Intense tissue eosinophilia is rare in the breast and has been described in three situations. Firstly, it is seen in association with parasitic infection, which should be excluded in all cases. Secondly, an inflammatory infiltrate consisting predominantly of eosinophils and centered on ducts and lobules may occur in the absence of any systemic manifestations and is probably a localized response to leakage of duct contents. Finally, a case has been described in which bilateral eosinophilic mastitis was the presenting manifestation of hypereosinophilic syndrome [55].

Idiopathic granulomatous mastitis

The term 'idiopathic' is employed here to contrast this well-defined condition of unknown etiology with specific granulomatous conditions, which may rarely present in the breast such as tuberculosis, sarcoidosis and Wegener's granulomatosis. Kessler and Wooloch described five cases in 1972 [56], and several further reports have since been described [57–61].

CONCEPTUAL APPROACH

Both the pathogenesis and etiology of this condition are unknown, although a number of observations have been made. For example, an association with recent pregnancy and hyperprolactinemia has been noted [59–62], although these are not absolute requirements for the development of the condition and the most recent pregnancy may have been several years previously [61]. An infective etiology is unlikely, given that organisms have never been identified, either histologically or following culture. However, such an etiology cannot be excluded. Finally, the possibility of an immune etiology has been suggested by Kessler and Wooloch as a result of the condition's morphological resemblance to granulomatous orchitis [56]. More recently, Axelsen and Reasbeck have described a case showing intense mononuclear cell infiltration of ductular epithelium associated with apoptotic bodies, suggesting cell-mediated destruction of mammary epithelium may play a role [63]. However, immunological abnormalities have not been identified in these patients to confirm this.

Fletcher and colleagues have suggested that the granulomatous response is a reaction to ductular epithelial damage of any sort (whether infective, chemical, traumatic or immunologically-mediated) that allows leakage of luminal contents into the lobular connective tissue [59].

CLINICAL FEATURES

Granulomatous mastitis generally occurs in women of reproductive age and has been associated with recent pregnancy, although Going et al. describe two cases in which the last pregnancy was 15 years prior to presentation [61]. Clinically, despite the relatively young age group affected, carcinoma may be suspected due to its presentation as a palpable mass, which is often but not always tender and may be associated with axillary lymphadenopathy. The disease may be bilateral.

Response to high-dose steroid treatment has been described [59, 64] but requires further evaluation. Currently, refractory cases require surgical excision. There is, however, a tendency for recurrence post surgery, and postoperative wound infection appears to be a particular problem [57–59].

PATHOLOGY

MACROSCOPY

The masses are generally ill-defined and several centimeters in size, ranging from 0.5 to 8 cm [61]. No characteristic gross features exist, but the cut surface of the tissue usually has a variable character and may appear fibrous, show features of fat necrosis with yellow areas or show evidence of microabscess formation with visible flecks of inflammatory exudate.

MICROSCOPY

Characteristically, a granulomatous inflammatory cell infiltrate including epitheliod histiocytes, occasional Langhans giant cells, lymphocytes, plasma cells and neutrophil leucocytes is centered on and distorts lobules with some extension into surrounding tissue in more advanced disease (Fig. 16.10). Microabscesses may also be seen in advanced cases. Specific etiological features are absent (apart from within the microabscesses), no necrosis or caseation is seen, and neither foreign material nor infective agents should be identifiable. Vasculitis has not been described, and if found should suggest an alternative diagnosis.

DIFFERENTIAL DIAGNOSIS

This diagnosis is essentially one of exclusion. An infective etiology should always be considered and fresh tissue obtained for culture whenever possible. For the same reason, special stains for mycobacteria and fungi should always be performed. Other differential diagnoses to be considered include sarcoidosis and Wegener's granulomatosis, and appropriate clinical information should be sought.

Sarcoidosis

Sarcoidosis rarely involves the breast, and when it does so is usually associated with extramammary

manifestations, thereby producing little diagnostic difficulty [65, 66]. Indeed, in some of earlier reports,

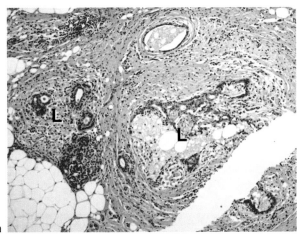

a

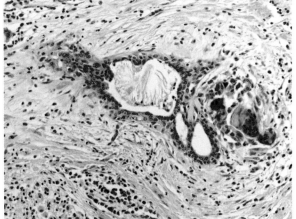

b

c

Fig. 16.10a–c Idiopathic granulomatous mastitis.

16.10a Low power view highlights the lobulocentric nature of this inflammatory process with involvement of two lobules (L). The cellular constituents are histiocytes, lymphocytes and plasma cells.

16.10b Another specimen from the same patient showing a lobule containing a dilated terminal ductule with inspissated secretory material and a well-developed granuloma with foreign-body giant cells in an otherwise edematous stroma containing lymphoplasmatic cellular infiltrates.

16.10c In this area the lobule is obliterated by an intense granulomatous reaction with epitheliod histiocytes and foreign-body giant cells. These changes are the result of an inflammatory reaction against inspissated secretory material.

confirmatory biopsy evidence of breast involvement was not obtained [67–69]. However, cases have been reported in which the disease has presented in the breast [70–72], although the diagnosis does not appear to have been substantiated clinically in all reported cases [71, 73].

Lesions in the breast present as single, multiple or bilateral nodules and may simulate carcinoma. The histological features are similar to those found in other sites, namely, noncaseating epitheliod granulomas with multinucleate giant cells, fibrosis and hyaliniza-tion (Fig. 16.11). The inflammatory response may be found in both the lobules and interlobular stroma. Diagnosis requires both exclusion of other causes of a granulomatous mastitis and confirmatory clinical evidence of sarcoidosis. If such confirmatory evidence is not found, an alternative diagnosis such as idio-pathic granulomatous mastitis should be considered. It is also worth noting at this point that sarcoid-like epitheliod granulomas may be seen in axillary lymph nodes in association with breast carcinoma [41].

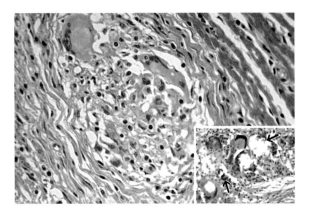

Fig. 16.11 Sarcoidosis of the breast. Specimen from a patient with widespread sarcoidosis and a mammographic mass in the breast. This noncaseating granuloma consists of epitheliod histiocytes and Langhans giant cells with intense fibrosis. Some-times cytoplasmic Schaumann bodies (arrows) are found in the giant cells, which consist of laminated secretions of calcium (inset).

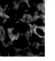

Lymphocytic mastopathy

This entity has been recognized under a variety of terms including fibrous mastopathy [74], fibrous disease of the breast [75] and, more recently, sclerosing lymphocytic lobulitis [76] and lymphocytic mastopathy [76–79], all reflecting its morphological features. Another recognized designation, diabetic mastopathy [80, 81], reflects the recognized association with diabetes mellitus. Despite reluctance to accept some of the earlier descriptions of predominantly sclerotic lesions as truly pathological, rather than as the result of an exaggerated involutional process, lymphocytic mastopathy is now emerging as a distinct clinicopathological entity strongly associated with autoimmune disease.

Palpable lumps are often resected but recurrences, often at different sites, are not uncommon. The morphological similarities with Hashimoto's thyroiditis and Sjögren's syndrome and the increased incidence of lymphoma in these conditions raise the possibility that lymphocytic mastopathy might precede the development of mammary lymphoma of MALT type. A recent study from Japan supports this assertion [79]. The authors examined 19 cases of primary non-Hodgkin's lymphoma of the breast, and in 11 of these they found histological evidence of lymphocytic mastopathy. Half of these lymphomas showed features of MALT type. Interestingly, no patients had any clinical history of autoimmune disease. The significance of their findings in terms of follow up and prognosis of women presenting with lymphocytic mastopathy has yet to be evaluated. It should be noted that this Japanese series of breast lymphoma appears to be different to two European series [85, 86]. A more recent case report has been published [87] in which lymphomas of predominantly high grade B-cell type without specific features of MALT lymphoma and occurring in older women have been associated with perilobular lymphoid infiltrates in which there is a predominance of T-cells. This is therefore not in keeping with lymphocytic mastopathy.

CONCEPTUAL APPROACH

Well-documented associations with diabetes mellitus, thyroiditis and arthropathy [75, 77, 80, 81] and some similarity between the histological features of lymphocytic mastopathy and those of pancreatic 'insulitis', Sjögren's syndrome and Hashimoto's thyroiditis suggest an autoimmune pathogenesis. This has been investigated further by Lammie et al. [76]. Three of the thirteen women in their series had type 1 diabetes mellitus, and one had Hashimoto's disease diagnosed five months after presenting

with bilateral lymphocytic mastopathy. These investigators were able to confirm previous findings of increased HLA-DR antigen expression in involved lobular epithelium [77] and an association with HLA-DR3 or -4 status [75], itself associated with autoimmune disease. Furthermore, autoantibodies were identified in four of seven patients investigated; two of the diabetic women were subsequently identified as having Hashimoto's disease, and in a fourth woman, who was not known to be suffering from an autoimmune disease, smooth muscle antibodies were found. Thus, although the pathogenesis of lymphocytic mastopathy is far from certain, autoimmunity appears to be strongly implicated.

CLINICAL FEATURES

This condition affects predominantly young and middle aged women but has an age range of 19–72 years. It presents as a firm, ill-defined, palpable mass, which is usually painless but may be tender. In some cases the masses are bilateral. The disease has also been described in men [81]. There may be a personal or familial history of autoimmune disease, particularly diabetes mellitus, as discussed above.

PATHOLOGY

MACROSCOPY

Resected mass lesions consist of ill-defined, firm, rubbery, gray-white tissue, reflecting the fibrosis, but are otherwise unremarkable. Reported cases range from 0.8 to 6 cm in size.

MICROSCOPY

Varying degrees of perivascular and lobulocentric lymphocytic infiltration and stromal fibrosis occur with obliteration of ducts and lobules (Fig. 16.12). Although endothelial cell swelling is described, there is no true vasculitis. There is an apparent morphological progression with an initial stage in which there is a dense lobular lymphoid infiltrate (Fig. 16.12d), followed by increasing lobular sclerosis and atrophy accompanied by reduction of the lymphoid infiltrate. The infiltrate is predominantly B-cell, is polyclonal and may include follicles containing germinal centers. Intraepithelial lymphocytes are common though not unusual in the breast, and lymphoepithelial lesions are reported. Lammie et al. [76] describe a case showing

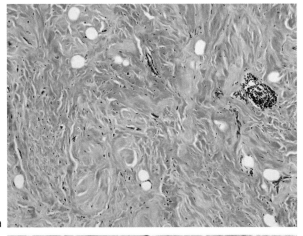

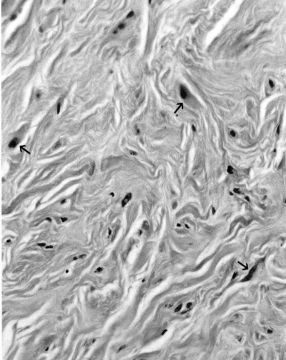

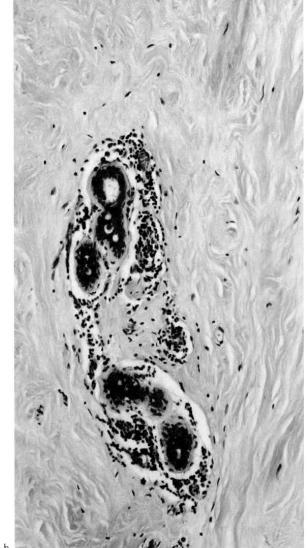

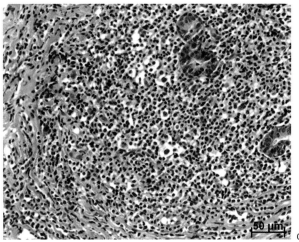

Fig. 16.12a–d Lymphocytic mastopathy. This lesion was obtained from a 54-year-old premenopausal woman with a palpable firm mass.
16.12a A low power view shows fibrosis and hyalinosis with prominent myofibroblasts and a focal perivascular lymphocytic infiltrate.
16.12b The figure shows a lobule with a lymphoid infiltrate.
16.12c The fibrous tissue contains prominent myofibroblasts (arrows).
16.12d Occasionally a more intense lymphocytic lobulitis may be seen.

epithelial destruction associated with a dense lympho-histiocytic infiltrate containing giant cells. Large epitheliod stromal cells have been noted by some, and may be dispersed as isolated cells or in clusters in the sclerotic stroma [81, 82]. They may be mistaken for infiltrating carcinoma but show negative immunohisto-chemical staining for cytokeratins and have been found to contain actin, favoring a myofibroblastic origin.

■ DIFFERENTIAL DIAGNOSIS

A number of breast lesions may be associated with marked lymphocytic infiltration and enter the differen-tial diagnosis. These include duct ectasia. However, in this disease the infiltrate is periductal rather than lobulocentric, and the infiltrate is predominantly T-cell rather than B-cell [83]. Dense lymphoid infiltrates may also accompany carcinoma, but again these tend to be periductal and to be predominantly T-cell [83]. However, lobular carcinoma in-situ may be associated with an intense lymphocytic mastopathy-like infiltrate, and a recent case report describes lymphocytic mastopathy in association with invasive lobular carci-noma [84]. Thus, careful attention should be given to the epithelial elements before interpreting a lobu-locentric lymphocytic infiltrate as lymphocytic mas-topathy.

Plasma cell granuloma

A single case of plasma cell granuloma or inflamma-tory pseudotumor has been reported [88] in a 29-year-old woman who presented with a 3.5 cm tender, mobile breast mass of one year's duration. As in similar lesions described elsewhere, histological examination revealed a prominent plasma cell infiltrate in a hyalinized fibrous stroma with scattered lymphocytes and fibroblasts. No recurrence was recorded 30 months after surgical excision.

Vasculitides

Wegener's granulomatosis [89–93], giant cell arteritis [94–98] and polyarteritis nodosa [99] have all, rarely, been described in the breast. The average age at presentation of the reported cases is in the mid-forties for Wegener's granulomatosis and in the mid-sixties for giant cell arteritis and polyarteritis nodosa. In each condition the disease may present as a breast mass, which may be tender and bilateral. The size of the reported lesions ranges from 1 to 8 cm with an average of 3 cm, and nipple retraction and skin tethering have been described. Often the clinical impression is of malignancy. Whereas systemic involvement is invariable in Wegener's granulomatosis, giant cell arteritis and polyarteritis nodosa can remain localized in the breast, and such localized disease appears to have an excellent prognosis based on the limited follow-up information available.

Fat necrosis

While commonly seen in association with duct ectasia and in the region of a recent biopsy site or following irradiation, isolated fat necrosis presenting as a clini-cally detectable mass is an unusual but well-recognized clinical entity, accounting for approximately 1 in 200 resected lesions in one series [101]. Most cases are believed to result from local trauma, although such a history is only obtained in a minority of patients and local ischemia may be a factor in some cases. Mammo-graphically, fat necrosis may show a characteristic benign ring-like calcification [102], representing calci-fication of an oil pseudo-cyst wall (Figs 16.13 and 16.14). However, the mammographic appearances may mimic almost any other type of pathology [103]. The associated inflammation and subsequent scarring may result in pain and tenderness and fixation to the over-lying skin. The clinical differential diagnosis thus includes both abscess and carcinoma.

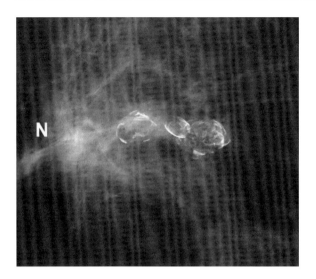

Fig. 16.13 Fat necrosis with architectural distortion and eggshell calcifications. Nipple (N).

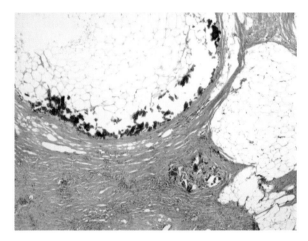

Fig. 16.14 Older fat necrosis showing a characteristic ring-like calcification and intense fibrosis with lymphoplasmacellular infiltration.

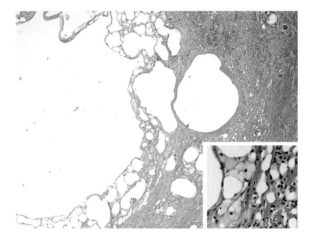

Fig. 16.15 Another area with one larger and smaller oil pseudocysts in the left field. The fibrosed stroma contains numerous foam cells (inset).

Most lesions are small, with an average size of less than 2 cm, firm and fixed to adjacent tissues. Slicing reveals a rounded outline with an indurated appearance, often with hemorrhage in early lesions and oily, cystic areas in older ones (Fig. 16.15). Eventually, the area may be replaced by a fibrous scar or transform into a thick-walled cyst, which may become calcified.

The histological appearance of fat necrosis has been well described. Foamy macrophages accumulate around the periphery of early lesions, and foreign-body giant cells surround fat globules. Hemosiderin, indicating previous hemorrhage, may be seen (Fig. 16.6). As the lesion ages, fibrosis becomes more prominent so that a tumor mass may be observed (Fig. 16.17) and dystrophic calcification may occur.

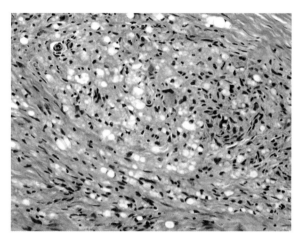

Fig. 16.16 A foreign-body granuloma from the same patient with numerous foam cells and foreign-body giant cells. Some of the histiocytes contain brown iron pigment as a result of a previous hemorrhage.

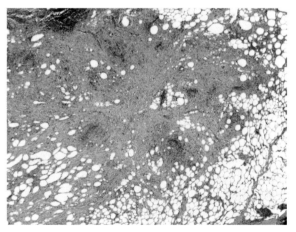

Fig. 16.17 Older fat necrosis with replacement of the necrotic tissue by fibrous tissue with a still intense inflammatory reaction and many small oil cysts in the right lower field. Radiographically such a lesion may be regarded as suspicious of malignancy.

Coumarin necrosis

Tissue necrosis is a rare but well-recognized complication of treatment with coumarin anticoagulants, which has a tendency to involve the breasts [104, 105] with bilateral involvement reported [106]. The pathophysiology of the condition appears to involve an imbalance between circulating clotting and anticoagulant factors, with initiation of the coumarin therapy reducing the anticoagulant, protein C, levels before the levels of the clotting factors prothrombin, Factor IX and Factor X fall, thereby inducing a hypercoaguable state [107].

Clinically, several days after initiation of the anticoagulant, local pain, swelling and echymoses appear, to be followed by blistering, ulceration and necrosis. Histologically, viable areas are interspersed with foci of hemorrhage and necrosis, associated with thrombosis of small veins and arteries and a variable inflammatory cell infiltrate. Although spontaneous healing may occur following conservative treatment and discontinuation of the anticoagulant [108], the majority of cases have required mastectomy.

Tissue reaction to breast implants

There is much controversy regarding the systemic effects associated with silicone implants, but the local effects are well described. The majority of implants are composed of silicone gel surrounded by a capsule composed of silicone elastomer. A fibrous capsule develops around the prosthesis, and in some cases contraction of this capsule is sufficient to require either capsulotomy or removal of the prosthesis and periprosthetic tissue. Histological examination of such specimens confirms the presence of fibrous scarring and capsule formation. Several recent studies have identified a cellular lining at the implant-tissue interface composed of cells with histological, immuno-histochemical and ultrastructural features of synovial cells [109–113]. Within the fibrous capsule itself, relatively large fragments of foreign material may be seen representing either silicone elastomer or birefringent talc granules. These elicit a typical foreign-body granulomatous response (Fig. 16.18). With time a dense fibrous capsule may be formed, which can undergo focal microcalcification. Peripheral to this is a zone of vacuoles and foamy macrophages filled with finely dispersed nonbirefringent silicone gel, much of which may have dissolved during processing.

Some modifications to this appearance may be seen with different types of implant. For example, Kasper has described a reaction to a saline implant surrounded by silicone elastomer: fibrous scarring and foreign-body reaction to silicone elastomer were seen as above but the peripheral zone of vacuolation and foamy macrophages were, not surprisingly, absent [113]. Capsules associated with polyurethane-covered implants contained nonpolarizing or partially polarizing geometrical crystals associated with a prominent foreign-body tissue response [113].

The foregoing descriptions refer to tissue responses associated with intact implants. Should a silicone gel implant rupture, large tumor-like silicone granulomas form, composed of lake-like accumulations of liquid silicone surrounded by sheets of foamy macrophages and foreign-body macrophages (Fig. 16.19). Clinically, these may be confused with carcinomas and may be sited some distance from the implant as a result of the tendency for liquid silicone to migrate through tissue.

The development of silicone granulomas following implant rupture is the result of a normal foreign-body inflammatory reaction. However, the fibrous scarring and tissue reactions associated with intact prostheses are less easy to explain. Silicone gel is known to migrate or 'bleed' from an intact bag-gel implant into periprosthetic tissue [114–116], and there is evidence to suggest that the extent of the tissue reaction is related to the amount of this silicone [117] bleed [118]. It has been postulated [117] that silicone gel enters the soft tissue surrounding the implant where it is ingested by macrophages, resulting in the release of a variety of cytokines trophic for fibroblasts and myofibroblasts among other cells. These in turn are responsible for collagen synthesis and capsular contracture.

The pathogenesis of the synovial-like metaplasia lining the fibrous capsules remains unknown, but similar changes have been described at other sites surrounding orthopedic prostheses: in skin following surgical procedures and in subcutaneous tissue following injection of air or oily fluids [109], suggesting it represents a fundamental biological phenomenon rather than a specific response to silicone implants.

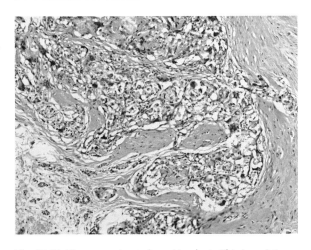

Fig. 16.18 Tissue reaction to breast implants. This is an intense foreign-body reaction with intensive fibrosis. The fibrous capsule, which usually develops around the prosthesis, is located in the right field.

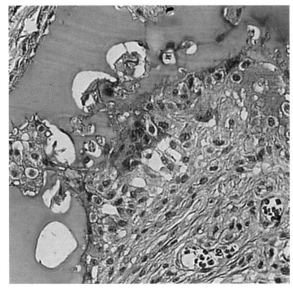

Fig. 16.19 A histiocytic and foreign-body giant cell reaction to hydrogel in the rat.

REFERENCES

1. Bloodgood JC. The clinical picture of dilated ducts beneath the nipple-The varicocoele tumour of the breast. Surg. Gynaecol. Obstet. 1923;36:486–495.
2. Payne RL, Straus AF, Glasser RE. Mastitis obliterans. Surgery 1943;14:719–727.
3. Tice GE, Dockerty MB, Harrington SW. Comedo-mastitis. A clinical and pathological study of data in 172 cases. Surg. Gynecol. Obstet. 1948;51:350–355.
4. Azzopardi JG. Cystic disease and duct ectasia. In: Problems in Breast Pathology. Philadelphia: W.B. Saunders, 1979: 72–87.
5. Haagensen CD. Mammary duct ectasia – a disease that may simulate carcinoma. Cancer 1951;4:749–761.
6. Hughes LE, Mansel RE, Webster DJT. Aberrations of normal development and involution (ANDI): A new perspective on pathogenesis and nomenclature of benign breast disorders. Lancet 1987;Dec 5:1316–1319.
7. Rees BI, Gravelle H, Hughes LE. Nipple retraction in duct ectasia. Br. J. Surg. 1977;64:577–580.
8. Abramson DJ. Mammary duct ectasia, mammillary fistula and subareolar abscess. Ann. Surg. 1969; 169:217–226.
9. Millis RR. Mammography. In: Azzopardi JG, ed. Problems in breast pathology. Philadelphia: WB Saunders, 1979: 437–459.
10. Davies JD. Pigmented periductal cells (ochrocytes) in mammary dysplasia: Their nature and significance. J. Pathol. 1974;114:205–216.
11. Haagensen CD. In: Diseases of the Breast. 3rd ed. Philadelphia: W.B. Saunders, 1986: 362.
12. Davies JD. Inflammatory damage to ducts in mammary dysplasia: A cause of duct obliteration. J. Pathol. 1975;117:47–54.
13. Bonser GM, Dossett JA, Jull JW. Human and Experimental Breast Cancer. London: Pitman Medical, 1961

14. Dixon JM, Anderson TJ, Lumsden AB, Elton RA, Roberts MM, Forrest APM. Mammary duct ectasia. Br. J. Surg. 1983;70:601–603.
15. Bundred NJ, Dover MS, Aluwihare N, Faragher EB, Morrison JM. Smoking and periductal mastitis. BMJ 1993;307:772–3.
16. Walker JC, Sandison AT. Mammary duct ectasia. A clinical study. Br. J. Surg. 1964;512:350–355.
17. Tedeschi LG, McCarthy PE. Involutional mammary duct ectasia and periductal mastitis in a male. Hum. Pathol. 1974;5:532–536.
18. Ashworth MT, Corcoran GD, Haqqani MT. Periductal mastitis and mammary duct ectasia in a male. Postgrad. Med. J. 1985;61:621–623.
19. Stringel G, Perelman A, Jimenez C. Infantile mammary duct ectasia: a cause of bloody nipple discharge. J. Pediat. Surg. 1986;21:671–674.
20. Haagensen CD. In: Diseases of the Breast. 3rd ed. Philadelphia: Saunders, 1986: 357–368.
21. Frantz VK, Pickren JW, Melcher GW, Auchincloss H. Incidence of cystic disease in so-called "normal breasts". A study based on 225 postmortem examinations. Cancer 1951;4:762–783.
22. Peters F, Schuth W. Hyperprolactinemia and nonpuerperal mastitis (duct ectasia). JAMA 1989;261:1618–20.
23. Shousha S, Backhouse CM, Dawson PM, Alaghband-Zadeh J, Burn I. Mammary duct ectasia and pituitary adenomas. Am J Surg Pathol 1988;12:130–3.
24. Leach RD, Eyken SJ, Phillips I, et al. Anaerobic subareolar breast abscess. Lancet 1979;1:35–37.
25. Walker AP, Edmiston CE, Krepel CJ, et al. A prospective study of microflora of non-peurperal breast abscess. Arch. Surg. 1988;123:908–911.
26. Aitken RJ, Hood J, Going JJ, Miles RS, Forrest AP. Bacteriology of mammary duct ectasia. Br J Surg 1988;75:1040–1.

27. Hughes LE. Non-lactational inflammation and duct ectasia. Br Med Bull 1991;47:272–83.

28. Young GB. Mammography in carcinoma of the breast. J. Royal College Surg. Edin. 1968;13:12–33.

29. Haagensen CD. In: Diseases of the Breast. 3rd ed. Philadelphia: W.B. Saunders Co., 1986: 384–393.

30. Rudoy RC, Nelson JD. Breast abscesses during the neonatal period. A review. Am. J. Dis. Child 1975; 129:1031–1034.

31. Habif D, Perzin K, Lattes R. Subareolar abscess associated with squamous metaplasia. Am. J. Surg. 1970;119:523–526.

32. Scholefield JH, Duncan JL, Rogers K. Review of a hospital experience of breast abscesses. Br J Surg 1987;74:469–70.

33. Sandison AT, Walker JC. Inflammatory mastitis, Mammary duct ectasia and mammillary fistula. Br. J. Surg. 1962;50:57–64.

34. Bundred NJ, Dixon JM, Chetty U, Forrest AP. Mammillary fistula. Br J Surg 1987;74:466–8.

35. Edmiston C, Jr., Walker AP, Krepel CJ, Gohr C. The nonpuerperal breast infection: aerobic and anaerobic microbial recovery from acute and chronic disease. J Infect Dis 1990;162:695–9.

36. Gottschalk FAB, Decker GAG, Schmaman A. Tuberculosis of the breast. S. Afr. J. Surg. 1976;14:19–22.

37. Apps MC, Harrison NK, Blauth CI. Tuberculosis of the breast. Br Med J 1984;288:1874–5.

38. Sharma PK, Babel AL, Yadav SS. Tuberculosis of breast (study of 7 cases). J Postgrad Med 1991;37:24–6.

39. Hartstein M, Leaf HL. Tuberculosis of the breast as a presenting manifestation of AIDS. Clin Infect Dis 1992;15:692–3.

40. Miller RE, Salomon PF, West JP. The coexistence of carcinoma and tuberculosis of the breast and axillary lymph nodes. Am. J. Surg. 1982;121:338–340.

41. Symmers WSC. The Breasts. In: Symmers WSC, ed. Systemic Pathology. Edinburgh: Churchill Livingstone, 1978: 1759–1861. vol 4).

42. Lefkowitz M, Wear DJ. Cat-scratch disease masquerading as a solitary tumour of the breast. Arch. Pathol. Lab. Med. 1989;113:473–475.

43. Symmers WSC, McKeown KC. Tuberculosis of the breast. Br. Med. J. 1984;289:48–49.

44. Symmers WSJ. Deep-seated fungal infections currently seen in histopathologic service of a medical school laboratory in Britain. Am. J. Clin. Pathol. 1966;46: 515–537.

45. Salfelder K, Schwarz J. Mycotic "pseudotumour" of the breast: Report of four cases. Arch. Surg. 1975;110:751–754.

46. Osborne BM. Granulomatous mastitis caused by Histoplasma and mimicking inflammatory breast carcinoma. Hum. Pathol. 1989;20:47–52.

47. Azzopardi JG. Miscellaneous entities. In: Problems in breast pathology. London: WB Saunders, 1979: 400.

48. Bocian JJ, Fahmy RN, Michas CA. A rare case of 'coccidioidoma' of the breast. Arch. Pathol. Lab. Med. (United States) 1991;115:1064–1067.

49. Jain BK, Sehgal VN, Jagdish S, Ratnakar C, Smile SR. Primary actinomycosis of the breast: a clinical review and a case report. J. Dermatol. 1994;21:497–500.

50. Whitaker HT, Moore RM. Gumma of the breast. Surg. Gynecol. Obstet. 1954;98:473.

51. Yuehan C, Qun X. Filiarial granuloma of the female breast: A histopathological study of 131 cases. Am. J. Trop. Med Hyg. 1981;30:1206–1210.

52. MacDougall LT, Magoon CC, Fritsche TR. Dirofilaria repens manifesting as a breast nodule. Diagnostic problems and epidemiologic considerations. Am. J. Clin. Pathol. 1992;97:625–630.

53. Tavassoli FA. Miscellaneous Lesions. In: Pathology of the Breast. Appleton and Lange, 1992: 621–622.

54. Juang YC, Wang LS, Chen CH, Lin CY. Mycobacterium fortuitum mastitis following augmentation mammaplasty: report of a case. Taiwan I Hsueh Hui Tsa Chih 1989;88:278–81.

55. Thompson AB, Barron MM, Lapp NL. The hypereosinophilic syndrome presenting with eosinophilic mastitis. Arch Intern Med 1985;145:564–5.

56. Kessler E, Wooloch Y. Granulomatous mastitis; a lesion clinically simulating carcinoma. Am. J. Clin. Pathol. 1972;58:642–646.

57. Koelmeyer TD, MacCormick DEM. Granulomatous mastitis. Aust. N. Z. J. Surg. 1976;46:173–176.

58. Brown LK, Tang PHL. Post-lactational tumoral granulomatous mastitis: a localised immune phenomenon. Am. J. Surg. 1979;138:326–329.

59. Fletcher A, Magrath IM, Riddel RH, Talbot IC. Granulomatous mastitis: A report of seven cases. J. Clin. Pathol. 1982;35:941–945.

60. Davies JD, Burton PA. Post-partum lobular granulomatous mastitis. J. Clin. Pathol. 1983;36:363.

61. Going JJ, Anderson TJ, Wilkinson S, Chetty U. Granulomatous lobular mastitis. J. Clin. Pathol. 1987;40: 535–540.

62. Rowe PH. Granulomatous mastitis associated with a pituitary prolactinoma. Br. J. Clin. Pract. 1984;38:32–34.

63. Axelsen RA, Reasbeck P. Granulomatous lobular mastitis: report of a case with previously undescribed histopathological abnormalities. Pathology 1988;20:383–9.

64. DeHertogh DA, Rossof AH, Harris AA, Economou SG. Prednisone management of granulomatous mastitis. N. Eng. J. Med. 1980;303:799–800.

65. Scadding JG. Sarcoidosis. In: London: Eyre and Spottiswoode, 1967: 335.

66. Ross MJ, Merino MJ. Sarcoidosis of the breast. Hum. Pathol. 1985;16:185–187.

67. Strandberg J. Contribution a la question de la clinique et de la pathologenie de la sarcoide de Boeck. Acta Derm Venereol 1921;2:253–257.

68. Reisner D. Boeck's sarcoid and systemic sarcoidosis: a study of 35 cases. Am Rev Tuberc 1944;437:462.

69. Longcope T, Freiman DG. A study of sarcoidosis. Medicine 1952;31:1–121.

70. Stallard HB, Tait CB. Boeck's sarcoidosis: a case record. Lancet 1939;1:440–442.

71. Fitzgibbons PL, Smiley DF, Kern WH. Sarcoidosis presenting initially as a breast mass: report of two cases. Hum. Pathol. 1985;16:851–852.

72. Banik S, Bishop PW, Ormerod LP, T.E.B. OB. Sarcoidosis of the breast. J. Clin. Pathol. 1986;39: 446–448.

73. Rigden B. Sarcoid lesion in breast after probable sarcoidosis in lung. Br. Med. J. 1978;2:1533–1534.

74. Minkowitz S, Hedayati H, Hiller S, Gardner B. Fibrous mastopathy: A clinical histopathologic study. Cancer 1973;32:913–916.

75. Soler NG, Khardori R. Fibrous disease of the breast, thyroiditis and cheiroarthropathy in type I diabetes mellitus. Lancet 1984;1:193–194.

76. Lammie GA, Bobrow LG, Staunton MD, Levison DA, Page G, Millis RR. Sclerosing lymphocytic lobulitis of the breast-evidence for an autoimmune pathogenesis. Histopathology 1991;19:13–20.

77. Schwartz IS, Strauchen JA. Lymphocytic mastopathy. An autoimmune disease of the breast? Am. J. Clin. Path. 1990;93:725–730.

78. Mills SE. Lymphocytic mastopathy, a "new" autoimmune disease? Am. J. Clin. Pathol 1990;93:834–835.

79. Aozasa K, Ohsawa M, Saeki K, Horiuchi K, Kawano K, Taguchi T. Malignant lymphoma of the breast. Immunologic type and association with lymphocytic mastopathy. Am J Clin Pathol 1992;97:699–704.

80. Byrd B, Jr., Hartmann WH, Graham LS, Hogle HH. Mastopathy in insulin-dependent diabetics. Ann Surg 1987;205:529–32.

81. Tomaszewski JE, Brook JSJ, Hicks D, Livolsi VA. Diabetic mastopathy: A distinctive clinicopathologic entity. Hum. Pathol. 1992;23:780–786.

82. Ashton MA, Lefkowitz M, Tavassoli FA. Epithelioid stromal cells in lymphocytic mastitis – a source of confusion with invasive carcinoma. Mod. Pathol. 1994;7:49–54.

83. Giorno R. Mononuclear cells in malignant and benign human breast tissue. Arch. Pathol. Lab. Med. 1983; 107:415–417.

84. Chetty R, Butler AE. Lymphocytic mastopathy associated with infiltrating lobular breast carcinoma. J Clin Pathol 1993;46:376–7.

85. Bobrow LG, Richards MA, Happerfield LC, et al. Breast lymphomas: a clinicopathological review. Hum. Pathol. 1993;24:274–278.

86. Hansen TG, Ottesen GL, Pedersen NT, Anderson JA. Primary non-Hodgkin's lymphoma of the breast (PLB): a clinicopathological study of seven cases. APMIS 1992;100:1089–1096.

87. Rooney N, Snead D, Goodman S, Webb AJ. Primary breast lymphoma with skin involvement arising in lymphocytic lobulitis. Histopathology 1994;24:81–84.

88. Pettinato G, Manivel JC, Insabato L, De Chiara A, Petrella G. Plasma cell granuloma (inflammatory pseudotumor) of the breast. Am J Clin Pathol 1988; 90:627–32.

89. Elsner B, Harper FB. Disseminated Wegener's granulomatosis with breast involvement. Arch. Pathol. 1969; 87:544–547.

90. Pambakian H, Tighe JR. Breast involvement in Wegener's granulomatosis. J. Clin. Pathol. 1971;24:343–347.

91. Oimoni M, Suehiro I, Mizuno N, Baba S, Okada S, Kanazawa Y. Wegener's granulomatosis with intracerebral granuloma and mammary manifestation. Arch. Intern. Med. 1980;140:853–854.

92. Deininger HZ. Wegener's granulomatosis of the breast. Radiology 1985;154:59–60.

93. Jordan JM, Rowe WT, Allen NB. Wegener's granulomatosis involving the breast. Report of three cases and review of the literature. Am J Med 1987;83:159–64.

94. Potter BT, Housley E, Thomson D. Giant-cell arteritis mimicking carcinoma of the breast. Br. Med. J. 1981; 282:1665–1666.

95. Thaell SF, Saue GL. Giant cell arteritis involving the breasts. J. Rheumatol. 1983;10:329–321.

96. Nirodi NS, Stirling WJI, White MFI. Giant cell arteritis presenting as a breast lump. Br. J. Clin. Pract. 1985; 39:84–86.

97. Stephenson TJ, Underwood JCE. Giant cell arteritis: An unusual cause of palpable masses in the breast. Br. J. Surg. 1986;73:105.

98. McKendry RJR, Guindi M, Hill DP. Giant cell arteritis (temporal arteritis) affecting the breast: report of two cases and review of published reports. Ann. Rheum. Dis. 1990;49:1001–1004.

99. Ng WF, Chow LTC, Lam PWY. Localized polyarteritis of the breast – report of two cases and a review of the literature. Histopathology 1993;23:535–539.

100. Cooper NE. Rheumatoid nodule in the breast. Histopathology. 1991;19:193–194.

101. Meyer JE, Silverman P, Gandbhir L. Fat necrosis of the breast. Arch. Surg. 1978;113:801–805.

102. Orson LW, Cigtay OS. fat necrosis of the breast: Characteristic xeromammographic appearance. Radiology 1983;146:35–38.

103. Roebuck EJ. Clinical Radiology of the Breast. (1st ed.) Oxford: Heinemann Medical Books, 1990

104. Nudelman HL, Kempson RL. Necrosis of the breast: A rare complication of anticoagulant therapy. Am. J. Surg. 1966;111:728–733.

105. Manstein CH, Steerman PH, Goldstein J. Sodium warfarin-induced gangrene of the breast. Ann Plast Surg 1985;15:161–2.

106. Lopez Valle CA, Herbert G. Warfarin-induced complete bilateral breast necrosis. Br. J. Plast. Surg. 1992;45:606–609.

107. Clouse LH, Comp PC. The regulation of haemostasis: The protein C system. N. Engl. J. Med. 1986;314: 1298–1304.

108. Mason JR. Haemorrhage induced breast gangrene. Br. J. Surg. 1970;57:700–702.

109. Chase DR, Oberg KC, Chase RL, Marlott RL, Weeks DA. Pseudoepithelialization of breast implant capsules. Int. J. Surg. Pathol. 1994;1:151–154.

110. Raso DS, Crymes LW, Metcalf JS. Histological assessment of fifty breast capsules from smooth and textured augmentation and reconstruction mammoplast prostheses with emphasis on the role of synovial metaplasia. Mod. Pathol. 1994;7:310–316.

111. del Rosario AD, Bui HY, Singh J, Petrocine S, Sheehan C, Ross JS. The synovial metaplasia of breast implant capsules: a light and electron microscopic study (Abstract). Lab. Invest. 1994;70:14A.

112. Hameed M, Erlanson R, Rosen PP. Capsular synovial metaplasia around mammary implants, similar to detritic synovitis: a morphologic and immunohistochemical study of 15 cases (Abstract). Lab. Invest. 1994;70:16A.

113. Kasper CS. Histologic features of breast capsules reflect surface configuration and composition of silicone bag implants. Am. J. Clin. Pathol. 1994;102:655–659.

114. Barker DE, Retsky MI, Schultz S. "Bleeding" of silicone from bag-gel implants and its clinical relation to fibrous capsule reaction. Plas. Reconstr. Surg. 1978;61:836–841.

115. Bergman RB, van der Ende AE. Exudation of silicone through the envelope of gel-filled breast prostheses. An in vitro study. Br. J. Plast. Surg. 1979;32:31–34.

116. Baker JL, LeVier RR, Spielvogel DE. Positive identification of silicone in human mammary capsular tissue. Plast. Reconstr. Surg. 1982;69:56.

117. Schnitt SJ. Tissue reactions to mammary implants: A capsule summary. Advances in Anatomic Pathology 1994;2:24–27.

118. Thomsen JL, Chrissensen L, Nielsen M, et al. Histologic changes and silicone concentrations in human breast tissue surrounding silicone breast prostheses. Plast. Reconstr. Surg. 1990;91:38–41.

Content

BASIC PRINCIPLES OF PRECURSOR LESIONS OF BREAST CANCER

WERNER BOECKER, HORST BUERGER, HERMANN HERBST AND THOMAS DECKER

The process of malignant tumorigenesis can be divided into two phases:

1. a noninvasive phase with growth of epithelial neoplastic cells in the confines of the ductal-lobular tree;
2. an invasive phase with invasion and destruction of the normal breast tissue by tumor cells and the potential for distant metastases.

Lesions that fulfill the first criteria represent 'precursor lesions'. **In this chapter a model of ductal and lobular precancerous biology is discussed. Emphasis is placed on the fact that most atypical epithelial proliferations arise de novo from transformations of glandular target cells of the TDLUs.** It will be shown that these lesions are characterized by a great variety of morphologies and that they develop along distinct genetic and morphological pathways.

The malignancy grade of the neoplastic proliferating cells and the stage of lesions within the ductal-lobular tree largely determine their outcome in terms of invasive malignancies.

A major part of this chapter will be dedicated to the discussion of the cellular components of malignant breast lesions as the basis of a new and better understanding of ductal and lobular neoplasia. **The overwhelming majority of breast malignancies display a purely glandular phenotype expressing Ck8/18 and lacking Ck5/14.** However, a smaller number of breast malignancies are characterized by expression of Ck5/14. Interestingly, such tumors may show a block in their differentiation or they may show differentiation characteristics comparable to normal breast epithelium. **In view of the currently available data, our contention is that the diversity of breast tumors can only be explained by assuming that different target cells of normal breast epithelium are the founding cells of malignant tumors. In the last paragraph of this chapter we propose a working formulation of a classification system of ductal and lobular neoplasia.**

Basic principles of precursor lesions of breast cancer

■ DEFINITION

'Precursor lesions' as defined by the WHO are biologically and clinically heterogeneous neoplastic lesions with the potential for direct progression to invasive breast cancer [1]. Precursor lesions include flat epithelial atypia (FEA), atypical ductal hyperplasia (ADH), ductal carcinoma in-situ (DCIS) and its subtypes, atypical lobular hyperplasia (ALH) and lobular carcinoma in-situ (LCIS) and its variants (Table 17.1) [1, 2]. While all these are precursor lesions, the potential for progression of these lesions to invasive breast carcinoma and thus the clinical implications of a given lesion vary considerably from entity to entity [3, 4]. This chapter addresses some basic principles of neoplastic transformation with the aim of defining and clarifying the above-mentioned entities in the context of breast carcinogenesis.

■ A MODEL OF DUCTAL PRECANCEROUS BIOLOGY

Despite considerable efforts aimed at elucidating the mechanisms of breast carcinogenesis, a unifying, generally accepted model has not yet been described [5–7]. The traditional model of linear progression to breast carcinoma implies a cascade of increasing malignancy from benign intraductal epithelial proliferations to invasive breast carcinoma (for a review see Lakhani [8]). According to this view the initial events of clonal selection and proliferation are identical in all forms of ductal breast carcinomas, with diversification among neoplastic lesions taking place at later stages. This paradigm still predominantes and revolves around benign intraductal epithelial proliferation as the central event and initial step in this process. However, the detection of striking differences between benign epithelial proliferation and most DCIS subtypes in terms of cellular composition, genetic changes and their respective status as precursors of invasive breast carcinoma has cast doubt on this concept. This has been addressed in more detail in Chapter 7.

Several lines of evidence support the status of DCIS as a genuine precursor of invasive breast carcinoma. First, when incompletely excised, DCIS bears a high risk of subsequently developing into invasive carcinoma in the region of the original biopsy [9–18]. Second, noninvasive lesions and their invasive counterparts are usually characterized by similar cellular morphologies [12, 19, 20]. Third, DCIS and invasive ductal carcinoma share distinct recurrent molecular and cytogenetic alterations as shown in comparative genomic hybridization (CGH) (Fig. 17.1) and loss of heterozygosity (LOH) studies [21–27].

Any approach to model tumorigenesis that acknowledges the precursor status of DCIS, nevertheless, must concede that DCIS consists of a group of biologically heterogeneous lesions. The degree of nuclear atypia has traditionally been used to address this hetero-

Tab. 17.1 Classification of benign and malignant proliferative breast disease

Benign proliferative breast disease lesions	Precursor lesions of invasive breast cancer*	Invasive breast carcinoma
Usual ductal hyperplasia	**Lobular neoplasia:**	Invasive lobular carcinoma (and subtypes)
Sclerosing adenosis	Atypical lobular hyperplasia	Invasive ductal carcinoma, no special type
Radial scar	Lobular carcinoma in-situ	Tubular carcinoma
Papilloma	Extensive lobular carcinoma in-situ	Cribriform carcinoma
Tubular adenoma	with comedonecrosis	Papillary carcinoma
Adenoma of the nipple	**Ductal neoplasia:**	Mucinous carcinoma
Adenomyoepithelial tumor	Flat epithelial atypia (FEA), standard-type and others	Medullary carcinoma
Fibroadenoma/phyllodes tumor	Atypical ductal hyperplasia (ADH), standard-type and others	Others
	Ductal carcinoma in-situ (DCIS) low, intermediate and high grade	

* Note that most of these precursors develop de novo from glandular cells of the TDLUs. The same precursor lesions may however also evolve against a background of benign proliferative breast disease lesions.

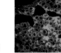

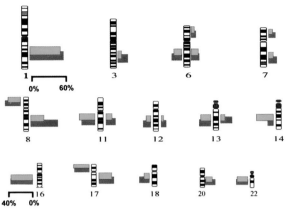

Fig. 17.1 Comparison of CGH results for DCIS (green bars) and invasive ductal carcinoma (red bars) in more than 900 breast carcinoma cases. Bars to the right indicate gains of chromosomal material, bars to the left losses; the size of the bars indicates the percentage of cases that show these genetic changes. Note the striking similarities between genetic changes in invasive and noninvasive lesions suggesting a causal relationship. The chromosomes not shown in this diagram do not display recurrent genetic gains or losses. The chromosome numbers are in black.

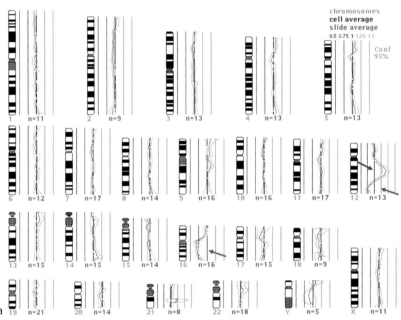

Fig. 17.2a–b Two figures summarizing the CGH results from a low grade DCIS and a high grade DCIS. This technique enables analysis of gross genetic imbalances. The CGH profiles indicate gains and losses of chromosomal material. The chromosome numbers are in green. The red curve to the right of each chromosome depicts the average ratio profile of a given tumor. Of the five lines to the right of each chromosome, the black line represents a normal ratio of 1.0. Extensions of the red curve to the right of the black line reflect gains, extensions to the left, losses of chromosomal material.

17.2a Low grade DCIS is typically characterized by few genetic changes. The most characteristic recurrent feature of these lesions is the loss of genetic material at 16q.

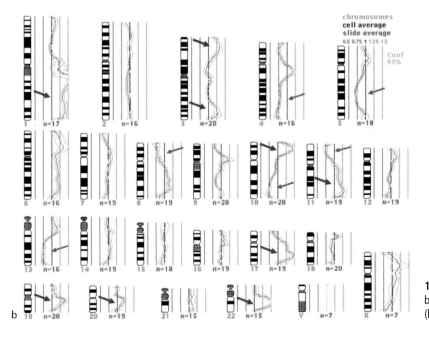

17.2b High grade DCIS is characterized by numerous losses (red arrows) and gains (blue arrows) at many chromosomal loci.

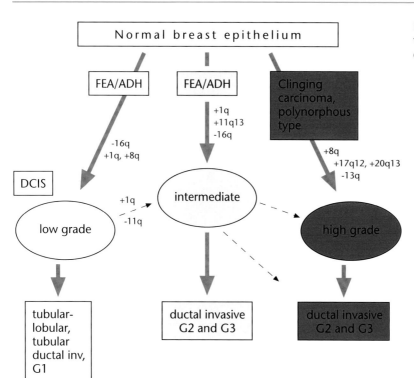

Fig. 17.3 Different genetic pathways in the development of ductal-type breast cancer.

geneity, in that it distinguishes DCIS subgroups of low, intermediate and high grade malignancy [11, 28–32]. Recent genetic data has provided further evidence to support this practical approach, revealing different genetic pathways in the development of breast carcinoma [21, 23, 25, 33, 34]. Thus, high grade DCIS is mainly characterized by gains of chromosomal material at 18q, 17q and 20q, whereas low grade DCIS usually shows losses at 16q (Fig. 17.2). Invasive carcinomas associated with either low grade or high grade DCIS often display similar morphological grades of malignancy and the same gross genetic imbalances as their respective in-situ counterparts [21–27, 35]. In conclusion this data support the theory that breast carcinoma comprises a heterogeneous group of diseases, with each entity having its own natural history and distinct pathway of development (Fig. 17.3).

Our progression model implies two central questions:
1. Can low grade lesions progress to high grade ones [21, 23, 25, 34, 36]?
2. Are there common progenitors of these different types of lesions?

In the daily experience of breast pathologists low grade in-situ lesions associated with their higher grade counterparts may occasionally be observed. Nevertheless, striking genetic differences between lesions of the low and high grade pathways preclude an obligate stepwise dedifferentiation of the low grade lesions [33, 36, 37]. This holds true even for a group of high grade lesions that, in addition to other genetic abnormalities, show losses of chromosomal material at 16q, a typical alteration of the low grade pathway. However, given the data from a recent study revealing different mechanisms for chromosomal 16q losses in high- and low grade lesions [38], it seems unlikely that even these high grade lesions can be regarded as morphological and genetic endpoints of a genetic and histological progression of low grade lesions. As we will see later, by no means less momentous is the conclusion that this pathway concept suggests, namely that a given malignant potential of lesions seems to be determined at a rather early stage and is usually retained over the various stages of the progression cascade [39, 40]. Low-, intermediate- and high grade DCIS and their invasive counterparts therefore represent developmental stages of different pathways.

The most important theoretical conclusion one could draw from the pathway concept is that the initial steps are not likely to be identical for all pathways, but rather that each pathway springs from its own early lesion (Fig. 17.3). Such a conception deviates considerably from the traditional and longstanding emphasis on benign intraductal proliferation of usual and atypical ductal hyperplasias as the general first steps in the development of breast cancer.

This theory, however, raises questions concerning the site of origin of these early lesions and, more importantly, their morphological status. A tentative answer to these questions can be gleaned from a proposal introduced by the British pathologist

Azzopardi as early as 1987. Using conventional histology he suggested that breast cancer usually develops de novo, with the earliest histologically recognizable lesions referred to in his terminology as 'clinging carcinoma'. He showed that two different types of early carcinoma may be distinguished: monomorphous and polymorphous types. In the light of our current knowledge, Azzopardi's notion of a de novo evolution of breast cancer from glandular cells of the normal lobular breast epithelium and the description of two subtypes of 'clinging carcinoma' must be regarded as an anticipation of early precursor lesions of the pathway model introduced here. Since the different types of clonal growth of precancerous

lesions may be extremely difficult to distinguish from one another and, at an early stage, sometimes even from benign breast epithelium, the reservations about Azzopardi's work were hardly surprising. Even to this day his insights into breast cancer development have not been duly acknowledged. It was, therefore, obvious that additional functional and genetic parameters were needed to better characterize the biology of proliferating cells of early neoplastic lesions [36, 40–44]. Molecular features assessing genetic changes in a given cell proliferation and/or immunostaining for differentiation markers are now available and have helped to develop a conceptual framework capable of putting the pathway model to the test.

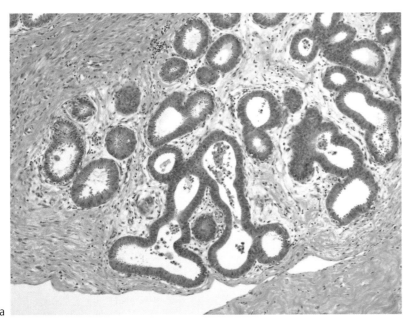

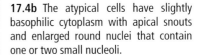

Fig. 17.4a–b Flat epithelial atypia, standard-type.
17.4a H&E-staining showing a lobule with cystically enlarged lobular ductules (acini) lined with monomorphic atypical cells.

17.4b The atypical cells have slightly basophilic cytoplasm with apical snouts and enlarged round nuclei that contain one or two small nucleoli.

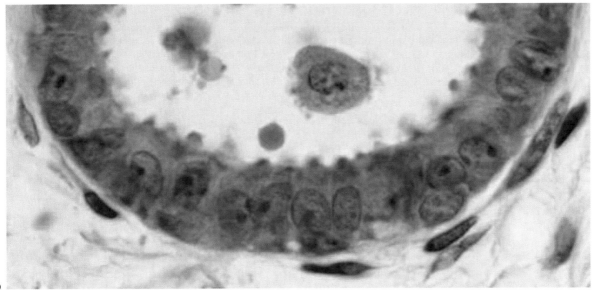

■ IMPLICATIONS OF THE PATHWAY
▦ CONCEPT ON THE DEVELOPMENT OF
EARLY NEOPLASTIC LESIONS

FEA, ADH AND GRADE 1 DCIS ARE PROBABLY STAGES ALONG THE LOW GRADE PROGRESSION PATHWAY

Some lesions such as FEA and ADH, which have been amply described in the literature, represent putative precursor lesions for the low grade pathway. These lesions share features such as cellular morphology, architecture, immunophenotype (Figs 17.4–17.7) and recurrent genetic alterations at certain genetic loci with low grade DCIS and tubular carcinoma [39, 40, 45–47]. In this book we use the terms 'standard-type-FEA' and 'ADH' to address these early, low grade lesions. The term 'flat epithelial atypia' (see Chapter 18) describes a lesion of the terminal ductal lobular unit whose acini are lined with one or a small number of layers of monomorphic atypical cells with slightly enlarged, round nuclei and a prominence of apical snouts [39, 40, 48–56]. Flat atypical proliferations may often coexist with ADH and/or with low grade DCIS, which is characterized by additional intraluminal proliferations of the same cell type, resulting in a more complex architecture. It must therefore be emphasized that the cells comprising FEA are cytologically identical to the cells of low grade DCIS [39, 54, 55, 57, 58]. With the recurrent 16q loss typical to these lesions [40], they are also strikingly similar in genetic terms; moreover they express glandular cytokeratins 8/18 in the absence of high molecular weight cytokeratins 5/14 [46], display intense nuclear expression of the estrogen receptor as well as strong cytoplasmic expression of the bcl-2 protein, and have a low proliferative activity [49, 57, 59, 60]. Last, but not least, FEA/ADH and low grade DCIS are the prototypical lesions associated with tubular carcinoma or grade 1 invasive carcinoma [45]. In view of such evidence, we consider these lesions to be elements and, more importantly, different stages along the low grade progression pathway.

One implication of our concept of a low grade pathway is, that the different stages are associated with variable progression potential; 'early' lesions such as FEA/ADH are relatively 'innocent' [51, 61–63], whereas the rate of invasive recurrences of fully developed low grade DCIS is as much as 50% over a follow-up period of 15–25 years [64–66].

This follow-up data may, however, be biased by standard surgical procedures. While there is a fair chance that FEA/ADH and even very small lesions of DCIS may be completely removed by diagnostic surgical biopsy, many of the DCIS cases originally

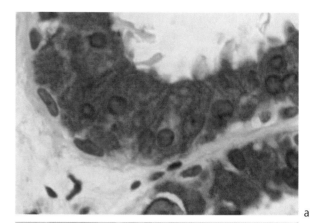

a

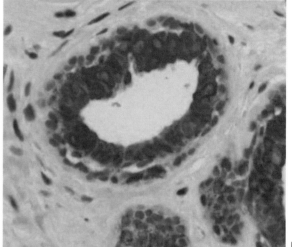

b

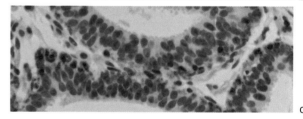

c

Fig. 17.5a–c Immunostaining for Ck8/18, 34βE12 and Ck5/6 of the case in Fig. 17.4
17.5a Immunostaining for Ck8/18 showing intense staining of all atypical cells.
17.5b Immunostaining with the 34βE12 antibody resulting in intense staining of the FEA lesion. This is not an uncommon finding.
17.5c Immunostaining for Ck5/6 showing positive staining of myoepithelial cells in contrast to the negativity of the neoplastic cells. The FEA remains completely unstained.

included in several studies as benign, and often not correctly diagnosed until many years later on histopathologic revision [65–68], were left with residual DCIS. Bearing this in mind, both the absence of local recurrences in ADH and FEA and the elevated local recurrence rate of low grade DCIS may be by no means surprising.

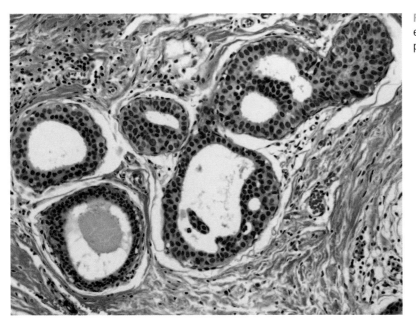

Fig. 17.6 Standard-type ADH. Part of an enlarged lobule with atypical epithelial proliferation and trabeculae.

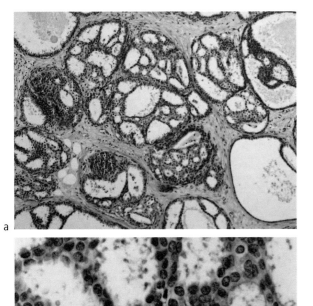

a

b

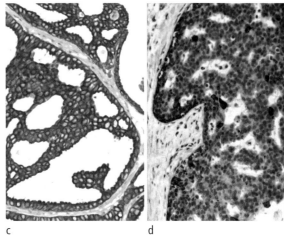

c   d

Fig. 17.7a–d Low grade ductal carcinoma in-situ.
17.7a The original lobular structures are unfolded to duct-like structures.
17.7b Higher magnification displays the same type of nuclear atypia as seen in FEA in 17.4a.
17.7c Immunostaining for Ck8/18 highlighting the glandular differentiation of the tumor cells.
17.7d Immunostaining for Ck5/6 highlighting expression of the basal-type cytokeratins in myoepithelial cells. The tumor cells do not express Ck5/6.

A closer look at some detailed follow-up data for subgroups of low grade DCIS extends the impression that standard-type ADH and DCIS represent individual points along a continuum of the low grade pathway [51]. After a central pathology review in the EORTC trial 10853, comparing excision alone with excision followed by radiotherapy, the recurrence rate was evaluated at a median follow-up of 5.4 years [62]. No recurrences were observed in the 59 patients with well-differentiated DCIS with a clinging architecture. A low rate of invasive recurrence was found in well-differentiated DCIS with a micropapillary growth pattern (7 out of 98 cases), whereas in well-differentiated cribriform DCIS the rate was similar to that in poorly differentiated DCIS.

In conclusion, the lesions of the low grade pathway seem to cover a wide morphological spectrum ranging from the relatively 'innocent-looking' clinging FEA-type lesions to those with a fully developed cribriform DCIS architecture. The evidence supports the conclusion that FEA/ADH and low grade DCIS are indeed stages in the progression pathway towards invasive grade 1 breast carcinoma, each stage having an increasing likelihood of developing into either invasive carcinoma or more extensive lesions [15, 69].

WHAT ARE THE PRECURSOR LESIONS OF THE HIGH GRADE PATHWAY?

Obvious links in terms of morphology, phenotype and molecular genetics also exist between the different stages of the high grade pathway. This is easily understood if we consider high grade DCIS and its grade 3 invasive counterparts and compare them with lesions of the low grade pathway. Thus they are characterized by their considerable number of different chromosomal alterations, which often include high-level amplification, by expression of c-erbB2 and p53, and by overtly malignant nuclear features on histology (Figs 17.8 and 17.9). Furthermore the genetic data indicates that, compared to lesions of the low grade pathway, these lesions are less stable clonal proliferations.

The most important feature of all high grade lesions is the presence of significant cytologic atypia with an overtly malignant nuclear morphology. This feature should be emphasized, because it is already present in the early lesions of this pathway. Such lesions were described as 'polymorphous type clinging carcinoma' or 'early comedo-type DCIS' by Azzopardi [70] in his textbook: 'Clinging type carcinoma arises sometimes as a variant of comedo cancer but the absence or sparcity of luminal debris and the paucity of neoplastic cells lining the lumen combine to make it easy for the whole lesions to be missed' [10]. Thus, these earliest lesions of the high grade pathway are rarely seen. They involve lobules or ductules that are often slightly distended and enlarged. The lobular ductules and terminal ducts are lined with a single or several layers of classic polymorphous tumor cells, that display a loss of polarity and a clear neoplastic anaplasia. The tumor cells often contain copious cytoplasm and large or polymorphous nuclei with more or less prominent nucleoli. Usually some ductules display an intraluminal growth with a solid or cribriform pattern. Similar changes may be seen in advanced comedocarcinomas, referred to as 'lobular cancerization', which are the result of retrograde tumor progression into lobules. Although the authors feel that distinguishing early clinging type polymorphous lesions from progressed comedocarcinomas is justified, there is now

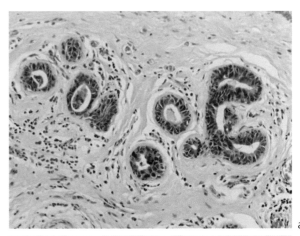

a

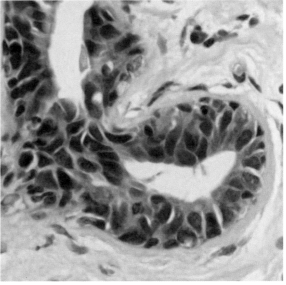

b

Fig. 18.8a–b Clinging carcinoma, polymorphous type.
17.8a This lesion probably represents a very early stage of the high grade pathway. From a conceptual point of view it would be preferable to use a term capable of denoting the developmental stage as, for example, in standard-type FEA. Currently, however, there is general agreement that even small lesions should be classified as high grade DCIS.
17.8b Higher magnification of a ductule with highly atypical cells, which are easily identified as malignant cells. This constellation has been described as 'clinging carcinoma, polymorphous type' by Azzopardi. Note focal comedonecrosis and psammomatous calcification in 17.8a.

general agreement that all in-situ malignancies with overtly malignant nuclear morphology should be termed high grade DCIS irrespective of their size [1] (Fig. 17.10).

PRECURSOR LESIONS OF AN INTERMEDIATE GRADE PATHWAY

As mentioned by Sloane [71], some forms of ADH appear to be characterized by proliferations composed

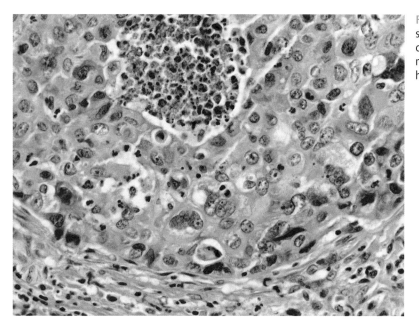

Fig. 17.9 Classic high grade DCIS of several centimeters in diameter with comedonecrosis. The cells show overtly malignant nuclei, one of the hallmarks of high grade lesions.

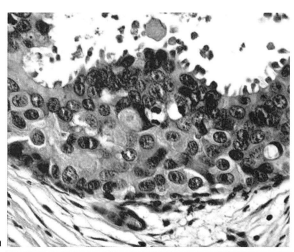

a

Fig. 17.10a–b High grade DCIS with Ck5/6 expression.
17.10a High power view of a high grade DCIS with overtly malignant nuclei. Even with H&E staining there is no doubt as to the malignant nature of the lesion.

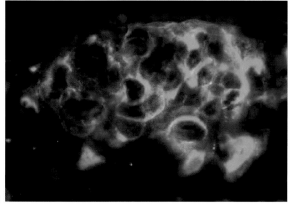

b

17.10b Immunofluorescence staining for Ck5/6 (red) and Ck8/18 (green) with a shift of the red color upwards, highlighting the expression of both cytokeratins. Three to five percent of DCIS are Ck5/14+, all of them high grade lesions.

of more pleomorphic cells, which cytologically and architecturally do not fit the classic definition of ADH or that of high grade ductal lesions.

Cytological and architectural features provide evidence that such lesions may be the earliest stages of an intermediate pathway. Therefore, we propose the terms non-standard-type FEA and ADH to address these early lesions. This conclusion is mainly supported by data obtained from immunohistochemical studies using cytokeratin antibodies. In contrast to

345

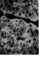

UDH, these lesions express Ck8/18 in the absence of Ck5/14, indicative of a purely glandular phenotype. In routine H&E-stained sections these proliferations can be easily distinguished from low grade lesions by their lack of a smooth geometry and cellular monotony. What sets them apart from high grade lesions, on the other hand, is their lack of overtly malignant nuclear features. However, based purely on morphology, such non-standard-type FEA/ADH lesions may be virtually indistinguishable from benign intraductal epithelial proliferations. Therefore, their detection cannot safely rely on routine histology alone (Figs 17.11–17.14).

Based on experience with other breast lesions, the most useful parameters to define neoplastic epithelial proliferations [44, 46] seem to be those derived from molecular studies. It is therefore important that similar studies be performed on these lesions. At the present time, the only reproducible criterion is the immunohistochemical demonstration of Ck5/14-negative cells.

The authors feel that the types of lesions illustrated by Page et al. 1988 [72] in figures 11.30 and 11.36 correspond to candidates for non-standard-type ADH as defined in this book. Moreover, in her chapter on

ADH, Tavassoli refers to an architectural variant, which she illustrates in figures 6.20a–c and 6.24 (1999) [73]. She characterizes this lesion as one that, starts as clusters of uniform cells in an area of IDH [usual ductal hyperplasia W.B.] and retains the IDH architecture. Although the authors agree that in-situ malignancies may rarely be observed in classic florid hyperplasia (Chapter 7) we propose that non-standard FEA/ADH is a de novo neoplastic growth similar to the early lesions described above for the low- and high grade pathway.

In conclusion the following general comments constitute a new conceptual approach to distinguishing benign epithelial proliferations and early neoplastic breast lesions:

1. Benign epithelial proliferations are characterized by heterogeneous epithelial proliferation of Ck5/14+ cells and their glandular progeny, expressing Ck8/18.
2. Most malignant lesions arise de novo from glandular cells of the terminal duct lobular unit. The vast majority are characterized by a glandular phenotype and lack expression of high molecular weight cytokeratins 5/14.

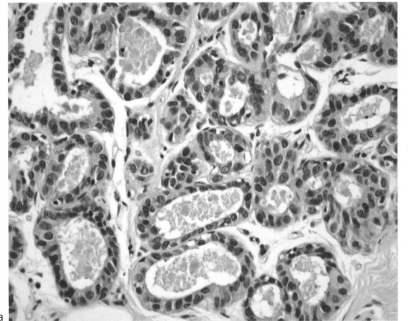

a

Fig. 17.11a–b Non-standard-type FEA.
17.11a Part of an enlarged lobule whose ductules are lined with more atypical polymorphous cells than normally seen in standard-type flat epithelial hyperplasia. The proliferating cells show neither the monotony of low grade lesions nor the overtly malignant features characteristic of polymorphous-type clinging carcinoma. The nuclei vary in size and have occasional nucleoli. Further criteria raising suspicion of a neoplastic proliferation are (1) the pallid to amphophilic cytoplasm of the cells and (2) the luminal detritus. Such lesions would probably be diagnosed as blunt duct adenosis by most pathologists. However, they differ from the latter by their lack of Ck5/14 expression.

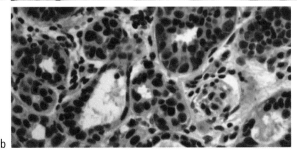

b

17.11b This is clearly shown in immunostains for Ck5/14, which indicate a clonal proliferation of CK5/14– cells. Only the myoepithelial cells and some residual normal luminal cells stain for Ck5/14. In our opinion these lesions can only be classified with the help of cytokeratin immunostaining. We strongly feel that these lesions may be the earliest stages along the intermediate pathway. Compare with 17.12 for distinction from blunt duct adenosis.

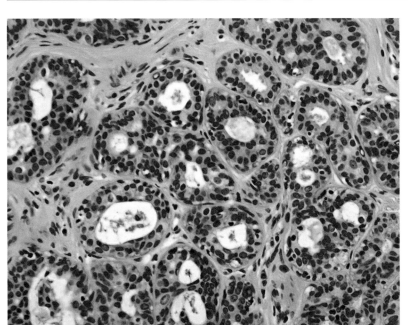

a

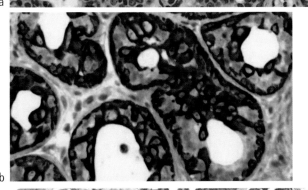

b

Fig. 17.12a–b Blunt duct adenosis.
17.12a H&E view of a lesion with hypertrophy and hyperplasia of a lobule. This lesion may cause problems whenever a clear distinction between a hyperplastic and neoplastic process is required. The epithelial cells contain several cell layers with loss of polarity and small mounds or tufts. The nuclei display some polymorphism, and the cytoplasm is pallid to amphophilic. Relying solely on H&E sections, it is impossible to decide whether this is a benign or neoplastic lesion.

17.12b Ck5/6 immunostaining highlights the typical Ck5/6 mosaicism of this lesion, indicating a benign epithelium.

Fig. 17.13a Non-standard-type ADH. Low power view of an H&E-section showing an enlarged lobule with epithelial proliferation. In routinely stained sections the cells contain round to oval, hyperchromatic nuclei with an uneven placement and a more solid growth.

Continuation

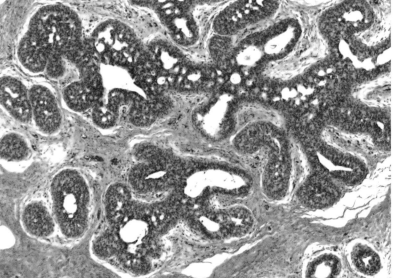

a

3. Early lesions of the low grade pathway (standard-type FEA and standard-type ADH) are highlighted by Ck5/14–, Ck8/18+, ERα+ cells with characteristic low grade nuclear atypia and/or smooth architecture. Based on the correlation with molecular findings, we have learnt to identify these lesions on a histological basis.

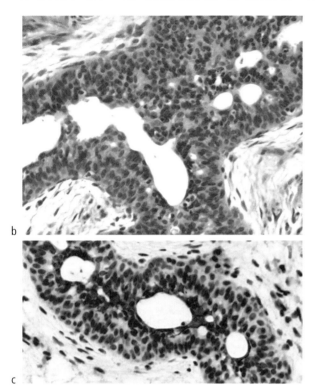

Fig. 17.13b–c Non-standard-type ADH.
17.13b Higher power view of the same lesion as shown in 17.13a. Some irregular secondary lumina with a fenestrated appearance can be seen. The nucleoli are regularly placed with a crowded appearance. Most pathologists would probably categorize this as benign epithelial hyperplasia.

17.13c The same lesion immunostained for Ck5/6. This staining highlights the Ck5/6– pagetoid proliferation with some residual normal attenuated luminal cells. These features clearly define the lesion as a neoplastic process, which we would classify as non-standard-type ADH.

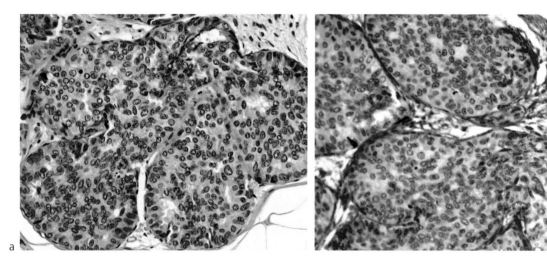

Fig. 17.14a–b Intermediate grade DCIS.
17.14a High power view shows a solid epithelial proliferation with unfolding of TDLUs. The neoplastic cells contain oval, euchromatic cells with some uneven placement. The growth pattern is solid with only a few small, barely visible, irregular lumina. This form of DCIS may be indistinguishable from UDH.
17.14b Immunostaining confirms a Ck5/14– clonal proliferation of ductal cells, thus the lesion meets the criteria of an intermediate grade DCIS.

4. Early lesions of the high grade pathway show an overtly malignant nuclear phenotype. Most of these lesions display a purely glandular phenotype (Ck8/18), but a small percentage show coexpression of Ck5/14. The earliest histologically recognizable form is the 'clinging carcinoma, polymorphous type' already described by Azzopardi [70]. Irrespec- tive of their size, these lesions are currently diagnosed as high grade DCIS.

5. Because of their indistinct intermediate cellular fea- tures, early lesions of the intermediate grade path- way are referred to as non-standard-type FEA/ADH. In H&E sections they may be indistinguishable from benign epithelial proliferations such as epithelial

hyperplasia. However, in contrast to benign epithelial proliferations with their Ck5/14 mosaicism, neoplastic intermediate grade lesions display a purely glandular phenotype, which lacks expression of basal cytokeratins 5 and 14. Cytokeratin immunostaining, therefore, is currently capable of improving interobserver reproducibility in the diagnostic process of such lesions.

■ LOBULAR NEOPLASIA AND INVASIVE LOBULAR CARCINOMA ARE CHARACTERIZED BY LOSS OF THE ADHESION MOLECULE E-CADHERIN

To this point we have been discussing precursor lesions of ductal-type. What are the features that characterize early lobular lesions? Even though the term 'lobular carcinoma in-situ' resonates with malignant potential, for almost two decades LCIS was regarded 'only' as a general risk indicator for the development of invasive breast cancer. Although the relationship between LCIS and invasive lobular carcinoma remains controversial, recent genetic data has improved our understanding of the biology of both lesions [74]. One of the most important genetic findings has been that deletions at chromosomal region 16q22.1 are found in a high percentage of invasive lobular carcinoma. This locus harbors the transmembrane adhesion molecule E-cadherin, which is not only involved in cell-to-cell contact but also in cell cycle regulation through the beta-catenin/Wnt pathway. Several recent studies have demonstrated a loss of the wild-type E-cadherin allele

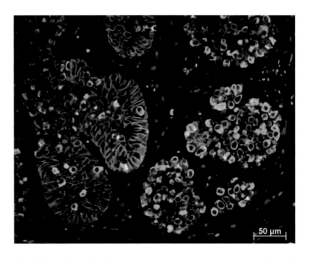

Fig. 17.16 Double fluorescence immunostaining of ADH and lobular neoplasia for E-cadherin (red signal) and cytokeratins 8/18 (green signal). Note the intense membrane-bound staining of the neoplastic cells of ADH and the loss of E-cadherin in the neoplastic cells of lobular neoplasia.

and point mutations in the other allele in both in-situ and invasive lobular tumors, resulting in a loss of function of E-cadherin [75, 76]. Moreover, Lu et al. [77] found striking homologies between atypical lobular hyperplasia (ALH), LCIS and lobular invasive carcinoma, clearly in support of a progression cascade within the lobular pathway.

The relationship between LCIS, DCIS and associated invasive carcinomas was for a long time poorly understood. It was assumed that 15–25% of DCIS cases were associated with invasive lobular carcinoma and that an equal percentage of patients diagnosed with LCIS would develop an invasive carcinoma of ductal subtype over the next 15–20 years [78]. Ductal carcinomas usually stain positive for E-cadherin, whereas the overwhelming majority of lobular carcinomas show a negative reaction [79]. Furthermore, genetic studies have revealed striking homologies of LCIS with FEA, ADH and well-differentiated DCIS, classified according to Holland et al. [29]. LOH studies identified recurrent 16q losses in all these lesions [33, 36, 77, 80, 81]. Given the observation that ALH and LCIS often coincide with early lesions of ductal neoplasia such as FEA and ADH in the same specimen and sometimes even in the same lobule [56], and with a view to the pathogenetic role of the E-cadherin gene, it is tempting to speculate that single cells of well-differentiated ductal neoplasia, already characterized by a loss of 16q material (i.e., loss of one E-cadherin allele) might exchange their ductal phenotype for a lobular one when mutation of E-cadherin occurs at a second allele (Fig. 17.15). Thus, the evolution of lobular neoplasia from ductal

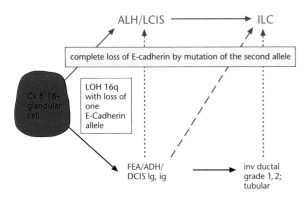

Fig. 17.15 Hypothetical model of the genetic evolution of lobular-type breast cancer. The inactivation of the E-cadherin gene seems to be responsible for the lobular phenotype. Single 'ductal' cells already characterized by a loss of one E-cadherin allele at 16q acquire a lobular phenotype after mutations of the E-cadherin gene occur at the second allele in subsequent divisions. Thus the point in time when the second hit occurs determines the phenotype(s) of a tumor observed in a given biopsy.

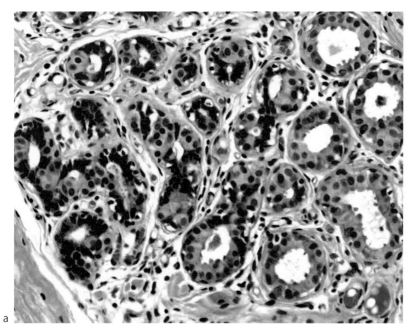

Fig. 17.17a–f Expansion of atypical ductal cells in FEA.

17.17a This lobule shows expansion of atypical cells that replace the normal cells. Residual normal cells are seen in the ductules (acini) in the left field. The atypical cells are easily identified due to their amphophilic cytoplasm and slightly enlarged nuclei, which contain small nucleoli (not visible at this magnification).

a

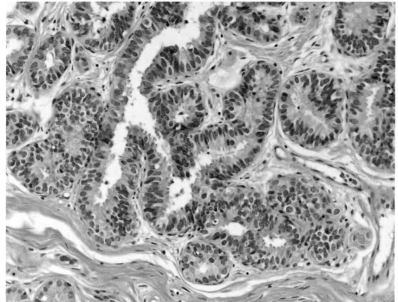

17.17b The normal glandular epithelium in this lobule is completely replaced by atypical cells that are characterized by their pallid cytoplasm and monotonous enlarged nuclei. There is only slight dilatation of the ductules. These subtle cytological changes that characterize FEA may be easily missed, since the normal lobular architecture is completely preserved and the alteration purely cytological.

Continuation

b

neoplastic cells with LOH at 16q that undergo a second hit in the E-cadherin gene might explain the occurrence of both ductal and lobular lesions in the same specimen [82] (Fig. 17.16). The inactivation of E-cadherin at a very early stage of breast carcinogenesis would lead to a monomorphous lesion with a lobular phenotype (lobular in-situ and/or invasive), while inactivation at a later stage, in the presence of ductal neoplasias such as FEA, atypical ductal carcinoma, DCIS or even grade 1 ductal invasive carcinoma, would probably result in a lesion of mixed ductal and lobular phenotype – either noninvasive, invasive or both. This hypothesis is also in line with the observation that lobular-type lesions are rare compared to ductal lesions, lobular carcinoma requiring the additional hit on the E-cadherin allele. Furthermore the fact that ALH and LCIS often coexist with early ductal neoplasia would also explain the development of invasive ductal carcinoma in cases diagnosed as LCIS.

The practical consequences of these findings are tremendous. The different treatment modalities of FEA, ADH, well-differentiated DCIS and LCIS are based on largely hypothetical differences in the biology of these lesions. These new findings require a re-evaluation of the treatment modalities currently in practice, as well as further clinicopathological studies to firmly establish the relationship between ductal and lobular neoplasias.

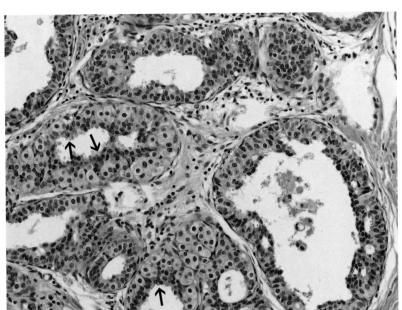

c

Fig. 17.17a–f Expansion of atypical ductal cells in FEA.
17.17c This figure shows part of a lobule with several layers of an atypical flat epithelium. The atypical cells contain a pallid cytoplasm with slightly enlarged nuclei. Some of the neoplastic cells are larger and grow in a pagetoid pattern (arrows) with compressed residual normal cells at the luminal border. Such lesions are also referred to as cylinder cell hyperplasia with atypia and may be misdiagnosed as blunt duct adenosis with epithelial hyperplasia.

Continuation

GROWTH PATTERNS AND SPREAD OF DUCTAL AND LOBULAR NEOPLASIA

One of the most important principles of histological growth patterns in proliferative breast pathology, based on more that 50 years of observations, is the dichotomy between ductal and lobular lesions. The definition of 'ductal' in this context confers to cellular growth patterns characterized by a cohesive proliferation of cells with close cell-to-cell contact. This can be observed in benign epithelial ductal proliferations, ductal in-situ malignancies and invasive ductal carcinomas and their subtypes [1]. This ductal growth pattern is in sharp contrast to lobular patterns that are characterized by discohesive cellular proliferation with typically round cellular shapes. These are observed in all forms of in-situ and invasive lobular malignancies. As discussed in the preceding paragraph, the adhesion molecule E-cadherin represents the molecular basis for the pattern of ductal versus lobular growth. This adhesion molecule is, however, not only responsible for the differences in growth pattern, but also for the differences in the spread of ductal and lobular in-situ neoplasias.

DUCTAL-TYPE SPREAD

The ductal-type lesion itself shows several patterns of cohesive neoplastic cell spread. In very early lesions, the **tumor cells may gradually replace the normal glandular cells** of single involved lobules. This growth pattern (Fig. 17.17) is associated with a distension of ductular spaces and enlargement of the whole lobule. These early changes are easily overlooked and require thorough assessment at high magnification. Characteristic clues as to the neoplastic nature of these cells are changes in their cytoplasmic staining patterns and subtle changes of their nuclei. Thus, the cytoplasm may display a striking pallor, amphophilia or more distinct granularity with increased eosinophilia. Furthermore, the cytoplasm may appear cloudy or vacuolated. Another characteristic feature of neoplastic cells is the truncation of the luminal margins. On the other hand the cells may show apocrine snouts or a hobnail appearance (see Chapter 18). The round to ovoid nuclei are enlarged and hyperchromatic and may have prominent nucleoli. In the literature these lesions have been described under a variety of names, including 'clinging carcinoma, monomorphic type', 'lobular cancerization', 'early ductal in-situ malignancies', 'atypical cystic lobules', 'columnar cell metaplasia/hyperplasia with atypia', and 'columnar alteration with prominent apical snouts and secretions' (CAPSS).

The **second type of proliferation is that of clearly intraluminal growth** with formation of tufts, micropapillae that lack a stromal component, bridges, arcades and bars as minute forms of a cartwheel pattern (Figs 17.18), of fully developed cribriform growth and, last but not least, of papillae. With the exception of tufts, micropapillae and papillae, which may also be seen in benign epithelial proliferations, these growth patterns are indicative of malignancy in ductal-type lesions [83], which is why they are constitutive features of even very early low grade malignant lesions usually located in terminal

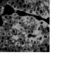

duct lobular units. As described by Wellings et al. [50] the intralobular tumor growth leads to unfolding of the lobular structure and formation of larger spaces with duct-like appearances. The usually widespread involvement of parts of the ductal system with a similar appearance is observed in more advanced neoplastic ductal growth patterns typical of DCIS.

The **third growth pattern is that of pagetoid spread**, more often seen in lobular neoplasia. In contrast to the latter, however, pagetoid spread of ductal-type tumor cells forms cell patterns that permeate the normal epithelium as a neoplastic cohesive cell group and dislodge the glandular normal cell layer from the myoepithelial layer towards the luminal surface. Thus the original inner and outer layers become compressed and attenuated, resulting in flattened Ck5/14+ cells in the basal and often in the luminal position (Fig. 17.17f). Azzopardi's notion that, the 'concept of a pagetoid appearance equates with malignancy' and is, 'never found in benign hyperplasia' is important for practical purposes [84]. Pagetoid spread may be seen in any type of DCIS and is usually easily recognized. In small ductal lesions of intermediate grade, however, it may be necessary to use Ck5/14 immunohistochemistry to recognize the neoplastic nature of the lesion. Pagetoid spread may be observed primarily in DCIS lesions with focal involvement of the ductal lobular system [85], but is also characteristic of Paget's disease of the nipple, where malignant cells of high grade DCIS spread into the epidermis of the nipple.

LOBULAR-TYPE SPREAD

The tumor cells of lobular neoplasia lack the adhesion molecule E-cadherin. This results in a **noncohesive growth pattern** markedly different from that found in ductal-type neoplasia. The neoplastic cells initially invade existing epithelial cells and original glandular cells, which may be displaced and interspersed with the neoplastic cells. Immunostains for Ck5/14 and sm-actin can highlight this type of spread since the tumor cells lack these markers (Fig. 17.19). The myoepithelial cells may be dislodged from the basement membrane to a more luminal position between single monomorphic tumor cells or whole clusters of them. Such changes are usually found in early lesions of ALH and in early stages of pagetoid spread into the ductal system, which is observed in about 75% of lobular neoplasia cases [86, 87]. In a second phase the neoplastic lobular cells coalesce and finally destroy and replace the normal epithelium. In contrast to the complete unfolding of lobules in ductal neoplasia, the lobular architecture is usually preserved in lobular neoplasia.

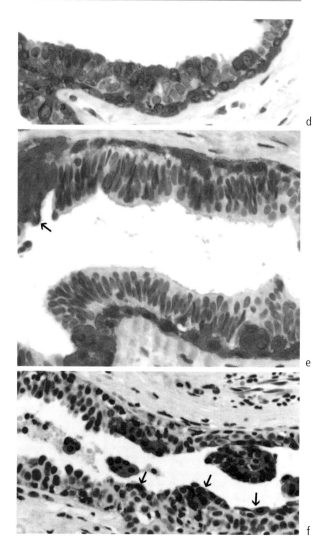

Fig. 17.17a−f Expansion of atypical ductal cells in FEA.
17.17d Normal breast epithelium of a small duct immunostained for Ck5/6, showing myoepithelial cells expressing Ck5/6. The luminal cells display the characteristic mosaic pattern. The luminal cells not expressing Ck5/6 are differentiated, Ck8/18+ glandular cells.
17.17e Normal glandular cells, which persist in one field (arrow), are replaced by clonal proliferation of the atypical cells.
17.17f In this case of FEA the neoplastic cohesive cell group has dislodged the normal glandular cell layer from the myoepithelial layer to the luminal surface. Thus the original inner and outer layer become compressed and attenuated, resulting in flattened Ck5/6+ cells (arrows).

◼ THE MYOEPITHELIAL CELL LAYER OF IN-SITU MALIGNANCIES

The myoepithelial cell layer of normal breast epithelium contains a heterogeneous population of cells, with few Ck5/14+ cells, many hybrid cells expressing both Ck5/15 and sm-actin and varying numbers of

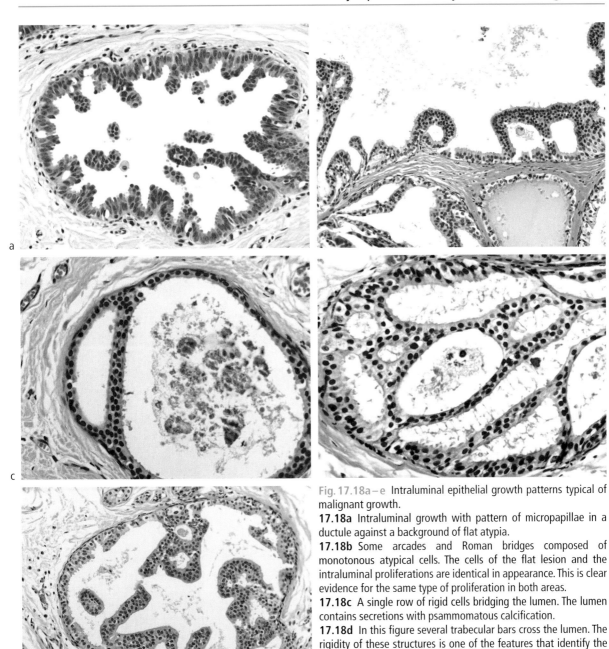

Fig. 17.18a–e Intraluminal epithelial growth patterns typical of malignant growth.

17.18a Intraluminal growth with pattern of micropapillae in a ductule against a background of flat atypia.

17.18b Some arcades and Roman bridges composed of monotonous atypical cells. The cells of the flat lesion and the intraluminal proliferations are identical in appearance. This is clear evidence for the same type of proliferation in both areas.

17.18c A single row of rigid cells bridging the lumen. The lumen contains secretions with psammomatous calcification.

17.18d In this figure several trabecular bars cross the lumen. The rigidity of these structures is one of the features that identify the lesion as neoplastic.

17.18e A ductule containing micropapillae and Roman bridges with the typical cytological features of neoplastic growth. Arcades and bridges are characterized by their robust and rigid structure. The atypical cells of the more complex structures and the flat epithelium display the same appearance.

differentiated cells expressing only sm-actin. Immunohistochemical studies suggest that these cells constitute a continuum from Ck5/14+ precursor cells to fully differentiated end cells (see Chapter 1). Of all the cellular constituents of breast epithelium, the cells of the myoepithelial lineage are the cell pool with the least proliferative potential [88, 89].

In ductal and lobular neoplasia the myoepithelial cell layer is usually well-preserved, although it may also be compressed and attenuated by the tumor growth [90]. Little is known about the myoepithelial reaction to, and its functioning within, in-situ malignancies [91–95]. The myoepithelial layer is likely to proliferate to a certain amount. Occasionally, however,

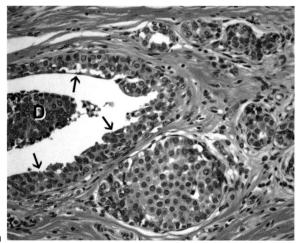

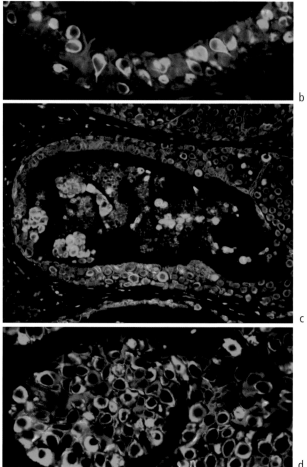

Fig. 17.19a–d Growth pattern of lobular neoplasia (LN).
17.19a Pagetoid growth pattern of a small duct (D) in LN. Note the typical discohesive monomorphic tumor cells, which compress and gradually replace the native cells. Note the pagetoid spread in the duct with attenuated luminal epithelium (arrows).
17.19b Immunostaining for E-cadherin (red signal) and Ck8/18 (green signal). The Ck8/18+ tumor cells infiltrate the native glandular epithelium which, in contrast to the neoplastic cells, stains intensely for E-cadherin. This early infiltration of normal epithelium by tumor cells is typical of 'lobular-type' neoplasias.
17.19c Immunostaining for Ck8/18 (green signal) and Ck5/6 (red signal). As the tumor cells grow, they coalesce and displace the normal epithelium. This ductule shows pagetoid growth of the Ck8/18+ cells with luminal displacement of the native Ck5/6+ cells.
17.19d Immunostaining for Ck8/18 (green signal) and Ck5/6 (red signal) of two ductules, showing infiltration and replacement of the native glandular cells.

identifying the myoepithelial layer on H&E-stained sections may be difficult.

Our present algorithm for myoepithelial cell identification in immunohistochemistry includes an antibody panel which may be helpful in the interpretation of staining patterns. It is important to bear in mind that the different antibodies immunostain only a part of the myoepithelial lineage. Thus, p63 [96–99] and Ck5/14 are mainly expressed in precursor cells and early myoepithelial cells, while sm-actin [100] and calponin [100–105] are seen in early myoepithelial cells, which coexpress Ck5/14 and p63, and in terminally differentiated end cells, which only express sm-actin (see Chapter 1).

In longstanding lesions of low grade DCIS, the myoepithelial cells may contain mainly differentiated end cells that lack p63 and Ck5/14 (Fig. 17.20), while in other lesions the myoepithelial layer may consist primarily of 'immature' myoepithelial cells that

express Ck5/14, p63 and sm-actin. This data must be taken into consideration when the presence of a myoepithelial layer is to be confirmed for diagnostic purposes. In our experience, in cases of DCIS with a long biological history, for example encysted papillary carcinoma, the myoepithelial cell layer may even vanish. This finding should not lead to a mistaken diagnosis of invasive carcinoma.

■ A NEW CONCEPT OF DUCTAL CARCINOMA ■ BASED ON THE CELLULAR COMPONENTS OF ▦ MALIGNANT BREAST LESIONS

In Chapter 7 we discussed the use of immunostains against cytokeratins expressed by the component cells of benign breast lesions. These markers serve to visually distinguish the various cells from one another. In view of the data obtained, we have reached the

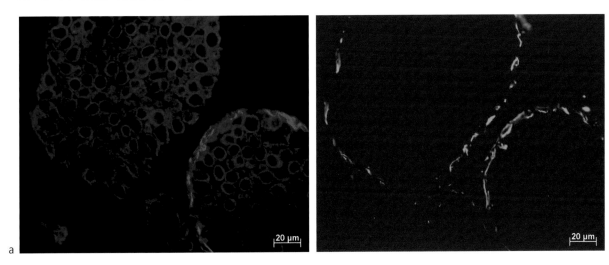
a   b

Fig. 17.20 Triple immunostaining for Ck5/6, Ck8/18 and sm-actin in low grade DCIS.
17.20a The tumor cells express Ck8/18 (blue signal), but display a complete lack of Ck5/6 (purple signal). Only the myoepithelial cells of the duct in the right field show a myoepithelial cell layer that expresses Ck5/6, contrasting with the Ck5/6-negative staining of the myoepithelial cells of the other duct.
17.20b Sm-actin (green signal) staining highlights the myoepithelial layer in both ducts, indicating a more differentiated status of the myoepithelial cells in the left duct.

conclusion that, with the exception of microglandular adenosis, all benign lesions contain Ck5/14+ progenitor cells and their glandular and/or myoepithelial progeny. In order to reveal their analogous features, this chapter will discuss the application of this tool to precursor lesions as well as their invasive counterparts. In addition to basal cytokeratins 5/14, glandular cytokeratins 8/18 and myoepithelial markers (sm-actin, p63 and calponin) are the most useful markers. In rare cases a squamous cell differentiation marker such as Ck10 may be needed to highlight the metaplastic capacity of neoplastic lesions.

Ck8/18+ BREAST CARCINOMAS

The overwhelming number of breast malignancies display a purely glandular phenotype, expressing Ck8/18 and lacking Ck5/14 expression in their tumor cells (Fig. 17.21). This phenotype is found in more than 90% of all invasive breast malignancies and in 95% of in-situ malignancies. It is observed in FEA, ADH, ALH, low, intermediate and most high grade DCIS as well as most invasive breast carcinomas of all grades [46, 106–108]. Thus, only a small percentage of all breast carcinomas express the basal cytokeratins 5/14 typically found in benign lesions.

Ck5/15+ BREAST CARCINOMAS

Pure Ck5/14+ PROGENITOR CELL CARCINOMAS

This is an extremely rare group of tumors that display Ck5/14 expression, but lack all of the lineage differen-
tiation markers of normal breast epithelium. In the largest series studied so far [106], only 0.8% of invasive breast carcinomas belonged to this group and all were considered basal cell carcinomas. We interpret them as pure Ck5/14+ progenitor cell carcinomas. Histologically, such cases are ductal-type carcinomas with grade 3 morphology and extensive central necrosis. Pure high grade DCIS of similar morphology (Fig. 17.22) are exceptionally rare.

Ck5/14+ TUMORS WITH ABORTIVE GLANDULAR DIFFERENTIATION

A second small group of breast carcinomas exists whose cells are characterized by the prevalence of Ck5/14+ neoplastic cells as an integral part of the tumor (Table 17.2). These cells show lineage differentiation to glandular cells coexpressing Ck8/18 (Fig. 17.10). This immunophenotype is observed in less than 5% of high grade DCIS and less than 10% of invasive carcinoma, most of them grade 3. The existence of such basal cell type tumors has been confirmed by immunohistochemical analyses, Western blotting experiments and gene expression studies [46, 106–109]. In addition to expressing Ck5/14, these neoplastic cells are also characterized by specific cytogenetic alterations and protein expression patterns, including a positive correlation with EGFR, p53 and Cyclin A expression and an inverse correlation with c-erbB2 expression [110, 111]. Interestingly, a large subgroup of these tumors seems to be associated with germline BRCA1 mutations [112, 113].

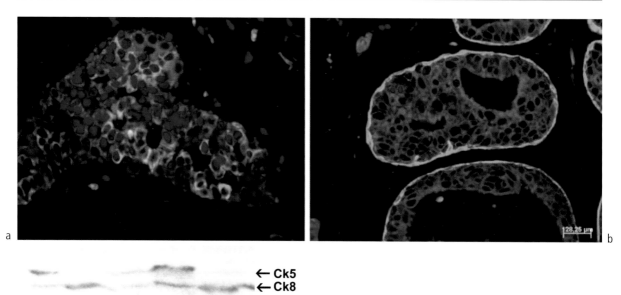

c   **A431**   **A549**   **Normal**   **UDH**   **DCIS**

Fig. 17.21a–c Comparison of UDH and DCIS using double immunostaining for Ck5/6 (green signal) and Ck8/18 (red signal).
17.21a Typical mosaicism of a benign epithelial proliferation (UDH).
17.21b In contrast, the Ck8/18+ tumor cells (red signal) of DCIS completely lack Ck5/6 (green signal) expression. In this example all the myoepithelial cells express Ck5/6, indicating the presence of intermediate myoepithelial cells. The myoepithelial cells were also positive for sm-actin (not shown here).
17.21c These findings were corroborated by Western blotting experiments, which show a single band of Ck8 in DCIS, whereas there are two bands corresponding to Ck8 and Ck5 in UDH. For comparison normal breast epithelium and two cell lines containing Ck5 and Ck8 (A431) and only Ck8 (A549).

The following tumors are all extremely rare tumors amounting to less than 1% of all tumors.

CK5/14+ CARCINOMAS WITH MYOEPITHELIAL DIFFERENTIATION (MYOEPITHELIAL CARCINOMA)

This is a neoplasm characterized by Ck5/14+ cells that differentiate along the myoepithelial pathway. Glandular lineage markers are not seen (see Chapter 14). Precursor lesions are not known.

CK5/14+ CARCINOMAS WITH BILINEAGE DIFFERENTIATION

Interestingly, a small number of malignant invasive breast tumors with Ck5/14+ cells may display a diversity of differentiations as seen in normal breast epithelium. Thus, adenoid cystic carcinoma and malignant adenomyoepithelial tumors (see Chapters 4 and 14) are composed of Ck5/14+ cells and cells with complete glandular (Ck8/18+) and myoepithelial differentiation (sm-actin+ or calponin+). Furthermore intermediate cells expressing Ck5/14 and only one of the lineage markers are also found, confirming the differentiating potential of Ck5/14+ cells into both lineages in these tumors. Precursor lesions are not known.

CK5/14+ CARCINOMAS WITH SQUAMOUS CELL METAPLASIA (SQUAMOUS CELL CARCINOMA)

The rare pure squamous cell carcinoma of the breast epithelium is a typical tumor in which Ck5/14+ cells show heterologous differentiation to keratinocytes (see Chapter 3). Adenosquamous carcinoma is another rare breast tumor in which Ck5/6+ cells differentiate along the squamous lineage in addition to the glandular lineage.

CK5/14+ METAPLASTIC TUMORS WITH MATRIX FORMATION

These Ck5/14+ tumors show mesenchymal transformation of tumor cells and matrix formation (see Chapter 3).

■ THE TARGET CELLS OF NORMAL BREAST EPITHELIUM IN BREAST TUMORIGENESIS

One of the most important questions concerning tumorigenesis still to be answered is whether breast cancer originates from normal epithelial (stem) progenitor cells or from a transit cell population of

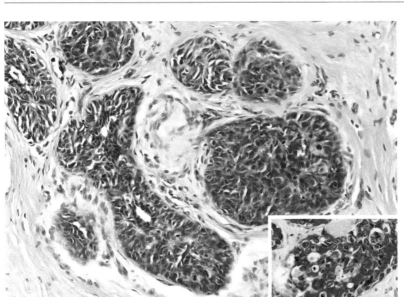

Tab. 17.2 Ck5/14+ malignant breast lesions (basal cell breast carcinomas)

Malignant breast lesion	Immunophenotype
Pure progenitor cell carcinomas, noninvasive or invasive (0.8%)	Ck5/14+, Ck8/18−, sm-actin−
Ck5/14+ grade 3 ductal lesions with glandular differentiation (less than 10% of all invasive and less than 5% of noninvasive carcinomas)	Ck5/14+, Ck8/18+, sm-actin−
Ck5/14+ carcinomas with bilineage differentiation (adenoid cystic carcinoma)*	Ck5/14+, Ck8/18+, sm-actin+
Ck5/14+ carcinomas with bilineage differentiation (adenomyoepithelial carcinoma)*	Ck5/14+, Ck8/18+, sm-actin+
Ck5/14+ carcinomas with only myoepithelial differentiation (myoepithelial carcinoma)*	Ck5/14+, sm-actin+ Ck8/18−
Ck5/14+ carcinomas with glandular and heterologous squamous differentiation (adenosquamous carcinoma)*	Ck5/14+, Ck6+, Ck10+, Ck8/18+, sm-actin−
Ck5/14+ carcinomas with only heterologous squamous differentiation (squamous cell carcinoma)*	Ck5/14+, Ck6+, Ck10+, Ck8/18− → +
Ck5/14+ carcinomas with mesenchymal differentiation and matrix formation	Ck5/14+, vimentin+, Ck8/18− → +

* Less than 1% of all breast carcinomas.

breast epithelium such as glandular cells. Experimental and theoretical evidence supports the hypothesis that epithelial stem cells are the primary targets for tumorigenesis in the adult mammary gland [114]. Stem cells are long-lived and have a large replication potential, allowing them to accumulate the mutations required for malignant potential. This is in line with the view of Dontu et al. [115, 116] and others [117] who have recently proposed a model in which estrogen receptor alpha (ER)+ stem cells and ER− stem cells or progenitor cells of normal breast epithelium are the founding cells of breast tumors. According to their model, the transformed cells then become 'cancer stem cells', that maintain the functional properties of differentiation present in normal stem cells. This theory would provide an explanation for the phenotypical diversity of breast tumors. However, in most tissues true stem cells are no more than a tiny fraction of the whole cell population, accounting for less than 1−2% [118]. Moreover, under normal conditions

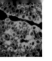

these stem cells cycle very slowly, thus protecting them from the genetic errors accumulated in the process of repeated DNA replication. Most primitive stem cells would seem, therefore, to be protected from transformation, they are few in number and proliferate only sporadically [118].

As discussed extensively in Chapter 1, using a small panel of immunohistochemical markers, substantial progress has been made in recent years identifying and characterizing subgroups of epithelial cells of the resting breast. In the last paragraph we have discussed the data from multiple in-situ staining techniques that have been used to identify the same various markers expressed by the component cells of both benign and neoplastic lesions. In contrast to biochemical analyses, such studies have the advantage of leaving the tissue intact and thus allow an insight into the architectural distribution of different cell subtypes. Based on the accumulated data, we propose a modified progenitor cell model of breast carcinogenesis (Fig. 17.23), which takes the analogies between normal breast epithelium and tumors into consideration [43]. We believe that the differentiation characteristics of various breast tumors provide a basis upon which to predict the possible target cells of malignant transformation. The balance of evidence detailed below indicates that the different breast tumors observed in the human female breast tend to recapitulate stages of normal epithelial differentiation so that, to a certain extent, they can be classified according to a corresponding normal stage.

The concept that breast carcinomas derive from different subtypes of the breast epithelium deviates considerably from current opinion on a possible stem cell origin. This model has important implications for understanding breast carcinoma development and may be integrated with the following data into a more consistent theory:

1. In the view of Dontu et al. [116] ER+ and ER− breast carcinomas are derived from ER+ and/or ER− target cells of normal breast epithelium. The problem with this theory, however, is that we do not yet know exactly which subset of normal cells actually expresses ER. Dontu et al. assume the existence of ER+ stem (progenitor) cells although they acknowledge that the origin of these cells in the normal breast epithelium has not been elucidated. Many immunohistochemical studies of normal TDLUs report the expression of ER, but only in a minority of luminal cells [119–122]. ER+ cells, while rarely expressing proliferation markers themselves, are often found in close proximity to proliferating cells [123]. The interpretation of these findings has been that ER+ cells have a paracrine or juxtacrine function triggered by estrogen signaling stimulating proliferation of the adjacent ER− cells. Clarke et al. [124] have modified this view and proposed a model in which cells expressing the estrogen receptor represent a slowly proliferating cell population usually found in close proximity to the more mitotically active, transit amplifying cells. In recent studies our group disclosed that ER expression is closely associated with colocalization of Ck8/18 in the resting breast epithelium of TDLUs. Thus, Ck8/18+ glandular cells of normal breast epithelium can be subdivided according to the presence or lack of ER expression into Ck8/18+/ER+ cells and CK8/18+/ER− cells (Fig. 17.24). The immunofluorescence data, moreover, indicates that the Ck8/18+/ER+ glandular cells do not express Ck5 or Ck14, or they do so only at a basal level. On the other hand, Ck5/14− cells are virtually always ER−.

2. At present, Ck8/18+ glandular cells of the resting breast epithelium are considered very mature differentiated cells. If we consider, however, the proliferation rate of the different subtypes of resting breast epithelium, the highest mitotic activity is found in the Ck8/18+ population [89]. Bearing in mind that in many organs slowly dividing stem cells give rise to transit/amplifying progenitor cells, which actively proliferate in response to specific stimuli [125], we hypothesize that the Ck8/18+ population of the resting breast epithelium might represent such a transit cell compartment and, what is more, that they may create sufficient daughter cells for the purpose of normal tissue generation over a long period of time.

3. To reconcile the data presented above with that of Iqbal et al., who showed a dissociation of ER expression and the proliferation marker Ki67 in normal breast epithelium, we propose the following explanation of the mechanisms that regulate normal glandular cell growth. Circumstantial evidence supports the view that Ck8/18+/ER+ cells are, at the most, a slowly proliferating cell population. More importantly, they seem capable of producing paracrine factors that influence and modulate the proliferative activity of the Ck8/18+/ER− cells. Thus the CK8/18+/ER+ cells and the CK8/18+/ER− cells are closely linked not only at a phenotypical but also on a functional level in terms of proliferation. The proliferative potential of these Ck8/18+ cells decreases irreversibly only with differentiation to lactating cells during pregnancy and lactation which represents the final stage of differentiation in breast epithelium. At present it is not known whether Ck8/18+/ER+ cells also adjust the proliferation of more immature progenitor cells such as the Ck5/14+/ER− cell population.

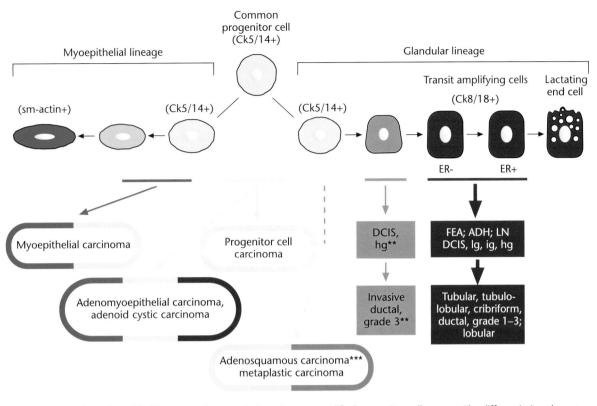

Fig. 17.23 Hypothetical model of breast carcinogenesis, based on our modified progenitor cell concept. The differentiation characteristics of specific tumors can be correlated with the different subtypes of the myoepithelial and glandular cell lineages (for details see text).

Accumulating evidence suggests that the different cells included in this progenitor cell model might be targets for malignant transformation and responsible for the diversity of breast cancer phenotypes (Fig. 17.23).

Our model predicts that different types of breast carcinomas derive from different target cells. 90% of all breast carcinomas express glandular Ck8/18 but not Ck5/14. Increased expression of ER is observed in about 75% of all noninvasive carcinomas [126] and in about 60% of invasive breast carcinomas, with the highest rates occurring in non-high grade lesions. We have seen ERα coexpressed in normal glandular epithelium of the resting breast and in breast carcinoma only in cells with Ck8/18, and not in those with CK5. The key role of estrogen and its receptor in normal breast regeneration and in the development of breast carcinoma is well-recognized [127, 128]. **Given the assumption that mitotically active cells of the normal breast epithelium are the most likely targets of malignant transformation and based on the foregoing observations, it is reasonable to conclude that the most likely target cells of malignant transformation are the CK8/18+/ER– transient cells** of normal breast epithelium – the cells which probably have the highest proliferation rate. Moreover, evidence discussed above supports the view that this malignant transformation is closely linked to the mechanisms that regulate ER expression within these cells. Arguments that support this view are (1) the predominance of the glandular phenotype and the high rate of ER+ carcinomas in the majority of breast carcinomas and (2) that even the earliest histologically recognizable epithelial malignancies such as FEA and ADH display exactly the same immunophenotype [46, 107]. This model predicts that the transformation of CK8/18+/ER– target cells could also result in tumors that show no or only a limited ER expression. Contrary to the view of Dontu et al., this model implies that the ER status of a Ck8/18+ tumor does not necessarily indicate whether the estrogen receptor of the target cell has had any impact in the pathogenesis of a given tumor.

Ck5/14+/ER– progenitor cells are the founding cells of a variety of rare malignancies.

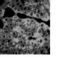

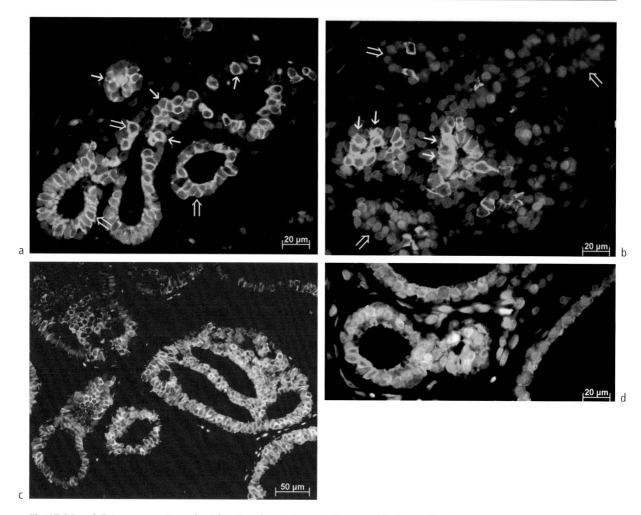

Fig. 17.24a–d Estrogen receptor and cytokeratin subtypes in normal breast epithelium and malignant tumors.
17.24a Part of a normal lobule with double immunostaining for Ck8/18 (green signal) and ERα (red signal). The Ck8/18+ cell population contains both an ER+ fraction (arrows) and an ER– fraction (double arrows). The myoepithelial cells lack estrogen receptor expression.
17.24b Part of a normal lobule. Double staining for Ck5/6 (green signal) and ERα (red signal). The Ck5/6+ cells (arrows) lack estrogen receptors in contrast to several ER+ luminal cells (double arrows) which lack Ck5/6 and represent Ck8/18+ cells (not shown here).
17.24c Atypical ductal hyperplasia. Double staining for Ck8/18 (green signal) and ERα (red signal). The atypical proliferating cells express both Ck8/18 and ER.
17.24d FEA. Double staining for Ck8/18 (green signal) and ERα (red signal). Note that this lesion consists of a Ck8/18+, ER+ clonal proliferation.

The broad diversity of breast tumors suggests that other cells should also be considered potential founding cells of tumor development within the progenitor cell concept. The most interesting tumors within this conceptual framework are carcinomas that display progenitor cell features with or without any of the differentiated characteristics observed in normal breast epithelium. Pure Ck5+ or Ck14+ tumors are characterized by a lack of lineage differentiation and are ER–. These tumors can best be explained when the target cells of transformation are Ck5/14+/ER– stem cells.

About 10% of breast carcinomas show an abortive differentiation to glandular cells, thus coexpressing the basal Ck5/14 and the lineage-specific glandular Ck8/18. We hypothesize that early Ck5/14+ glandular progenitor cells are the founding cells of these tumors, which normally lack ER expression. Recently, Weinberg and co-workers [129, 130] showed that Ck14+/CK18+ human mammary epithelial cells can be transformed into carcinoma cells through the introduction of three genes encoding the SV40 large T-antigen, the telomerase catalytic subunit and an H-Ras oncoprotein. These cells lacked expression of the estrogen receptor and were suggested to provide a model for the development of ER-negative carcinomas with basal cell characteristics [129–131]. Interestingly the phenotype of the target cells was preserved in the tumor. Thus the experiments established a new system for understanding the molecular mechanisms of malignant cell growth in this cell population.

A few extremely rare groups of breast carcinomas such as adenoid cystic carcinomas and malignant adenomyoepithelial tumors show the full range of the two differentiated cell lineages of normal breast epithelium. The most likely explanation for these types of tumors is that the Ck5+ precursor cells are the target cells of malignant transformation which retain some or all of their 'physiological differentiation potential' at transformation. Another subgroup of progenitor cell carcinomas – namely adenosquamous carcinomas – undergoes glandular and/or heterologous squamous cell differentiations (see Chapter 4). Finally, occasional myoepithelial carcinomas are characterized by Ck5/14+ cells that only differentiate to myoepithelial cells. The normal target cell of transformation is probably an early Ck5/14+ myoepithelial progenitor cell with fixed differentiation potential (all sm-actin+, these tumors are not discussed in Dontu's classification).

In conclusion, we believe that the differentiated characteristics of a tumor depend on the nature of the founding cell and its genetic alterations. Breast tumors may thus mimic all the different types of normal cell populations found in breast epithelium. The differentiation potential of the malignant tumor seems to be determined by the position of the target cell in the precursor cell hierarchy of normal breast epithelium.

There is sound evidence that genetic alterations determine the tumor biology (malignancy grade) within a given target cell population.

If most breast carcinomas do indeed derive from the same target cell population of Ck8/18+ cells, then which mechanisms are responsible for their diverse clinical features and malignancies? Data on the macrogenetic fingerprints of breast tumors obtained in CGH studies affords a preliminary answer. This data suggests that different genetic events within the Ck8/18+ target cell may determine the malignancy of the resultant tumor. As discussed above, loss of genetic material at chromosomal position 16q is a characteristic feature of low grade ductal in-situ lesions, LCIS and grade 1 invasive carcinomas, whereas high grade ductal lesions and grade 3 invasive carcinomas are mainly characterized by amplification of several oncogenes. These findings are in accordance with observations from gene expression and immunohistochemical studies showing amplification and overexpression of c-erbB2 in many high grade lesions

in contrast to the very low rate of expression in low grade lesions [126].

Another finding that may be surprising at first sight is that Ck5/14+ invasive tumors such as progenitor cell carcinomas, adenoid cystic, adenomyoepithelial and myoepithelial carcinomas usually display a lower number of genetic abnormalities than classic grade 3 carcinomas. A possible explanation is that Ck5/14+ cells may already have an inherent capacity for self-renewal and even active invasion so that fewer mutations are needed to disrupt the tight control of functions leading to deregulation of proliferation and invasion.

These views are supported by experimental transgenic studies using various activated oncogenes or targeted deletions of tumor suppressor genes in diverse target cells of the epidermis, which have shown that both the target cell and genes involved in the tumorigenesis process are determinants of its phenotype. Furthermore it was shown that individual cell types are selectively susceptible to particular oncogenes [132, 133]. Thus, the ras oncogene leads to a carcinoma when selectively expressed in the basal cells of the epidermal hair follicle, whereas it induces benign papillomas in keratinocytes during terminal differentiation.

In conclusion, as in other tissues, genetic mutational events may occur in any target cell of malignant transformation, from stem cells to transit amplifying glandular cells of the breast epithelium. The cell involved will ultimately determine the observed histological phenotype. Furthermore, the genetic mutations acquired may be fundamental in determining the malignancy of a transformed target cell [129–131]. This cell model opens a new field in which distinct target cell subtypes can be appraised in terms of their potential to generate lineage-specific tumors. It provides a rational, cell biological framework within which to better understand tumor development. We have begun to analyze the differential expression of factors that may influence the various subsets of target cells. If we were to understand the regulatory mechanisms that govern growth and differentiation [134], we might be able to design chemopreventative strategies to eradicate early transformed cells [135] or even cells of noninvasive breast cancer.

CLASSIFICATION OF DUCTAL AND LOBULAR NEOPLASIA

Several classification systems of ductal intraepithelial neoplasia have been proposed over the years. The most common, traditional classification systems include FEA, ADH, and ductal carcinoma and its subtypes. Recently Tavassoli [1, 136, 137] in adopting a proposal of Rosai [138] proposed a new classification, using the term 'ductal intraepithelial neoplasia', with a subdivision into three grades.

Ductal intraepithelial neoplasia (DIN)

DIN 1a Corresponding to UDH

DIN 1b Corresponding to FEA

DIN 1c Corresponding to ADH and small grade 1 DCIS

DIN 2 Corresponding to larger grade 1 DCIS and grade 2 DCIS

DIN 3 Corresponding to grade 3 DCIS

From a conceptual point of view, the hallmark of this classification is that both UDH (DIN 1a) and DCIS (DIN 1c, DIN2 and DIN3) are included under DIN. This is understandable in terms of the diagnostic difficulties one may occasionally encounter in distinguishing UDH and certain forms of DCIS. However, since cell biological criteria and molecular data currently suggest a sharper separation than histological evidence allows and in view of the fact that UDH and all grades of DCIS indicate completely different management systems, we regard this classification as unacceptable. As Rosai [139] noted, 'linking these conditions in a graded system that presupposes a nosologic unity might be unwarranted and misleading'. The authors' view is also in keeping with that of the majority of participants in the WHO working group who felt that, at the time of writing, there was not sufficient evidence to regard UDH as a precursor lesion of breast carcinoma [1]. For this reason the WHO committee felt that the original DIN classification should be modified: FEA was introduced instead of UDH as DIN 1a. Moreover, considering the likelihood of new advances in the fields of molecular and especially cell biology, the group decided for the time being to retain the traditional terminology in the official WHO classification rather than adopting a new one. Therefore the traditionally used terms are retained in this book, notwithstanding the refinements that have been made to cell biological insights and diagnostic criteria for some entities.

While any future official WHO reclassification of neoplastic intraductal proliferations will most likely be postponed until our molecular and cell biological understanding of the various subtypes is more firmly established than it is today, we would like to propose a working hypothesis based on the new data described in

Tab. 17.3 Classification of atypical ductal proliferations

Traditional classification (WHO) +	Ductal intraepithelial neoplasia (DIN) terminology ++	Working formulation, modified traditional terms°	Mammary intraductal neoplasia, ductal-type (MIN-D)****
FEA	DIN 1a	Standard-type FEA*	MIN-D 1a
ADH	DIN 1b	Standard-type ADH *	
Low grade DCIS	DIN 1c	Low grade DCIS	MIN-D 1b
		Non-standard-type FEA ** Non-standard-type ADH	MIN-D 2a
Intermediate grade DCIS	DIN 2	Intermediate grade DCIS	MIN-D 2b
		Early high grade carcinoma (clinging carcinoma, polymorphous type) ***	MIN-D 3a
High grade DCIS	DIN 3	High grade DCIS	MIN-D 3b

+ The WHO has adopted the traditional classification.

++ The original Tavassoli classification included UDH under DIN 1a, as discussed in some detail in Chapters 7 and 17. However, from the data available we conclude that there is currently no evidence of UDH being a precursor lesion. The committee of the WHO therefore replaced UDH with FEA.

* This refers to the classic description of FEA/ADH, as defined by the WHO.

** This does not include special types such as apocrine lesions.

*** This refers to early high grade lesions confined to a TDLU. It does not include clinging carcinoma caused by retrograde extension of high grade DCIS into the lobules.

° In the working formulation ductal neoplasias are subdivided according to grade (nuclear appearance) and to stage (extension) of the disease. Stage 'a' refers to focal (lobular) confinement of the lesion, and stage 'b' to ductal-segmental extension of the atypical epithelial proliferation.

**** A similar classification could be used in lobular neoplasia. Mammary intraepithelial neoplasia of lobular-type (MIN-L) could be divided into traditional ALH and lobular carcinoma in-situ as stage 'a' and extensive lobular neoplasia with comedo type necrosis as stage 'b'.

this book. Table 17.3 comprises a list of distinctive clinicopathological entities that can usually be recognized on H&E-stained sections, but at least after immunostains.

We propose a three-tiered grading system, which corresponds to the three pathways, combined with a two-tiered staging system referring to the extension of the lesion of in-situ neoplasias (Table 17.3). Employing the term mammary intraepithelial neoplasia, ductal-type (MIN-D) for all neoplastic ductal in-situ lesions, one could thus subdivide them as follows: low grade pathway lesions include standard-type FEA/ADH as MIN-D 1a and low grade DCIS as MIN-D 1b; intermediate grade pathway lesions include non-standard-type FEA/ADH as MIN-D 2a and intermediate grade DCIS as MIN-D 2b; and high grade pathway lesions include small clinging polymorphous type carcinoma as MIN-D 3a and high grade DCIS as MIN-D 3b. The numbers 1–3 thus refer to grades low to high, respectively, of the lesion; the lowercase letters 'a' (focal/lobular confinement) and 'b' (ductal-segmental extension) refer to the stages of intraductal proliferation. As usually more than one individual lesion of FEA/ADH is found in such specimens, a letter (m) may indicate the presence of multiple lesions. It should be evident from the description above that the rationale for this classification is the theoretical and empirical evidence that each pathway has its own early precursor lesions. The modifications to the DIN-classification of Tavassoli are obvious: First, we differentiate in-situ lesions only as those confined to the terminal duct lobular units and those with ductal segmental distribution ('a' vs. 'b'), and second, we classify each lesion according to its nuclear malignancy grade. We are convinced that, for the time being, these are the most distinguishing two features for management of patients and prognostic purposes. For example, the common clinical denominator for all early lesions such as FEA and ADH is necessarily, that the diagnostic approach has excluded a possible DCIS. In contrast the common clinical denominator of all lesions with ductal segmental extension (DCIS) is the therapeutic approach, whether to remove the whole lesion either by breast-conserving therapy or mastectomy, or to use radiotherapy in certain conditions. Further subdivision between FEA (DIN 1a) and ADH (DIN 1b) seems, to the authors, merely an academic exercise.

The clinical implications of correctly identifying lobular neoplasias justify extending a similar classification to this entity by introducing terms such as MIN-L a and MIN-L b, the former including the classic ALH and LCIS, and the latter extended LCIS with comedonecrosis. We feel that such a working hypothesis emphasizes the biological features of the various neoplasias, reducing our dependence on a purely size-oriented approach. Moreover, the persistent use of various classification systems for precursor lesions creates communication problems, and thus hinders advances of knowledge in the field. Faced with the tremendous increase in precursor lesions detected in daily practice, coming to a consensus in this field will be a major task in the near future.

REFERENCES

1. Tavassoli FA, Hoefler H, Rosai J, et al. Intraductal proliferative lesions. In: Tavassoli FA, Devilee P, editors. Tumours of the Breast and Female Genital Organs. Lyon: IARC-Press; 2003. p.63–73.
2. Tavassoli FA, Millis RR, Boecker W, Lakhani SR. Lobular neoplasia. In: Tavassoli FA, Devilee P, editors. Tumours of the Breast dn Female Genital Organs. Lyon: IARC Press; 2003. p.60–2.
3. Page DL, Dupont WD. Anatomic markers of human premalignancy and risk of breast cancer. Cancer 1990;66:1326–35.
4. Page DL, Dupont WD. Premalignant conditions and markers of elevated risk in the breast and their management. Surg Clin North Am 1990;70:831–51.
5. Going JJ. Stages on the way to breast cancer. J Pathol 2003;199:1–3.
6. Walker RA. Are all ductal proliferations of the breast premalignant? J Path 2001;195:401–3.
7. Haber D. Roads leading to breast cancer. N Engl J Med 2000;343:1566–8.
8. Lakhani SR. The transition from hyperplasia to invasive carcinoma of the breast. J Pathol 1998;187:272–8.
9. Silverstein MJ, Lagios MD, Groshen S, et al. The influence of margin width on local control of ductal carcinoma in-situ of the breast. N Engl J Med 1999; 340:1455–61.
10. Lagios MD. Heterogeneity of ductal carcinoma in-situ of the breast. J Cell Biochem Suppl 1993;17G:49–52.
11. Lagios MD, Margolin FR, Westdahl PR, Rose MR. Mammographically detected duct carcinoma in-situ. Frequency of local recurrence following tylectomy and prognostic effect of nuclear grade on local recurrence. Cancer 1989;63:618–24.
12. London SJ, Connolly JL, Schnitt SJ, Colditz GA. A prospective study of benign breast disease and the risk of breast cancer [published erratum appears in JAMA 1992 Apr 1;267(13):1780]. JAMA 1992;267:941–4.
13. Palli D, Rosselli-Del TM, Simoncini R, Bianchi S. Benign breast disease and breast cancer: a case-control study in a cohort in Italy. Int J Cancer 1991;47:703–6.
14. Marshall LM, Hunter DJ, Connolly JL, et al. Risk of breast cancer associated with atypical hyperplasia of lobular and ductal-types. Cancer Epidemiol Biomarkers Prev 1997;6:297–301.
15. Dupont WD, Page DL. Risk factors for breast cancer in women with proliferative breast disease. The New England Journal of Medicine 1985;312:146–51.
16. Dupont WD, Parl FF, Hartmann WH, et al. Breast cancer risk associated with proliferative breast disease and atypical hyperplasia [see comments]. Cancer 1993; 71:1258–65.

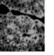

17. Fitzgibbons PL, Henson DE, Hutter RV. Benign breast changes and the risk for subsequent breast cancer: an update of the 1985 consensus statement. Cancer Committee of the College of American Pathologists. Arch Pathol Lab Med 1998;122:1053–5.

18. Page DL, Rogers LW, Schuyler PA, Dupont WD, Jensen RA. The natural history of ductal carcinoma in-situ of the breast. In: Silverstein MJ, Recht A, Lagios MD, editors. Ductal carcinoma in-situ of the breast. 2nd ed. Philadelphia: Lippincott Williams & Wilkins; 2002. p.17–21.

19. Holland R, Faverley D. The local distribution of ductal carcinoma in-situ of the breast: whole-organ studies. In: Silverstein MJ, Recht A, Lagios MD, editors. Ductal Carcinoma In-Situ of the Breast. 2nd ed. Philadelphia: Lippincott Williams & Wilkins; 2003. p.240–8.

20. Bijker N, Peterse JL, Duchateau L, et al. Histological type and marker expression of the primary tumour compared with its local recurrence after breast-conserving therapy for ductal carcinoma in-situ. Br J Cancer 2001;84:539–44.

21. Buerger H, Otterbach F, Simon R, et al. Different genetic pathways in the evolution of invasive breast cancer are associated with distinct morphological subtypes. J Pathol 1999;189:521–6.

22. Waldman FM, DeVries S, Chew KL, et al. Chromosomal alterations in ductal carcinomas in-situ and their in-situ recurrences. J Natl Cancer Inst 2000;92:313–20.

23. Boecker W, Buerger H, Schmitz K, et al. Ductal epithelial proliferations of the breast: a biological continuum? Comparative genomic hybridisation and high-molecular-weight cytokeratin expression patterns. J Path 2001; 195:415–21.

24. Aubele M, Mattis A, Zitzelsberger H, et al. Extensive ductal carcinoma In-situ with small foci of invasive ductal carcinoma: evidence of genetic resemblance by CGH. Int J Cancer 2000;85:82–6.

25. Buerger H, Schmidt H, Beckmann A, et al. Genetic characterisation of invasive breast cancer: a comparison of CGH and PCR based multiplex microsatellite analysis. J Clin Pathol 2001;54:836–40.

26. Shen CY, Yu JC, Lo YL, et al. Genome-wide search for loss of heterozygosity using laser capture microdissected tissue of breast carcinoma: an implication for mutator phenotype and breast cancer pathogenesis. Cancer Res 2000;60:3884–92.

27. Farabegoli F, Champeme MH, Bieche I, et al. Genetic pathways in the evolution of breast ductal carcinoma in-situ. J Pathol 2002;196:280–6.

28. Sloane JP, Lakhani SR, Stratton MR. Terminology for carcinoma-in-situ of the breast. Lancet 1996;347:1259–60.

29. Holland R, Peterse JL, Millis RR, et al. Ductal Carcinoma in-Situ: A Proposal for a New Classification. Semin Diagn Pathol 1994;11:167–80.

30. Poller DN, Silverstein MJ, Galea M, et al. Ductal Carcinoma in-Situ of the Breast: A Proposal for a New Simplified Histological Classification Association Between Cellular Proliferation and c-erbB2 Protein Expression. Mod Pathol 1994;7:257–62.

31. Silverstein MJ, Lagios MD, Craig PH, et al. A prognostic index for ductal carcinoma in-situ of the breast. Cancer 1996;77:2267–74.

32. Ottesen GL, Graversen HP, Blichert-Toft M, Zedeler K, Andersen JA. Ductal Carcinoma in-Situ of the Female Breast. Short-Term Results of a Prospective Nationwide Study. Am J Surg Pathol 1992;16:1183–96.

33. Vos CB, ter Haar NT, Rosenberg C, et al. Genetic alterations on chromosome 16 and 17 are important features of ductal carcinoma in-situ of the breast and are associated with histologic type. Br J Cancer 1999;81:1410–8.

34. Roylance R, Gorman P, Hanby A, Tomlinson I. Allelic imbalance analysis of chromosome 16q shows that grade I and grade III invasive ductal breast cancers follow different genetic pathways. J Pathol 2002;196:32–6.

35. Stratton MR, Collins N, Lakhani SR, Sloane JP. Loss of heterozygosity in ductal carcinoma in-situ of the breast. J Pathol 1995;175:195–201.

36. Buerger H, Otterbach F, Simon R, et al. Comparative genomic hybridization of ductal carcinoma in-situ of the breast-evidence of multiple genetic pathways. J Pathol 1999;187:396–402.

37. Buerger H, Mommers EC, Littmann R, et al. Ductal invasive G2 and G3 carcinomas of the breast are the end stages of at least two different lines of genetic evolution. J Pathol 2001;194:165–70.

38. Cleton-Jansen AM, Buerger H, Haar N, et al. Different mechanisms of chromosome 16 loss of heterozygosity in well- versus poorly differentiated ductal breast cancer. Genes Chromosomes Cancer 2004;41:109–16.

39. Goldstein NS, O'Mally BA. Cancerization of Small Ectatic Ducts of the Breast by Ductal Carcinoma in-Situ Cells with Apocrine Snouts. A Lesion associated with Tubular Carcinoma. Am J Clin Pathol 1997;107:561–6.

40. Moinfar F, Man YG, Bratthauer GL, Ratschek M, Tavassoli FA. Genetic abnormalities in mammary ductal intraepithelial neoplasia-flat type ("clinging ductal carcinoma in-situ"): a simulator of normal mammary epithelium. Cancer 2000;88:2072–81.

41. Lakhani SR, Collins N, Stratton MR, Sloane JP. Atypical ductal hyperplasia of the breast: clonal proliferation with loss of heterozygosity on chromosomes 16q and 17p. J Clin Pathol 1995;48:611–5.

42. Allred DC, O'Connell P, Fuqua SAW, Kent Osborne C. Immunohistochemical studies of early breast cancer evolution. Breast Cancer Res Treat 1994;32:13–8.

43. Boecker W, Moll R, Poremba C, et al. Common Adult Stem Cells in the Human Breast Give Rise to Glandular and Myoepithelial Cell Lineages: A New Cell Biological Concept. Lab Invest 2002;82:737–46.

44. Boecker W, Moll R, Dervan P, et al. Usual ductal hyperplasia of the breast is a committed stem (progenitor) cell lesion distinct from atypical ductal hyperplasia and ductal carcinoma in-situ. J Pathol 2002;198:458–67.

45. Weidner N. Malignant breast lesions that may mimic benign tumors. Semin Diagn Pathol 1995;12:2–13.

46. Otterbach F, Bankfalvi A, Bergner S, et al. Cytokeratin 5/6 immunohistochemistry assists the differential diagnosis of atypical proliferations of the breast. Histopathol 2000;37:232–40.

47. Lakhani SR, Collins N, Stratton MR. Loss of heterozygosity in lobular carcinoma in-situ of the breast. J Clin Pathol: Mol Pathol 1995;48:M74–M78.

48. Tsuchiya S. Atypical ductal hyperplasia, atypical lobular hyperplasia and interpretation of a new borderline lesion. Jpn J Cancer Res 1998;44:548–55.

49. Oyama T, Iijima K, Takei H, et al. Atypical cystic lobule of the breast: an early stage of low grade ductal carcinoma in-situ. Breast Cancer 2000;7:326–31.

50. Wellings SR, Jensen HM, Marcum RG. An atlas of subgross pathology of the human breast with special reference to possible precancerous lesions. J Natl Cancer Inst 1975;55:231–73.

51. Eusebi V, Feudale E, Foschini MP, et al. Long-term follow-up of in-situ carcinoma of the breast. Semin Diagn Pathol 1994;11:223–35.

52. Fraser JL, Raza S, Chorny K, Connolly JL, Schnitt SJ. Columnar alteration with prominent apical snouts and secretions: a spectrum of changes frequently present in breast biopsies performed for microcalcifications. Am J Surg Pathol 1998;22:1521–7.

53. Page DL, Kasami M, Jensen RA. Hypersecretory hyperplasia with atypia in breast biopsies. What is the proper level of clinical concern? Pathol Case Rev 1996;1:36–40.

54. Rosen PP. Columnar cell hyperplasia is associated with lobular carcinoma in-situ and tubular carcinoma. Am J Surg Pathol 1999;23:1561.

55. Schnitt SJ, Vincent-Salomon A. Columnar cell lesions of the breast. Adv Anat Pathol 2003;10:113–24.

56. Schnitt SJ. Flat epithelial atypia. In: Boecker W, editor. Preneoplasia of the Breast. München: Elsevier; 2005.

57. Fraser JL, Raza S, Chorny K, Connolly JL, Schnitt SJ. Immunophenotype of columnar alteration with prominent apical snouts and secretions (CAPSS) [abstract]. Lab Invest 2000;80:21A.

58. Schnitt SJ. The diagnosis and management of pre-invasive breast disease: Flat epithelial atypia – classification, pathologic features and clinical significance. Breast Cancer Res 2003;5:263–8.

59. Allred DC, Mohsin SK, Fuqua SA. Histological and biological evolution of human premalignant breast disease. Endocr Relat Cancer 2001;8:47–61.

60. Oyama T, Maluf H, Koerner F. Atypical cystic lobules: an early stage in the formation of low grade ductal carcinoma in-situ. Virchows Arch 1999;435:413–21.

61. van de Vijver MJ, Peterse H. The diagnosis and management of pre-invasive breast disease: pathological diagnosis – problems with existing classifications. Breast Cancer Res 2003;5:269.

62. Bijker N, Peterse JL, Duchateau L, et al. Risk factors for recurrence and metastasis after breast-conserving therapy for ductal carcinoma-in-situ: analysis of European Organization for Research and Treatment of Cancer Trial 10853. J Clin Oncol 2001;19:2263–71.

63. Rosen PP. Tubular Carcinoma. In: Rosen's Breast Pathology. 2nd ed. Philadelphia: Lippincott Williams & Wilkins; 2001. p.365–80.

64. Betsill WL, Jr., Rosen PP, Lieberman PH, Robbins GF. Intraductal carcinoma. Long-term follow-up after treatment by biopsy alone. JAMA 1978;239:1863–7.

65. Page DL, Dupont WD, Rogers LW, Landenberger M. Intraductal carcinoma of the breast: follow-up after biopsy only. Cancer 1982;49:751–8.

66. Page DL, Dupont WD, Rogers LW, Jensen RA, Schuyler PA. Continued local recurrence of carcinoma 15–25 years after a diagnosis of low grade ductal carcinoma in-situ of the breast treated only by biopsy. Cancer 1995;76:1197–200.

67. Farrow JH. Current concepts in the detection and treatment of the earliest of the early breast cancers. Cancer 1970;25:468–77.

68. Rosen PP, Braun DW, Jr., Kinne DE. The clinical significance of pre-invasive breast carcinoma. Cancer 1980;46:919–25.

69. Alpers CE, Wellings SR. The Prevalence of Carcinoma in-Situ in Normal and Cancer-associated Breasts. Hum Pathol 1985;16:796–807.

70. Azzopardi JG. The Histogenesis of 'Early' Carcinoma. In: Problems in Breast Pathology. 1st ed. London: W.B. Saunders; 1979. p.92–112.

71. Sloane JP. Atypical ductal hyperplasia. In: Sloane JP, Lakhani SR, editors. Biopsy Pathology of the Breast. 2nd ed. London: Arnold; 2001. p.105–9.

72. Page DL, Anderson TJ, Rogers LW. Epithelial hyperplasia. In: Page DL, Anderson TJ, editors. Diagnostic Histopathology of the Breast. Edinburgh: Churchill Livingstone; 1988. p.120–56.

73. Tavassoli FA. Ductal intraepithelial neoplasia 1B & C (Atypical intraductal hyperplasia). In: Pathology of the Breast. 2nd ed. Stanfort, Connecticut: Appleton & Lange; 1999. p.226–60.

74. Cleton-Jansen A-M. E-cadherin and loss of heterozygosity at chromosome 16 in breast carcinogenesis: different genetic pathways in ductal and lobular breast cancer. Breast Cancer Res 2002;4.

75. Berx G, Cleton-Jansen AM, Nollet F, et al. E-cadherin is a tumour/invasion suppressor gene mutated in human lobular breast cancers. EMBO J 1995;14:6107–15.

76. Vos CB, Cleton-Jansen AM, Berx G, et al. E-cadherin inactivation in lobular carcinoma in-situ of the breast: an early event in tumorigenesis. Br J Cancer 1997;76:1131–3.

77. Lu YJ, Osin P, Lakhani SR, et al. Comparative genomic hybridization analysis of lobular carcinoma in-situ and atypical lobular hyperplasia and potential roles for gains and losses of genetic material in breast neoplasia. Cancer Res 1998;58:4721–7.

78. Millikan R, Dressler L, Geradts J, Graham M. The need for epidemiologic studies of in-situ carcinoma of the breast. Breast Cancer Res Treat 1995;35:65–77.

79. Gillett CE, Miles DW, Ryder K, et al. Retention of the expression of E-cadherin and catenins is associated with shorter survival in grade III ductal carcinoma of the breast. J Pathol 2001;193:433–41.

80. Buerger H, Mommers EC, Littmann R, et al. Correlation of morphologic and cytogenetic parameters of genetic instability with chromosomal alterations in in-situ carcinomas of the breast. Am J Clin Pathol 2000;114:854–9.

81. Buerger H, Simon R, Schafer KL, et al. Genetic relation of lobular carcinoma in-situ, ductal carcinoma in-situ, and associated invasive carcinoma of the breast. Mol Pathol 2000;53:118–21.

82. Devilee P, Cleton-Jansen AM, Cornelisse CJ. Ever since Knudson. Trends Genet 2001;17:569–73.

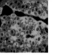
83. Azzopardi JG. Epitheliosis and In-Situ Carcinoma. In: Problems in Breast Pathology. 1st ed. London: W.B. Saunders; 1979. p.113–49.

84. Azzopardi JG. The concept of pagetoid spread. In: Problems in Breast Pathology. London: W.B. Saunders; 1979. p.214–6.

85. Toker C. Some observations on Paget's disease of the nipple. Cancer 1961;14:653–72.

86. Andersen JA, Fechner RE, Lattes R, Rosen PP, Toker C. Lobular Carcinoma in-Situ: A Symposium. Pathol Annu 1980;193–223.

87. Haagensen CD. Diseases of the Breast. 3rd ed. Philadelphia: W.B. Saunders; 1986.

88. Lakhani SR, O'Hare MJ. The mammary myoepithelial cell – Cinderella or ugly sister. Breast Cancer Res 2001;3:1–4.

89. Bankfalvi A, Ludwig A, de Hesselle B, et al. Different proliferative activity of the glandular and myoepithelial lineages in benign proliferative and early malignant breast diseases. Mod Pathol 2004;17:1051–61.

90. Gusterson BA, Warburton MJ, Mitchell D, et al. Distribution of myoepithelial cells and basement membrane proteins in the normal breast and in benign and malignant breast diseases. Cancer Res 1982;42:4763–70.

91. Sternlicht MD, Kedeshian P, Shao ZM, Safarians S, Barsky SH. The human myoepithelial cell is a natural tumor suppressor. Clin Cancer Res 1997;3:1949–58.

92. Rudland PS, Fernig DG, Smith JA. Growth factors and their receptors in neoplastic mammary glands. Biomed Pharmacother 1995;49:389–99.

93. Shao ZM, Nguyen M, Alpaugh ML, O'Connell JT, Barsky SH. The human myoepithelial cell exerts antiproliferative effects on breast carcinoma cells characterized by p21WAF1/CIP1 induction, G2/M arrest, and apoptosis. Exp Cell Res 1998;241:394–403.

94. Gomm JJ, Browne PJ, Coope RC, et al. A paracrine role for myoepithelial cell-derived FGF2 in the normal human breast. Exp Cell Res 1997;234:165–73.

95. Slade MJ, Coope RC, Gomm JJ, Coombes RC. The human mammary gland basement membrane is integral to the polarity of luminal epithelial cells. Exp Cell Res 1999;247:267–78.

96. Damiani S, Ludvikova M, Tomasic G, et al. Myoepithelial cells and basal lamina in poorly differentiated in-situ duct carcinoma of the breast. An immunocytochemical study. Virchows Arch 1999;434:227–34.

97. Reis-Filho JS, Schmitt FC. Taking advantage of basic research: p63 is a reliable myoepithelial and stem cell marker. Adv Anat Pathol 2002;9:280–9.

98. Ribeiro-Silva A, Zamzelli Ramalho LN, Garcia SB, Zucoloto S. Is p63 reliable in detecting microinvasion in ductal carcinoma in-situ of the breast? Pathol Oncol Res 2003;9:20–3.

99. Barbareschi M, Pecciarini L, Cangi MG, et al. p63, a p53 homologue, is a selective nuclear marker of myoepithelial cells of the human breast. Am J Surg Pathol 2001;25:1054–60.

100. Lazard D, Sastre X, Frid MG, et al. Expression of smooth muscle-specific proteins in myoepithelium and stromal myofibroblasts of normal and malignant human breast tissue. Proc Natl Acad Sci U S A 1993;90:999–1003.

101. Di Tommaso L, Pasquinelli G, Damiani S. Smooth muscle cell differentiation in mammary stromo-epithelial lesions with evidence of a dual origin: stromal myofibroblasts and myoepithelial cells. Histopathol 2003;42:448–56.

102. Zhang RR, Man YG, Vang R, et al. A subset of morphologically distinct mammary myoepithelial cells lacks corresponding immunophenotypic markers. Breast Cancer Res 2003;5:R151–R156.

103. Dabbs DJ, Gown AM. Distribution of calponin and smooth muscle myosin heavy chain in fine-needle aspiration biopsies of the breast. Diagn Cytopathol 1999;20:203–7.

104. Werling RW, Hwang H, Yaziji H, Gown AM. Immuno-histochemical distinction of invasive from noninvasive breast lesions: a comparative study of p63 versus calponin and smooth muscle myosin heavy chain. Am J Surg Pathol 2003;27:82–90.

105. Mosunjac MB, Lewis MM, Lawson D, Cohen C. Use of a novel marker, calponin, for myoepithelial cells in fine-needle aspirates of papillary breast lesions. Diagn Cytopathol 2000;23:151–5.

106. Abd El-Rehim DM, Pinder SE, Paish CE, et al. Expression of luminal and basal cytokeratins in human breast carcinoma. J Pathol 2004;203:661–71.

107. Wetzels RHW, Holland R, van Haelst UJGM, et al. Detection of Basement Membrane Components and Basel Cell Keratn 14 in Noninvasive and Invasive Carcinomas of the Breast. Am J Pathol 1989;134:571–9.

108. Wetzels RHW, Kuijpers HJH, Lane EB, et al. Basal Cell-specific and Hyperproliferation-related Keratins in Human Breast Cancer. Am J Pathol 1991;138:751–63.

109. Perou CM, Sorlie T, Eisen MB, et al. Molecular portraits of human breast tumours. Nature 2000; 406:747–52.

110. Korsching E, Packeisen J, Agelopoulos K, et al. Cytogenetic alterations and cytokeratin expression patterns in breast cancer: integrating a new model of breast differentiation into cytogenetic pathways of breast carcinogenesis. Lab Invest 2002;82:1525–33.

111. Wang X, Southard RC, Kilgore MW. The increased expression of peroxisome proliferator-activated receptor-gamma1 in human breast cancer is mediated by selective promoter usage. Cancer Res 2004;64:5592–6.

112. Foulkes WD, Stefansson IM, Chappuis PO, et al. Germline BRCA1 mutations and a basal epithelial phenotype in breast cancer. J Natl Cancer Inst 2003; 95:1482–5.

113. van der Groep P., Bouter A, van der ZR, et al. Re: Germline BRCA1 mutations and a basal epithelial phenotype in breast cancer. J Natl Cancer Inst 2004; 96:712–3.

114. Boulanger CA, Smith GH. Reducing mammary cancer risk through premature stem cell senescence. Oncogene 2001;20:2264–72.

115. Dontu G, Al Hajj M, Abdallah WM, Clarke MF, Wicha MS. Stem cells in normal breast development and breast cancer. Cell Prolif 2003;36 Suppl 1:59–72.

116. Dontu G, El Ashry D, Wicha MS. Breast cancer, stem/progenitor cells and the estrogen receptor. Trends Endocrinol Metab 2004;15:193–7.

117. Pardal R, Clarke MF, Morrison SJ. Applying the principles of stem-cell biology to cancer. Nat Rev Cancer 2003;3:895–902.

118. Alison MR, Poulsom R, Forbes S, Wright NA. An introduction to stem cells. J Pathol 2002;197:419–23.

119. Potten CS, Watson RJ, Williams GT, et al. The effect of age and menstrual cycle upon proliferative activity of the normal human breast. Br J Cancer 1988;58:163–70.

120. Schmitt FC. Multistep progression from an oestrogen-dependent growth towards an autonomous growth in breast carcinogenesis. Eur J Cancer 1995;31A:2049–52.

121. Allegra JC, Lippman ME, Green L, et al. Estrogen receptor values in patients with benign breast disease. Cancer 1979;44:228–31.

122. Ricketts D, Turnbull L, Ryall G, et al. Estrogen and progesterone receptors in the normal female breast. Cancer Res 1991;51:1817–22.

123. Iqbal M, Davies MP, Shoker BS, et al. Subgroups of non-atypical hyperplasia of breast defined by proliferation of oestrogen receptor-positive cells. J Pathol 2001;193:333–8.

124. Clarke RB, Anderson E, Howell A, Potten CS. Regulation of human breast epithelial stem cells. Cell Prolif 2003;36 Suppl 1:45–58.

125. Singh SK, Clarke ID, Terasaki M, et al. Identification of a cancer stem cell in human brain tumors. Cancer Res 2003;63:5821–8.

126. Allred C. Biologic Characteristics of Ductal Carcinoma in-Situ. In: Silverstein MJ, Recht A, Lagios MD, editors. Ductal Carcinoma in-Situ of the Breast. Lippincott Williams & Wilkins; 2002. p.37–48.

127. Mohsin SK, Hilsenbeck SG, Allred DC. Estrogen receptors and growth control in premalignant breast disease. Mod Pathol 2000;28A:#145.

128. Henderson BE, Ross R, Bernstein L. Estrogens as a cause of human cancer: the Richard and Hinda Rosenthal Foundation award lecture. Cancer Res 1988;48:246–53.

129. Elenbaas B, Spirio L, Koerner F, et al. Human breast cancer cells generated by oncogenic transformation of primary mammary epithelial cells. Genes Dev 2001;15:50–65.

130. Hahn WC, Counter CM, Lundberg AS, et al. Creation of human tumour cells with defined genetic elements. Nature 1999;400:464–8.

131. Hanahan D, Weinberg RA. The hallmarks of cancer. Cell 2000;100:57–70.

132. Owens DM, Romero MR, Gardner C, Watt FM. Suprabasal alpha6beta4 integrin expression in epidermis results in enhanced tumourigenesis and disruption of TGFbeta signalling. J Cell Sci 2003;116:3783–91.

133. Owens DM, Watt FM. Contribution of stem cells and differentiated cells to epidermal tumours. Nat Rev Cancer 2003;3:444–51.

134. Siziopikou KP, Schnitt SJ. MIB-1 Proliferation Index in Ductal Carcinoma In-Situ of the Breast: Relationship to the Expression of the Apoptosis-Regulating Proteins bcl-2 and p53. Breast J 2000;6:400–6.

135. Dooley WC, Ljung BM, Veronesi U, et al. Ductal lavage for detection of cellular atypia in women at high risk for breast cancer. J Natl Cancer Inst 2001;93:1624–32.

136. Bratthauer GL, Tavassoli FA. Lobular intraepithelial neoplasia: previously unexplored aspects assessed in 775 cases and their clinical implications. Virchows Arch 2002;440:134–8.

137. Tavassoli FA. Ductal carcinoma in-situ: introduction of the concept of ductal intraepithelial neoplasia. Mod Pathol 1998;11:140–54.

138. Rosai J. Borderline Epithelial Lesions of the Breast. Am J Surg Pathol 1991;15:209–21.

139. Rosai J. Breast. In: Rosai and Ackerman's Surgical Pathology. 9th ed. Edinburgh: Mosby; 2004. p.1762–876.

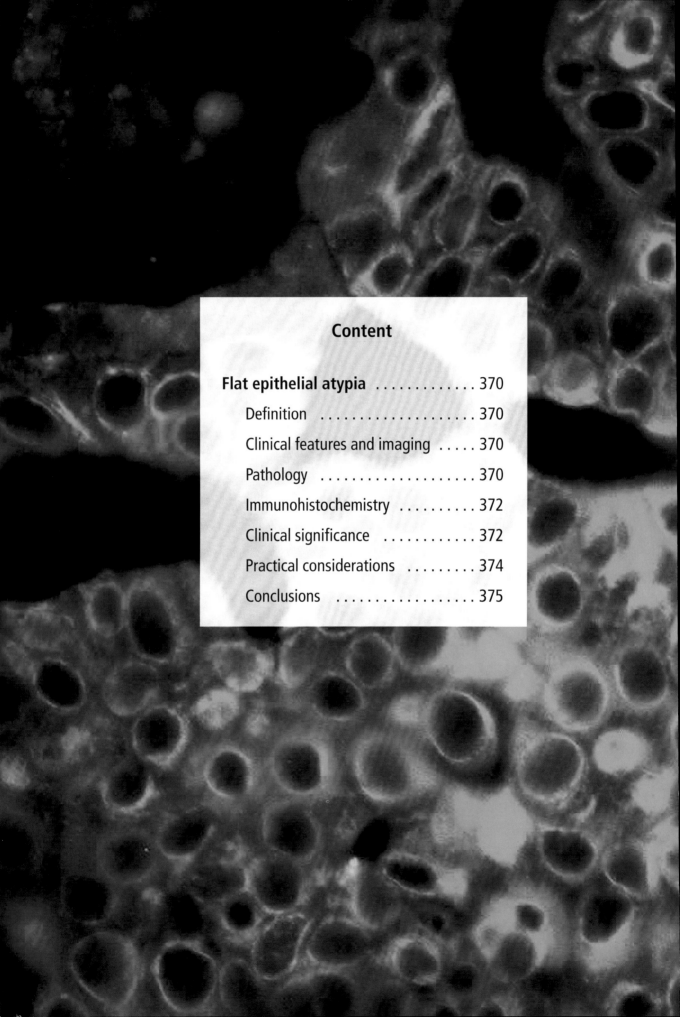

Content

18

FLAT EPITHELIAL ATYPIA

Stuart J. Schnitt

The term 'flat epithelial atypia' (FEA) has only been introduced in recent years. It refers to a proliferation of slightly atypical cells within the lobular compartment. Its pathological features and clinical significance will be described in this chapter.

Flat epithelial atypia

■ DEFINITION

Flat epithelial atypia is the term preferred by the World Health Organization Working Group on the Pathology and Genetics of Tumors of the Breast [1] for a lesion of the terminal duct lobular units (TDLUs) in which the native epithelial cells are replaced by one to several layers of epithelial cells that show low grade cytologic atypia. This lesion has previously been described by a wide assortment of other names, most notably 'clinging carcinoma of the monomorphic type' [2, 3], columnar cell change with atypia [4], and columnar cell hyperplasia with atypia [4] (Table 18.1).

■ CLINICAL FEATURES AND IMAGING

Flat epithelial atypia most often presents as mammographic microcalcifications, which are typically round and non-branching and have an appearance more similar to those seen in benign lesions and low grade DCIS than high grade DCIS [5]. Less often, these lesions are encountered as incidental microscopic

Tab. 18.1 Other names used to describe lesions currently categorized as flat epithelial atypia (in alphabetical order)

Atypical cystic duct [23]
Atypical cystic lobules [10]
Atypical lobules type A [17]
Clinging carcinoma (monomorphic type) [2, 3]
Columnar alteration with prominent apical snouts and secretions (CAPSS) with atypia [5]
Columnar cell change with atypia [22]
Columnar cell hyperplasia with atypia [22]
Ductal intraepithelial neoplasia (DIN) of the flat monomorphic type [6]
Hypersecretory hyperplasia with atypia [15]
Pretubular hyperplasia [16]
Small ectatic ducts lined by atypical ductal cells with apocrine snouts [14]

findings in breast biopsies removed for another abnormality. These lesions are not infrequently seen in association with low grade DCIS and tubular carcinoma, as will be discussed in more detail below.

■ PATHOLOGY

Flat epithelial atypia is characterized by TDLUs that display variably dilated acini lined by one to several layers of epithelial cells of cuboidal to columnar shape. The cells show low grade cytologic atypia characterized by the presence of relatively monomorphic round to ovoid nuclei that are not regularly oriented perpendicular to the basement membrane, with a slight increase in the nuclear/cytoplasmic ratio (Figs 18.1–18.4). Cellular and nuclear stratification is seen in some cases. The nuclear chromatin may be evenly dispersed or slightly marginated, and nucleoli are variably prominent. Mitotic figures may be seen but are uncommon. In some cases, the cells cytologically resemble those comprising the tubules of tubular carcinoma. The epithelial cells in these lesions may form small mounds, tufts or short, abortive micropapillae. However, complex architectural patterns, such as well-developed micropapillae, rigid cellular bridges, bars and arcades, or sieve-like fenestrations, with evidence of cellular polarization within the micropapillae and bars or around the fenestrations, are absent. Thus, it should be apparent that 'flat' in this context is a relative term, simply denoting the absence of complex architectural patterns as described above. Exaggerated apical cytoplasmic snouts and abundant flocculent intraluminal secretions are often present, and some of the cells comprising such lesions may have a hobnail appearance. These lesions frequently show intraluminal calcifications, which in some instances may have the configuration of psammoma bodies.

In some cases of flat epithelial atypia, the lesion may be overlooked entirely on low power microscopic examination due to the lack of significant cellular proliferation and the subtle nature of the cytologic atypia [6]. In fact, TDLUs exhibiting this alteration are often misinterpreted on low power microscopic examination as either normal or as showing only microcysts, and it is only after examination of such foci under high magnification that the subtle cytologic atypia becomes evident.

It should be noted that high grade cytologic atypia with nuclear pleomorphism of the type seen in high grade DCIS is not a feature of lesions included in the category of flat epithelial atypia [4]. The presence of such high grade nuclear features merits the designation of high grade DCIS, even if the cells comprise only a single cell layer [3]. However, such lesions are rarely seen in the absence of high grade DCIS exhibiting other architectural patterns (for instance comedo and solid patterns).

While flat epithelial atypia may be observed in isolation, this lesion often coexists with intraductal proliferative lesions that are composed of cytologically identical cells but show sufficient architectural complexity to warrant a diagnosis of ADH or DCIS. In fact, the presence of flat epithelial atypia should prompt a diligent search for areas diagnostic of ADH or DCIS.

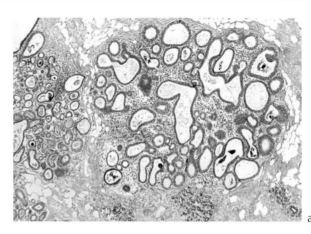

a

Fig. 18.1a−c Flat epithelial atypia.

18.1a Low power view demonstrates enlarged terminal duct lobular units with dilated acini. Flocculent intraluminal secretions and calcifications are evident.

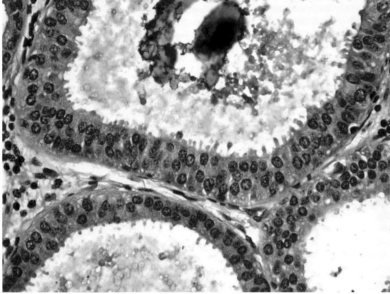

b

18.1b Higher power view shows that the acini are lined by one to several layers of columnar epithelial cells with apical snouts. The nuclei are relatively uniform in size and shape.

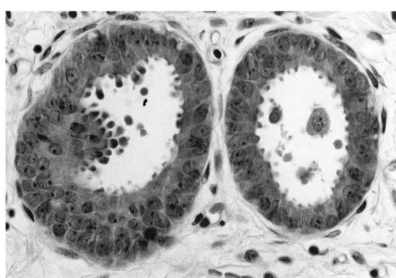

c

18.1c Higher power view to demonstrate cytologic detail.

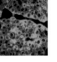

IMMUNOHISTOCHEMISTRY

Studies of the expression of various biological markers in flat epithelial atypia are fairly limited. Available data have indicated that the majority of the cells comprising these lesions exhibit expression of cytokeratin 19 [7] and consistently lack expression of high molecular weight cytokeratins as defined by antibody 34βE12 and antibodies to cytokeratin 5/6 [8, 9]. In addition, they typically show intense nuclear expression of estrogen receptor [10–12] and progesterone receptor [7] in the majority of the cells. These cells also show strong cytoplasmic expression of the bcl-2 protein [11] and variable expression of cyclin D1 [7]. In most examples of flat epithelial atypia, very few of the cells show staining for the Ki67 antigen, indicating that the cells comprising these lesions have a low proliferative rate [11].

CLINICAL SIGNIFICANCE

Assessment of the clinical significance of flat epithelial atypia has been hampered by variations in the terminology used to describe these lesions and the limited number of cases that have been studied in a systematic fashion. There have been two types of studies that have addressed the potential clinical importance of these lesions: observational studies and clinical outcome studies.

OBSERVATIONAL STUDIES

A number of authors have noted that flat epithelial atypia is often seen in association with DCIS and with some types of invasive breast carcinoma, particularly tubular carcinoma. Oyama et al. studied 21 cases of the flat lesion they termed 'atypical cystic lobules' [10] and found these lesions to be more common in specimens containing DCIS (36%) than in specimens without DCIS (3%). They also noted geographic proximity between the flat lesion and the DCIS. Weidner described a lesion composed of small ectatic ducts lined by one or two layers of columnar cells with apical snouts similar to those seen in tubular carcinoma [13]. He considered this flat lesion to represent an example of low grade DCIS. In a more detailed analysis, Goldstein and O'Malley found an association between a similar lesion they called 'small ectatic ducts lined by atypical cells with apocrine snouts' with both low grade DCIS and tubular carcinoma [14]. Other authors have also noted an association between various flat atypical lesions and DCIS and/or invasive carcinoma [15–17] (Fig. 18.5).

In addition, cytologic, immunophenotypic, and genetic similarities between flat epithelial atypia and DCIS and/or tubular carcinoma have been described by various authors.

Among 16 cases with both atypical cystic lobules and low grade DCIS, Oyama et al. noted that the cells comprising the atypical cystic lobules were cytologically similar to the cells of the fully developed DCIS present in the same specimen [10]. Other investigators have also noted that the cells comprising some flat atypical lesions are cytologically similar or identical to the cells comprising some forms of DCIS or to the cells comprising the glands of tubular carcinoma [3, 6, 14, 16, 18]. Oyama et al. further noted immunophenotypic identity in their 16 cases between atypical cystic lobules and coexistent low grade DCIS (the cells of both lesions being positive for estrogen receptor,

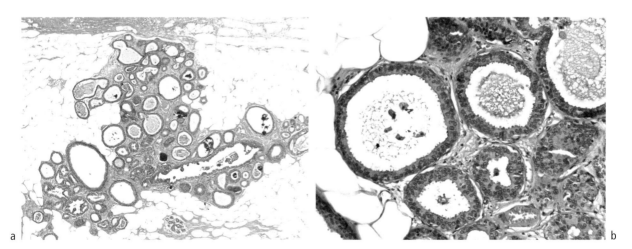

Fig. 18.2a–b Flat epithelial atypia.
18.2a The enlargement of this terminal duct lobular unit is evident at low power, as are the intraluminal secretions and calcifications.
18.2b Higher power view to demonstrate the acinar lining cells, which are cuboidal to columnar in shape, exhibit apical snouts and have round, uniform nuclei.

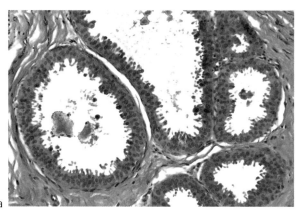
a

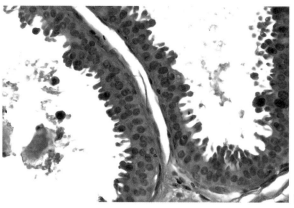
b

Fig. 18.3a–b Flat epithelial atypia.
18.3a In this example of flat epithelial atypia, apical snouts are particularly prominent and exaggerated. Some of the cells have a hobnail appearance.
18.3b High power view demonstrates cytologic detail.

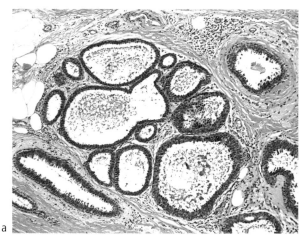
a

Fig. 18.4a–b Flat epithelial atypia.
18.4a Medium power view demonstrates dilated acini and flocculent luminal secretions. Apical snouts are evident even at this power.

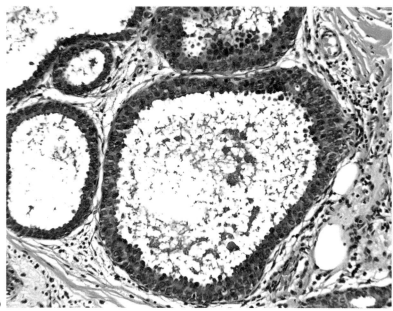
b

18.4b The acini are lined by one to several layers of cells with round, monomorphic nuclei.

progesterone receptor, keratin 19 and cyclin D1) [10]. In a genetic study of 13 cases of the flat atypical lesion designated 'DIN-flat monomorphic type', Moinfar et al. found that 70% showed LOH at one or more of the eight loci evaluated and further, that the genetic alterations in these columnar cell lesions were the same as those in the associated DCIS or invasive cancer [6].

Based on the foregoing observations, it is reasonable to conclude that at least some flat epithelial atypias are likely neoplastic proliferations that may well represent either a precursor of, or the earliest morphologic manifestation of, low grade DCIS as well as a precursor to invasive carcinoma, in particular tubular carcinoma. While this is of great interest from a biological point of view, the clinical implications of these observations can only be determined from follow-up studies. Unfortunately there is a paucity of data on this subject, and the few available studies are characterized by very small numbers of patients.

CLINICAL OUTCOME STUDIES

To date, only two follow-up studies have directly addressed the clinical significance of flat epithelial atypia. In a review of over 9,000 breast biopsies that were initially considered benign, Eusebi et al. retrospectively identified 25 patients with so-called 'clinging carcinoma' of the flat, monomorphic (low nuclear grade) type [3] (these lesions would currently be categorized as flat epithelial atypia). Only one of these patients (4%) is reported to have developed a 'local recurrence' after an average follow-up period of 19.2 years. However, the 'local recurrence' in this patient consisted of a 'clinging carcinoma' lesion

histologically identical to the original lesion, and it is not possible to determine whether this simply reflected persistence of the original lesion due to inadequate excision or if this represented a true local recurrence. Of note, none of these 25 patients developed an invasive breast cancer within the follow-up period. In another study, 59 patients with 'clinging carcinoma' of the low nuclear grade type were identified among the patients entered into European Organization for Research and Treatment of Cancer (EORTC) trial 10853, a randomized clinical trial comparing excision and radiation therapy and excision alone for the treatment of women with DCIS [19]. None of these 59 patients has developed a local recurrence or an invasive breast cancer with a median follow-up period of 5.4 years. Thus, the very limited available data suggest that among patients with 'clinging carcinoma' of the low nuclear grade/monomorphic type the likelihood of local recurrence or progression to invasive breast cancer is exceedingly low, at least with the available follow-up (Table 18.2). However, additional clinical follow-up studies are clearly needed to better understand the relationship between these flat epithelial atypias and the risk of subsequent breast cancer.

■ PRACTICAL CONSIDERATIONS

The appropriate pathology work-up and clinical management of patients whose biopsy specimens show flat epithelial atypia are evolving as information regarding these lesions begins to accumulate. The limited available data suggest that when flat epithelial atypia is encountered in a **core needle biopsy specimen**, subsequent ex-

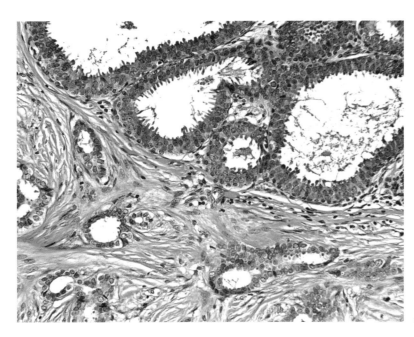

Fig. 18.5 Flat epithelial atypia present in association with tubular carcinoma.

	Eusebi et al. [3]	EORTC 10853 [19]
Number of patients	25	59
Type of study	Retrospective review of breast biopsies originally considered benign	Prospective, randomized clinical trial
Treatment	Diagnostic biopsy; no attempt at excision	Excision alone or excision and radiation therapy**
Follow-up	19.2 years (mean)	5.4 years (median)
Number (%) with local recurrence	1 (4%)*	0
Number with subsequent invasive breast cancer	0	0

Tab. 18.2 Outcome of patients with 'clinging carcinoma' (flat type, with low nuclear grade/monomorphic nuclei)

* The 'local recurrence' in this case consisted of a 'clinging carcinoma' lesion histologically identical to the original lesion; it is, therefore, not possible to determine whether this simply reflected persistence of the original lesion due to inadequate excision or if this represents a true local recurrence.

** Number of patients in each treatment arm with pure 'clinging carcinoma' are not provided.

cision shows a more advanced lesion in about one-third of cases, which is sufficiently frequent to recommend excision in such cases as a matter of routine [20, 21].

The presence of flat epithelial atypia in an **excisional biopsy specimen** should prompt a careful search for areas with diagnostic features of ADH or DCIS by examining additional sections from the block or blocks containing the lesion and by the submission of the remainder of the tissue for histological examination. There are several other considerations regarding the identification of flat epithelial atypia in excisional biopsy specimens that merit discussion. When a proliferation that fulfills the diagnostic criteria for ADH or DCIS is found to arise against a background of flat epithelial atypia, it seems most prudent to manage the patient as one would manage ADH or DCIS in any other setting. However, there are two issues that remain to be resolved when the flat atypia is found to coexist with diagnostic areas of DCIS, particularly in cases in which the cytologic features of the cells comprising the flat atypia are similar to those of the cells comprising the diagnostic areas of DCIS. The first is whether or not the flat atypia should be taken into consideration in determining the size or the extent of the DCIS lesion, and the second is whether or not the presence of flat atypia at the excision margins is sufficient to render the margins 'positive', requiring further surgical resection. As noted above, the limited clinical data available suggest that flat atypia is associated with a very low risk of recurrence or progression to invasive carcinoma. Therefore, we believe that these lesions

should not be taken into consideration when determining the size of a coexistent DCIS lesion or in the evaluation of the status of the margins of excision, even when they are composed of cells that are cytologically similar to those in the diagnostic areas of DCIS [22].

Another problem is the management of patients whose breast biopsies, after thorough examination, show flat epithelial atypia without diagnostic areas of ADH or DCIS. Again, pathologists that consider these flat lesions to represent 'cancerization of lobules' by the cells of low grade DCIS or 'clinging carcinoma' would argue that they should be considered variants of DCIS and managed as such [14]. Others would argue that despite the fact that these flat lesions may well be neoplastic and may even be composed of cells that are identical to those seen in some forms of DCIS or even tubular carcinoma, the few available clinical follow-up studies suggest that they are associated with a risk of subsequent breast cancer that is considerably lower than that seen with fully developed forms of low grade DCIS. The concern, therefore, is that managing patients with such lesions as if they had DCIS would result in overtreatment of many patients.

■ CONCLUSIONS

Flat epithelial atypia is being encountered with increasing frequency due to the widespread use of screening mammography. Recent studies have begun

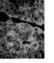

to provide insights into the biological and clinical significance of these lesions. However, additional morphologic, immunophenotypic and genetic studies are needed to better define the relationships between flat atypical lesions and DCIS/invasive breast cancer. Emerging data suggest that flat epithelial atypias may be neoplastic lesions that represent the earliest form of low grade DCIS. Despite this, the limited available clinical follow-up data suggest that the risk of local recurrence or progression of these lesions to invasive cancer is quite low, supporting the notion that categorizing such lesions as 'clinging carcinoma' and managing them as if they were fully developed DCIS will result in overtreatment of many patients. Thus, at this time, the appropriate management of patients whose breast biopsies show flat epithelial atypia in the absence of diagnostic areas of ADH or DCIS is unknown and requires evaluation in further clinical outcome studies.

REFERENCES

1. Tavassoli FA, Hoefler H, Rosai J, Holland R, Ellis I, Schnitt S, Lakhani, SR, Boecker W, Heywang-Kobrunner SH, Moinfar F, Peterse J. Intraductal proliferative lesions. In: Tavassoli FA, Devilee, P., ed. Pathology and Genetics of Tumours of the Breast and Female Genital Organs. Lyon: IARC Press, in press.

2. Azzopardi JG. Problems in Breast Pathology. Philadelphia: WB Saunders, 1979.

3. Eusebi V, Feudale E, Foschini MP, et al. Long-term follow-up of in-situ carcinoma of the breast. Semin Diagn Pathol 1994; 11:223–35.

4. Schnitt SJ, Vincent-Salomon A. Columnar cell lesions of the breast. Adv Anat Pathol 2003; 10:113–124.

5. Fraser JL, Raza S, Chorny K, Connolly JL, Schnitt SJ. Columnar alteration with prominent apical snouts and secretions: a spectrum of changes frequently present in breast biopsies performed for microcalcifications. Am J Surg Pathol 1998; 22:1521–7.

6. Moinfar F, Man YG, Bratthauer GL, Ratschek M, Tavassoli FA. Genetic abnormalities in mammary ductal intraepithelial neoplasia-flat type ("clinging ductal carcinoma in-situ"): a simulator of normal mammary epithelium. Cancer 2000; 88:2072–81.

7. Oyama T, Maluf H, Koerner F. Atypical cystic lobules: an early stage in the formation of low grade ductal carcinoma in-situ. Virchows Arch 1999; 435:413–21.

8. Otterbach F, Bankfalvi A, Bergner S, Decker T, Krech R, Boecker W. Cytokeratin 5/6 immunohistochemistry assists the differential diagnosis of atypical proliferations of the breast. Histopathology 2000; 37:232–40.

9. Carlo VP FJ, Pliss N, Connolly JL, Schnitt SJ. Can absence of high molecular weight cytokeratin expression be used as a marker of atypia in columnar cell lesions of the breast? Mod Pathol 2003; 16:24A.

10. Oyama T, Iijima K, Takei H, et al. Atypical cystic lobule of the breast: an early stage of low grade ductal carcinoma in-situ. Breast Cancer 2000; 7:326–31.

11. Fraser JL RS, Chorny K, Connolly JL, Schnitt SJ. Immunophenotype of columnar alteration with prominent apical snouts and secretions (CAPSS). Lab Invest 2000; 80:21A.

12. Allred DC, Mohsin SK, Fuqua SA. Histological and biological evolution of human premalignant breast disease. Endocr Relat Cancer 2001; 8:47–61.

13. Weidner N. Malignant breast lesions that may mimic benign tumors. Semin Diagn Pathol 1995; 12:2–13.

14. Goldstein NS, O'Malley BA. Cancerization of small ectatic ducts of the breast by ductal carcinoma in-situ cells with apocrine snouts: a lesion associated with tubular carcinoma. Am J Clin Pathol 1997; 107:561–6.

15. Page DL KM, Jensen RA. Hypersecretory hyperplasia with atypia in breast biopsies. What is the proper level of clinical concern? Pathol Case Reviews 1996; 1:36–40.

16. Rosen PP. Columnar cell hyperplasia is associated with lobular carcinoma in-situ and tubular carcinoma. Am J Surg Pathol 1999; 23:1561.

17. Wellings SR, Jensen HM, Marcum RG. An atlas of subgross pathology of the human breast with special reference to possible precancerous lesions. J Natl Cancer Inst 1975; 55:231–73.

18. Rosen PP. Rosen's Breast Pathology. Philadelphia, PA: Lippincott-Raven, 2001.

19. Bijker N, Peterse JL, Duchateau L, et al. Risk factors for recurrence and metastasis after breast-conserving therapy for ductal carcinoma-in-situ: analysis of European Organization for Research and Treatment of Cancer Trial 10853. J Clin Oncol 2001; 19:2263–71.

20. Brogi E, Tan LK. Findings at excisional biopsy (EBX) performed after identification of columnar cell change (CCC) of ductal epithelium in breast core biopsy (CBX). (Meeting abstract. Mod Pathol 2002; 15:29A–30A.

21. Harigopal M YD, Hoda SA, DeLellis RA, Vazquez MF. Columnar cell alteration diagnosed on mammotome core biopsy for indeterminate microcalcifications: Results of subsequent mammograms and surgical excision. Mod Pathol 2002; 15:36A.

22. Allred DC, Clark GM, Molina R, et al. Overexpression of HER-2/neu and its relationship with other prognostic factors change during the progression of in-situ to invasive breast cancer. Hum Pathol 1992; 23:974–9.

23. Tsuchiya S. Atypical ductal hyperplasia, atypical lobular hyperplasia, and interpretation of a new borderline lesion. Jpn J Cancer Clin 1998; 44:548–555.

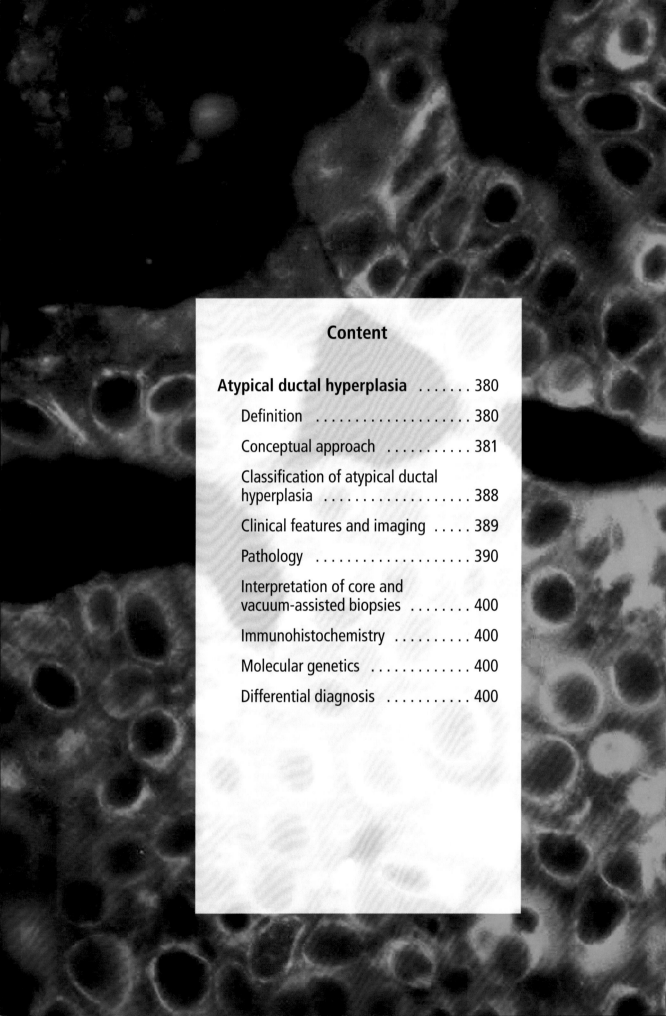

Content

19

ATYPICAL DUCTAL HYPERPLASIA

WERNER BOECKER, HORST BUERGER, HERMANN HERBST AND THOMAS DECKER

Atypical ductal hyperplasia (ADH) has become one of the key lesions of early breast cancer development. Its typical defining features are:
1. a proliferation of monotonous atypical cells; and
2. a smooth architecture.

Other important features are its lobular location and confinement, which can be used as differential diagnostic criterium to distinguish the lesion from DCIS. **This standard-type ADH must be set apart from several other ADH lesions,** one of which is characterized by a more polymorphic cell morphology and a growth pattern that may mimic the micropapillary and fenestrating growth of benign epithelial proliferations. The distinguishing feature of the latter is a positive immunoreaction to Ck5/14, in contrast to the Ck5/14-proliferation of the cells of nonstandard-type ADH. Early high grade lesions should be classified as DCIS. **From a conceptual and practical viewpoint, we distinguish such de novo developments from atypical ductal proliferations that arise in clearly benign proliferative breast disease lesions (atypical ductal proliferations ex benign proliferative breast disease) and from atypical lesions with apocrine differentiation. In conclusion, we propose that ADH should be regarded as a heterogeneous group of early neoplastic disorders rather than as a single entity. Their diagnostic implications in daily routine pathology and their clinical consequences are discussed below.**

Atypical ductal hyperplasia

■ DEFINITION

Synonyms: ductal intraepithelial neoplasia 1b (DIN 1b), atypical intraductal hyperplasia

THE PROBLEM OF DEFINITION

Over a period of almost two decades the term 'atypical ductal hyperplasia' has been used to designate a borderline epithelial proliferation between DCIS and common mammary hyperplasia. Thus Page, who defined ADH in 1987, noted that 'ADH is recognized within the series of usual hyperplasia when there are some of the qualitative histological features which characterize DCIS,' and that, 'ADH has some of these features, but lacks the full measure of these criteria for DCIS' [1]. In addition, he described ADH as usually unifocal and small, often less than 1 mm in size [2]. The introduction of such a borderline category of intraductal epithelial neoplasia was a great step ahead in the classification of precursor lesions. It specifically separated a subgroup with a much better prognosis from the general group of ductal in-situ malignancies [2, 3]. However, the authors also conceded that such a definition by exclusion did not meet the requirements for reliable classification of any lesion in daily practice. In their subsequent definition Page and Rogers [4] therefore suggested more positive criteria for ADH including:

1. a constellation of cytological and architectural features; and
2. the extent of lesions.

'The cells comprising the lesion have rounded hyperchromatic nuclei and are evenly spaced producing the micropapillary or cribriform pattern known of DCIS, well-differentiated, but comprise only a part of the cell population in any given basement-bound space with a maximum of two ducts involved.' In 1990, Tavassoli and Norris emphasized similar cytologic features as imperative for the diagnosis of ADH. With the 2 mm aggregate diameter they also introduced an upper size limit [5]. In spite of those refined criteria, the current definition still raises a number of conceptual and practical problems that are closely interlinked:

1. Many experts in the field still regard ADH as one step in a progressive cascade of changes with UDH located at the lower end. This is exemplified by the definitions of ADH in two current textbooks on breast pathology: 'The lower boundary of ADH is defined by examples of florid hyperplasia with focal areas of cellular uniformity and even placement of cells' [6]. The definition given by Tavassoli who stated that, 'ADH is found either focally in a background of florid usual ductal hyperplasia or is present as an isolated lesion' distinguished two types of ADH, one of them displaying transitions from UDH to DCIS [7]. Although the WHO Working Group commissioned with the most recent version of *Pathology and Genetics, Tumors of the Breast and Female Genital Organs* felt, 'that at the time of the meeting, there was insufficient genetic evidence to classify it [usual ductal hyperplasia – W.B.] as a precursor lesion', nevertheless retained the same defining features, namely that, 'ADH is diagnosed when characteristic cells coexist with patterns of UDH, and/or there is partial involvement of TDLU by classic morphology' [8].

   In contrast to these definitions Azzopardi noted, that 'one of the more striking findings was the absence of any evidence of transition from areas of epitheliosis [usual ductal hyperplasia – W.B.] to cancer, except perhaps in a single case' [9].
2. Several authors have proposed quantitative criteria to distinguish ADH from low grade DCIS [4, 7]. These take into account the size and/or the number of ductules involved by the neoplastic cell population. The quantitative criteria introduced by Page to distinguish ADH from DCIS stipulated that the lesion should involve less than two basement-bound spaces. Tavassoli et al. [5] proposed the quantitative definition that ADH involved an atypical cell population in one or several lobular ductules of less than 2 mm in sum total diameter. However, even if the positive and seemingly precise criteria of Page and Rogers or Tavassoli are applied, diagnostic consistency still remains unacceptably low [10]. Furthermore, these two different approaches to defining the size of lesions do not even always recognize identical cases [11].
3. The cytological and architectural criteria currently associated with ADH are monomorphic small cells with a smooth, geometrical architecture. Sloane pointed out that such a definition may be too narrow and prone to exclude other histological variants with non-high grade morphologies [12].
4. The current definition of ADH resulted in an interobserver consistency of no more than 0.25 with kappa statistics, which is unacceptably low for any diagnostic entity [13–16]. This poor result may either be attributed to the definition's shortcomings or the pathologists' failure to learn to recognize the characteristic features of ADH – or a mixture of

both. At the time of writing no convincing solution exists to the dilemma of inconsistency in the diagnosis of ADH.

CONCEPTUAL APPROACH

As discussed above, one of the main difficulties facing the pathologist in identifying ADH lesions is the lack of a universally accepted definition of early lesions.

In order to render the concept of ADH more precise, three requirements must be met. To begin with, the concept must be cohesive and noncontradictory – it should be consistent with our current knowledge of molecular and cell biological data. Secondly, it must fulfill the criteria of demarcation with other diagnostically related lesions. And finally, the pathologist must be able to apply the concept and its implicit conclusions to daily practice.

It is evident from histological, cell biological and molecular observations that breast cancer is a heterogeneous disease. Nevertheless most experts still instinctively favor the idea of a common precursor lesion that precedes the formation of a clinically detectable and finally metastasizing tumor. As discussed in Chapter 17, there is, however, good reason to believe that even early precursor lesions of breast cancer can be subdivided into different subgroups that are correlated with distinct genetic pathways [17–26].

Thus, the most important implication of the pathway concept is that it requires abandoning the notion of a universal precursor lesion for all subtypes of DCIS, and thus for all pathways. Instead, we conclude that every pathway has its own particular early neoplastic precursor lesions from the onset of its clonal process. Putative candidates for the three different pathways have been discussed in Chapter 17. Here we will focus on the spectrum of those lesions which we feel should be referred to as ADH.

STANDARD-TYPE ATYPICAL DUCTAL HYPERPLASIA

The presence of focal proliferation of atypical uniform ductal-type cells with rounded or oval hyperchromatic nuclei and even spacing of cells is now universally recognized as indicating ADH [4, 32, 8] (Fig. 19.1). In this book we refer to this type of proliferation as 'standard-type ADH'. There is evidence to support the idea that standard-type ADH is a lesion, which incurs an increased risk of breast carcinoma anywhere in both breasts [11, 27–30]. Moreover, it is a lesion of the low grade pathway (for details see Chapter 17) [31]. We agree with Page [4] and Tavassoli [32] that the following cytological and architectural criteria are essential for a diagnosis of standard-type ADH.

1. The most important feature of standard-type ADH is a proliferation of small uniform cells [33]. Sometimes, differences in cytoplasmic staining and/or differences in

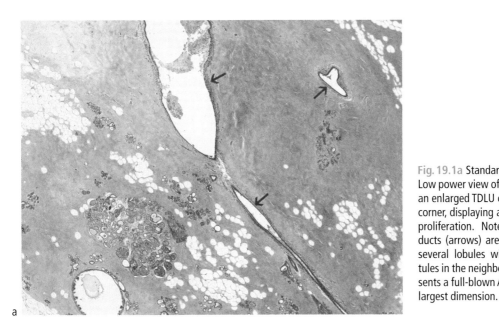

Fig. 19.1a Standard-type ADH.
Low power view of standard-type ADH with an enlarged TDLU complex in the lower left corner, displaying an epithelial intraluminal proliferation. Note that the interlobular ducts (arrows) are not involved. There are several lobules with slightly dilated ductules in the neighborhood. This lesion represents a full-blown ADH of about 3 mm in its largest dimension.

Continuation

a

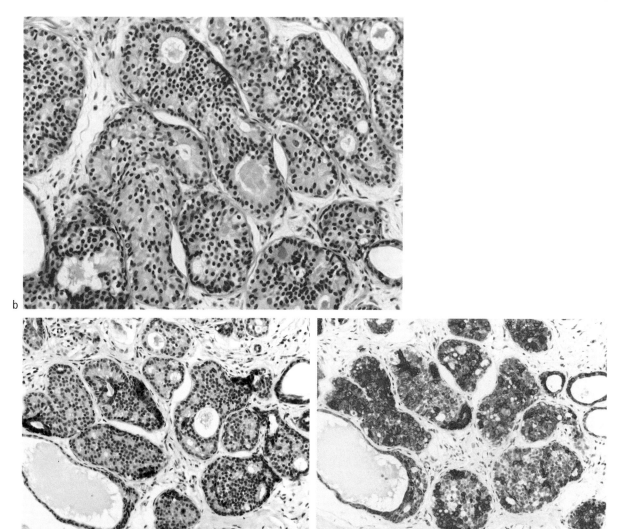

b

c

d

Fig. 19.1a–d Standard-type ADH.

19.1b High power view of the same lesion with several ductules showing an atypical monotonous cell proliferation with darkly staining nuclei and cribriform growth pattern.

19.1c Immunostaining for Ck5 shows the residual luminal cells. The tumor cells lack Ck5. This staining pattern is in clear contrast to the Ck5/14 mosaicism of benign epithelial proliferations. The myoepithelial cells are not or only weakly stained, contrasting with the intense sm-actin immunostaining (not shown here).

19.1d Immunostaining for Ck1, 5, 10, 15 (34βE12). Note the intense reactivity of most of the tumor cells to this antibody. Since in our experience 10 to 20% of atypical ductal proliferations stain positively for 34βE12, this antibody does not help in distinguishing between different ductal-type cell proliferations.

size and polarization of proliferating cells, even in the same location, may occur, giving the observer an impression of a two-cell type differentiation. Taking into account the immunophenotype of such lesions (expression of Ck8/18/19 alone without Ck5/14) it becomes clear, however, that such a dimorphic pattern is caused by the glandular cells phenotype (Fig. 19.2b–c).

2. Architectural features with a complex morphology are characterized by a smooth and rigid geometry of micropapillae, arcades, Roman bridges, bars and cribri-

form growth. Published descriptions and illustrations suggest that ADH lesions of the breast represent lesions of TDLUs. Azzopardi [34] was the first to clearly describe these early forms of ductal neoplastic growth patterns. Even in minute amounts, such features are inevitable evidence of neoplastic growth (Fig. 19.3). These growth patterns are essential for a diagnosis of ADH, in contrast to benign epithelial proliferations.

3. As size is not a criterion that can be reliably used to demarcate ADH from low grade DCIS in daily routine prac-

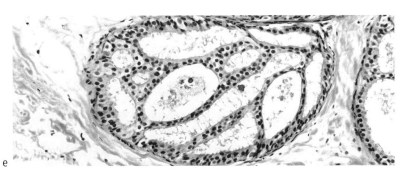

e

DEMARCATION OF STANDARD-TYPE ADH AT THE LOWER AND UPPER LIMITS

Within the theoretical framework proposed in this book, standard-type ADH constitutes the link between FEA on the one hand and low grade DCIS on the other. This concept is, however, beset with two problems, namely to find criteria which enable the pathologist to distinguish ADH lesions both at the lower and the upper limits.

SOLVING THE PROBLEM OF DEMARCATION AT THE LOWER LIMIT

A theory of how breast cancer develops is of utmost importance in solving the problem of the lower limit. As discussed in Chapters 7 and 17, in FEA/ADH it is rare to see direct transitions from benign epithelial proliferation; on the contrary, these lesions appear to arise de novo from glandular cells of the TDLU. Normal luminal cells are first replaced by atypical ones in a flat pattern, which may proliferate subsequently to show a form of intraluminal growth pattern. Such transitions are easily recognized in daily routine practice. Thus the demarcation line at the lower end lies between FEA and the different forms of intraluminal growth. We therefore classify as ADH any type of atypical intraluminal proliferation of a lobular ductule (such as micropapillae, Roman bridges and bar or sieve-like cribriform growth patterns), irrespective of whether such proliferations partially or completely involve one or all of the ductules of a lobule. This is based on the circumstantial evidence that intraluminal growth indicates a qualitative change of the proliferative process compared to FEA, although from a cytological and even molecular point of view no sharp dividing line between FEA and ADH exists. In daily routine practice, we recommend further sectioning of paraffin blocks with FEA lesions to exclude ADH or even DCIS in such tissue.

THE PROBLEM OF DEMARCATION AT THE UPPER LIMIT

Here we are concerned with distinguishing ADH from low grade DCIS. It should be emphasized that the size considerations introduced by several authors provide guidelines rather than precise biological definitions [37]. As discussed above, there are several objections that may be raised against such size criteria. The most serious, perhaps, is that size does not provide a suitable tool for demarcation in routine practice since it is associated with an unacceptably low interobserver consistency.

Based on the hypothesis that ADH is a neoplastic lesion of the TDLU, we propose a biologically-founded definition of standard-type ADH as a small atypical ductal-type epithelial proliferation (usually about 2–5 mm in diameter) involving individual TDLU structures, but with no, or only minor, ductal involvement, thus leaving the interlobular ducts untouched (Figs 19.1 and 19.7). In this concept, therefore, ADH sharply contrasts with DCIS, which is characterized by its spread into the ductal system in a segmental manner. In the authors' experience two or even more separate individual lobules in different locations of an excision biopsy may be affected by such atypical cell growth. In all these cases the lobular extension criterion of ADH can be fully appreciated only if the entire lesion is present. Thus adequate sampling is required to rule out a more advanced (ductal-segmental) process, which would indicate a DCIS.

It must be acknowledged that the extension of an otherwise classic low grade DCIS into lobules (lobular cancerization) should be regarded as part of the DCIS, and thus included into any size considerations. This is in line with the observations of Goldstein et al. [40] who found that DCIS with 'ADH' at the periphery of the lesion was associated with recurrences at the same location. Thus DCIS may be inadequately excised if these lobular extensions are not regarded as part of the DCIS. In this context the additional diagnosis of 'ADH' may be misleading to the clinician and hence may be dangerous for the patient.

This approach is also in line with the observation that lesions of ADH have been proven to indicate an increased risk of developing cancer anywhere in the breast [2, 4, 41], in contrast to the local risk associated with DCIS due to its segmental spread [3, 42–46]. The presence of such atypical ductal epithelial proliferations therefore represents a general risk factor for subsequent development of both ductal and lobular-type carcinoma of the breast. Such data can be attributed to the assumption that lesions of ADH may be multifocal in the breast under scrutiny or even in both breasts, as is the case with lobular neoplasias. However, the increased general risk of women with such lesions may also be caused by the fact that ADH indicates a general genetic instability of breast epithelium.

We are confident that this pragmatic approach to standard-type ADH, which, in addition to the cytological and architec-

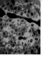

tural criteria, recognizes the site of origin and the confinement to individual lobule(s) of these early ductal neoplasias as one of their most characteristic and determining features, will be of help in diagnosing these lesions more consistently. Our criteria of demarcation at the lower and upper limits are intended as a proposal for a pragmatic approach. In conclusion we regard the following histological criteria as constitutive for a diagnosis of standard-type ADH.

1. Focal proliferation of atypical uniform ductal-type cells with rounded or oval hyperchromatic nuclei usually originating and confined to the TDLU.
2. Architectural features with a complex morphology characterized by micropapillae, arcades, Roman bridges, bars, or complete cribriform patterns.
3. No involvement of the ductal system or only minor involvement of terminal ducts.

NONSTANDARD-TYPE ATYPICAL DUCTAL HYPERPLASIA

NONSTANDARD-TYPE ADH OF INTERMEDIATE NUCLEAR GRADE

As discussed in Chapter 17 and below, we agree that small lesions with atypical epithelial proliferation of a more polymorphous morphology exist that can be clearly distinguished from standard-type ADH (Fig. 19.4). Diagnostically, these lesions are problematical. In contrast to the low and high grade pathways, reliably distinguishing such lesions from benign epithelial proliferations (UDH and some forms of adenosis) using routine histology alone is extremely difficult. In all these lesions routine histology shows epithelial proliferation with some crowding, pseudostratification and loss of

orientation of the nuclei. Based on their histological appearance and, more importantly, on the fact that they are constituted by Ck5/14-negative clonal epithelial proliferations (Fig. 19.4b), we assume that these ADH lesions are elements of the intermediate pathway, contrasting sharply with the Ck5/14 mosaicism of small UDH lesions. This view is also supported by their histological and immunohistochemical similarity to intermediate grade DCIS.

It is tempting to speculate that those cases of 'UDH' described by Shoker et al. [47–49] in which all cells of the lesions express ER might correspond to the lesions described here. This view is supported by the fact that, in the authors' experience, these lesions may show ER+ and Ck8/18+ cells that lack Ck5/14 expression.

In this context, the rule of thumb according to which benign epithelial proliferations are characterized by their Ck5/14 mosaicism, whereas cells of ductal neoplasia are characterized by their glandular phenotype and lack expression of Ck5/14 [50–52], is indispensable in understanding these lesions. Ck5/14 negativity of the proliferating cells thus provides the most important objective measure of clonal growth at the expense of normal cells and is thus indicative of an atypical proliferation of this type.

The authors have the impression, that some of the ADH cases described by Page [1, 6] and some of the lesions classified as type 1 ADH by Tavassoli [7] could be included under nonstandard-type ADH. There are rare cases where the atypical proliferation evolves against a background of UDH [7, 53]. Such cases will be discussed in more detail in the paragraph 'Atypical ductal proliferation ex benign proliferative breast disease'. In the authors' opinion, such lesions clearly differ from nonstandard-type ADH as described here.

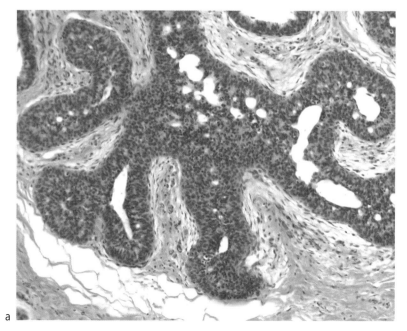

Fig. 19.4a−b Nonstandard-type ADH of intermediate nuclear grade, mimicking a benign epithelial proliferation.
19.4a TDLU with solid and slightly fenestrating proliferation of cells with a tendency towards nuclear uniformity, but uneven spacing (compare Fig. 17.13a). Typical criteria such as streaming and differences in cytoplasmic staining are not recognizable. Such an appearance may be the result of a more monotonous benign proliferation or of malignant cell growth. In such a case H&E sections do not provide sufficient clues to reach a final diagnosis.

Continuation

a

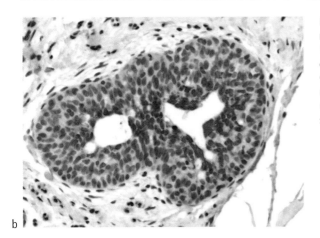

b

Fig. 19.4b Nonstandard-type ADH of intermediate nuclear grade, mimicking a benign epithelial proliferation.
Immunostaining for Ck5/6 highlights the Ck5/6-negative clonal cell proliferation with a pagetoid growth pattern. Some residual Ck5/6+ luminal cells remain. This staining clearly indicates a neoplastic cell proliferation. The lesion was localized close to uninvolved interlobular ducts so that the diagnosis of non-standard-type ADH appears to be appropriate.

The clinical significance of these lesions is not yet known. Further studies are needed to gauge their frequency and biological/clinical implications. Studies, for instance, along the lines of Eusebi et al. [54] on clinging carcinoma or, preferably, prospective studies might come up with answers to these questions. It follows that a consistent terminology to classify the various lesions of the different pathways according to their stage is required.

EARLY MINUTE DUCTAL IN-SITU LESIONS WITH HIGH GRADE MORPHOLOGY

Characteristic morphology, phenotype and molecular genetics also connect the different stages of the high grade pathway. As early as 1979, Azzopardi described 'clinging carcinoma, polymorphous type' as an early variant of comedo cancer, thus representing the lower end of this pathway (Fig. 19.5) [33]. Although these early lesions are reminiscent of FEA/ADH in the low and intermediate grade pathway, most experts in the field currently feel that all malignant lesions with high nuclear grade morphology should be termed high grade DCIS irrespective of their size [8, 53].

FURTHER SUBTYPES OF ADH

These include lesions such as
1. atypical apocrine hyperplasia,
2. atypical ductal proliferations that develop within a pre-existing benign proliferative lesion such as sclerosing adenosis, UDH or papilloma, and
3. extremely rare lesions with a monotonous Ck5/14+ cell proliferation.
These are described below.

In conclusion we propose that ADH should be regarded as a heterogeneous group of early neoplastic disorders rather than a single entity [53]. Currently, a distinction is made between early precursor lesions of the low grade (FEA/ADH) and the high grade pathways (clinging carcinoma, polymorphous type), which seem to develop de novo in terminal ductal lobular units. We propose that the intermediate grade pathway has its own specific early lesions composed of Ck5/14-negative cell proliferations that are distinct from benign epithelial proliferation.

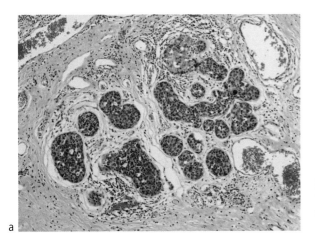

a

Fig. 19.5a–b Early high grade ductal in-situ malignancy.
19.5a Single lobule with slightly distended ductules which are filled with tumor cells with overtly malignant features.

Continuation

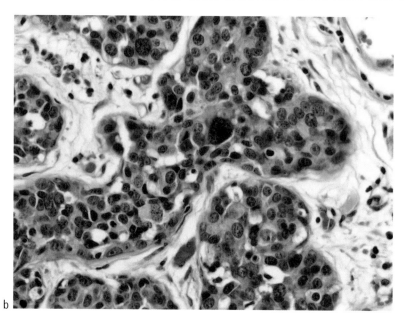

Fig. 19.5b Early grade 3 ductal in-situ malignancy.
Higher magnification view showing enlarged nuclei and variations in nuclear size and shape.

b

THE RELATIONSHIP OF FEA/ADH AND LCIS

As discussed in Chapter 17 the most important feature distinguishing non-high grade ductal lesions from lobular neoplasia is the loss of the adhesion molecule E-cadherin. The presence or absence of this molecule results, respectively, in the typical ductal or lobular growth patterns. The former is characterized by its cohesive growth, the latter by its discohesive growth and its typical change of cell shape to round tumor cells, easily recognizable on H&E sections. Double immunofluorescence studies using Ck8/18 and E-cadherin antibodies further highlight these changes. Moreover, the presence of E-cadherin has a tremendous impact on the spread of the tumor cells, as discussed in Chapter 17. In one of the authors' experience (W.B.), FEA/ADH is more often associated with lobular neoplasia than might be expected (Fig. 19.6). This coincidence is currently under investigation.

In conclusion:
1. Ductal and lobular malignancies appear to arise de novo in the TDLUs. These early stages may affect one or even several lobules.
2. FEA/ADH and LCIS may be observed coexisting in adjacent lobules and even in the same lobule.

◾ CLASSIFICATION OF ATYPICAL DUCTAL
◾ HYPERPLASIA

In this chapter we use the concept developed by Page and Rogers [4] as a basis for defining the classic form of ADH (which we term 'standard-type ADH').

However, we enhance this concept to include further ADH morphologies within the spectrum of ADH lesions. As already mentioned, these include non-standard-type ADH lesions of intermediate grade, ductal malignancies on the ground of benign epithelial proliferations such as papillomas and atypical apocrine hyperplasia. Finally, we include very rare neoplastic lesions of bland-looking Ck5/14+ cells that, so far, have not yet been described in the literature. To summarize, the following morphological types are described.
1. Standard-type ADH (mainly Page's criteria).
2. Nonstandard-type ADH with intermediate grade morphology. These lesions can only be reliably diagnosed by Ck5/14 immunostaining.
3. Atypical ductal proliferations (ADH/DCIS) ex benign proliferative breast disease lesions.
4. Atypical apocrine hyperplasia.
5. Atypical ductal proliferations of Ck5/14+ progenitor cell type (extremely rare).

We are aware that, so far, a specific link between morphological criteria and epidemiologically determined risk of invasive breast cancer has only been established for standard-type ADH [6]. This caveat should be kept in mind when applying the definitions used below in daily practice. However, we strongly feel that this conceptual approach may lead to a better understanding of benign and malignant proliferative cell growth and thus overcome a number of diagnostic difficulties.

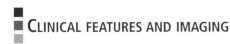

CLINICAL FEATURES AND IMAGING

CLINICAL FEATURES

The frequency of ADH diagnosis has multiplied with the advent of mammographic screening. In biopsies from mass lesions identified in screening programs, ADH is only found in 2–4% of specimens. However, in biopsies that were performed due to the presence of microcalcifications this percentage rises to 12–17% [54, 55].

IMAGING

With the exception of occasional punctuate lobular calcifications, no mammographic abnormalities are associated with the lesion.

THERAPY AND PROGNOSIS

CLINICAL IMPACT OF FEA/ADH

What action should be undertaken when FEA or ADH are diagnosed in vacuum-assisted biopsies or in a diagnostic biopsy? The NHSBSP guidelines for nonoperative diagnostic procedures [56] suggest that, if a low or intermediate grade atypical epithelial proliferation is found in a vacuum-assisted biopsy that is insufficient in extent or degree of ductal/lobular involvement to be classified as DCIS, the lesion should be categorized as B3 and an indication for a diagnostic biopsy to exclude DCIS should be made. In practice, we modify these guidelines for cases in which sufficient material is available to show that the atypical epithelial proliferation is clearly confined to lobules and spares the interlobular ducts, as well as in cases where the mammogram shows only minor changes that have been removed by the procedure. Follow-up of these patients with annual control mammography seems a reasonable management option. The same holds true for ADH in diagnostic biopsies. In contrast, if interlobular ducts are involved in the atypical proliferations, which usually indicates low grade DCIS, we prefer further diagnostic and, if necessary, therapeutic procedures. In patients with non high grade DCIS, we perform wide excision and, if necessary, even breast ablation.

It would, of course, be premature to draw any conclusions in terms of biology concerning nonstandard-type lesions. Many of these early lesions are likely to have the same clinical course as those currently interpreted as FEA/standard-type ADH. Further studies are needed to gain a better insight into their biology.

In lesions with micropapillary and more solid growth, however, it is vital to distinguish neoplastic lesions from UDH and to exclude a potential DCIS in daily practice.

Tab. 19.1 Atypical ductal hyperplasia

Standard-type ADH	Usually confined to one or several individual TDLU(s), lacking the ductal segmental spread of low grade DCIS. It shows the characteristic cellular monomorphism and the smooth geometrical growth pattern of the proliferating cells, which are per se indicative of neoplastic growth. In such cases the distinction from low grade DCIS may be problematic.
Nonstandard-type ADH of intermediate nuclear grade	This form mimics UDH. In the authors' experience it can only reliably be recognized by using Ck5/14 immunostaining, which displays a Ck5/14– clonal proliferation in contrast to the Ck5/14+ mosaicism of UDH. Nonstandard-type ADH shows the same lobular involvement as standard-type ADH.
Atypical ductal proliferation (ADH/DCIS) ex benign proliferative breast disease	These lesions constitute the third distinctive subtype. Development of an atypical epithelial proliferation in a primarily benign proliferative breast lesion is probably the exception, which is why the clinical significance of this lesion is still largely unknown. These lesions are, however, important as malignancy may also be found outside the confines of the benign lesion.
Atypical apocrine hyperplasia	These rare variant forms are characterized by their characteristic complex growth pattern, combined with only slight to moderate cytological apocrine atypia. To distinguish these lesions from DCIS, apocrine type, the same criteria should be used as in standard-type ADH.
Atypical ductal hyperplasia of Ck5/14+ progenitor cell type	This is a very rare type of atypical cell proliferation. It is characterized by proliferation of monotonous cells that homogeneously stain for Ck5/14, but not for Ck8/18. Electron microscopy reveals the cytoplasm contains only a few organelles such as mitochondriae or endoplasmic reticulum, and is filled with intermediate filaments, which are probably cytokeratins in view of the positive Ck5/14 immunohistochemistry.

■ PATHOLOGY

MACROSCOPY

ADH is not associated with any specific macroscopic features.

MICROSCOPY

In order to assess the precancerous potential and other features of ADH subtypes, five distinct types of histology must be distinguished. Failure to do so has contributed to the confusion and conflicting views on this subject. The different forms of pathology are listed in Table 19.1.

STANDARD-TYPE ADH

Standard-type ADH is characterized by a proliferation of evenly spaced monotonous cells producing the familiar growth patterns of low grade DCIS. Lesions are confined to one or several individual TDLU(s), lacking the ductal segmental spread of low grade DCIS (Figs 19.6 and 19.7). Compared to normal cells, the nuclei are enlarged, normochromatic to hyperchromatic and show little variability. The growth patterns

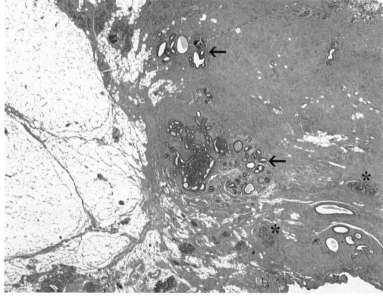

a

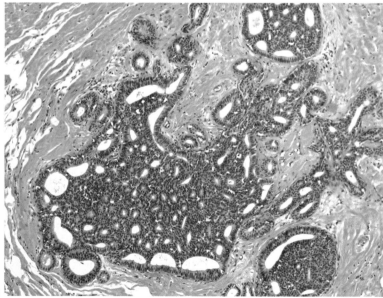

b

Fig. 19.6a–b Ductal and lobular neoplastic cell growth in the same excision biopsy.

19.6a Standard-type ADH in the center of the figure. Other TDLUs can also be seen that show cylinder cell change with psammomatous calcification (arrows) and several foci of lobular neoplasia (asterisks).

19.6b Higher magnification showing a distorted TDLU. This lesion shows typical monotonous cell proliferation with cribriform growth and expansion of an extralobular terminal duct and adjacent ductules.

Continuation

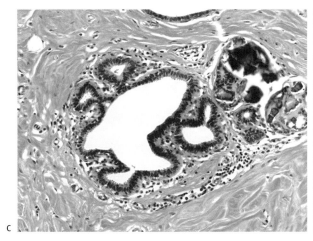

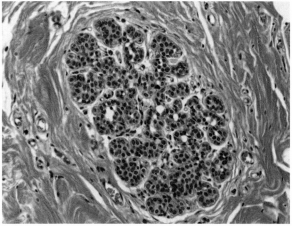

Fig. 19.6c–d Ductal and lobular neoplastic cell growth in the same excision biopsy.

19.6c Another lobule in the same slide showing cylinder cell change without atypia. Such lesions probably represent a clonal proliferation of glandular cells. The lesion is associated with psammomatous calcifications, which were the cause of the biopsy. These changes should be interpreted as benign.

19.6d Yet another lobular lesion from the same specimen. This lesion is characterized by a proliferation of monotonous cells with round nuclei and meets the criteria of atypical lobular hyperplasia. We feel that such lesions are more often associated with FEA/ADH than mere coincidence might account for.

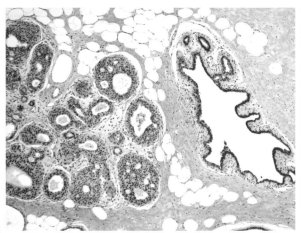

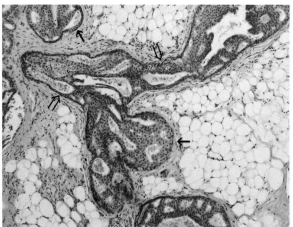

Fig. 19.7a–b Comparison of standard-type ADH and low grade DCIS.

19.7a ADH is a lobular lesion. This medium power view shows a standard-type ADH involving a lobule with ductal-type cell growth of cribriform pattern. The interlobular duct in the right field is not involved. This feature distinguishes ADH most clearly from DCIS.

19.7b Low grade DCIS involving unfolded lobules (arrows) and medium sized ducts (double arrows).

include micropapillae, epithelial columns of atypical cells lacking fibrovascular cores, arcades, Roman bridges, bars crossing the glandular space and full-blown lesions with solid or cribriform patterns (Figs 19.7 and 19.8). In some lesions the cells comprising the flat growth in the background – and sometimes even a part of the intraductal population – are cytologically different from those of the main neoplastic cell growth, so that a dimorphic cytology may emerge (Figs 19.3 and 19.8b).

In the literature, the cells showing flat growth have often been regarded as ordinary breast epithelial cells, due to a certain amount of variation in size (more cytoplasm), shape (tapering of arches or bars), polarization (apical snouts) and variation in type of nuclei (more vesicular nuclei), compared to the cellular population in the center of the space (Fig. 19.3). However, when these lesions are immunostained for cytokeratins it becomes obvious that the cells display the same glandular phenotype:

expression of Ck8/18, lack of expression of basal Ck5/14 and, usually, ER-positivity of the nuclei. Moreover, recent studies have shown that genetic alterations in FEA are identical to those observed in ADH [19]. The obvious conclusion, therefore, is that the dimorphic cytological patterns in those lesions are indicative of subtle changes in the glandular phenotype of ultimately identical neoplastic disease processes, rather than of any type of normal epithelium or epithelial hyperplasia.

From a practical point of view we thus diagnose ADH whenever

1. there is (partial or complete) involvement of TDLU(s) in classic morphology; and
2. the ductal system is not, or only to a minute degree, involved in the neoplastic process.

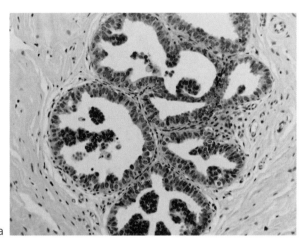
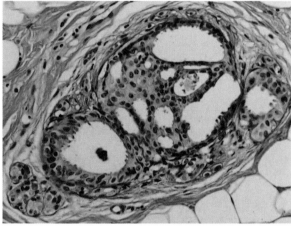

a
b

Fig. 19.8a–c Standard-type ADH.

19.8a Part of a TDLU with several cystically dilated ductules containing a uniform cell proliferation forming epithelial tufts and micropapillae against a background of flat epithelial atypia. If size criteria were to be used in this case, which ductule should be regarded as completely involved? Both in Page's and Tavassoli's classification such a decision would govern whether the lesion was classified as ADH or DCIS. This case clearly demonstrates the problem with size criteria in daily practice (compare also Fig.19.3a and Fig.19.3b).

19.8b This is a very small lobular lesion of ADH. The specific stroma of the lobule is still visible. The ductules are variably dilated and contain a proliferation of atypical cells with pallid cytoplasm and monotonous nuclei against a background of FEA.

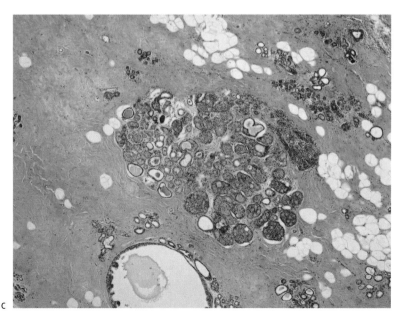

c

19.8c This is a full-blown lesion of ADH with a size of about 5 mm (same case as Fig.19.1). The slightly dilated ductules contain a monotonous atypical cell proliferation with solid to cribriform growth pattern. The lack of involvement of interlobular ducts (compare Fig.19.1) in the excision biopsy indicates this lesion should be classified as ADH rather than DCIS.

These criteria seem to be of special practical relevance as they can be assessed more reliably than the size criterion. Furthermore the subjective criterion partial versus complete can be abandoned.

Psammomatous-type microcalcifications may be absent, focal or extensive within the lumen of involved ductal lobular units; their presence has no impact on diagnosis.

NONSTANDARD ADH OF INTERMEDIATE GRADE (ADH MIMICKING UDH)

As discussed above, these lesions cannot be readily assigned to the 'classic type' category of Page and Rogers as they lack the cellular and architectural features of such lesions. The histological features of this type of lesion resemble intermediate grade DCIS and consist of more polymorphous cells with usually oval nuclei and irregular spacing (Figs 19.4 and 19.9). Thus they may mimic small lesions of benign epithelial proliferation. The growth patterns may be micropapillary, solid or fenestrating with cells lining small irregular secondary lumina. The most important feature distinguishing these lesions from benign epithelial proliferations is the Ck8/18-positivity and the Ck5/14-negativity, indicative of a clonal cell proliferation. Nonstandard-type ADH as defined here may correspond to Tavassoli's [7] 'type 1 ADH'. The criteria to distinguish these lesions from corresponding

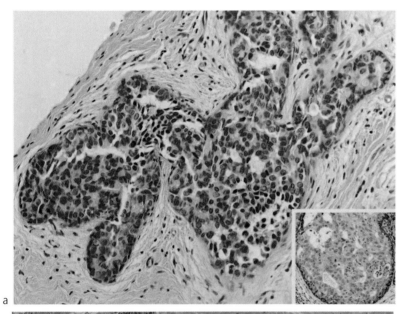

a

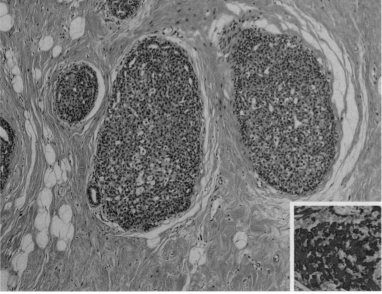

b

Fig. 19.9a–b A comparison of nonstandard-type ADH of intermediate grade with UDH.

19.9a View of a part of a lobule showing a cell proliferation at first sight reminiscent of a benign proliferation. The inset, however, shows the Ck5-negativity of the tumor cells.

19.9b View of a lesion showing a mainly solid epithelial cell growth. Although there is some irregularity in cell spacing, this is an ambivalent lesion. The inset shows Ck5 mosaicism indicative of a benign epithelial proliferation.

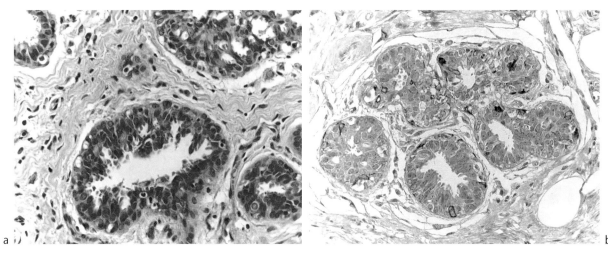

Fig. 19.10a – b Nonstandard FEA of intermediate grade mimicking benign epithelial hyperplasia.

19.10a View showing an epithelial growth, which at first sight is likely to be classified as benign epithelial hyperplasia. The lesion shows variation in cells, nuclear size and shape as well as irregular placement of cells. In such a context, routine histology is not helpful in distinguishing benign from malignant epithelial growth, which is why cytokeratin immunostaining is required.

19.10b Ck5 immunostaining of this lesion highlights the Ck5– atypical cell proliferation, thus indicating a neoplastic cell growth. Some residual Ck5+ cells are seen. This is not the type of mosaicism normally observed in benign epithelial proliferations. The Ck5-negativity in this context is a surrogate for clonal cell growth.

nonstandard-type flat atypical lesions and intermediate DCIS are the same as those used to demarcate standard-type ADH from its corresponding lesions at the lower and upper limit, as previously discussed.

ATYPICAL DUCTAL PROLIFERATION (ADH/DCIS) EX BENIGN PROLIFERATIVE BREAST DISEASE

In rare cases, atypical ductal proliferation (ADH/DCIS) may evolve from primarily benign proliferative breast lesions, such as papilloma, radial scar, sclerosing adenosis, and fibroadenoma. With the exception of peripheral papillomas, all other benign lesions rarely undergo malignant transformation. In such instances identifying an underlying benign lesion is important for an appropriate diagnosis. It should be emphasized that the same cytological and architectural criteria used for the identification of atypical ductal proliferations discussed above are also applied in this context. There are two main problems in this setting. These are related
1. to the extent or size of the atypical proliferation; and
2. to the clinical impact of such findings.

At the time of writing there was no generally accepted solution to these problems [6, 57].

ATYPICAL DUCTAL PROLIFERATION (ADP) EX BENIGN PAPILLARY LESIONS (SEE CHAPTERS 11 AND 20)

We define ADP in benign papillary lesions as partial involvement of an otherwise typically benign papillary lesion with areas of atypical proliferation having features of low grade DCIS (Fig. 19.11). A possible DCIS

outside the papillary lesion should be excluded. The lesions are composed of typical papillary lesions with one or more areas of a monotonous proliferation of cells usually involving less than 50% of the entire papillary lesion [58]. The number of myoepithelial cells in these atypical areas may be reduced. In difficult cases the neoplastic growth pattern may be highlighted by Ck5/14 immunostaining (Fig. 19.11b) (see Chapter 8).

At times, atypical cell proliferation of cylinder cell type with formation of tufts or micropapillary growth, and only occasional rigid bars and bridges, may merge with normal papillary epithelium. It is therefore hardly surprising that these lesions may be difficult to diagnose.

The presence of atypical ductal proliferation in papillary lesions seems to indicate an increased general risk of developing breast cancer [58, 59].

ATYPICAL DUCTAL PROLIFERATION EX RADIAL SCAR (SEE CHAPTER 10)

We diagnose any partial involvement of radial scar by an atypical proliferation with features of non-high grade DCIS as atypical ductal proliferation ex radial scar. According to Sloane [60] atypical ductal proliferation may involve a very variable percentage of the lesion with mean values for 'ductal carcinoma in-situ' of 32% and for ADH of 25%. In the series investigated by Sloane there was a clear relationship between the presence of atypical ductal proliferation and the size of the lesion, the cut-off point being approximately 6–7 mm, above which ADH was common. As there is no data on

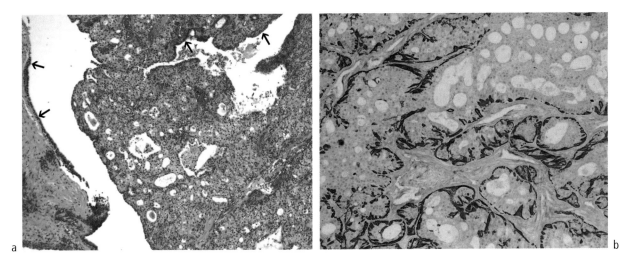

Fig. 19.11a–b Atypical ductal proliferation ex papilloma.
19.11a Normal epithelium lining the duct wall and residual benign papillary structures (arrows). Note the central proliferation of monotonous tumor cells with a cribriform growth pattern.
19.11b Ck5 immunostaining highlights the myoepithelial cells. The atypical cell proliferation is Ck5-negative.

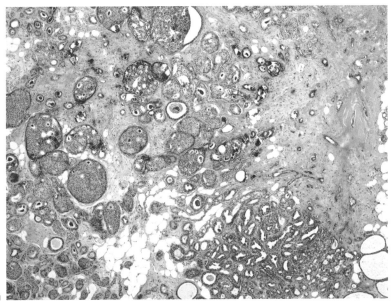

Fig. 19.12a–b Atypical ductal proliferation ex sclerosing adenosis.
19.12a Low power view highlighting the background of sclerosing adenosis in the lower and right fields. Most of the area shows glands with an atypical ductal proliferation of monotonous cells. Note the intense psammomatous calcification in the middle of the field.

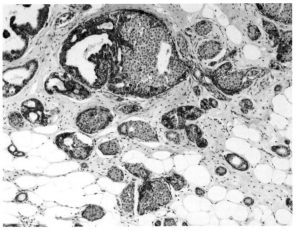

19.12b Ck5/6 immunostaining highlighting the myoepithelial cells and some residual normal luminal cells. The tumor cells, however, lack Ck5/6.

the clinical significance of the degree to which radial scar is involved by the atypical cellular proliferation, the authors would, for the time being, categorize any lesion as atypical ductal proliferation ex radial scar provided that the atypical proliferation is genuinely confined to the benign lesion and, in addition, that the underlying benign lesion is clearly visible.

ATYPICAL DUCTAL PROLIFERATION EX USUAL DUCTAL HYPERPLASIA (SEE CHAPTER 8)

Convincing examples of transitions of florid UDH to malignant growth patterns are exceptionally rare (see Chapters 7, 8 and 17). According to the data of Shoker et al. [48, 61] some cases of ductal hyperplasia apparently fulfilling the Page criteria show expression patterns of ER and MIB1 that are similar to those seen in low grade DCIS.

ATYPICAL DUCTAL PROLIFERATION EX SCLEROSING ADENOSIS (SEE CHAPTER 9)

Atypical ductal proliferation ex sclerosing adenosis is a malignant transformation in a preexisting sclerosing adenosis. Histologically, the malignant component usually exhibits the cytological and architectural features of a low grade lesion with cribriform growth pattern (Fig. 19.12). Less commonly, the lesion shows high grade features or apocrine change.

The underlying architecture of sclerosing adenosis can be either obvious or difficult to identify [62]. In difficult cases immunostains for myoepithelial markers such as sm-actin, sm-myosin heavy chain, p63, calponin and Ck5/14 highlight the dual glandular-myoepithelial differentiation of the lesion.

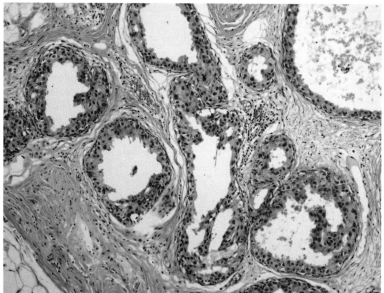

a

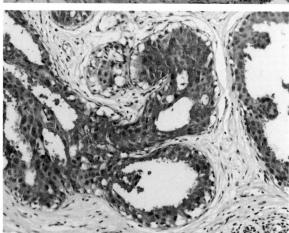

b

Fig. 19.13a–b Atypical apocrine hyperplasia.
19.13a Part of an involved lobule showing a clinging and atypical micropapillary epithelial proliferation. The cells are smaller than in classic benign apocrine change and display a more basophilic cytoplasm and a relative monotony of the nuclei. Nucleoli are not evident.

19.13b Immunostaining for gross cystic disease fluid protein-15, which was positive in both areas.

ATYPICAL DUCTAL PROLIFERATION 'EX OTHER' BENIGN LESIONS

Fibroadenoma see Chapter 15.

Cystic hypersecretory hyperplasia see Chapters 2 and 20.

Mucocele-like lesions see Chapters 2 and 20.

ATYPICAL APOCRINE HYPERPLASIA

Rare morphological variations of atypical-ductal proliferations include cases with apocrine-type morphology [63–69]. An attempt to define apocrine lesions was undertaken by O'Malley [69] and Raju et al. [65]. O'Malley uses cytological criteria (usual apocrine, borderline features, and 'as in DCIS') and extension criteria (< 4 mm, 4–8 mm, > 8 mm) to distinguish between benign, borderline and malignant categories. According to Raju et al. [58] the criteria of atypical apocrine hyperplasia are met whenever a lesion shows features of low grade DCIS and is of small size. Atypical apocrine features may occur partially or diffusely in ADH [58].

While we certainly agree with O'Malley's view that the extension of atypical apocrine lesions may be important with respect to their prognosis, we nevertheless feel that, for the time being, a simplified system might be more appropriate (Table 19.2). Generally speaking, we are convinced that the same fundamental criteria used to define atypical ductal proliferations of non-specific type (distinguishing such lesions from ductal carcinoma) also apply to lesions with apocrine proliferation. Thus, lobular confinement and/or the restriction of atypical apocrine cells to the boundaries of a given benign lesion, as discussed above, and complex growth patterns of atypical cell proliferation, such as atypical bridges, rigid arcades, micropapillary

Tab. 19.2 Distinguishing features of apocrine proliferations

	Atypical apocrine hyperplasia	Atypical apocrine proliferation ex BPBD lesions	Apocrine DCIS	Apocrine change and apocrine hyperplasia
Site	TDLUs.	Sclerosing adenosis, papilloma, radial scars etc.	Segmental growth with involvement of ducts and lobules.	TDLUs, sclerosing adenosis, papilloma, UDH, radial scar.
Cytology	Small cells with eosinophilic cytoplasm, but paler than in classic benign apocrine cells. More monotonous nuclei with inconspicuous nucleoli. Or: Enlarged cells with eosinophilic granular cytoplasm, enlarged nuclei with coarse chromatin and enlarged nucleoli.	Small cells with eosinophilic cytoplasm, but paler than in classic benign apocrine cells. Or: Enlarged cells with eosinophilic granular cytoplasm and enlarged nuclei with coarse chromatin and enlarged nucleoli.	Small to enlarged cells with eosinophilic cytoplasm, but paler than in classic benign apocrine cells. Proliferation of overtly malignant cells with eosinophilic granular cytoplasm and enlarged polymorphous nuclei with coarse chromatin and prominent nucleoli, irrespective of the size of the lesion.	Heavily enlarged cells with strongly eosinophilic granular cytoplasm. Variant: clear cells containing enlarged nuclei with prominent nucleoli.
Architecture	Complex architecture with rigid bars, arcades, Roman bridges and a cribriform pattern.	Identical to atypical apocrine hyperplasia, but a background of benign lesion must be recognized.	Identical to atypical apocrine hyperplasia.	Single cell larger, which may contain simple tufts of papillary growth pattern. May even be more complex, however, with classic benign apocrine morphology.
Clinical implications	Not known.	Not known*.	If not completely excised, local recurrence.	No increased cancer risk.
Differential diagnosis	Apocrine change, apocrine DCIS.	Apocrine DCIS, invasive apocrine carcinoma.	Invasive carcinoma.	Atypical apocrine lesion.

* See Chapter 9

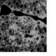

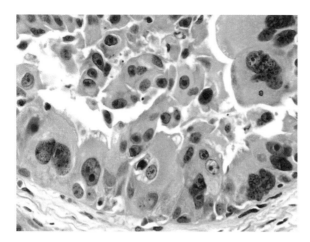

Fig. 19.14 Small apocrine DCIS of high grade. High power view showing an enlarged ductule with apocrine cell growth and overtly malignant nuclear features. Note the variation in nuclear size, the coarse granularity of the chromatin and the large nucleoli, all features of malignant apocrine cells.

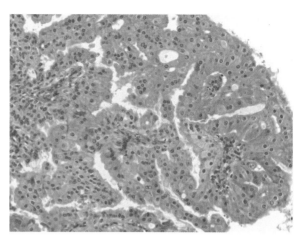

Fig. 19.15 Benign apocrine proliferation with complex growth pattern in a lesion of so-called 'juvenile papillomatosis' with prominent papillary and benign epithelial cell growth of usual type. Higher power view highlighting the more complex growth pattern. However, the cells display characteristic benign features with abundant, deeply eosinophilic and granular cytoplasm. We would classify this lesion as benign apocrine hyperplasia.

buds and cribriform pattern, should be key features in its identification.

However, in contrast to the ductal lesions of non-specific type discussed above, cytological criteria capable of distinguishing benign from malignant lesions are not readily applicable and much more difficult to define for this group of cells. This is due to the fact that even cells of clearly benign lesions of apocrine change usually display enlarged nuclei with prominent nucleoli. Among the cytological hallmarks of low grade apocrine lesions are a smaller cell size, cytoplasmic eosinophilia or pallor with less coarse granularity than in classic benign apocrine cells, and moderately stained regular nuclei with usually small nucleoli and a higher nucleus-to-cytoplasm ratio. Low grade lesions can easily be distinguished from their high grade counterparts. High grade DCIS is defined by pleomorphic, hyperchromatic nuclei, coarse chromatin and prominent nucleoli [8].

We therefore classify lesions confined to individual lobules and containing a proliferation of atypical apocrine cells as atypical apocrine hyperplasia (Fig. 19.13), while any atypical apocrine proliferation arising in a benign lesion and clearly confined to it qualifies as atypical apocrine proliferation ex BPBD lesion. Atypical apocrine proliferations extending into ducts or expanding beyond the confines of a benign lesion and overtly malignant apocrine proliferations of any size (Fig.19.14) should be classified as apocrine DCIS (Table 19.3).

All lesions that contain a proliferation of classic benign apocrine cells should be categorized as benign, including benign apocrine papillary lesions and even those with focal complex growth pattern (Fig. 19.15). While cases have been reported showing the whole sequence from benign apocrine change to in-situ malignancies and invasive apocrine carcinoma, they are probably extremely rare in view of the frequency of benign apocrine metaplasia.

ADH OF CK5/14+ PROGENITOR CELL TYPE

Exceptionally rare cases of intraductal epithelial proliferations with a homogeneous Ck5/14 positivity may be observed.

We (W.B.) encountered three such cases in recent years. Two cases were microscopic findings associated with other disease processes. In one patient a small well-circumscribed lesion had been discovered on mammography. The ages of the women were 39, 62, and 63 years. Two of the lesions were focal papillary lesions of 7 and 9 mm size, while one lesion was found in a TDLU with more solid growth, measuring 5 mm.

Two lesions (one of the papillary lesions and the solid lesion) were characterized by a monomorphic proliferation of epithelial cells with round-to-oval cells and bland-looking nuclei. This epithelial proliferation was covered by cells reminiscent of the umbrella cells of the urothelium (Fig. 19.16). In contrast to the Ck5/14+ mosaicism of UDH, the proliferating cells of these lesions homogeneously expressed Ck5/14. Glandular cytokeratins such as Ck8/18 were not expressed. In terms of immunohistochemistry, these lesions differ from urethelial tumors, which express glandular, but not basal, cytokeratins. Comparative genomic hybridization only revealed subtle chromosomal alterations in the two lesions.

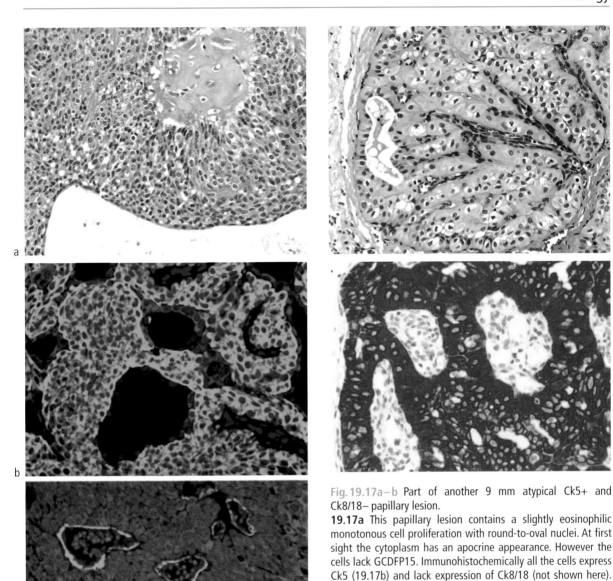

a

b

c

Fig. 19.16a−c ADH of Ck5/14+ cell type.
19.16a Part of a 7 mm papillary lesion with a monotonous proliferation of cells covered by umbrella-like cells. Even in ordinary histology there is no doubt as to the neoplastic nature of this process.
19.16b Double staining for Ck5 (green signal) and Ck8/18 (red signal), highlighting the proliferation of cells only expressing Ck5, while the umbrella-like cells are residual glandular cells. This is an exceptionally rare lesion, the biology of which is unknown.
19.16c Double staining for Ck5 and sm-actin again displays the C5+ proliferation. The basal myoepithelial layer is preserved.

a

b

Fig. 19.17a−b Part of another 9 mm atypical Ck5+ and Ck8/18− papillary lesion.
19.17a This papillary lesion contains a slightly eosinophilic monotonous cell proliferation with round-to-oval nuclei. At first sight the cytoplasm has an apocrine appearance. However the cells lack GCDFP15. Immunohistochemically all the cells express Ck5 (19.17b) and lack expression of Ck8/18 (not shown here). A myoepithelial cell layer was absent. Based on immunohistochemistry we interpret this lesion as a neoplastic Ck5 progenitor cell lesion. The biology is again unknown.

The second papillary lesion was characterized by a well-defined papillary growth pattern. The large cells covering the delicate fibrovascular stalks showed a pale, finely granular cytoplasm. Immunohistochemically they expressed only cytokeratins 5 and 14, and no other cytokeratins (Fig. 19.17a). The Ki67 proliferation index was less than 2%. Myoepithelial cells were not detected. Electron microscopy revealed the cells contained only a few organelles such as rough endoplasmic reticulum and a few mitochondriae. Abundant filaments reminiscent of intermediate filaments corresponding to basal cytokeratins were seen.

All these lesions were clearly distinct from standard-type ADH and classic low grade DCIS (characterized by the growth of Ck8/18+, Ck5/14– cells) as well as from Ck5/14+ high grade DCIS and UDH.

The clinical significance of these lesions is currently unknown. Based on morphology and CGH results, however, we regard these extremely rare lesions as Ck5/14+ precursor lesions without any sign of differentiation and probably with a very low malignant potential. They may therefore represent yet another rare form of ADH.

INTERPRETATION OF CORE AND VACUUM-ASSISTED BIOPSIES

Atypical epithelial proliferations of varying severity may be found in core biopsies, ranging from lesions insufficient for a definite diagnosis of DCIS, but where suspicion of DCIS is high, to those that only show a minor, usually architectural degree of atypia, requiring further assessment. Thus appropriate categorization such as B3 or B4 is required. These proliferations must be clearly distinguished from benign epithelial proliferations (see Chapter 8, 'Differential diagnosis').

The definition of ADH is derived from surgical resection specimens. Due to the limited amount of tissue, ADH cannot be reliably diagnosed on core biopsy because the atypical intraductal epithelial proliferative foci in the core biopsies may form part of an established in-situ neoplastic lesion, with or without associated invasion. Thus in 12–62% of needle core biopsies with a diagnosis of ADH, surgical excision biopsy showed either in-situ or invasive carcinoma [70–84]. The limited tissue sampling that can be undertaken by core biopsy guns (often by stereotactic methods for foci of microcalcification) usually provides insufficient material for a definitive diagnosis of low grade DCIS, if only a few 'ductal' spaces are obtained. ADH or DCIS can be more accurately diagnosed using vacuum-assisted biopsy devices, which reveal more contiguous tissue than a core biopsy needle. The reported rate of DCIS and invasive breast cancers ranges from 0 to 38% [79–82, 85–89]. In our experience the involvement of interlobular ducts by an atypical proliferation of ductal-type in vacuum biopsies is a good surrogate marker for DCIS, contrasting with the absence of such a finding in ADH. Despite these improvements, however, the prevalence of carcinoma in these lesions is still sufficiently high to warrant surgical excision if any ADH-like finding is detected. **In the event of such ADH-like findings in minimal invasive biopsy specimens, the *European Working Group for Breast Screening Pathology* has, therefore, recommended abandoning the term ADH in favor of 'atypical proliferation, ductal-**

type' (Wells CA et al., *European Guidelines for Quality Assurance in Mammography Screening – Fourth Edition*, Office for Official Publications of the European Communities, 2005).

IMMUNOHISTOCHEMISTRY

Standard-type ADH represent Ck8/18+, ER+ and Ck5/14– lesions [51, 90]. This may be helpful in the differential diagnosis of small lesions. Overexpression of c-erbB2 is absent in normal ducts and rare in ADH. Increasing levels of cyclin D1 expression were recently described in 27–57% of ADH lesions. Nuclear accumulation of the TP53 protein is absent in ADH and low grade DCIS [91].

MOLECULAR GENETICS

Several studies have analyzed the molecular features of standard-type ADH using loss of heterozygosity [92–94] and comparative genomic hybridization [94]. In all studies [20] losses at 16q and 17p were the most frequent changes in ADH. Interestingly, similar findings were obtained in low grade DCIS, in grade 1 invasive ductal carcinoma and also in lobular neoplasia (LCIS and ALH) [95–98]. The causal relationship between ADH and invasive carcinoma is supported by the fact that 50% of such lesions share the same LOH pattern when occurring in the same breast [91]. The data indicates a high genetic stability with only a few genomic alterations.

DIFFERENTIAL DIAGNOSIS

Low grade neoplasias are easily identified by their monotonous cell population with its smooth and rigidly geometrical architecture, whereas high grade lesions are characterized by their overtly malignant nuclear appearance. However, as discussed above, nonstandard ADH of intermediate nuclear grade is virtually indistinguishable from more monomorphous types of UDH. In this context it is helpful to use Ck5/14 immunohistochemistry to obtain a more objective feature as to the nature of these cells. Epithelial proliferations of benign lesions display the characteristic Ck5/14+ mosaicism, in contrast to the Ck5/14– neoplastic growth pattern of ADH. Lesions with overtly malignant features are currently diagnosed as high grade DCIS, irrespective of the lesion's size.

ADH is a rare condition found in about 4% of symptomatic benign biopsies [99]. A higher rate of ADH has been reported for screening-detected benign microcalcifications, most commonly as an incidental finding independent of the biopsy target. This rate ranges from less than 10% [100] to more than 31% [101]. One must bear in mind that ADH is rarely the correlate of an abnormality found on imaging. Decision-making is therefore fraught with two problems: the biopsy may contain only a very small amount of atypical proliferation of ductal-type or it may show an intraductal proliferation that cannot be easily classified as either neoplastic or hyperplastic in nature (Table 19.3). Whenever a definitive diagnosis

Tab. 19.3 Comparison of histological features of UDH, standard-type ADH and low grade DCIS*

Histological features	UDH	Standard-type ADH	Low grade DCIS
Size	Variable size but rarely extensive, unless associated with other benign processes such as papilloma or radial scar.	Usually lobular lesion with involvement of ductules, unless associated with other benign processes such as papilloma or radial scar.	Ductal-lobular involvement, may be very extensive.
Cellular composition	Mixed. Epithelial cells and spindle-shaped cells** present. Mosaicism of Ck5/14+ cells, Ck8/18+ cells and intermediate cells. Myoepithelial cells around the periphery.	Single cell population. Ck8/18+ glandular cells, lacking Ck5/14. Residual normal Ck5/14+ cells, usually attenuated and in a luminal position.	Single cell population of Ck8/18+ glandular cells. Myoepithelial cells usually in normal location around the ductal periphery but may be attenuated.
Architecture	Variable.	Micropapillae, bars, Roman bridges, arcades, cribriform or solid pattern.	Micropapillae, cribriform or solid patterns.
Lumina	Irregular, often ill-defined peripheral slit-like spaces are common and a useful distinguishing feature.	May be distinct well-formed rounded spaces in cribriform type. In less developed forms bridges and bars. Irregular, ill-defined lumina may also be present.	Well-delineated, regular punched-out lumina of cribriform type.
Cell orientation	Streaming pattern common with long axes of nuclei arranged parallel to the direction of cellular bridges, which often have a 'tapering' appearance.	Cell nuclei may be at right angles to bridges in cribriform type, forming 'rigid' structures.	Micropapillary structures with indiscernible fibrovascular cores or smooth, well-delineated geometric spaces. Cell bridges 'rigid' in cribriform type with nuclei orientated towards the luminal space.
Nuclear spacing	Uneven.	Even, occasionally uneven.	Even.
Epithelial/ tumor cell character	Small ovoid but showing variation in shape.	Small uniform or medium-sized monotonous population. Some cases may show variation in cell size (Ck5/14–).	Small uniform monotonous population with cell borders often visible.
Nucleoli	Indistinct.	Often single, small.	Often single, small.
Mitoses	Infrequent with no abnormal forms.	Infrequent, abnormal forms rare.	Infrequent, abnormal forms rare.
Necrosis	Rare.	Rare.	If present, confined to small particulate debris in cribriform and/or luminal spaces.

* Modified version of the table in *European Guidelines for Quality Assurance in Mammography Screening* – Fourth Edition, Office for Official Publications of the European Communities, 2005.

** These cells are usually called myoepithelial cells but immunohistochemical studies have shown that they have characteristics of basal keratin-type epithelial cells.

cannot be reached this should be indicated, rather than prematurely diagnosing the lesion as ADH. Pathologists should refrain from using ADH as a blanket term for indecisive findings, and should instead seek external consultation.

When in doubt, the pathologist should try to reconcile clinical, radiological and pathological findings by discussing them in a multidisciplinary team. In clinical practice, such an approach will often resolve the problem or at least lead to a practical approach to clinical management.

Some experienced breast pathologists would go so far as to question the validity of the ADH category on the grounds that is scientifically unfounded and does not help to resolve the problem of interobserver variability in classifying intraductal breast lesions [31].

In preexisting benign lesions the same strict qualitative criteria should be used for atypical proliferations as discussed for intraductal proliferations in Chapter 8. The atypical proliferation should be clearly confined to the benign lesion.

The differential diagnosis of atypical apocrine hyperplasia is another problem area due to the presence of 'atypical' nuclei even in benign apocrine metaplasia. The problem is further addressed in the corresponding chapters (4 and 20).

Atypical proliferations of Ck5/14+, Ck8/18– cells are exceptionally rare. They are easily distinguished from Ck5/14+ high grade lesions due to their bland cytology and from UDH due to their monotony and homogeneous Ck5/14 staining pattern.

For practical reasons, we recommend that the diagnostic criteria discussed above be used very restrictively. Provided that these conditions are met, the ADH category will be helpful in avoiding overtreatment.

References

1. Page DL, Anderson TJ, Rogers LW. Epithelial hyperplasia. In: Page DL, Anderson TJ, editors. Diagnostic Histopathology of the Breast. Edinburgh: Churchill Livingstone; 1988. p.120–56.
2. Page DL, Dupont WD, Rogers LW, Rados AM. Atypical Hyperplastic Lesions of the Female Breast. A Long-Term Follow-Up Study. Cancer 1985;55:2698–708.
3. Dupont WD, Page DL. Risk factors for breast cancer in women with proliferative breast disease. The New England Journal of Medicine 1985;312:146–51.
4. Page DL, Rogers LW. Combined Histologic and Cytologic Criteria for the Diagnosis of Mammary Atypical Ductal Hyperplasia. Human Pathology 1992;23:1095–7.
5. Tavassoli FA, Norris HJ. A Comparison of the Results of Long-Term Follow-Up for Atypical Intraductal Hyperplasia and Intraductal Hyperplasia of the Breast. Cancer 1990;65:518–29.
6. Jensen RA, Page DL. Epithelial hyperplasia. In: Elston CW, Ellis IO, editors. The Breast. Edinburgh: Churchill Livingstone; 1998. p.65–89.
7. Tavassoli FA. Ductal intraepithelial neoplasia 1B &C (Atypical intraductal hyperplasia). In: Pathology of the Breast. 2nd ed. Stanfort, Connecticut: Appleton & Lange; 1999. p.226–60.
8. Tavassoli FA, Hoefler H, Rosai J, et al. Intraductal proliferative lesions. In: Tavassoli FA, Devilee P, editors. Tumours of the Breast and Female Genital Organs. Lyon: IARC-Press; 2003. p.63–73.
9. Azzopardi JG. Study of minute ductal carcinomas. In: Problems in Breast Pathology. London: W.B. Saunders; 1979. p.107–12.
10. Sloane JP, Amendoeira I, Apostolikas N, et al. Consistency achieved by 23 European pathologists from 12 countries in diagnosing breast disease and reporting prognostic features of carcinomas. European Commission Working Group on Breast Screening Pathology. Virchows Arch 1999;434:3–10.
11. Page DL, Dupont WD, Rogers LW, Jensen RA, Schuyler PA. Continued local recurrence of carcinoma 15–25 years after a diagnosis of low grade ductal carcinoma in-situ of the breast treated only by biopsy. Cancer 1995;76:1197–200.
12. Sloane JP. Benign intraductal proliferations. In: Lakhani SR, editor. Biopsy Pathology of the Breast. 2nd ed. London: Arnold; 2001. p.101–18.
13. Swanson Beck J, members of the Medical Research Council Breast Tumour Pathology Panel. Observer variability in reporting of breast lesions. J Clin Pathol 1985;38:1358–65.
14. Sloane JP, Ellman R, Anderson TJ, et al. Consistency of histopathological reporting of breast lesions detected by screening: findings of the U.K. National External Quality Assessment (EQA) Scheme. U. K. National Coordinating Group for Breast Screening Pathology. Eur J Cancer 1994;30A:1414–9.
15. Wells WA, Carney PA, Eliassen MS, Tosteson AN, Greenberg ER. Statewide study of diagnostic agreement in breast pathology. J Natl Cancer Inst 1998;90:142–5.
16. Elston CW, Sloane JP, Amendoeira I, et al. Causes of inconsistency in diagnosing and classifying intraductal proliferations of the breast. European Commission Working Group on Breast Screening Pathology. Eur J Cancer 2000;36:1769–72.
17. Lagios MD. Practical pathology of ductal carcinoma in-situ: how to derive optimal data from the pathologic examination. In: Silverstein MJ, Recht A, Lagios MD, editors. Ductal carcinoma in-situ of the breast. 2nd ed. Philadelphia: Lippincott Williams & Wilkins; 2002. p.207–21.
18. Buerger H, Otterbach F, Simon R, et al. Comparative genomic hybridization of ductal carcinoma in-situ of the breast-evidence of multiple genetic pathways. J Pathol 1999;187:396–402.
19. Moinfar F, Man YG, Bratthauer GL, Ratschek M, Tavassoli FA. Genetic abnormalities in mammary ductal intraepithelial neoplasia-flat type ("clinging ductal carcinoma in-situ"): a simulator of normal mammary epithelium. Cancer 2000;88:2072–81.

20. O'Connell P, Pekkel V, Fuqua SA, et al. Analysis of loss of heterozygosity in 399 premalignant breast lesions at 15 genetic loci. J Natl Cancer Inst 1998;90:697–703.

21. Holland R, Peterse JL, Millis RR, et al. Ductal Carcinoma in-Situ: A Proposal for a New Classification. Semin Diagn Pathol 1994;11:167–80.

22. Lagios MD. Duct carcinoma in-situ. Pathology and treatment. Surg Clin North Am 1990;70:853–71.

23. Bijker N, Peterse JL, Duchateau L, et al. Histological type and marker expression of the primary tumour compared with its local recurrence after breast-conserving therapy for ductal carcinoma in-situ. Br J Cancer 2001;84:539–44.

24. Douglas-Jones AG, Gupta SK, Attanoos RL, Morgan JM, Mansel RE. A critical appraisal of six modern classifications of ductal carcinoma in-situ of the breast (DCIS): correlation with grade of associated invasive carcinoma. Histopathol 1996;29:397–409.

25. Patchefsky AS, Schwartz GF, Finkelstein SD, et al. Heterogeneity of intraductal carcinoma of the breast. Cancer 1989;63:731–41.

26. Vos CB, ter Haar NT, Rosenberg C, et al. Genetic alterations on chromosome 16 and 17 are important features of ductal carcinoma in-situ of the breast and are associated with histologic type. Br J Cancer 1999;81:1410–8.

27. Betsill WL, Jr., Rosen PP, Lieberman PH, Robbins GF. Intraductal carcinoma. Long-term follow-up after treatment by biopsy alone. JAMA 1978;239:1863–7.

28. Page DL, Dupont WD, Rogers LW, Landenberger M. Intraductal carcinoma of the breast: follow-up after biopsy only. Cancer 1982;49:751–8.

29. Silverstein MJ, Cohlan BF, Gierson ED, et al. Duct carcinoma in-situ: 227 cases without microinvasion [see comments]. Eur J Cancer 1992;28:630–4.

30. Lagios MD. Heterogeneity of ductal carcinoma in-situ of the breast. J Cell Biochem Suppl 1993;17G:49–52.

31. van de Vijver MJ, Peterse H. The diagnosis and management of pre-invasive breast disease: pathological diagnosis – problems with existing classifications. Breast Cancer Res 2003;5:269.

32. Tavassoli FA. Ductal intraepithelial neoplasia. In: Pathology of the Breast. 2nd ed. Stanford, Connecticut: Appleton & Lange; 1999. p.260–323.

33. Azzopardi JG. The Histogenesis of 'Early' Carcinoma. In: Problems in Breast Pathology. 1st ed. London: W.B. Saunders; 1979. p.92–112.

34. Azzopardi JG. Epitheliosis and In-Situ Carcinoma. In: Problems in Breast Pathology. 1st ed. London: W.B. Saunders; 1979. p.113–49.

35. Wellings SR, Jensen HM, Marcum RG. An atlas of subgross pathology of the human breast with special reference to possible precancerous lesions. J Natl Cancer Inst 1975;55:231–73.

36. Azzopardi JG. Problems in Breast Pathology. 1st ed. London: W.B. Saunders; 1979.

37. Page DL, Rogers LW, Schuyler PA, Dupont WD, Jensen RA. The natural history of ductal carcinoma in-situ of the breast. In: Silverstein MJ, Recht A, Lagios MD, editors. Ductal carcinoma in-situ of the breast. 2nd ed. Philadelphia: Lippincott Williams & Wilkins; 2002. p. 17–21.

38. Page DL, Jensen RA, Simpson JF. Premalignant and Malignant Disease of the Breast: The Roles of the Pathologist. Mod Pathol 1998;11:120–8.

39. Page DL, Simpson JF. Ductal carcinoma in-situ – the focus for prevention, screening, and breast conservation in breast cancer. N Engl J Med 1999;340:1499–500.

40. Goldstein NS, O'Mally BA. Cancerization of Small Ectatic Ducts of the Breast by Ductal Carcinoma in-Situ Cells with Apocrine Snouts. A Lesion associated with Tubular Carcinoma. Am J Clin Pathol 1997;107:561–6.

41. Schnitt SJ, Conolly JL, Tavassoli FA, et al. Interobserver Reproducibility in the Diagnosis of Ductal Proliferative Breast Lesions Using Standardized Criteria. Am J Surg Pathol 1992;16:1133–43.

42. London SJ, Connolly JL, Schnitt SJ, Colditz GA. A prospective study of benign breast disease and the risk of breast cancer [published erratum appears in JAMA 1992 Apr 1;267(13):1780]. JAMA 1992;267:941–4.

43. Palli D, Rosselli-Del TM, Simoncini R, Bianchi S. Benign breast disease and breast cancer: a case-control study in a cohort in Italy. Int J Cancer 1991;47:703–6.

44. Marshall LM, Hunter DJ, Connolly JL, et al. Risk of breast cancer associated with atypical hyperplasia of lobular and ductal-types. Cancer Epidemiol Biomarkers Prev 1997;6:297–301.

45. Dupont WD, Parl FF, Hartmann WH, et al. Breast cancer risk associated with proliferative breast disease and atypical hyperplasia [see comments]. Cancer 1993; 71:1258–65.

46. Fitzgibbons PL, Henson DE, Hutter RV. Benign breast changes and the risk for subsequent breast cancer: an update of the 1985 consensus statement. Cancer Committee of the College of American Pathologists. Arch Pathol Lab Med 1998;122:1053–5.

47. Shoker BS, Jarvis C, Sibson DR, Walker C, Sloane JP. Oestrogen receptor expression in the normal and pre-cancerous breast. J Path 1999;188:237–44.

48. Shoker BS, Jarvis C, Clarke RB, et al. Estrogen receptor-positive proliferating cells in the normal and precancerous breast. Am J Pathol 1999;155:1811–5.

49. Iqbal M, Davies MP, Shoker BS, et al. Subgroups of non-atypical hyperplasia of breast defined by proliferation of oestrogen receptor-positive cells. J Pathol 2001;193: 333–8.

50. Boecker W, Moll R, Dervan P, et al. Usual ductal hyperplasia of the breast is a committed stem (progenitor) cell lesion distinct from atypical ductal hyperplasia and ductal carcinoma in-situ. J Pathol 2002;198:458–67.

51. Otterbach F, Bankfalvi A, Bergner S, et al. Cytokeratin 5/6 immunohistochemistry assists the differential diagnosis of atypical proliferations of the breast. Histopathol 2000;37:232–40.

52. Wetzels RHW, Holland R, van Haelst UJGM, et al. Detection of Basement Membrane Components and Basel Cell Keratn 14 in Noninvasive and Invasive Carcinomas of the Breast. Am J Pathol 1989;134:571–9.

53. Sloane JP. Biopsy Pathology of the Breast. Vol. 24, 2nd edition ed. London: Arnold; 2001.

54. Eusebi V, Foschini MP, Cook MG, Berrino F, Azzopardi JG. Long-term follow-up of in-situ carcinoma of the

breast with special emphasis on clinging carcinoma. Semin Diagn Pathol 1989;6:165–73.

55. Scott MA, Lagios MD, Axelsson K, et al. Ductal carcinoma in-situ of the breast: reproducibility of histological subtype analysis. Hum Pathol 1997;28:967–73.

56. Guidelines for non-operative diagnostic procedures and reporting in cancer screening. [no. 50]. 2001. NHSBSP Publications. Ref Type: Serial (Book,Monograph)

57. Raju UB, Lee MW, Zarbo RJ, Crissman JD. Papillary neoplasia of the breast: immunohistochemically defined myoepithelial cells in the diagnosis of benign and malignant papillary breast neoplasms. Mod Pathol 1989;2:569–76.

58. Raju U, Vertes D. Breast papillomas with atypical ductal hyperplasia: a clinicopathologic study. Hum Pathol 1996;27:1231–8.

59. Page DL, Dupont WD, Jensen RA. Papillary apocrine change of the breast: associations with atypical hyperplasia and risk of breast cancer. Cancer Epidemiol Biomarkers Prev 1996;5:29–32.

60. Sloane JP, Mayers MM. Carcinoma and atypical hyperplasia in radial scars and complex sclerosing lesions: importance of lesion size and patient age. Histopathol 1993;23:225–31.

61. Shoker BS, Jarvis C, Clarke RB, et al. Abnormal regulation of the oestrogen receptor in benign breast lesions. J Clin Pathol 2000;53:778–83.

62. Rosen PP. Rosen's Breast Pathology. 2nd ed. Philadelphia: Lippincott Williams & Wilkins; 2001.

63. O'Malley FP, Page DL, Nelson EH, Dupont WD. Ductal Carcinoma In-Situ of the Breast With Apocrine Cytology. Definition of a Borderline Category. Hum Pathol 1994;25:164–8.

64. Bussolati G, Cattani MG, Gugliotta P, Patriarca E, Eusebi V. Morphologic and Functioanl Aspects of Apocrine Metaplasia in Dysplastic and Neoplastic Breast Tissue. Ann NY Acad Sci 1986;464:262–74.

65. Raju U, Zarbo RJ, Kubus J, Schultz DS. The Histologic Spectrum of Apocrine Breast Proliferations: A Comparative Study of Morphology and DNA Content by Image Analysis. Hum Pathol 1993;24:173–81.

66. Carter DJ, Rosen PP. Atypical Apocrine Metaplasia in Sclerosing Lesions of the Breast: A Study of 51 Patients. Mod Pathol 1991;4:1–5.

67. Seidman JD, Ashton M, Lefkowitz M. Atypical apocrine adenosis of the breast: a clinicopathologic study of 37 patients with 8.7-year follow-up. Cancer 1996;77:2529–37.

68. Moriya T, Sakamoto K, Sasano H, et al. Immunohistochemical analysis of Ki-67, p53, p21, and p27 in benign and malignant apocrine lesions of the breast: its correlation to histologic findings in 43 cases. Mod Pathol 2000;13:13–8.

69. O'Malley FP, Bane AL. The spectrum of apocrine lesions of the breast. Adv Anat Pathol 2004;11:1–9.

70. Harvey J, Sterrett GF, Frost FA. Indeterminate results in core biopsies of breast from mammographically detected lesions: outcomes of excision biopsy. Pathology International 2001;51.

71. Jackman RJ, Nowels KW, Rodriguez-Soto J, et al. Stereotactic, automated, large-core needle biopsy of nonpalpable breast lesions: false-negative and histologic underestimation rates after long-term follow-up. Radiology 1999;210:799–805.

72. Jackman RJ, Nowels KW, Shepard MJ, Finkelstein SI, Marzoni F-AJ. Stereotaxic large-core needle biopsy of 450 nonpalpable breast lesions with surgical correlation in lesions with cancer or atypical hyperplasia. Radiology 1994;193:91–5.

73. Mendez I, Andreu FJ, Saez E, et al. Ductal carcinoma in-situ and atypical ductal hyperplasia of the breast diagnosed at stereotactic core biopsy. Breast J 2001;7:14–8.

74. Zhao L, Freimanis R, Bergman S, et al. Biopsy needle technique and the accuracy of diagnosis of atypical ductal hyperplasia for mammographic abnormalities. Am Surg 2003;69:757–62.

75. Liberman L, Cohen MA, Dershaw DD, et al. Atypical ductal hyperplasia diagnosed at stereotaxic core biopsy of breast lesions: an indication for surgical biopsy [see comments]. AJR Am J Roentgenol 1995;164:1111–3.

76. Liberman L, Dershaw DD, Glassman JR, et al. Analysis of cancers not diagnosed at stereotactic core breast biopsy. Radiology 1997;203:151–7.

77. Burbank F. Mammographic findings after 14-gauge automated needle and 14-gauge directional, vacuum-assisted stereotactic breast biopsies. Radiology 1997;204:153–6.

78. Liberman L, Smolkin JH, Dershaw DD, et al. Calcification retrieval at stereotactic, 11-gauge, directional, vacuum-assisted breast biopsy. Radiology 1998;208:251–60.

79. Brem RF, Behrndt VS, Sanow L, Gatewood OM. Atypical ductal hyperplasia: histologic underestimation of carcinoma in tissue harvested from impalpable breast lesions using 11-gauge stereotactically guided directional vacuum-assisted biopsy. AJR Am J Roentgenol 1999;172:1405–7.

80. Philpotts LE, Shaheen NA, Carter D, Lee CH. Comparison of rebiopsy rates after stereotactic breast core biopsy with 11-gauge vacuum suction probe vs. 14-gauge needle and automated gun. AJR Am J Roentgenol 1999;170 (Suppl.):83 (abst.).

81. Jackman RJ, Burbank FHPSH. Atypical ductal hyperplasia diagnosed by 11-gauge, directional, vacuum-assisted breast biopsy: how often is carcinoma found at surgery [abstract]? Radiology 1997;205(P):325.

82. Meyer JE, Smith DN, Lester SC, et al. Large-core needle biopsy of nonpalpable breast lesions. JAMA 1999;281:1638–41.

83. Brown TA, Wall JW, Christensen ED, et al. Atypical hyperplasia in the era of stereotactic core needle biopsy. J Surg Oncol 1998;67:168–73.

84. Lin PH, Clyde JC, Bates DM, et al. Accuracy of stereotactic core-needle breast biopsy in atypical ductal hyperplasia. Am J Surg 1998;175:380–2.

85. Burbank F. Stereotactic breast biopsy of atypical ductal hyperplasia and ductal carcinoma in-situ lesions: improved accuracy with directional, vacuum-assisted biopsy. Radiology 1997;202:843–7.

86. Philpotts LE, Lee CH, Horvath LJ, et al. Underestimation of breast cancer with II-gauge vacuum suction biopsy. AJR Am J Roentgenol 2000;175:1047–50.

87. Darling ML, Smith DN, Lester SC, et al. Atypical ductal hyperplasia and ductal carcinoma in-situ as revealed by large-core needle breast biopsy: results of surgical excision. AJR Am J Roentgenol 2000;175:1341–6.

88. Jackman RJ, Burbank F, Parker SH, et al. Atypical ductal hyperplasia diagnosed at stereotactic breast biopsy: improved reliability with 14-gauge, directional, vacuum-assisted biopsy. Radiology 1997;204:485–8.

89. Gal-Gombos ED, Esserman LE, Said E. Accuracy of image-directed large core needle biopsy in atypical intraductal hyperplasia of the breast [abstract]. Breast J 2000;6:342.

90. Kersting C, Tidow N, Schmidt H, et al. Gene dosage PCR and fluorescence in-situ hybridization reveal low frequency of egfr amplifications despite protein over-expression in invasive breast carcinoma. Lab Invest 2004;84:582–7.

91. Lakhani SR. The transition from hyperplasia to invasive carcinoma of the breast. J Pathol 1998;187:272–8.

92. Lakhani SR, Collins N, Stratton MR, Sloane JP. Atypical ductal hyperplasia of the breast: clonal proliferation with loss of heterozygosity on chromosomes 16q and 17p. J Clin Pathol 1995;48:611–5.

93. Amari M, Suzuki A, Moriya T, et al. LOH analyses of premalignant and malignant lesions of human breast: frequent LOH in 8p, 16q, and 17q in atypical ductal hyperplasia. Oncol Rep 1999;6:1277–80.

94. Gong G, DeVries S, Chew KL, et al. Genetic changes in paired atypical and usual ductal hyperplasia of the breast by comparative genomic hybridization. Clin Cancer Res 2001;7:2410–4.

95. Buerger H, Schmidt H, Beckmann A, et al. Genetic characterisation of invasive breast cancer: a comparison of CGH and PCR based multiplex microsatellite analysis. J Clin Pathol 2001;54:836–40.

96. Nishizaki T, Chew K, Chu L, et al. Genetic alterations in lobular breast cancer by comparative genomic hybridization. Int J Cancer 1997;74:513–7.

97. Lakhani SR, Collins N, Stratton MR. Loss of heterozygosity in lobular carcinoma in-situ of the breast. J Clin Pathol: Mol Pathol 1995;48:M74–M78.

98. Nayar R, Zhuang Z, Merino MJ, Silverberg SG. Loss of heterozygosity on chromosome 11q13 in lobular lesions of the breast using tissue microdissection and polymerase chain reaction. Hum Pathol 1997;28:277–82.

99. Bartow SA, Pathak DR, Black WC, Key CR, Teaf SR. Prevalence of benign, atypical, and malignant breast lesions in populations at different risk for breast cancer. A forensic autopsy study. Cancer 1987;60:2751–60.

100. Yeh IT, Dimitrov D, Otto P, et al. Pathologic review of atypical hyperplasia identified by image-guided breast needle core biopsy. Correlation with excision specimen. Arch Pathol Lab Med 2003;127:49–54.

101. Stomper PC, Cholewinski SP, Penetrante RB, Harlos JP, Tsangaris TN. Atypical hyperplasia: frequency and mammographic and pathologic relationships in excisional biopsies guided with mammography and clinical examination. Radiology 1993;189:667–71.

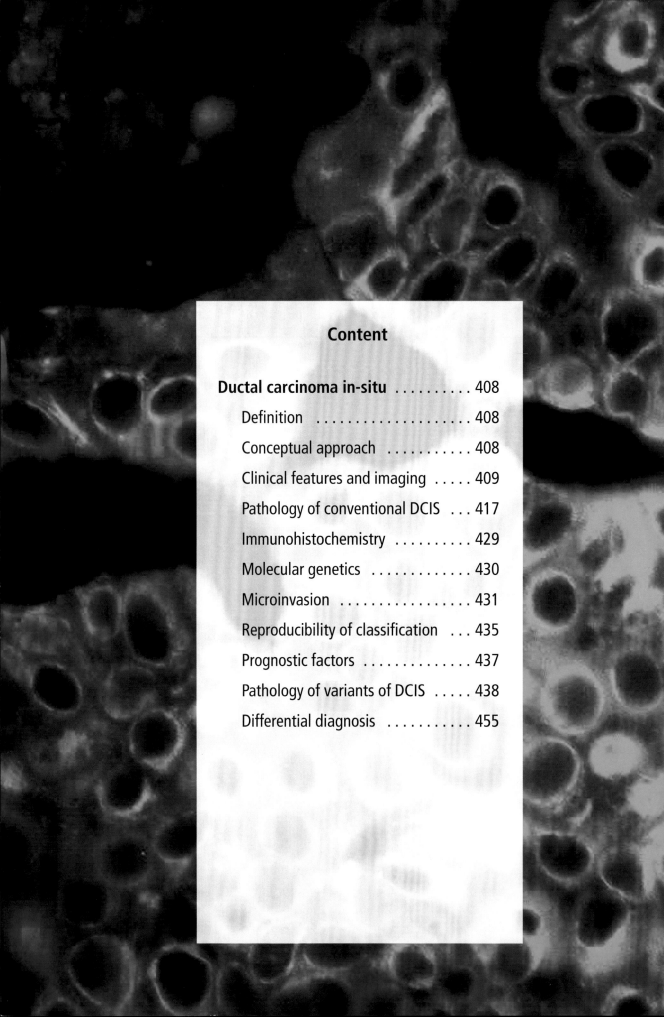

Content

DUCTAL CARCINOMA IN-SITU

WERNER BOECKER, STEVE PARKER, RUEDIGER SCHULZ-WENDTLAND,
STUART SCHNITT AND HORST BUERGER

Ductal carcinoma in-situ (DCIS) refers to a malignant epithelial proliferation of ductal-type within the ductal lobular system. The incidence of DCIS has increased six to seven times during the past decades, chiefly as a result of early detection efforts such as improved radiology and screening mammography. DCIS is divided into three grades (low, intermediate and high grade). Although there is evidence that all these lesions are direct precursor lesions of invasive carcinoma, it is important to emphasize that the different subtypes are, biologically, inhomogeneous proliferative disease processes. Whereas the traditional paradigm proposes a linear progression model with increasing malignancy of intraductal epithelial proliferations and stepwise 'dedifferentiation' from low to high grade lesions, there is increasing evidence to support the idea that the development of breast cancer follows different and distinct pathways, which are reflected in different types of DCIS and their invasive counterparts.

Thus DCIS is not a single disease entity but a heterogeneous group of noninvasive malignant proliferations that vary in cytology, architecture, genetic alterations, radiological features and clinical outcome. The diagnostic issues for pathologists are compounded both by the increase in the incidence of DCIS and by a number of recent events that have increased the difficulty in interpretation. Firstly, many patients undergo core biopsies due to microcalcifications while having no other clinical evidence of cancer. This results in an enormous number of biopsies that may only contain small suspicious foci of an intraductal epithelial proliferation. Secondly, the pathologist has not only to recognize the lesions in the core biopsy; he or she must also make sure that these lesions correlate to radiological findings. Although this correlation should be assured in interdisciplinary conferences, it requires a basic knowledge of the imaging findings on the side of the pathologist and pathological knowledge on the side of the radiologist. Thirdly, a number of diagnostic pitfalls and lesions mimicking DCIS have been described. Thus the pathologist has, for example, to distinguish DCIS from benign epithelial proliferations such as usual ductal hyperplasia (UDH) and papilloma. Fourthly, the pathologist today plays a decisive role in the disease management of patients with DCIS, as he or she has to provide accurate pathological diagnoses and prognostically significant information both on core and excisional biopsies of DCIS lesions. This has been discussed in more detail in Chapters 5 and 6. This chapter aims to provide a guide to diagnostic issues surrounding DCIS to practicing pathologists and radiologists, who are confronted with those intraductal epithelial proliferations on a daily basis.

Ductal carcinoma in-situ

■ DEFINITION

Synonyms: intraductal carcinoma, ductal intraepithelial neoplasia

WHO: Ductal carcinoma in-situ (DCIS)

ICD-O code: 8500/2

ICD-O code: 8503/2: (intraductal papillary carcinoma)

ICD-O code: 8504/2 (intracystic papillary carcinoma)

ICD-O code: 8540/3: (Paget's disease of the nipple)

The term ductal carcinoma in-situ encompasses a clinically, pathologically and biologically heterogeneous group of noninvasive malignancies. The introduction of screening mammography has led to a remarkable increase in the incidence of DCIS. The age-adjusted rate of DCIS rose from 2.3 to 15.8 cases per 100,000 women/year seen between 1973 and 1992 [15].

The hallmark of ductal carcinoma in-situ is a proliferation of malignant epithelial cells of ductal-type within the boundaries of the ductal lobular tree. Careful three-dimensional reconstruction of DCIS reveals that most DCIS cases show a unifocal, segmental growth within the ductal lobular network [1-9]. Histological, epidemiological and molecular studies furnished ample evidence that this type of epithelial proliferation is associated with an elevated risk of subsequent invasion, which is why DCIS is conceived of as the ultimate precursor lesion of invasive breast carcinoma [8, 10-14]. The cells comprising DCIS vary markedly in cytological appearance, architectural pattern, and extent of the lesion, adding to the heterogeneity of these lesions. Recent classification systems stratify DCIS lesions into three grades.

In some cases, the intraductal proliferation of DCIS may pose difficulties in distinguishing them from benign proliferative counterparts.

■ CONCEPTUAL APPROACH

Current knowledge derived from recent studies provides sound evidence that DCIS lesions are direct precursors of invasive breast cancer. This conclusion is supported by:

1. data on local recurrences after diagnostic biopsy or attempted excision [2, 3, 5-7];
2. evidence that DCIS and associated invasive breast carcinoma usually share grade and tumor markers [10, 11]; and
3. genetic studies showing striking similarities between the genetic changes in DCIS and invasive breast carcinoma (compare also Chapter 17).

On a cytogenetic level, comparative genomic hybridization (CGH) showed an almost complete homology of chromosomal alterations in DCIS and associated invasive cancers.

However, in contrast to the prevailing linear concept of breast carcinogenesis [20], data obtained by means of CGH analyses gave rise to a new interpretation of breast cancer development with multiple different parallel pathways (Chapters 17 and 23). A key marker for this new hypothesis is the loss of chromosomal locus 16q, which has been detected in two-thirds of well-differentiated DCIS lesions, whereas it was present in only a quarter of poorly differentiated lesions. In addition, it could be shown that other mechanisms led to the 16q loss of heterozygosity in well-differentiated as opposed to poorly differentiated breast cancer lesions [21].

Given this data, a progression or dedifferentiation from low grade towards high grade DCIS is probably the exception.

In our progenitor cell model, breast carcinomas may broadly be divided into two categories. The large majority of breast carcinomas (> 90% of invasive, > 95% of noninvasive) is of purely glandular phenotype (CK8/18+, Ck5/14–), whereas a small proportion (< 10% of invasive, < 5% of noninvasive) displays a basal phenotype recognizable by their nuclear features (Fig. 12.2a–e). As discussed in more detail in Chapter 17, it seems likely that the phenotypic diversity of human breast carcinomas is largely dependent on the intrinsic biology of the target cells of origin (Fig. 20.1). Research is currently being undertaken to analyze the mechanisms of such factors that might perturb the subsets of

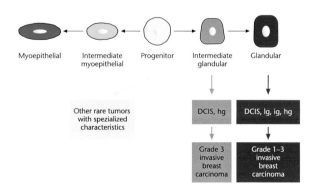

Fig. 20.1 Illustration of the hypothetical concept correlating the differentiated characteristics of epithelial breast tumors with different cell subtypes of the progenitor cell model.

cells that comprise the different phenotypes. If we were able to understand the regulatory mechanisms that govern growth and differentiation of these tumors [26], we might be able to design new diagnostic or even therapeutic strategies. From a practical point of view, the present knowledge of the component cells of benign and malignant breast lesions already provides the rationale behind a number of immunohistochemical applications in routine diagnostic work.

CLINICAL FEATURES AND IMAGING

CLINICAL FEATURES

In current clinical practice, DCIS is most often detected as a mammographic abnormality, although the lesion may also present as a palpable mass, as pathologic nipple discharge, as Paget's disease of the nipple, or as an incidental microscopic finding in breast tissue removed as the result of another abnormality. The most frequent mammographic presentation of DCIS is as microcalcifications. However, up to 30% of DCIS lesions may present with other mammographic findings, or an area of architectural distortion [28]. Many of these mammographically detected DCIS lesions are quite small and of uncertain clinical significance.

IMAGING

Ductal carcinoma in-situ (DCIS) is a diagnosis that is now made far more frequently, thanks to the advent of widespread screening. Before mammography, DCIS was relatively rare. The percentage of total breast malignancies that is now represented by DCIS is approximately 30% in populations undergoing screening mammography. Of the total number of

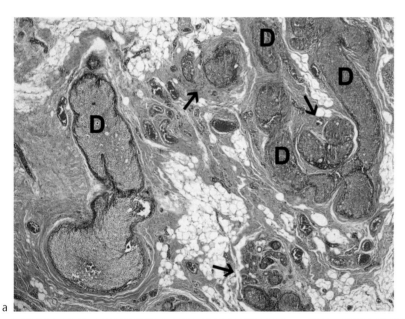

a

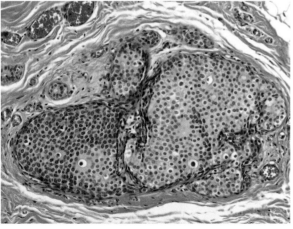

b

Fig. 20.2a–f DCIS.
20.2a Low power view of a DCIS showing the typical ductal (D)-lobular (arrows) growth pattern.
20.2b DCIS, low grade, with mainly solid growth of a monomorphic population of atypical cells.

c

20.2c Ck5/6 immunostaining shows a complete lack of basal cytokeratins in the tumor cells. *Continuation*

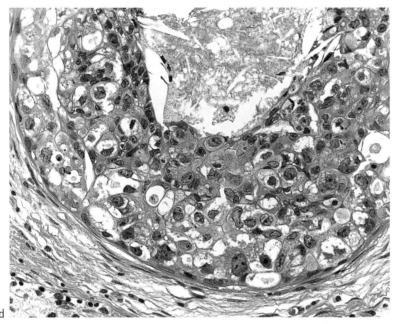

d

Fig. 20.2a−f DCIS.

20.2d High grade DCIS consisting of highly pleomorphic tumor cells.

20.2e−f High grade DCIS. Ck5/6 immunostaining showing no expression in the tumor cells in the majority of cases (e) or strong and diffuse expression in rare cases (f).

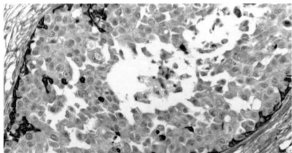

e

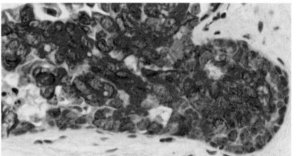

f

malignancies diagnosed at the Sally Jobe Breast Center (SJBC) in 2002, this percentage was 35% (including the three other intraepithelial neoplasias – atypical ductal hyperplasia [ADH], lobular carcinoma in-situ [LCIS], and atypical lobular hyperplasia [ALH]). In contrast, only 2–3% of all breast malignancies in the premammographic era were diagnosed as DCIS. Although DCIS is and was occasionally detected at clinical examination, it is now almost always detected as a result of the presence of microcalcifications on a mammogram. With the expanding use of breast ultrasound and magnetic resonance imaging (MRI), however, DCIS is also increasingly detected with these techniques.

MAMMOGRAPHY

The earliest mammographic evidence of DCIS was provided by Leborgne and Egan in the 1950s [29]. These investigators noted that microcalcifications were sometimes associated with breast malignancy and commonly the process was observed to be DCIS.

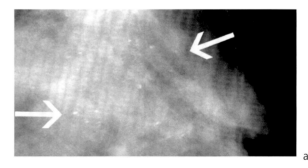

a

Fig. 20.3a−e Benign calcifications.

20.3a Scattered calcifications, mainly round and smooth.

Continuation

Standard film screen mammography improved over the ensuing two decades and more detailed analysis of the various types of microcalcifications ensued. The most important analyses using modern film screen technique were probably those performed by Dr László Tabár in Falun, Sweden. In the late 1970s and early

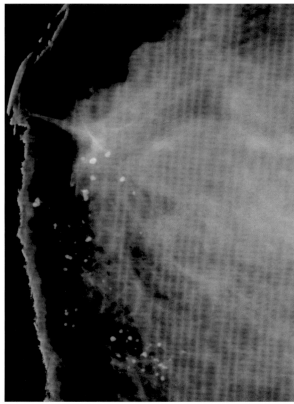

b

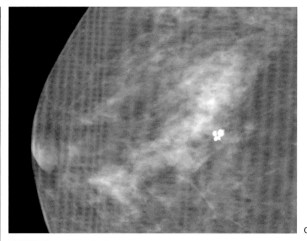

c

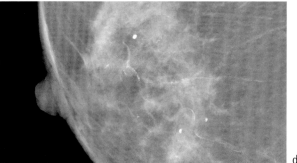

d

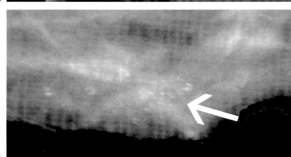

e

Fig. 20.3a – e Benign calcifications.
20.3b Dense, coarse calcifications.
20.3c Fibroadenoma with coarse, popcorn-like calcifications.
20.3d Vascular calcifications.
20.3e 'Milk of calcium' calcifications, 'teacup'-like.

1980s, Dr Tabár and others began advocating micro-focus magnification views for microcalcifications seen on standard mammography. This approach allowed the character and morphology of the calcifications to be more easily evaluated. Dr Tabár, working in conjunction with the late pathologist Dr Adel Gad and later on with Dr Tibor Tot in Falun, recognized that distinct patterns of microcalcifications existed based on the pathologic subtype of DCIS [30]. Breast imagers working with the American College of Radiology also came up with a classification system for mammographic microcalcifications but did not attempt to correlate them with specific histology. Recently, they have provided a classification system in radiology, which is shown in Chapter 5, Table 5.1.

At the SJBC, we use a straightforward approach to the classification of microcalcifications. We categorize microcalcifications into one of three broad types:
1. clearly benign calcifications,
2. clustered, indistinct/granular calcifications,
3. dense, distinct/pleomorphic calcifications.

When considering whether biopsy is indicated when calcifications are discovered during a mammographic work-up, only the second and third types delineated above need to be considered. Calcifications in the first group may be recognized as clearly benign on the screening mammogram alone or after appropriate magnification mammography. In either case, no further intervention is required if the calcifications are categorized as clearly benign.

BENIGN CALCIFICATIONS

Calcifications can be classified as clearly benign if they fall into the following categories:

1. smooth, round calcifications,
2. dense, large, coarse calcifications (sometimes associated with fat necrosis),
3. 'popcorn' calcifications,
4. vascular calcifications,
5. 'milk of calcium' calcifications.

Smooth, round calcifications are commonplace and are sometimes referred to as 'involutional' calcifications. These are generally scattered and not tightly clustered (Fig. 20.3a). Dense, large, coarse calcifications can be round or somewhat irregular but are easily distinguished from their smaller, more worrisome, dense, pleomorphic cousins (Fig. 20.3b). The usually dense 'popcorn' calcifications are almost always associated with a benign fibroadenoma that has undergone degeneration (Fig. 20.3c). Vascular calcifications are usually easy to classify as such except when only one wall of the vessel undergoes calcification (Fig. 20.3d). 'Milk of calcium' calcifications can sometimes be problematic on standard mammographic imaging since they can appear clustered. On 90 degree magnification views, however, these calcifications are noted to layer, indicating that they are in solution and therefore benign (Fig. 20.3e).

CALCIFICATIONS REQUIRING BIOPSY

Automated core biopsy is currently the technique of choice for the majority of breast biopsies performed due to calcifications of the breast (see also Chapter 5). For detailed analyses of calcification of benign and malignant breast lesions the reader is referred to the literature [8, 31–36].

In the simplified calcification classification system used at the SJBC, only two categories of calcifications require biopsy: clustered indistinct calcifications and dense pleomorphic calcifications. **Clustered indistinct calcifications** have a fairly low probability of association with DCIS (Fig. 20.4). Only approximately 15% of these biopsies yield DCIS. The remainder of these biopsies yield some form of benign fibrocystic change (FCC) or benign proliferative breast disease. When DCIS is found to be associated with these indistinct/granular calcifications, it is usually a low grade DCIS. Therefore, this type of biopsy-inducing calcification carries with it the lowest probability of associated DCIS and, when DCIS is present, it is the least worrisome histology of all mammographic findings. According to current standards in the United States, however, an imaging lesion that carries with it a greater than 2% chance of malignancy should undergo biopsy. In Europe and many other countries, only BI-RADS 4 lesions, which are

lesions with an indefinite or suspect abnormality, and BI-RADS 5 abnormalities, suggestive of cancer, are thought to need microscopic analysis (Wells CA et al., *European Guidelines for Quality Assurance in Mammography Screening – Fourth Edition*, Office for Official Publications of the European Communities [2005]).

On the other hand, **dense pleomorphic calcifications** are generally more ominous. These calcifications can manifest in two ways: clustered in a lobular distribution or linearly distributed along the path of a duct. Those that are clustered in a lobular distribution are associated with DCIS approximately 50% of the time (Fig. 20.5). When they are associated with DCIS, it is generally an intermediate grade DCIS. The other 50% of lesions associated with this category of calcifications tend to be benign fibroadenomas that did not calcify in the classic fashion. Occasionally, one can see clustered, dense, pleomorphic calcifications that are not associated with a DCIS or a fibroadenoma, but are instead associated with a benign dystrophic process or some form of benign proliferative breast disease. When this type of lesion is evaluated histo-

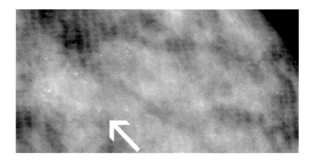

Fig. 20.4 Calcification requiring biopsy. Clustered indistinct calcification (arrow) associated with benign fibrocystic change.

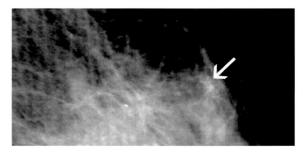

Fig. 20.5 Calcification requiring biopsy. Clustered, slightly polymorphic calcification (arrow) associated with low grade ductal carcinoma in-situ.

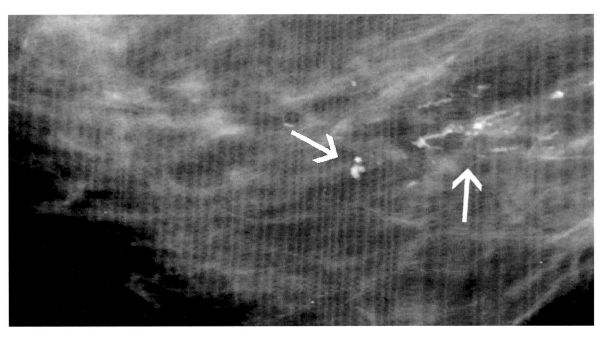

Fig. 20.6 Calcification requiring biopsy. Large, pleomorphic and linear branching calcification typical of high grade ductal carcinoma in-situ.

logically after a stereotactic biopsy, it is important that the pathologist sees these relatively large calcifications in their slide preparations before a diagnosis of fibrocystic change can be accepted. Not infrequently, the pathologist can see very small microcalcifications that the radiologist was not targeting and render an erroneous diagnosis of FCC. If the pathologist does not identify large pleomorphic calcifications histologically, it is imperative that the block should be further sectioned to identify those calcifications and the pathologic process associated with them (see Chapter 5).

Dense pleomorphic calcifications that are ductal in distribution are almost always associated with DCIS (Fig. 20.6). In addition, the DCIS is almost always high grade. Therefore, these calcifications are associated with the most nefarious form of DCIS, and, if not recognized, could result in the untimely demise of the patient. The few cases of benign histology associated with this type of calcification usually represent benign secretory disease or vascular calcifications in which only one wall of the vessel calcifies. If the benign linear calcifications are associated with a vessel, it usually does not take long to recognize this fact early in the process of a stereotactic biopsy.

FULL-FIELD DIGITAL MAMMOGRAPHY AND DCIS

As noted earlier, the microfocus magnification film screen technique has been the standard technique for evaluating screen-detected microcalcifications over the past two decades. This may change as full-field digital (FFD) mammography assumes a larger role in breast screening and diagnosis. FFD only became available for routine clinical use at the start of the 21st century. Although small field of view digital mammography had been used for almost a decade previously, technical and regulatory issues prevented FFD from coming to fruition for far too long. It was always clear from experience with digital stereotactic mammography used for breast biopsy that contrast resolution was substantially improved in digital techniques compared to film screen techniques. This fact has been confirmed in our experience of FFD mammography. Since calcification conspicuity is highly dependent on contrast resolution, it should not be surprising that FFD detects and displays calcification character and morphology better than the standard film screen technique. At the SJBC, we have shown that work-up of microcalcifications using FFD reduces the number of stereotactic biopsies performed for what ultimately prove to be benign lesions. Thus, the positive predictive value of FFD mammography in the setting of microcalcifications is greater than that for the standard film screen magnification technique (33% vs. 22%).

The major drawback of FFD mammography is cost. The cost of an FFD mammography unit is approximately four times that of a film screen unit

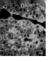

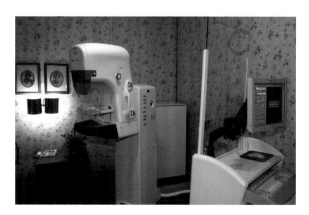

Fig. 20.7 Fischer Imaging Senoscan full-field digital mammography unit.

($ 200,000). If, in addition, one considers that one technician FTE (Full Time Equivalent) can be saved for each digital machine employed, then one can save an additional $ 100,000 in salary and benefits over a two-year period. This, then, brings the true cost of an FFD unit down to $ 100,000, nearly the same as a film screen unit. In addition, there are other savings in terms of decreased space requirements, and decreased clerical, filming, storage and mailing costs.

If the cost can be justified, it would seem clear that most breast screening and diagnostic programs around the world would convert to FFD as their preferred mammography modality. As breast centers and hospitals start to adopt FFD, it would be best to convert all mammography machines to FFD at the same time in order to move to 'soft copy' reading and PACS storage without having to deal with a hybrid transitional period (Fig. 20.7). With FFD screening in place, it is our belief that the call-back rate for calcifications will decrease. For those patients who are recalled for diagnostic magnification views, the positive predictive value of the diagnostic FFD will increase compared with film screen techniques. If automated whole breast ultrasound could become integrated into FFD machines so that women could have both screening mammography and correlative ultrasound in one visit, then the call-back rate could be reduced further. In cases where calcifications suspicious enough for call-back and possible biopsy are detected, the correlative ultrasound could determine if a particular area is suspicious for invasive carcinoma, in which case the biopsy could be targeted accordingly. The future of FFD, then, would seem promising for both screening and diagnostic breast imaging.

($ 400,000 vs. $ 100,000). On the surface, this would seem to make it impossible to afford such systems in the average clinical setting. However, if one considers the increased throughput of digital systems compared with film screen, then the actual cost is comparable. In our experience, one can double patient throughput using the digital system (providing that the images are interpreted in a 'soft copy' fashion at a work station rather than printing the digital images on film and hanging them on a view box to be read). Therefore, if one digital machine can replace two film screen units, then the cost is effectively cut in half, making the cost of the digital equipment twice that of film screen

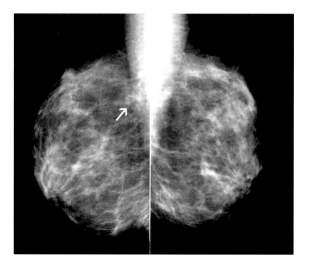

Fig. 20.8 Mammography. Small mass (arrow) with mammographic calcifications.

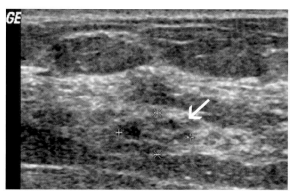

Fig. 20.9 Ultrasound. Same mass as in Fig. 20.8 (arrow).

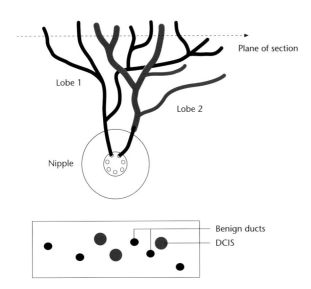

Fig. 20.17 Schematic drawing of the segmental distribution of DCIS. In this example DCIS involves one lobe. In two-dimensional sampling intervening benign ducts in a tissue sample suggest two separate foci of DCIS. Three-dimensional studies have, however, shown a continuous ductal distribution.

5 mm in 82% of cases), and the likelihood of finding such gaps was related to the histologic type of the lesion. Whereas 90% of the cases of poorly-differentiated DCIS grew in a continuous ductal pattern without gaps, only 30% of well-differentiated and 45% of intermediately-differentiated lesions were continuous [45].

MACROSCOPY

Most DCIS lesions detected as a result of mammographic microcalcifications present no macroscopic abnormalities. However, examples of palpable DCIS, even those detected mammographically, exist that appear as a firm, tan tumor mass with cords of pasty material exuding from the cut surface of the specimen or readily expressed from involved ducts by specimen palpation or compression (Fig. 20.18).

HISTOLOGICAL CLASSIFICATION

The traditional method of classifying DCIS was based primarily on the architectural features or growth patterns of the lesions and essentially recognized five major types: comedo, micropapillary, cribriform, solid and papillary. While this classification scheme was perfectly acceptable at a time when all cases of DCIS, regardless of histologic appearance, were treated by mastectomy, this scheme proved to be unsatisfactory for several reasons in the era of breast-conserving therapy. Firstly, while small lesions may be of a uniform pattern, larger lesions frequently show

considerable variability with growth patterns changing from slide to slide, within the same slide, and even, occasionally, within a single involved terminal duct lobular unit. Furthermore, the criteria defining those architectural patterns are somewhat subjective and imprecise, and considerable interobserver variation exists. This is reflected by considerable variation in the incidence of the different subtypes in reported series of DCIS and probably, at least in part, also accounts for the persisting differences in the reported incidence of subsequent invasive carcinoma for the various subtypes of DCIS treated with breast-conserving therapy. Therefore, a reproducible classification system is urgently needed, possibly with the added dimension of prognostic significance so vital to patients eligible for breast-conserving therapy.

A number of alternative classification schemes for DCIS have been proposed in an attempt to overcome the limitations of the traditional, architecturally-based model [9, 46–57]. Initial attempts to improve classification divided DCIS into two broad groups termed variously comedo and noncomedo, high grade and low grade, or large cell and small cell. There is, however, increasing evidence that division into two categories is an oversimplification, and most recently proposed classification systems stratify DCIS lesions into three grades, primarily on the basis of nuclear grade and/or necrosis, with architectural pattern given secondary or no consideration [58]. Lagios et al. were the first to propose a system based primarily on nuclear grade and necrosis, rather than on architecture [7]. The most recent modification of this system recognizes three major categories of DCIS: high, intermediate and low grade [59]. Investigators in Nottingham, England, developed a classification system based primarily on the presence or absence of necrosis [49]. This group divides DCIS into three categories: pure comedo (lesions in which involved spaces show centrally necrotic debris surrounded by large, pleomorphic tumor cells in solid masses); DCIS with necrosis, also called non-pure comedo (lesions with necrotic neoplastic cells but with a micropapillary or cribriform pattern); and DCIS without necrosis (lesions with a micropapillary, cribriform, solid, or papillary pattern and no necrosis). A classification system proposed by Tavassoli, similar to the Lagios system, used nuclear grade and necrosis to stratify DCIS into three grades: low, moderate and high [60]. The classification scheme proposed by Silverstein et al. [50] is essentially a modification of the Nottingham system in which DCIS lesions are classified based on nuclear grade as either high grade or non-high grade. The non-high grade lesions are further stratified by the presence or absence of comedo type necrosis. This essentially creates a three-tiered system in which DCIS is classified as either high grade, non-high grade with necrosis, or non-high grade without necrosis. A group of European pathologists have proposed classifying DCIS, in addition, as well, intermediately or poorly-differentiated. This system, frequently referred to as the Holland system, is based primarily on cytonuclear differentiation and cell polarization [51]. Pathologists associated with the 'United Kingdom National Breast Cancer Screening Programme' utilize a classification scheme for DCIS based solely on nuclear grade, recognizing high, inter-

Tab. 20.1 Summary of various three-tiered classification systems for DCIS

Classification system	Low grade	Intermediate grade	High grade
Tavassoli [60]	Low grade. Cribriform and micropapillary patterns. Uniform population of cells lacking necrosis or nuclear pleomorphism.	Moderate-grade. DCIS lacking cellular atypia and forming solid, cribriform or micropapillary patterns with either moderate atypia or central necrosis, or minimal amounts of both. Many special types of DCIS also fall in this category due to moderate nuclear atypia.	High grade. DCIS showing severe cytological atypia with or without necrosis. Includes all comedo carcinomas and signet-ring cell variants of intraductal carcinoma and many intraductal apocrine carcinomas.
European Pathologists Working Group (EPWG) [51]	Well-differentiated. Evenly spaced, markedly polarized nuclei of uniform size and regular contour with uniformly dispersed fine chromatin, inconspicuous nucleoli and rare mitotic figures. Necrosis absent or minimal. Laminated and rarely amorphous calcifications may be present.	Intermediately-differentiated. Mildly or moderately pleomorphic nuclei with some polarization and variation in size, contour and distribution. Fine to coarse nuclear chromatin and small nucleoli. Occasional mitotic figures. Variable central or individual cell necrosis. Calcifications amorphous or laminated.	Poorly-differentiated. Highly pleomorphic, poorly polarized nuclei with irregular contour and distribution. Coarse, clumped chromatin and prominent nucleoli. Mitotic figures common. Central and individual cell necrosis often present. Amorphous calcifications common.
Nottingham [49]	DCIS without necrosis. No necrosis or only a few necrotic or desquamated cells within ductal lumens. A majority of classical cribriform, papillary and micropapillary subtypes fall into this category.	DCIS with necrosis (non-pure comedo). While necrotic cells are present within duct lumens, they lack a pure comedo pattern, often displaying a cribriform or micropapillary architecture.	DCIS with necrosis (pure comedo). Abundant necrotic debris in duct lumens surrounded by a solid proliferation of large pleomorphic tumor cells.
Van Nuys [50]	Non-high grade without necrosis. The proliferating cells have low or intermediate grade nuclei. No comedonecrosis.	Non-high grade with necrosis. Low grade nuclei (1–1.5 red blood cells in diameter) with inconspicuous nucleoli and diffuse chromatin or intermediate grade nuclei (1–2 red blood cells in diameter) with occasional nucleoli, coarse chromatin and comedo-type necrosis. Individual necrotic cells not accepted.	High grade. High grade nuclei (> 2 red blood cells in diameter) with several nucleoli. Comedonecrosis is surrounded by either large pleomorphic cells or cribriform and micropapillary patterns. Necrosis may be absent.
European Working Group on Breast Screening Pathology (EWGBSP) [61]	Low grade. The proliferating cells have low grade nuclei, few mitotic figures *and* absent or rare single cell necrosis.	Intermediate grade. The nuclei are mildly to moderately pleomorphic.	High grade. The nuclei may be pleomorphic and there are a large number of mitotic figures. Necrosis is not essential.
Scott et al., 1997 (modified Lagios system) [59]	Low grade. Non-comedo histology, low nuclear grade and no necrosis.	Intermediate grade. Intermediate histology (admixture of noncomedo patterns), intermediate nuclear grade and no necrosis.	High grade. Comedo histology, higher nuclear grade and extensive necrosis.

mediate, and low grade types [61]. This classification system has been adopted also by the European Breast Screening Pathology Working Group chaired by the late John Sloane and now by Clive Wells (*European Guidelines for Quality Assurance in Mammography Screening* – Fourth Edition, Office for Official Publications of the European Communities [2005]). Further classification systems have been proposed by other authors [41, 46, 52, 53]. The details of several of these classification schemes are summarized in Table 20.1.

Recent international consensus conferences have recommended that grading of DCIS be primarily based on cytonuclear features (Fig. 20.19a–b) [7, 54, 63, 64]. There is common agreement that the highest grade subgroup of all classification systems has as its

most important and defining feature the overtly malignant morphology of the nuclei, irrespective of the presence or absence of comedonecrosis. Moreover accumulating molecular, histological and epidemiological data seem to indicate that ductal neoplastic lesions in the low grade spectrum are in a category of their own, characterized by cells with small, monotonous, usually hyperchromatic nuclei and a growth pattern of extreme rigidity and smoothness. These two features are easily recognized on histological grounds. We therefore feel that a classification system of DCIS should contain these two categories as cornerstones of the classifying principle. All other DCIS cases should be classified as intermediate grade. This is probably the least well-defined category with different biological potential, which currently can only

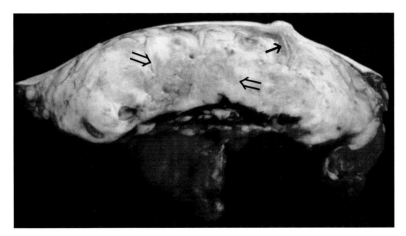

Fig. 20.18 Macroscopy of comedo-type DCIS. This is a typical macroscopic view of an extended grade 3 DCIS with typical comedonecrosis. Multiple, 'stacked', distended ducts responsible for the mass can be recognized. Even the outlines and size of this DCIS lesion can be determined macroscopically (double arrows). The retroareolar ducts form yellow streaks (arrow), making it likely that they are also involved.

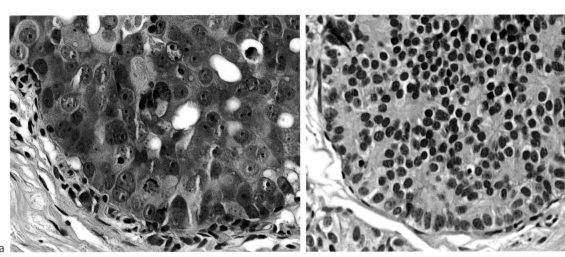

a   b

Fig. 20.19a–b DCIS, high grade versus low grade.
20.19a DCIS, high grade, showing the typical cytonuclear features of this solid tumor growth. The distended glandular space contains large tumor cells with basophilic cytoplasm and large nuclei. Moderately enlarged, single or multiple nucleoli are present in nearly all tumor cells. An occasional apoptotic body is seen in the upper field. Lymphocytes or red blood cells in the periductal stroma are useful in measuring the size of the nuclei of the tumor cells. Nuclei of high grade lesions usually measure more than 3 red blood cells in diameter.
20.19b The same magnification of a DCIS with cytonuclear features of a low grade lesion. The hyperchromatic nuclei are characterized by their even size and regular placement, the size of nuclei being approximately 2 red blood cells or less in diameter.

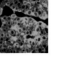

be further subclassified by use of molecular techniques. In line with the above-mentioned recommendations, we regard comedonecrosis as an additional histological feature which – although usually seen in high grade comedo-type DCIS tumors – may be found associated with any of the subgroups.

Thus we propose the following grading system (Table 20.2).

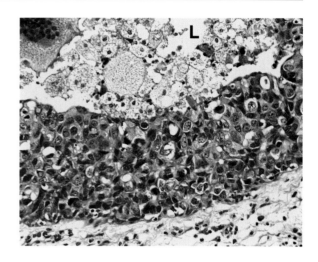

Fig. 20.20 High grade DCIS. The tumor cells contain large, polymorphous nuclei with small nucleoli. The lumen (L) contains cellular debris and foam cells. The nuclei of high grade lesions should be more than 3-times the diameter of a red blood cell. This may be helpful in assessing the grade of a DCIS.

Tab. 20.2 Ductal carcinoma in-situ, three-tier grading system used in this book

Grade/feature	High grade (grade 3)	Low grade (grade 1)	Intermediate grade (grade 2)
Definition	Proliferation of overtly malignant epithelial cells of ductal-type within the boundaries of the ductal lobular tree. Usually unifocal and segmental growth.	Proliferation of monomorphous malignant epithelial cells of ductal-type within the boundaries of the ductal lobular tree. Usually unifocal and segmental growth.	Proliferation of mildly to moderately polymorphous cells of ductal-type within the boundaries of the ductal lobular tree. Usually unifocal and segmental growth.
Tumor forming	Some (classic progressed comedo-type and occasional rare papillary-type DCIS).	Usually not, exception papillary-type.	Usually not, exception papillary-type.
Nuclei	Overtly malignant, large, pleomorphic or blastic nuclei with mitotic figures. Nucleoli may be large. Often coarse chromatin pattern. Size of nuclei usually more than three red blood cells in diameter.	Usually small, monotonous and hyperchromatic nuclei, regular in size and contour, usually round or oval. Diffuse chromatin. Mitotic figures rare. Size of nuclei usually less than two red blood cells in diameter.	Mildly to moderately pleomorphic nuclei, some irregularities in size, shape and contour, fine to coarse chromatin, occasional mitotic figures. Size usually 2 – 3 red blood cells in diameter.
Spacing of nuclei	Indistinct.	Evenly spaced.	Often unevenly spaced.
Nucleoli	May be prominent.	Inconspicuous.	Small.
Comedo type necrosis	Often present, but not required for diagnosis.	Rare, but may be seen.	Rare, but may be seen.
Calcification	Amorphous (polymorphous) with ductal branching pattern.	Psammomatous (laminated), rarely amorphous.	May be psammomatous or amorphous.
Cytokeratins	Ck8/18+, Ck5/14 usually negative, but may be positive	Ck8/18+, Ck5/14–	Ck8/18+, Ck5/14–
Growth pattern	Mostly solid, sometimes clinging; micropapillary or cribriform; papillary-type rare.	Mostly micropapillary or cribriform (bridges, bars, arcades), solid or papillary.	Solid to fenestrated, micropapillary or papillary.
Polarization of cells	Usually not present.	Often present.	May be present to some extent.

HIGH GRADE DCIS

High grade DCIS is comprised of cells with cytological pleomorphism and large pleomorphic nuclei with vesicular or coarse chromatin and one or more nucleoli (Fig. 20.19–20). The cytoplasm may be abundant with a marked pallor, and may be amphophilic or eosinophilic with a slight granularity. Mitotic figures may be numerous. Central comedo-type necrosis is often present but is not required for the diagnosis of a high grade DCIS lesion. Necrosis is occasionally so extensive that only a few cells are present at the periphery of the involved space (Fig. 20.21a–b). Occasionally, the malignant cells produce a solid sheet filling the duct lumen without central necrosis. Alternatively, the cells may grow in a cribriform or micropapillary pattern. In contrast to well-differentiated DCIS, polarization is usually not seen. The central necrotic material often becomes calcified forming amorphous and polymorphous calcifications. These calcifications are irregular in form, size and density usually with a large, triangular or elongated shape. They normally produce a typical ductal, branching, linear, or casting pattern, which is readily seen on mammograms and specimen radiographs and

which is diagnostic of malignancy (Fig. 20.22a–b) [51, 65]. The involved spaces may be very distended, and this type of DCIS may be quite large and result in a palpable abnormality in the breast. This is due to the distension of the whole ductal lobular tree involved in the process, but partly also to the surrounding stromal reaction, which is usually more evident in this pattern of DCIS than in others. Involvement of lobules is frequent. The lobular architecture may be preserved (lobular cancerization), which may lead to an appearance that mimics invasive growth (Fig. 20.23). Usually, however, the involved lobules are distended to become duct-like structures and are no longer recognized as lobules.

According to the WHO, Paget's disease of the nipple is defined by the 'presence of malignant glandular

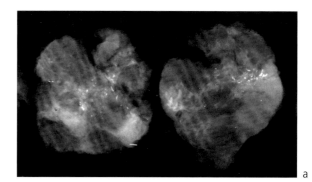
a

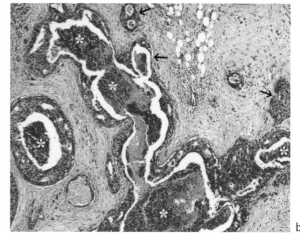
b

Fig. 20.22a–b High grade DCIS. Specimen radiography and histology.
20.22a An example of malignant-type amorphous calcification on specimen radiography. The calcifications differ in size, density and shape and are irregular in outline. They display a typical branching or casting-type calcification with segmental distribution.
20.22b Lower power view of high grade DCIS, with typical comedonecrosis. Distended glandular spaces contain solid tumor masses with centrally located necrotic debris, which shows amorphous calcification (asterisks). The periductal stroma shows a slight inflammatory reaction. The lobular structures are unfolded by tumor cell growth (arrows).

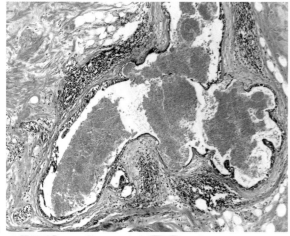
a
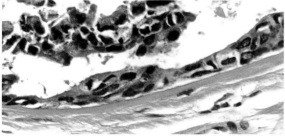
b

Fig. 20.21a–b DCIS, high grade with clinging growth pattern.
20.21a Lower power view of DCIS with massive comedonecrosis and only a few layers of polymorphic tumor cells. The fibrous stroma contains numerous lymphocytes.
20.21b High power view showing polymorphic tumor cells with overtly malignant nuclei.

cells within the squamous epithelium of the nipple' [66]. Paget's disease of the nipple is almost invariably associated with an underlying high grade DCIS with or without infiltration. It is characterized by a chronic eczema-like skin lesion in the region of the nipple. Histologically it is defined by the presence of secretory glandular neoplastic cells in the epidermis. The tumor cells appear as large, round to oval cells with copious cytoplasm and polymorphic, hyperchromatic nuclei (Fig. 20.24). The cells lie singly, or in clusters and nests, in the lower portion of the epidermis and may extend to the epidermal surface. Skin appendages may also be involved. Immunostains for low molecular weight cytokeratins 8/18/19 and erbB2 oncoprotein highlight the tumor cells contrasting with the negativity of the epidermal cells [67]. Based on cell culture

studies, it seems likely that heregulin-α, produced and released by normal epidermal cells, binds to tyrosine kinase receptors of tumor cells such as erbB2 oncoproteins, EGFR 3 and 4, resulting in increased motility with a chemotactically-induced migration of the tumor cells into the epidermis [68].

LOW GRADE DCIS

This type of DCIS lies at the other end of the spectrum of the classification based primarily on nuclear grade. The nuclei are usually small, with diffuse darkly stained chromatin and inconspicuous nucleoli (Fig. 20.19b). The cells are evenly spaced. There may be prominent, uniform cell polarization (architectural differentiation), sometimes with apocrine snouts (Fig. 20.25b). The majority of cases of 'Van Nuys non-

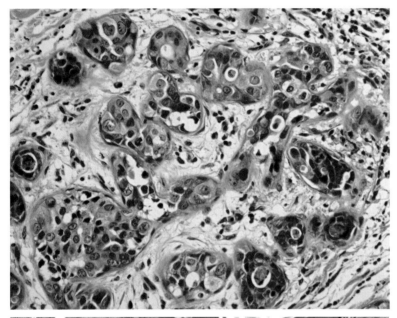

Fig. 20.23 High grade DCIS with lobular cancerization. The normal ductular epithelium is replaced by large tumor cells with overtly malignant nuclei showing prominent nucleoli. This may lead to an erroneous diagnosis of invasion. However even the single cells in the center of the figure are surrounded by myoepithelial cells.

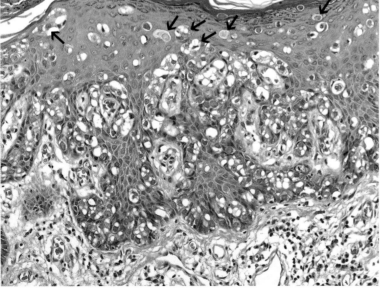

Fig. 20.24 Paget's disease of the nipple. This figure illustrates the typical features. Tumor cells are aggregated in the deep parts of the epidermis and scattered in the superficial part (arrows). The cells have abundant cytoplasm and polymorphic nuclei.

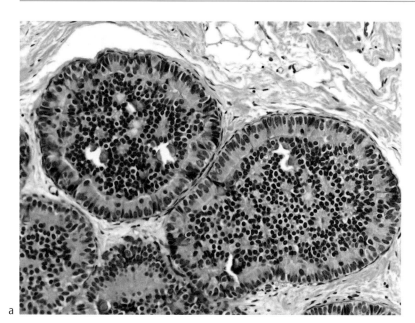

Fig. 20.25a–f Low grade DCIS.

20.25a In this case there is a more solid growth pattern with small, incompletely formed intercellular spaces and polarization of the surrounding cells, resulting in a microacinar or rosette-like appearance. The nuclei are monotonous and hyperchromatic.

a

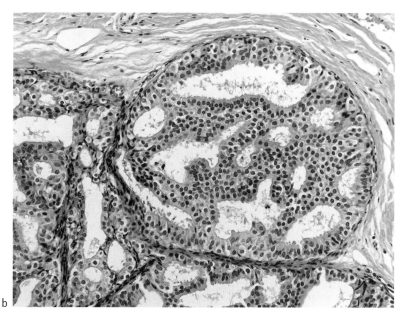

20.25b This DCIS is characterized by a cribriform growth pattern. There is polarization of cells with recognizable apical snouts in some areas. The one-cell type composition clearly indicates malignancy.

b

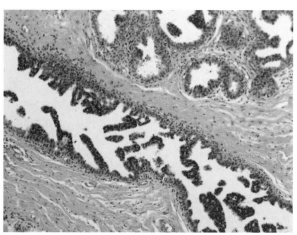

20.25c A low grade DCIS with typical micropapillary growth. The proliferating cells extend into the lumen of the glandular structure, but without a fibrovascular stalk. The micropapillae frequently have a club-like and finger-like appearance, with even distribution of the cells within the papillae. The distinction from benign micropapillary epithelial growth may be difficult, necessitating Ck5/14 immunostaining. *Continuation*

c

high grade DCIS without necrosis' and 'Nottingham DCIS without necrosis' probably also fall into this category. The growth pattern of most lesions of this group is micropapillary, cribriform, papillary or, less frequently, solid- or clinging-type (Fig. 20.25a–f). In the classical cribriform pattern, intercellular lumina between the proliferating cells are geometric, punched out, rigid, and rounded and they are usually evenly distributed within the cell masses. Simple arcades, Roman bridges and bars may be regarded as miniature versions of cribriform growth pattern. The cells within the center of the proliferating strands forming the bridges and arcades are arranged regularly and usually lie at right angles to the plane of the cellular strands. In the micropapillary pattern, proliferating cells extend

into the lumen of the glandular structure but without a fibrovascular stalk (Fig. 20.25c). The micropapillae frequently have a club-like appearance with even distribution of the cells within the papillae. Small rosettes of cells with surface polarization, apparently separated from the papillae, are often seen floating free within the duct lumen. When the growth pattern is solid, there are usually small, incompletely-formed intercellular spaces with polarization of the surrounding cells, resulting in a microacinar or rosette-like appearance (Fig. 20.25a). Necrosis is rarely associated with cells of low grade. Calcification, when present, is usually rounded and laminated or psammomatous and is deposited within the secretions (Fig. 20.26a–b). The secretions in the lumen of low

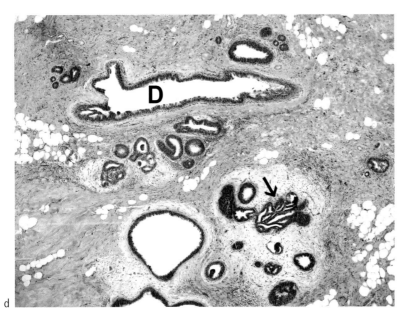

d

Fig. 20.25a–f Low grade DCIS.
20.25d–e Low grade DCIS with extensive flat growth pattern. This lesion is diagnosed as malignant due to its ductal-segmental spread of atypical cells. Lobules and inter-lobular ducts (D) are equally involved. Note the focal cribriform pattern (arrow). The data in the literature indicate that these lesions have a better prognosis than those with full-blown solid or cribriform growth (see also Chapter 17). *Continuation*

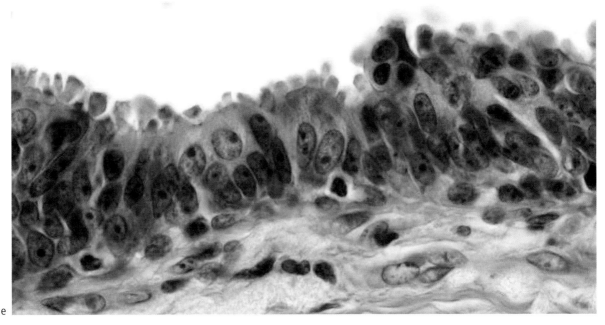

e

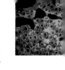

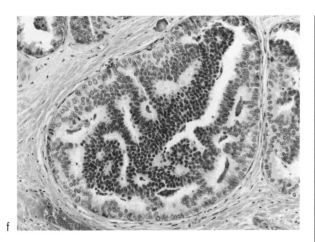

f

Fig. 20.25a–f Low grade DCIS.
20.25f DCIS, low grade, with dimorphic cell pattern.

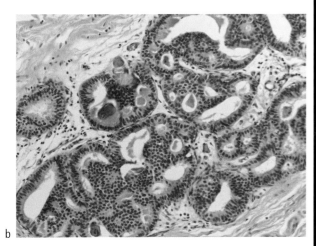

b

Fig. 20.26a–b Psammomatous calcifications in low grade DCIS.
20.26a Specimen radiography showing clustered small, moderately polymorphic calcifications. These are calcifications that can also be seen in a number of benign breast lesions.
20.26b Higher power view showing several psammomatous calcifications. The individual calcifications are too small to be recognized on mammograms, but the summation of several of these can be seen as clustered microcalcification.

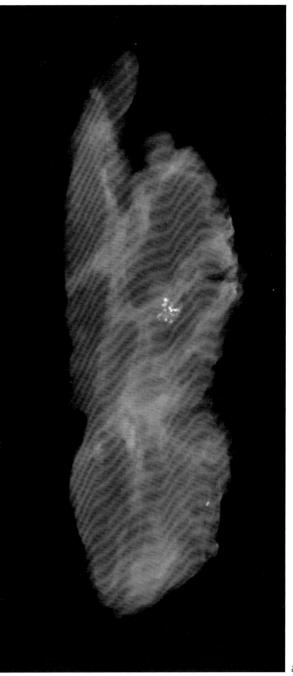

a

grade DCIS may calcify as small laminated bodies. These clustered psammoma-like calcifications are seen in mammograms as monomorphous, small, powdery calcifications only when they are numerous, similar to those seen in some benign proliferative breast disease lesions. It should be noted that calcifications can be detected mammographically only if they are at least 100 microns in diameter (either the individual calcification or the calcifications in sum diameter).

INTERMEDIATE GRADE DCIS

The third type of DCIS in classifications based primarily on a three-tier nuclear grade system is composed of cells with intermediate grade nuclei (Fig. 20.27). The nuclei are mildly to moderately polymorphic with some variation in size, outline and spacing. The growth pattern varies and may be solid, micropapillary or fenestrating, with formation of irregular slit-like lumina. The cellular features lie in between those of high grade and low grade types. In the classification of Holland and coworkers [35],

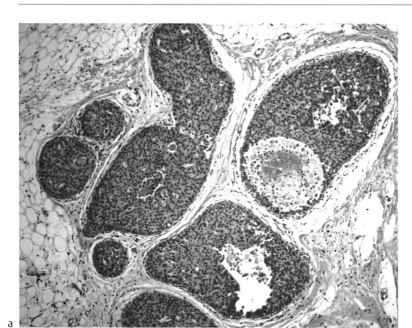

Fig. 20.27a – c Intermediate grade DCIS.
20.27a Lower magnification showing a lobule with ductular structures distended by a solid proliferation of cells with formation of some irregular secondary lumina. The central lumina contain histiocytes and some type of comedonecrosis.

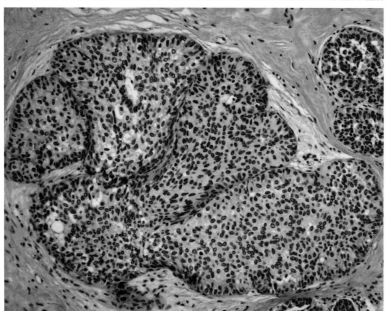

20.27b Higher magnification of an area of the same lesion highlighting the variation in size and placing of the nuclei of the proliferating cells. Due to the one-cell type nature of these lesions the overall picture is more that of a DCIS than of a ductal hyperplasia. However, this lesion has been classified both as benign and malignant by experienced breast pathologists. The only means of arriving at a more objective diagnosis in such a case is to resort to the use of Ck5/14 immunostaining.

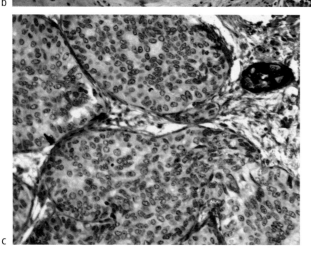

20.27c Immunostaining for Ck5/14 (same case). The complete lack of Ck5/14 in the proliferating cells is clearly indicative of the malignancy of this lesion. Note the normal gland with Ck5/14+ myoepithelial and luminal cells.

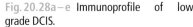

the presence of cell polarization is mentioned, although this is not as prominent and uniform as in the well-differentiated type. Necrosis may or may not be present. Calcification, when present, may be psammomatous or amorphous. The cellular composition in combination with the ductal lobular growth patterns, however, usually allows a clear diagnosis of DCIS to be made. However, the differences of size and shape of nuclei and a more irregular spacing and staining of the neoplastic cells with fenestrating growth may lead to difficulties in recognizing small lesions as neoplastic and in differentiation from UDH. In rare cases Ck5/14 immunostaining may help in arriving at a solution.

■ IMMUNOHISTOCHEMISTRY

Ninety-five percent of all DCIS show a purely glandular phenotype with expression of low molecular weight cytokeratins 8/18/19, but not of high molecular weight cytokeratins 5/14 (Fig. 20.28). A subset of high grade DCIS with expression of cytokeratins 5 and 14 [22] has however also been detected (Fig. 20.29). Similarly, nearly all low and intermediate grade DCIS that one of the authors (WB) was so far able to examine did not express Ck5/14 in their neoplastic cells. A number of extremely rare pitfalls are discussed in the differential diagnostic section.

A substantial subset of tumors, 75% of all DCIS lesions, expressed the estrogen receptor (Fig. 20.28e). These lesions were mainly of the low and intermediate grade DCIS subgroups [69]. A difference between ER-α and ER-β could not be detected.

C-erbB2 is among the most thoroughly investigated prognostic factors in DCIS. Expression has been described in up to 40% of all DCIS lesions, almost always associated with an amplification of the gene. The highest frequencies were seen in high grade DCIS (amounting to 70%). It is worth mentioning that the expression and amplification of c-erbB2 is signifi-

Fig. 20.28a–e Immunoprofile of low grade DCIS.
20.28a Higher power view of low grade DCIS with cribriform growth pattern.
20.28b Ck8/18 immunostaining, highlighting the extensive expression of this glandular cytokeratin.
20.28c Ck5/14 immunostaining shows lack of expression in the tumor cells. Note that in this area myoepithelial cells lack Ck5/14.   *Continuation*

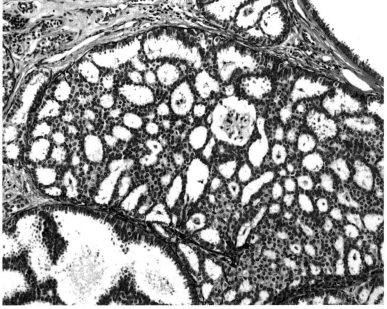

a

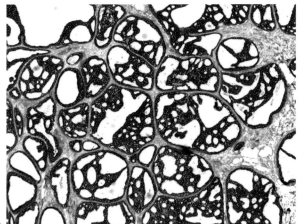

b

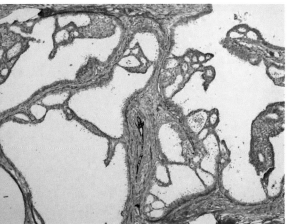

c

cantly lower in invasive breast cancer. Similar staining patterns have been observed for c-erbB3 and EGFR [70–73].

Expression of nuclear p53, often associated with a gene mutation, has almost exclusively been detected in high grade DCIS with comedonecrosis, where it is seen in about a third of cases [73–79]. Done and coworkers [74] could furthermore demonstrate that all cases of invasive carcinomas displayed the same p53 mutation observed in associated DCIS, thus supporting the view that this mutation is an early event of this progression pathway. The expression of p53 and members of the erb-gene family were constantly associated with a high cellular proliferation and high apoptotic indices. TUNEL assays and immunohistochemical investigations used to detect apoptosis revealed similar findings [80–83]. Sporadic studies showed a comparable tendency for c-met/SF [83] and a larger series of investigations demonstrated a greater degree of DNA aneuploidy [84–86].

■ MOLECULAR GENETICS

On the genomic level, microsatellite analyses have been repeatedly used to recognize chromosomal regions involved in the pathogenesis of DCIS. Based on the inherent limitations of this technique, only a limited number of chromosomal regions containing putative tumor suppressor genes could be investigated. Nevertheless, the observations have enhanced our insight into the mechanisms of breast carcinogenesis,

even though the polymorphic markers applied in those studies vary considerably [87, 88]. Interestingly, the involvement of distinct genetic regions could be consistently reproduced. Thus chromosomal loci on 6q, 9p, 11q, 13q, 16q, 17p, and 17q were recurrently affected by LOH with frequencies amounting to 60% [87, 89, 90]. Such elevated ratios point to the presence of several tumor suppressor genes at these loci. The LOH data of DCIS with synchronous invasive carcinoma components provide clear evidence that DCIS must be regarded as a precursor of invasive breast carcinoma [88, 91]. Nevertheless, these authors also demonstrated a large degree of intratumoral genetic heterogeneity, sometimes even more extensive in DCIS than in invasive breast cancer [89]. Some authors also aimed at defining 'early markers' in breast carcinogenesis such as LOH on 16q [92], which are often associated with unbalanced chromosomal translocations such as t(1;16) [93, 94] and LOH on 17p [95] and 8p [96, 97], since these regions seemed to be affected by LOH in DCIS with low grade. In contrast, other authors could find LOH on 8p in invasive breast cancer only [98]. Similar results have also been reported for amplifications of 17q12 with c-erbB2 as the major component of the amplicon [99]. The interpretation of these findings is unfortunately hampered by the use of various morphological classification schemes. Irrespective of these problems the overwhelming majority of all studies were able to show for other markers (1, 6q, 11q13, 9p) [100–103] that the frequency of LOH within DCIS was raised significantly with increasing nuclear grade. It was also

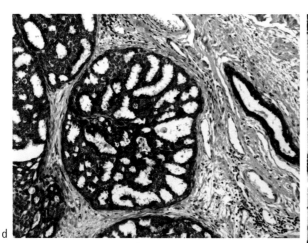
d

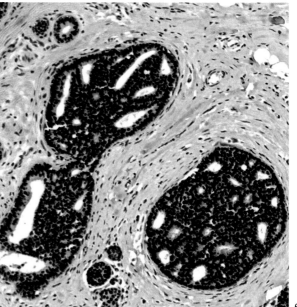
e

Fig. 20.28a–e Immunoprofile of low grade DCIS.
20.28d 34βE12 (Ck1, 5, 10, 14) immunostaining showing intense staining of the tumor cells with some variability in staining reaction in contrast to 20.28c. In our experience this antibody is not useful in the differential diagnosis of intraductal epithelial proliferations.
20.28e Estrogen immunostaining shows an intense reaction of nearly all tumor cells.

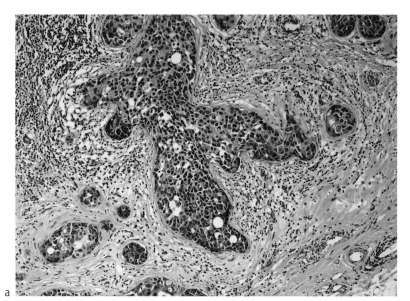

Fig. 20.29a–b High grade DCIS.
20.29a Medium magnification of a high grade DCIS lesion.

a

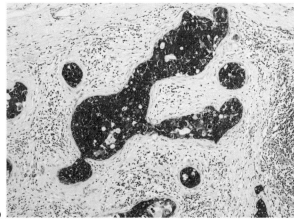

b

20.29b Ck5/6 immunostains highlight the expression of basal cytokeratins in tumor cells.

evident that at least some markers have the potential to distinguish between hyperplastic and neoplastic lesions such as 11q13, which is mainly amplified/overexpressed in DCIS, whereas it is absent in atypical hyperplasias [104].

First studies using CGH gave further evidence that DCIS shares a high degree of cytogenetic homology with invasive breast cancer. This substantiated the hypothesis that the most common genetic changes of invasive carcinoma are already present at the in-situ level [19, 105]. A direct comparison between DCIS and its invasive counterpart within one patient underlined this point of view. In addition, CGH analysis also underlines the LOH data indicating an intratumoral cytogenetic heterogeneity already within in-situ carcinomas [19, 89].

MICROINVASION

One of the most important goals in the histological examination of DCIS lesions is the identification

of foci of stromal invasion, since the therapeutic algorithm for patients with pure DCIS differs from that of patients with DCIS and associated invasive breast cancer. A frequently encountered problem in examinations of such specimens is identifying the smallest foci of invasive carcinoma, so-called microinvasion. In fact, while this diagnosis often appears in surgical pathology reports, this term has not been applied in a consistent, standardized manner. Furthermore, the histological diagnosis of microinvasion is not straightforward and is often problematical for the pathologist. Finally, studies of patients with microinvasion have been limited by small numbers of cases and variable degrees of tissue sampling. As a consequence, the diagnosis and clinical significance of microinvasion remain a matter of debate, if not confusion.

DEFINITION

In the 5th edition of the *AJCC Cancer Staging Manual* [106], microinvasion was defined as, 'the extension of cancer cells beyond the basement membrane into the adjacent tissues with no focus more than 0.1 cm in greatest dimension' (Fig. 20.30). Lesions that fulfill this definition are staged as T1mic, a subset of T1 breast cancer. The staging manual further states that, 'when there are multiple foci of microinvasion, the size of only the largest focus is used to classify the microinvasion', and that the size of the individual foci should not be added together. The European Breast Screening Pathology Working Group has adopted this definition [107]. Note that invasive carcinomas without a DCIS component are always classified as invasive [107].

Unfortunately, widely varying definitions of microinvasion have been used in the past, and some of these definitions differ substantially from that offered in the *AJCC Staging Manual* (Table 20.3).

The article by Silver and Tavassoli uses yet another definition for microinvasion: DCIS with, 'a single focus of invasive carcinoma < 2 mm or up to three foci of invasion, each < 1 mm in greatest dimension' [113]. This lack of a uniform definition for microinvasion has clearly contributed to the confusion regarding this entity.

PATHOLOGICAL DIAGNOSIS OF MICROINVASION

Identifying microinvasion in a lesion that is primarily DCIS can be difficult for the pathologist due to a variety

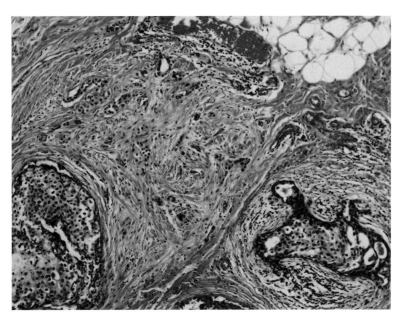

Fig. 20.30 Low grade DCIS with a focus of microinvasion.
Low grade DCIS with a small area of an invasive ductal carcinoma in the center field. The maximum size of the invasive lesion is less than one millimeter. It must therefore be classified as microinvasion.

Tab. 20.3 Definition of microinvasion

DCIS with 'evidence of stromal invasion' [108].

'DCIS with limited microscopic stromal invasion below the basement membrane, but not invading more than 10% of the surface of the histologic sections examined' [109].

'Breast cancer cells confined to the duct system of the breast with only a microscopic focus of malignant cells invading beyond the basement membrane of the duct as determined by light microscopy' [110].

'Predominantly intraductal carcinoma with maximal extent of invasion of < 2 mm or invasive carcinoma comprising < 10% of the tumor' [111].

'Mainly a DCIS showing focal microinvasion below the basement membrane in one or several individual ducts, but in not more than 10% of the surface of the histologic sections examined' [112].

Tab. 20.4 Lesions commonly mistaken for microinvasion [114–120]

DCIS involving lobules ('cancerization of lobules').

Branching of ducts.

Distortion or entrapment of involved ducts or acini by fibrosis.

Inflammation present in association with, and obscuring, involved ducts or acini.

Crush artifact.

Cautery effect.

Artifactual displacement of DCIS cells into the surrounding stroma or adipose tissue due to tissue manipulation or a prior needling procedure.

DCIS involving benign sclerosing processes such as radial scars, complex sclerosing lesions or sclerosing adenosis, or papilloma.

of DCIS patterns that may be misconstrued as stromal invasion. According to Fisher, microinvasion, 'represents one of if not the most commonly overdiagnosed events in the pathology of breast cancer' (compare Fig. 20.31) [114]. Most pathologists with large breast pathology consultation practices would likely concur with this sentiment. Lesions that are commonly mistaken for microinvasion are listed in Table 20.4.

A variety of methods exist which can help in distinguishing such lesions from true stromal invasion. Obtaining further levels through the block is often useful in defining the nature of the process. Histochemical stains, such as PAS and reticulin, have been used to help delineate basement membrane material around nests of tumor cells, which defines the process as noninvasive. Most recently, immunohistochemical (IHC) stains for basement membrane (for example, collagen IV, laminin) and myoepithelial cells have been employed to help determine whether a process represents in-situ carcinoma or stromal invasion [121–124]. In our experience as well as that of others,

IHC stains for collagen IV and laminin are often associated with technical problems in formalin-fixed, paraffin-embedded tissue and we have not found these stains to be reliable in this context. Therefore, at the present time, IHC stains for myoepithelial cells appear to be the most useful adjunct in this setting.

A variety of markers have been used to detect myoepithelial cells including S-100 protein, smooth muscle actin, calponin, p63, and smooth muscle myosin heavy chain (SMM-HC) [125]. It should be noted, however, that these markers vary in their sensitivity and specificity. For example, S-100 protein is a nonspecific marker also expressed by the epithelial cells of in-situ and invasive breast carcinomas as well as by benign breast epithelial cells. Therefore, expression of S-100 protein cannot be relied upon to define cells in the breast as being myoepithelial. Sm-actin, calponin, and SMM-HC are sensitive myoepithelial cell markers. However, all of these proteins are also expressed to some degree in myofibroblasts (actin > calponin > SMM-HC), and this can create problems

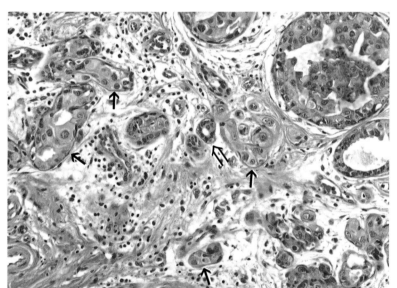

a

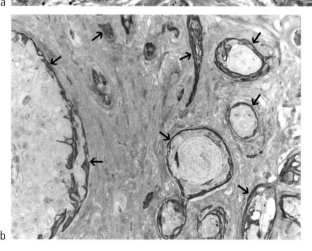

b

Fig. 20.31a–c Mimickers of invasion.
20.31a High grade DCIS with worrisome cancerization of lobular structures. Higher magnification showing distended ductules containing atypical cells. The ductules are lined in part by a thickened basement membrane (arrows) and, in part, by clearly recognizable myoepithelial cells so that invasion can be excluded. Some of the ductules contain atrophic glandular cells (double arrow). The fibrous stroma shows a moderate inflammatory response.

20.31b Ck5/6 immunostain displaying positivity of the original benign ductular structures. The tumor cells, however, lack Ck5/6 expression. Myoepithelial cells also stain positively for Ck5/6 (arrows). *Continuation*

433

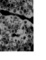

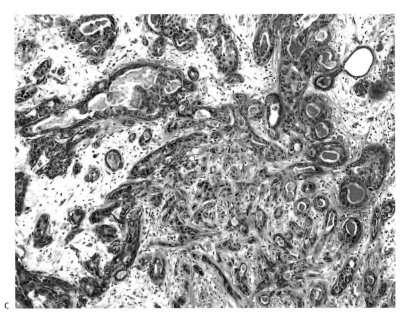

c

Fig. 20.31a–c Mimickers of invasion.
20.31c DCIS involving a benign sclerosing lesion.
Lower power view with a high grade DCIS and comedonecrosis in the left and upper right field, involving a pre-existing sclerosing lesion in the right lower field. The tubular structures of sclerosing adenosis can be highlighted by Ck5/6 or p63 immunostaining (compare 20.31b).

in interpretation. For example, we have seen cases of invasive breast cancer in which myofibroblasts staining for one or more of these markers were closely apposed to nests of invasive breast cancer cells, giving the illusion that these were myoepithelial cells. In such cases, interpretation of these cells as myoepithelial cells rather than myofibroblasts would result in a lesion being erroneously categorized as benign or in-situ, when in fact invasive.

Several recent studies have described additional markers that may be used to identify myoepithelial cells and may, in turn, be diagnostically useful in distinguishing benign or in-situ lesions from invasive breast cancer. These include maspin, a member of the serpin family of protease inhibitors [126] which is expressed in both the cytoplasm and nuclei of myoepithelial cells; p63, a member of the p53 gene family [127] which is expressed exclusively in the nuclei of myoepithelial cells; and CD10, which was recently found to be consistently positive in breast myoepithelial cells [128]. It should be noted however that while most cases can be resolved with the use of additional levels and/or adjunctive stains, the unequivocal identification of microinvasion sometimes remains problematical, even with the use of these ancillary techniques.

What, then, are the minimum criteria for identifying bona fide stromal invasion in the setting of DCIS? The criteria used at our institutions to distinguish true invasion from the lesions mimicking invasion described above take into consideration all of these recommendations. In order to diagnose unequivocal stromal invasion or microinvasion in the setting of DCIS, the worrisome area should be present clearly beyond the immediate periductal and perilobular

region and should consist of a recognized type of invasive cancer. The clinical significance of a few single tumor cells or tumor cell clusters admixed with inflammatory cells in the immediate periductal region, as illustrated by Silver and Tavassoli (Figure 1) [113] is unclear. In such cases, we register the presence of such foci, but indicate that we are uncertain about their clinical importance. It should be noted that, while the presence of stromal desmoplasia and inflammation should heighten the suspicion of invasion, these phenomena are so often present in association with high grade DCIS without demonstrable invasion that their presence cannot be depended upon to make this distinction.

Another potential problem with the pathological diagnosis of microinvasion relates to tissue sampling. Previous published studies of microinvasion have generally failed to indicate how much of a given specimen was submitted for microscopic evaluation. Thus, some lesions categorized as microinvasive based on limited tissue sampling could in truth represent frankly invasive carcinomas in which the largest area of invasion was not submitted for histological evaluation or was not represented on the slides because the cancer was deeper in the blocks. Even when an entire specimen is submitted for histological evaluation, only a fraction of the tissue is ultimately examined microscopically. For example, if a 6 cm excision specimen is sectioned grossly at 3 mm intervals (producing 20 slices), each of these slices is embedded in a separate paraffin block and one 5 micron section is cut from each block, less than 1% of the entire specimen will be examined microscopically.

In addition, the suspicious area should clearly not be seen in a benign sclerosing lesion (Fig. 20.31c).

CLINICAL SIGNIFICANCE OF MICROINVASION

Given the problems with both the definition and pathologic diagnosis of 'microinvasion', it should not be surprising that the clinical significance of this lesion is controversial. The reported incidence of axillary lymph node involvement in patients given a diagnosis of microinvasion ranges from 0% to 20% [108–113, 129–136] (Table 20.3). Furthermore, there are few available data on the outcome of patients with microinvasion treated with either mastectomy or breast-conserving therapy. In one small retrospective study, local recurrence, disease-free survival and overall survival rates for 21 patients with DCIS with microinvasion were similar to those of 622 patients with DCIS without identifiable microinvasion [129]. In the Silver and Tavassoli study of 33 patients treated by mastectomy, there were no instances of local recurrence or metastatic disease with a mean follow-up of 7.5 years [113]. In a study of 21 patients with microinvasive carcinoma followed for a median of 28 months, Prasad et al. [132] reported local recurrence in two patients, one in the breast following breast-conserving therapy and one in the chest wall following mastectomy. No incidents of distant metastases or death from disease were reported. Padmore et al. [134], in a study of 11 patients with microinvasion, reported a 5-year recurrence-free survival rate of 91% (one local recurrence following breast conserving treatment) and a 5-year cause-specific survival rate of 100%. Mann et al. [135], in a study of 18 patients with microinvasive carcinoma, reported no local or distant recurrences at 6-year follow-up. Of note is also a recent follow-up study of 243 patients in which de Mascarel et al. found that the outcome of patients whose microinvasion was characterized by the presence of a few scattered tumor cells in the stroma was similar to patients with pure DCIS [137]. Given the paucity and conflicting nature of the clinical outcome data, some clinicians view DCIS lesions with microinvasion no differently than DCIS of equivalent size and grade without demonstrable microinvasion, and manage patients in these two groups in a similar fashion. In contrast, others consider lesions with microinvasion a subset of invasive breast cancer and treat them as they would any other invasive breast cancer, which may include the use of axillary dissection (or sentinel node biopsy) and/or consideration of adjuvant systemic therapy.

Ideally the term microinvasion in the breast should be used in a manner similar to that used for lesions of the cervix: to identify those invasive lesions of limited extent that have virtually no risk of metastasis. Unfortunately, at the present time, the available data is inadequate to permit the reproducible identification of such a subset due to differences among studies with

Tab. 20.5 Axillary lymph node involvement in patients diagnosed with microinvasion

Study	No. of patients	No. * of node-positive patients (percent)
Wong [110]	33	0
Silverstein [129]	17	0
Akhtar [130]	25	0
Padmore [134]	11	0
Mann [135]	18	0
Silver [113]	38	0
Rosner [109]	34	1 (3)
Solin [111]	39	2 (5)
Penault-Llorca [131]	58	3 (5)
Klauber-DeMore [136]	31	3 (10)
Patchefsky [112]	16	2 (12)
Prasad [132]	15	2 (13)
Zavotsky [133]	14	2 (14)
Schuh [108]		6 (20)

* Determined by sentinel node biopsy.

regard to the definition of microinvasion, variations in the extent of tissue sampling, small patient numbers and limited follow-up. Additional clinicopathological studies using a standardized definition of microinvasion are clearly needed to address this important question. While the definition of microinvasion in the *AJCC Cancer Staging Manual* [106] may ultimately be modified, it represents an important step toward standardization, and its use in both clinical research and clinical practice should be encouraged. Based on our current level of understanding, it is likely that patients categorized as having microinvasive carcinoma using this definition will have an extremely low rate of axillary nodal involvement (less than 5%) and a cure rate approaching 100% with appropriate local treatment alone.

REPRODUCIBILITY OF CLASSIFICATION

To attain widespread clinical use, any classification system has not only to be clinically relevant, but must also be reproducibly applicable by different observers.

Although some authors have claimed that their system is or should be easy to use, relatively few studies have formally addressed the issue of interobserver agreement in the classification of DCIS. The studies vary with regards to the number of classification schemes evaluated (2–6), number of DCIS cases examined (6–180), methodology used (for example, glass slides or 35 mm transparencies), statistical analysis (kappa statistic vs. percentage agreement), number of participating pathologists (2–23), and experience of the pathologists (expert breast pathologists vs. general surgical pathologists). A teaching set of slides was not provided for any of the studies, and learning mainly relied on the original scientific papers describing the classification schemes, with the exception of one study which provided illustrated tutorials for participants [48].

In the study of Douglas-Jones et al. [47], two expert pathologists independently classified the DCIS component of 180 invasive carcinomas using six different published classification schemes. The six classification schemes used were:

1. traditional architecture-based (comedo, solid, cribriform, micropapillary, mixed);
2. based on nuclear grade (similar to that used by the UKNBCSP);
3. the Van Nuys classification;
4. the Holland classification;
5. the Nottingham classification; and
6. based on extent of necrosis (divided into three categories: extensive necrosis, DCIS with necrosis and DCIS without necrosis).

The total overall agreement was 54% between the two pathologists for all the classification schemes. When classifying by extent of necrosis, the interobserver agreement was 82%. The authors found the lowest interobserver disagreement for the Van Nuys (21%) and Nottingham (22%) classifications, and the highest disagreement when using a traditional architectural classification (34%). The UKNBCSP (cytonuclear grade) and Holland classifications were intermediate in disagreement (29% and 30% respectively).

In the paper by Scott et al. [59], only 16 cases were studied, but six pathologists were involved. Interestingly, the participating pathologists reviewed color 35 mm slides (transparencies) of each case (and not glass microscope slides), on two separate occasions. Pathologists first classified lesions using a two-tier system into low or high grade lesions (noncomedo vs. comedo). A second review was made using a three-tier system (modified Lagios classification). The agreement was only 56% with the two-tier system, but increased to 94% with the three-tier system (there was disagreement over one case regarding intermediate vs. high grade). It should be noted that the authors

purposefully included cases which would provide difficulty arriving at a consensus using a two-tier (dichotomous) system such as comedo vs. non-comedo, possibly influencing the final analysis.

In another study, 23 European pathologists (associated with the European Commission Working Group on Breast Screening Pathology) categorized 33 cases of DCIS using five classification systems [61]. Three of the classification schemes were three-tier (Holland, Van Nuys, and UKNBCSP) and two were two-tier (the same classification as UKNBCSP but using only presence or absence of high nuclear grade and a classification based on presence or absence of comedonecrosis). A teaching set of slides was not distributed, but participants were given the articles in which the classification schemes were described. Amongst the classification schemes using three categories, the Van Nuys gave highest overall kappa statistic (0.42 or moderate agreement), while the Holland and UKNBSP classifications had similar kappa statistics of 0.37 and 0.35, respectively (or fair agreement). The authors concluded from their data that adding cell polarization (for instance to the Holland classification) did not improve reproducibility. The middle category in all the three-tier classifications had the worst kappa statistic: 0.25 (fair) and 0.19 (slight) and 0.17 (slight) for Van Nuys, Holland and UKNBSP classifications, respectively. When the two-tier classifications were utilized, the classification based on nuclear grade (modified UKNBCSP) had a higher kappa statistic than that based on comedonecrosis (0.46 vs. 0.34, respectively). The authors concluded that the most reliable histological feature was nuclear grade (high vs. low) and necrosis (as long as recognition of comedonecrosis was not a requirement). Nonetheless, the highest kappa statistic was only 0.46 (considered moderate).

In another study from New Zealand, 11 pathologists examined 25 cases of DCIS [48]. The Holland, Van Nuys and traditional architectural classifications were compared. All pathologists received a tutorial and photomicrographs for training prior to studying the test cases. These investigators found that interobserver agreement was worst in architectural classification, mainly due to the difficulty in classifying lesions with more than one pattern, with a kappa statistic of 0.13 (slight) for cases with more than one architectural type. The best agreement was achieved using the Van Nuys scheme (kappa statistic of 0.66 or substantial), with most discordances due to difficulty in classifying luminal necrosis. The Holland classification achieved a kappa statistic of 0.57 (or moderate).

Sneige et al. assessed interobserver reproducibility in the classification of DCIS using the Lagios grading system [138]. In that study, 125 DCIS cases were reviewed by six pathologists following review of a training set of 12 cases and of written criteria. Complete agreement among the six observers was seen in 35% of cases, and five of six agreed on 71% the cases. Pairwise kappa values ranged from fair to substantial (0.30 to 0.61). Generalized kappa value indicated moderate agreement (0.46). The authors concluded that further refinements are needed, particularly if grading is to influence future therapy.

The most recent study of interobserver agreement is by Wells et al. [139]. This study is unique in that seven general surgical pathologists without expertise in breast pathology participated, and their interpretations were compared to those of three expert breast pathologists. Three classification schemes were studied: Holland, modified Lagios and Van Nuys. Forty cases of DCIS were utilized (six had associated invasive carcinoma). Diagnostic accuracy (non-expert vs. expert), interobserver agreement (between non-experts), and intraobserver reproducibility (for individual non-expert pathologists) were analyzed using kappa statistics. Overall, the best interobserver agreement amongst non-experts was achieved using the Holland classification (kappa = 0.46 or moderate), compared to the modified Lagios and Van Nuys classifications (kappa statistic = 0.26 or fair for both). The Holland classification also showed the best overall agreement between experts and non-experts (kappa statistic = 0.53) compared to the modified Lagios and Van Nuys classifications (both 0.29). The Holland classification was also best for assessing nuclear grade with a kappa statistic of 0.49 between expert and non-expert, and kappa statistic of 0.45 among non-experts. Interestingly, the best interobserver agreement for the non-experts was achieved with the modified Lagios classification (kappa statistic of 0.57) and the worst with the Van Nuys classification (kappa statistic of 0.29).

In 1997, a consensus conference was convened in an attempt to reach agreement on the classification of DCIS [54]. While the panel did not endorse any one system of classification, there was agreement that certain features be routinely documented in pathology reports of DCIS lesions. These include nuclear grade (low, intermediate or high grade), the presence of necrosis (comedo or punctate), cell polarization, and architectural pattern(s). In fact, if these individual features are recorded, there will be sufficient information available to permit the categorization of a DCIS lesion according to virtually all of the recently proposed, three-tiered classification schemes.

PROGNOSTIC FACTORS

Numerous retrospective studies have identified a variety of features associated with local recurrence of

DCIS or progression to invasive breast cancer following breast-conserving therapy (for example, excision with or without radiation therapy). Results from these studies are difficult to compare due to differences in patient selection, extent of surgery, details of radiation therapy, histological classification, and length of follow-up. Features that have been most consistently reported to be associated with a higher risk of local recurrence or progression to invasive breast cancer are high grade, the presence of comedonecrosis, larger tumor size and, in particular, involved margins of excision [140, 141]. However, the relative importance of these factors is poorly understood and has varied among these studies [55]. The status of the margins of excision is arguably the most important of these factors. For example, in one large, retrospective study, neither size, nuclear grade, nor comedonecrosis were significant prognostic factors for local recurrence if the lesion was excised with margins of 10 mm or more [5]. These factors may, however, be of importance with smaller margin widths [5].

The need to consider length of follow-up in evaluating the potential prognostic importance of histologic features is emphasized by the results of the study of Solin and colleagues [111]. In that study, patients whose DCIS showed a combination of comedo architecture and grade 3 nuclei had a significantly higher 5-year local recurrence rate after conservative surgery and radiotherapy than patients whose DCIS did not show this combination of features (11% vs. 2%, respectively; p = 0.009). However, at 10 years, this difference was no longer statistically significant (18% vs. 15%, respectively, p = 0.15).

Silverstein et al. have suggested that the histological type of DCIS, size of the lesion, and width of the margins can be combined into a prognostic index to predict the likelihood of local recurrence after breast-conserving therapy and to select treatment options, for instance excision alone, excision plus radiation therapy or mastectomy [142]. Although all of the factors included in the so-called Van Nuys Prognostic Index (VNPI) are likely to be important considerations in the selection of treatment options for patients with DCIS, their relative importance and the interactions among them are not well understood [55]. In fact, the group that initially proposed the VNPI subsequently reported that, for DCIS lesions excised with a negative margin ≥ 10 mm, neither nuclear grade nor lesion size were significant prognostic factors for local recurrence in patients treated with excision and radiation therapy or excision alone [5]. Thus, margin status appears to be the overriding prognostic factor in this population. Nevertheless, whether or not margin width by itself can identify a subset of patients who do not benefit from postoperative radiation therapy remains an unresolved issue. Most recently, Silverstein

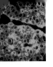

has added age to histological type, size, and margin status in the development of a revised University of Southern California/Van Nuys prognostic index [143].

Data from the pathological analysis of patients enrolled in two prospective randomized clinical trials of breast-conserving therapy for DCIS have also indicated that certain pathological features appear to be associated with an increased risk of local recurrence. In the NSABP B-17 trial, nuclear grade, comedonecrosis, margin status and histological type were significant prognostic variables for local recurrence in univariate analysis [114]. However, in multivariate analysis, the presence of comedonecrosis and margin status were the only independent pathological features associated with local recurrence [114]. In contrast, in an analysis of data from the EORTC 10853 trial, the presence of solid and cribriform architectural patterns and involved margins were significantly associated with local recurrence in multivariate analysis [10].

Currently, the only biological marker that appears to provide clinically useful information in DCIS is estrogen receptor status. In a recent analysis of data from the NSABP-B24 trial, designed to evaluate the role of tamoxifen in the treatment of patients with DCIS treated with breast-conserving surgery and radiation therapy, the use of tamoxifen was associated with a significantly reduced risk of local recurrence, but only for patients whose DCIS was estrogen receptor-positive [144]. As a result of this study, determination of the estrogen receptor status of DCIS is now becoming a routine part of the pathologic evaluation of these lesions.

One clinical feature that appears to be an important prognostic factor for local recurrence following breast-conserving therapy for DCIS is patient age at diagnosis. In several studies, young patient age has been associated with a significantly increased risk of local recurrence [145]. While this may in part be explained by a higher frequency of adverse pathologic prognostic factors in the DCIS of younger patients, the possibility that this could also be due to differences in treatment factors such as extent of surgical excision, or to inherent biological differences in DCIS in younger and older patients cannot be excluded.

■ PATHOLOGY OF VARIANTS OF DCIS

Variants of DCIS possess either special types of growth pattern, for instance papillary type, or special cellular differentiation of neoplastic cells, such as apocrine change. Moreover, there is a small group of precursor lesions which are rarely seen and typically only observed associated with their invasive counterparts, such as adenoid cystic carcinoma.

PAPILLARY DCIS

DEFINITION

Synonym: noninvasive papillary carcinoma
ICD-O code: O8503/2
Variant: intracystic papillary carcinoma, ICD-O code: 8504/2

Like its benign counterpart this tumor is characterized by its papillary growth pattern. However, in contrast to papillomas the fibrovascular cores are covered by a malignant epithelium. Keys to correct diagnosis are, therefore, identifying the tumor's papillary structures as well as recognizing their malignant epithelium. We would like to emphasize that many papillary in-situ carcinomas have additional DCIS of nonpapillary-type in the adjacent breast tissue (Chapter 6). Papillary-type carcinoma is predominantly grade 1 or 2.

CLINICAL FEATURES

Papillary DCIS comprises less than 2% of all breast carcinomas [38, 146]. The lesion usually occurs in older patients, with an average age of 65 years [146–152]. Papillary DCIS presents clinically as serosanguinous nipple discharge and/or as mammographic mass or, less frequently, as microcalcification [153]. Furthermore, papillary DCIS can present as a solitary, circumscribed nodule, which may be partially or completely cystic (encysted papillary carcinoma). Clinical findings are similar to benign papillomas and cannot be employed in differentiating between benign and malignant lesions. Half of all cases are located centrally, the other half peripherally. Papillary DCIS usually has an excellent prognosis [150, 154].

MACROSCOPY

Papillary DCIS is typically circumscribed and sometimes nodular with a fibrous margin (Fig. 20.32a). The lesions are tan or gray and may show varying degrees of hemorrhage. Some tumors exhibit cystic change. Peripheral papillary DCIS may present as fibrotic lesions with nodular or microcystic areas. The size of the lesions varies, the average size being 2–3 cm. Rare cystic cases may measure up to 5–10 cm. Papillary DCIS is regarded as a variant of intraductal carcinoma and should be treated in the same way.

MICROSCOPY

The key features of papillary DCIS are its papillary structure and its malignant epithelium. The prototypical lesion contains arborizing papillae with delicate fibrovascular cores, a single glandular cell population with nuclear hyperchromasia and striking nuclear uniformity. These papillations usually lack a myoepithelial cell layer [155] (Fig. 20.32c–d). They may be broad with cores that show extensive sclerosis. The epithelium covering the fibrovascular cores is the feature determining the malignancy of lesions. The principal growth patterns of the neoplastic cells are the same as in classical DCIS (described above). Thus micropapillary and cribriform growth (with its variants) or even solid patterns may be seen [150, 154, 156–159]. Solid growth of tumor cells may completely fill the lumina between the papillary fibrovascular

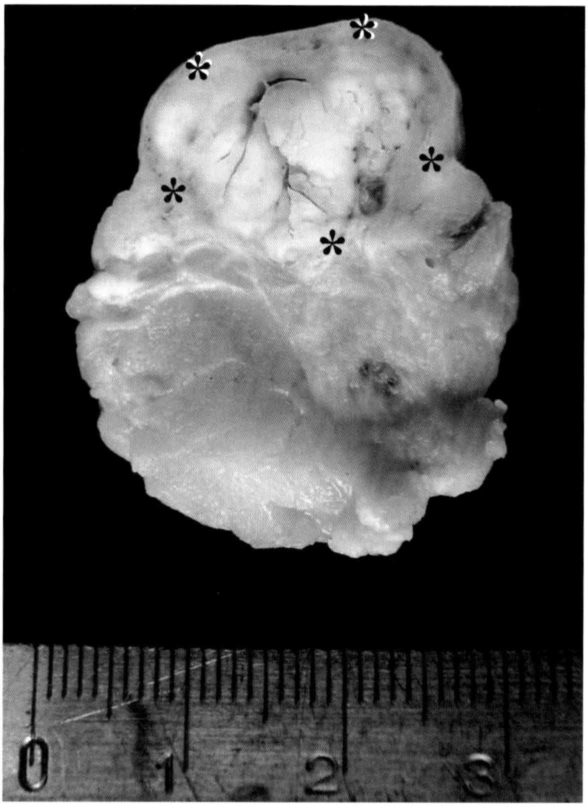

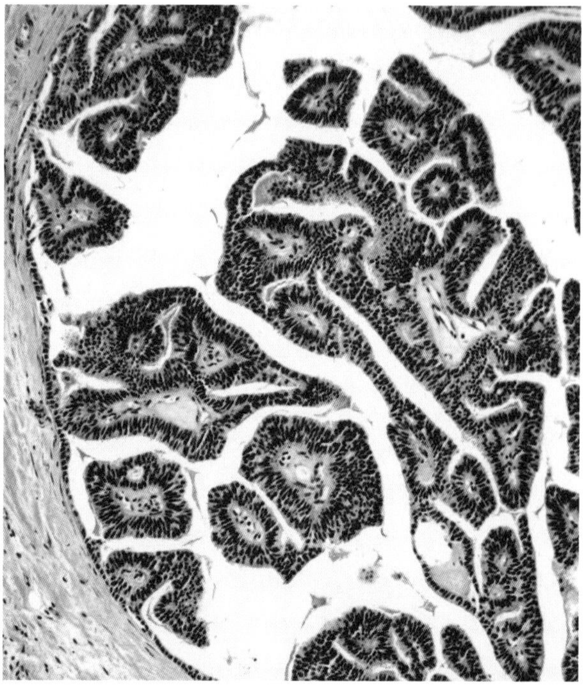

Fig. 20.32a–f Low grade DCIS, papillary type.

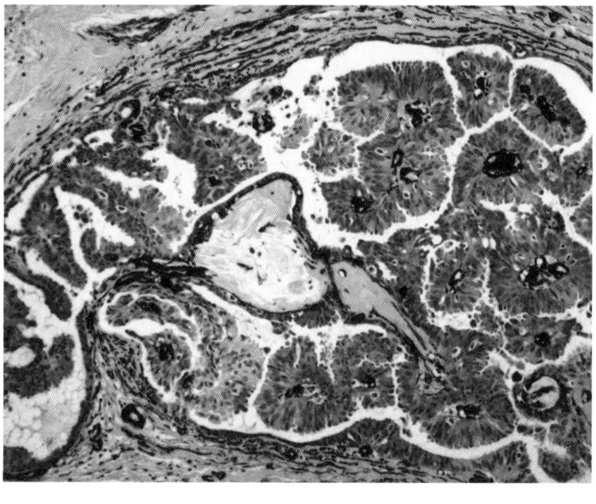

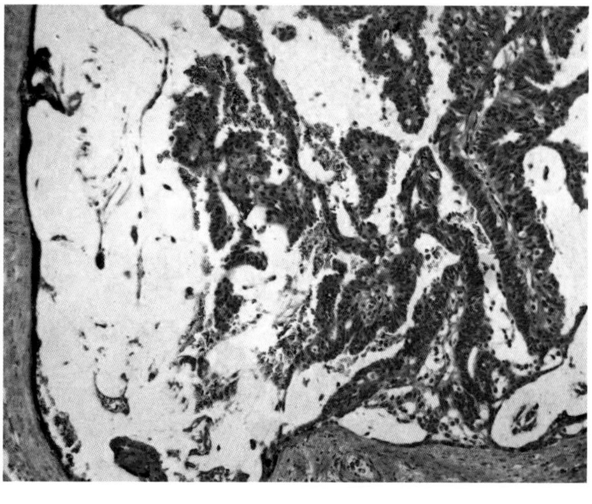

20.32a Macroscopic view of a central DCIS, papillary type. Note the fibrous capsule (asterisks). In the lower field normal fibrofatty breast tissue (courtesy of Dr. Kellner, Minden).

20.32b H&E section demonstrating the atypical monotonous cell population with oval, dark, multilayering staining of nuclei. The fibrovascular stroma of the papillae contains many small blood vessels. A myoepithelial cell layer is not seen.

20.32c Sm-actin immunostaining shows positivity of 'blood vessels' and myofibroblasts in the surrounding stroma. Because the blood vessels are very close to the atypical epithelium, it is impossible to exclude the presence of myoepithelial cells. The lack of a myoepithelial layer can be demonstrated using immunostaining for p63 or calponin, which do not react with smooth-muscle cells or myofibroblasts.

20.32d Ck5 immunostaining showing some residual normal epithelium on the left. The papillary lesions lack any positivity. As p63 was also negative, the presence of myoepithelial cells could be ruled out. This confirms the diagnosis of a low grade DCIS, papillary-type.

Continuation

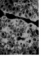

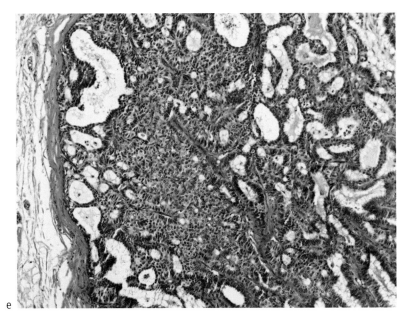

e

Fig. 20.32a–f Low grade DCIS, papillary type.
20.32e Another low grade papillary-type DCIS. H&E section showing a solid to cribriform growth pattern of monotonous cells.

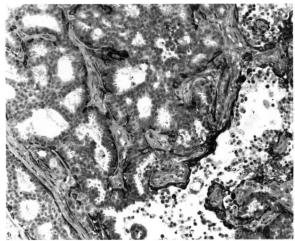

f

20.32f Ck5/6 immunostaining with positive staining of the well-developed myoepithelial cell layer. Note that the features that define DCIS are atypical glandular cells despite the presence of the myoepithelial cell layer.

cores so as to obliterate the papillary pattern [160]. The neoplastic cells are usually polygonal to cuboidal, with the cytoplasm being lightly eosinophilic to amphophilic in character. Neuroendocrine features, signet-ring, plasmacytoid, spindle or clear cell cytological variants of papillary carcinoma have all been described [159, 161–164]. The most common is the apocrine variant. Using gross cystic disease fluid protein-15 (GCDFP) stains, Papotti [165] found apocrine changes in 50% of papillary carcinomas. Cytoplasmic and extracellular mucin can sometimes be observed [159]. Most lesions can be classified as low or intermediate grade DCIS (Figs 20.32 and 20.34), however high grade variants occur (Fig. 20.33).

Some papillary DCIS have cores which are covered by a pavement-like cylindrical epithelium, which is dome-shaped or highly columnar and usually shows some tufting. The apical border of the cells may show apocrine snouts, or they may be truncated, hobnailed

(Fig. 20.34a), or display blurring (Fig. 20.34b). The oval nuclei are enlarged and appear crowded and irregularly placed due to an 'up-and-down' placement (Fig. 20.34b). Sometimes the basal neoplastic cells show a pagetoid appearance with a dimorphic glandular cell type [150], which, if it consists of only two layers, may be mistaken for a normal double layer (Fig. 20.35a–b). The tumor cells show a faintly eosinophilic polygonal cytoplasm and contrast against the luminal neoplastic columnar tumor cells. By excluding the myoepithelial nature of the basal neoplastic cells through immunostaining for sm-actin, S-100 and cytokeratins, Lefkowitz et al. [150] concluded that both 'cell differentiations' are glandular in nature. Thus, both are phenotypes of the same neoplastic glandular cell proliferation.

Although papillary DCIS usually lacks the normal myoepithelial cell layer within the papillae, the presence of such a layer does not exclude this

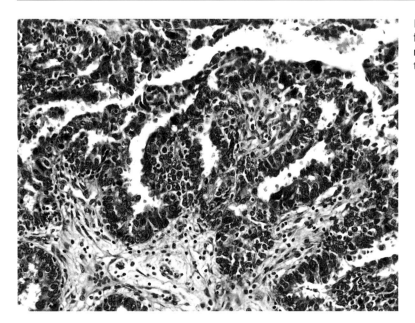

Fig. 20.33 High grade papillary DCIS. This figure shows polymorphous, hyperchromatic nuclei with uneven placement, so that grade 3 seems appropriate.

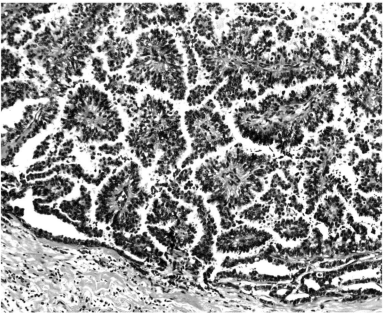

a

Fig. 20.34a–c Central, papillary, intermediate grade DCIS, cylinder cell type.
20.34a Papillary lesion with slender arborizing papillae in a dilated duct and its ramifications. Note the periductal fibrosis and a slight inflammatory reaction.
20.34b High magnification of another case with slender papillae paved by a malignant cylindrical epithelium with blurring of the apical cell border. The oval nuclei are enlarged and appear crowded and irregularly placed due to an 'up-and-down' placement. Compared to low grade the nuclei are enlarged with a coarser chromatin, so that a grade 2 seems appropriate.
20.34c Ck5/6 immunostaining highlights the well-developed myoepithelial layer.

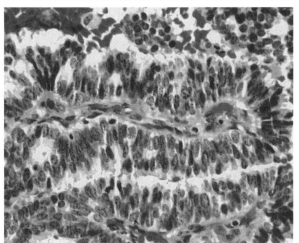

b

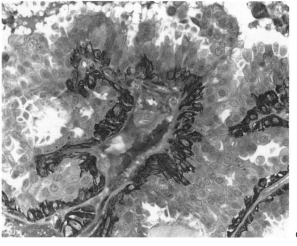

c

diagnosis [147, 156, 165–169]. A complete absence of the myoepithelial layer usually indicates malignancy. There are, however, cases that contain a myoepithelial layer in parts or even throughout the lesion [165, 168]. The diagnosis of malignancy in these cases is made with reference to the cytological and/or architectural features of the proliferating epithelial cells. The myoepithelial layer is best identified by means of cytokeratin 5/14 (Figs 20.32f and 20.34c) or specific myoepithelial markers such as calponin, maspin or by p63.

As in its benign counterpart, papillary carcinoma may demonstrate a marked fibrosis with entrapment of epithelial structures. Care should be taken not to consider this as invasion. Only a small proportion of papillary DCIS displays foci of invasive carcinoma

[148, 170]. The most reliable evidence of invasion is the demonstration of tumor in the surrounding parenchyma or fibro-fatty tissue (Fig. 20.36). Finally, in a recent study of cystic papillary carcinomas, the authors were unable to demonstrate a delimiting layer of myoepithelial cells around the periphery of the lesion using any of five sensitive myoepithelial cell markers [171]. While this may be the result of myoepithelial cell compression and atrophy caused by an expansile intraductal lesion, this finding raises the possibility that at least some papillary carcinomas considered to be in-situ lesions based on conventional morphologic criteria actually are, after all, circumscribed, expansile nodules of invasive carcinoma.

For details of atypical ductal proliferation ex papilloma see Chapter 11.

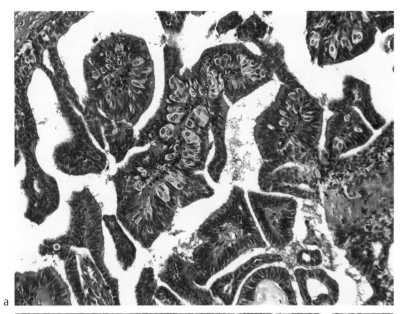

a

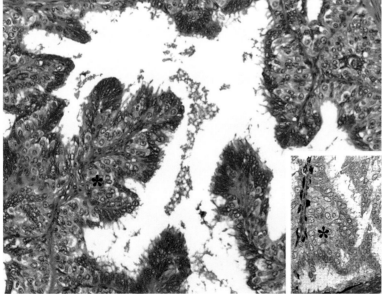

b

Fig. 20.35a–c Papillary-type dimorphic DCIS.

20.35a Low power view showing the dimorphic glandular cell type, which consists of two layers. These may be mistaken for a normal double layer. Immunostaining for P63 showed the absence of a myoepithelial cell layer.

20.35b Another case with dimorphic glandular cell type. The basal tumor cells show a faintly eosinophilic polygonal cytoplasm and stand out against the neoplastic luminal tumor cells which are coboidal and have a more basophilic cytoplasm. Ck5 immunostaining (insert) shows some residual myoepithelial cells. The basal tumor cells lack Ck5 (asterisks).

Continuation

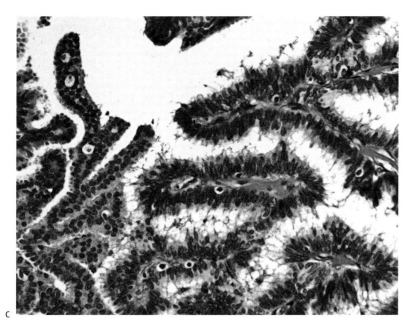

c

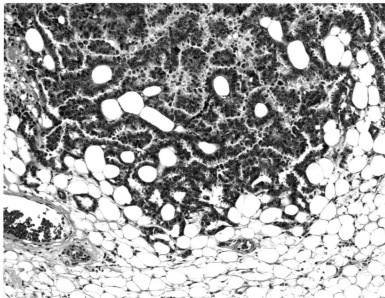

Fig. 20.35a–c Papillary-type dimorphic DCIS.
20.35c An area of another lesion at higher magnification showing a different type of dimorphic pattern. On the right the cylindrical cell type, on the left a more monomorphic cell growth with round, even nuclei that per se would be classified as grade 1.

Fig. 20.36 Papillary carcinoma with clear invasion of fatty tissue.

IMMUNOHISTOCHEMISTRY

Papillary DCIS consists of an atypical, usually monomorphic single glandular cell proliferation which in histology is the most important feature in diagnosing malignancy. Thus the tumor cells stain for glandular cytokeratins 8/18, but not for basal cytokeratins 5/14. Furthermore the non-high grade variants are usually strongly positive for both estrogen and progesterone. The tumors usually lack a myoepithelial layer thus showing a negative staining for calponin and p63. But this is an inconsistent feature as some papillary carcinomas contain a well-developed myoepithelial layer (Fig. 20.34c) [168, 172, 173]. It should be noted that sm-actin immunostaining decorates myofibroblasts and pericytes surrounding small blood vessels of the fibro-vascular stalks, which may misleadingly be interpreted as indicative of the presence of myoepithelial cells.

DIFFERENTIAL DIAGNOSIS

See Chapter 11.

APOCRINE CELL DCIS

DEFINITION

Apocrine DCIS denotes lesions composed of cells with apocrine features [174–176]. The incidence of apocrine DCIS is probably low, since the incidence of apocrine invasive carcinoma is only 0.3–4.0% of all breast carcinomas [174, 177, 178].

CLINICAL FEATURES

There are no clinical or radiological features that are typical of apocrine DCIS [179]. However, apocrine proliferations may present mammographically with intensive polymorphic microcalcification. The clinical course of patients with these lesions seems to be similar to those with nonapocrine DCIS [174]. Thus assessment of the excision margins and treatment by complete removal of the tumor are of great importance.

MACROSCOPY

There are no characteristic features. As in nonapocrine lesions the comedo type lesions may show the characteristic pattern on the cut surface and form a tumor mass.

MICROSCOPY

The most characteristic feature of apocrine tumor cells is the cytoplasm, which is eosinophilic and usually granular in appearance due to the accumulation of mitochondria. The cytoplasm may show more homogeneous eosinophilia or clearing due to the ballooning of cell organelles [180]. Furthermore tumor cells may be interspersed with cells with intracytoplasmic lumina or cytoplasmic mucin production with formation of signet-ring cells. Apocrine DCIS shows the same growth pattern as nonapocrine DCIS. All growth patterns may be found. The most important features for making a diagnosis of apocrine DCIS are its complex architecture and its segmental growth pattern with involvement of ducts and lobules (Fig. 20.37).

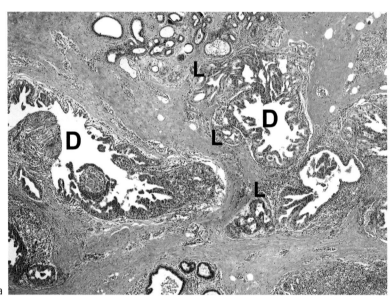

a

Fig. 20.37a – b Low grade apocrine DCIS. **20.37a** Low power view demonstrating the micropapillary growth of the apocrine tumor with involvement of interlobular ducts (D) and lobules (L).

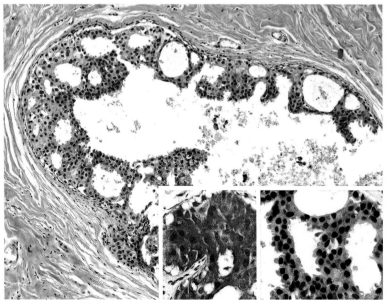

b

20.37b Higher magnification showing the micropapillary-cribriform growth pattern. Note the relatively small cells with eosinophilic cytoplasm which is, however, paler than in classic benign cells. The nuclei are dark and monotonous with inconspicuous nucleoli. The insets highlight the expression of GCDFP-15 (left) and androgen receptor in the nuclei (right) respectively.

In-situ carcinomas with apocrine differentiation are usually categorized as grade 3. This classic type is characterized by marked nuclear polymorphism with nuclear size two to three times that of usual cells (Fig. 20.38) [181], mitoses and central comedonecrosis. Nuclear membranes are prominent, and there is usually a coarse granular chromatin. The nucleoli are heavily enlarged and prominent with either basophilic or eosinophilic staining. These lesions often display a periductal inflammatory reaction and fibrosis. Grade 3 carcinomas are not generally difficult to diagnose [90, 182].

Low grade apocrine DCIS usually has darker and more monotonous nuclei with inconspicuous nucleoli. The cells are smaller and have a paler cytoplasm than their benign apocrine counterparts (Fig. 20.38a and c) [183]. The classification of in-situ lesions at the lower end of the spectrum is still an area of controversy (see Chapter 19) [158, 176, 181, 184].

IMMUNOHISTOCHEMISTRY

The apocrine tumor cells immunostain for the glandular cytokeratins 8/18, but not for basal cytokeratins 5 and 14. Immunostaining with antibody 34βE12 (against Ck1, 5, 10, 14 and others) shows a mixed reaction with intensively stained positive and completely negative cells, even in the same lesion. Apocrine DCIS usually expresses androgen receptors and is negative for estrogen and progesterone receptors [175, 185]. GCDFP-15 has been reported to be expressed in about 75% of invasive breast tumors with apocrine features [186, 187] (Fig. 20.37b). This ratio, however, could not be reproduced by other authors [188]. Moreover, the apocrine tumor cells do

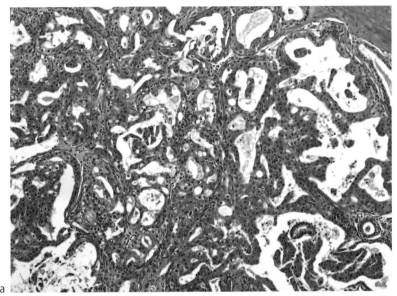

a

b

Fig. 20.38a–c Apocrine DCIS vs. benign apocrine hyperplasia.
20.38a Low grade apocrine DCIS. The solid to cribriform growth pattern of cells with pale eosinophilic cytoplasm, dark nuclei and inconspicuous nucleoli classifies this lesion as low grade apocrine DCIS.

20.38b High grade DCIS with large apocrine cells containing overtly malignant nuclei. Note the variation in size of nuclei and the large nucleoli. *Continuation*

not express the bcl-2 proto-oncogene product, a 25 kDa protein located at the inner mitochondrial membrane [189]. The bcl-2 protein prolongs the survival of cells by interfering with the mechanisms of programmed cell death.

ATYPICAL APOCINE HYPERPLASIA/APOCRINE DCIS VS. APOCRINE CHANGE AND HYPERPLASIA

Apocrine metaplasia and hyperplasia must be distinguished from neoplastic apocrine cell growth [183, 190]. Because they both frequently demonstrate distension of lobular units and may even be found in several lobules, the differential diagnostic criteria have to include both the cytology and architecture of the lesion. Benign apocrine cells reveal abundant eosinophilic cytoplasm with a granular appearance and large uniform vesicular nuclei with prominent nucleoli [191]. These lesions may display a growth pattern with micropapillary and papillary structures, and sometimes display an even more complex architecture (Fig. 20.38c). Care is needed here to avoid overdiagnosing the benign lesions as atypical.

The cells of low grade malignant apocrine proliferations usually have a paler cytoplasm and are smaller than benign apocrine cells. They may display select apical cytoplasmic snouts. In addition, the nuclei are usually minimally hyperchromatic and generally have inconspicuous or small nucleoli. All these features lend the lesion a bland appearance so that atypical apocrine hyperplasia and low grade apocrine DCIS may be underdiagnosed [183].

As can be seen from benign apocrine change, the presence of large vesicular nuclei with prominent nucleoli of apocrine cells is not in itself indicative of malignancy [183, 192]. Thus, distinguishing benign lesions from high grade apocrine DCIS of small size

may also be difficult and requires strict criteria. High grade malignant apocrine lesions show a greater degree of polymorphism, larger nucleoli, an elevated nuclear cytoplasmic ratio and usually a greater degree of cytoplasmic basophilia. The overall context in which the lesions are found, the extent of the apocrine proliferation and an assessment of nuclear and architectural features usually help in reaching a final diagnosis.

Grade 1 apocrine DCIS vs. atypical apocrine hyperplasia (see Chapter 19)

Atypical apocrine proliferation in benign proliferative breast disease (see Chapters 9, 11 and 19)

CYSTIC HYPERSECRETORY DCIS

This variant was first described in 1984 by Rosen and Scott and later by other authors [184, 193, 194]. It is characterized by an accumulation of abundant colloid-like, deeply eosinophilic material in cystically dilated TDLUs, which are usually lined by a clinging-type or micropapillary malignant epithelium, grade 2 or 3. Clinically, these lesions present as a mass or palpable lesion. Macroscopically, cystic hypersecretory lesions usually form a mass 1–10 cm in diameter, containing multiple cystic spaces with a gelatinous material (Fig. 20.39). Histologically, the hallmarks of cystic hypersecretory DCIS are cysts filled with colloid-like secretory material that stains heavily with eosin, and a malignant epithelium (Fig. 20.40b). The tumor forms a clinging-type malignant epithelium associated with micropapillary tufts, both of which consist of crowded cells with hyperchromatic, enlarged and clearly malignant nuclei. The malignant cells show frayed apical borders. The cytoplasm is eosinophilic and may have a vacuolated appearance due to secretory vacuoles. The

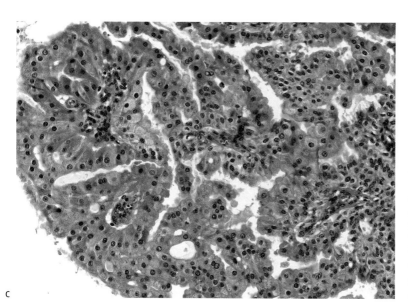

c

Fig. 20.38a–c Apocrine DCIS vs. benign apocrine hyperplasia.
20.38c Benign apocrine hyperplasia in a case of usual hyperplasia showing typical apocrine cells with abundant eosinophilic granular cytoplasm and large nuclei with prominent nucleoli. Notice that, due to the typical benign apocrine cell appearance, the more complex growth pattern alone does not justify classification of this lesion as atypical.

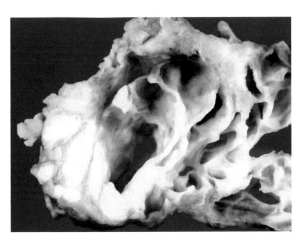

Fig. 20.39 Cystic hypersecretory DCIS. Macroscopic appearance of a cystic hypersecretory DCIS. Note multiple cystic structures aggregated to a tumor-forming mass (courtesy of Prof. Pfeifer, Bonn).

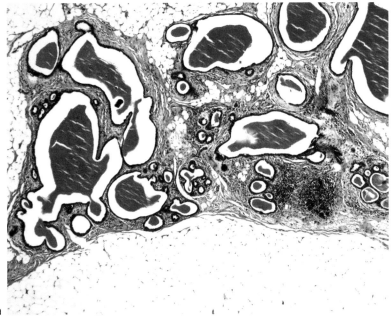

Fig. 20.40a–c High grade cystic hypersecretory DCIS.

20.40a Low power view, demonstrating the colloid-like, deeply eosinophilic material within the cystic spaces. Note the flat, micropapillary epithelium.

20.40b Medium power view. At this level a micropapillary tufting of the lining epithelium can be seen. Furthermore there is a small invasive carcinoma.

20.40c High power view. It is only at this magnification level that the high grade nuclei of the flat epithelium of the cysts are evident. The cells of the infiltrating component display the same nuclear features. Based on the overtly malignant nuclei of the flat/micropapillary epithelium, the in-situ lesion must be classified as grade 3 DCIS.

a

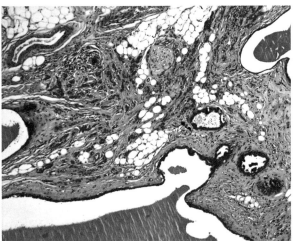

b

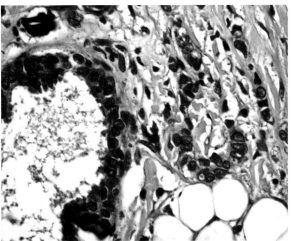

c

cytoplasm is immunoreactive for lactalbumin and carcinoembryonic antigen. Furthermore, the tumor cells may stain for S-100 and cytokeratin 5. Most cases are intermediate to high nuclear grade. As the lesions may also contain areas with invasive growth, extensive sampling is mandatory [184] to exclude an associated invasive carcinoma, which, if present, is usually of high grade ductal-type.

In core needle biopsy cystic hypersecretory lesions can be identified due to their characteristic secretory material. Depending on the type of epithelium seen in the core lesions they should be classified as B3 or B4. Excisional biopsy is required to make a definite diagnosis. The differential diagnosis should consider cystic hypersecretory hyperplasia, which, by definition, only contains epithelium with a bland appearance (see Chapter 3), periductal mastitis usually with irregularly dilated ducts, fibrosis/hyalinosis of duct walls along with inspissated eosinophilic material and, finally, fibrocystic change.

SECRETORY(JUVENILE)-TYPE DCIS

These lesions are characterized by intra- and extracellular secretion with formation of pale pink and vacuolated milk-like material (Fig. 20.41). The tumor cells have small monotonous nuclei. Their cytoplasm is pale to clear and sometimes vacuolated due to the formation of cytoplasmic membrane bound vacuoles [195, 196]. The tumor cells stain for alpha-lactalbumin and S-100 [196–198]. These tumors are usually negative for estrogen receptor. In secretory tumors, typical features of apocrine differentiation are often evident [199]. DCIS of either secretory- or low-grade-type may be seen.

MUCINOUS DCIS

This rare variant of DCIS is characterized by the formation of extracellular mucin (Fig. 20.42). Usually a conventional ductal cell type with varying growth patterns [159] may be seen. The mucinous material is generally far less conspicuous than in invasive mucinous carcinoma. Several authors have demonstrated the relationship between mucin production, papillary growth pattern and neuroendocrine differentiation [160, 200–204]. As applies to other variants of DCIS, this type should be classified by nuclear grade, size, and adequacy of excision [107].

MUCOCELE-LIKE DCIS

Mucocele-like DCIS can be regarded as a subtype of mucinous DCIS characterized by an abundance of extracellular mucin that can even spill into the surrounding stroma (Fig. 20.43). Clinically, the lesions may present as a palpable mass. Mammographically mucocele-like DCIS presents as a nodular lesion, which may have coarse calcifications. On ultrasound the lesion is usually a hypoechoic, round to lobulated mass [205, 206]. Macroscopically, mucocele-like DCIS appears as an aggregation of mucin-filled cysts. The histological hallmarks are large amounts of extracellular mucin in cystically dilated TDLUs and the presence of a malignant epithelium. The epithelial lining is usually monomorphic or cuboidal with occasional micropapillary growth patterns. In other parts of the aggregated cysts the epithelium may be completely absent. The cysts are segregated by fibrous stroma. Several authors have shown the association of

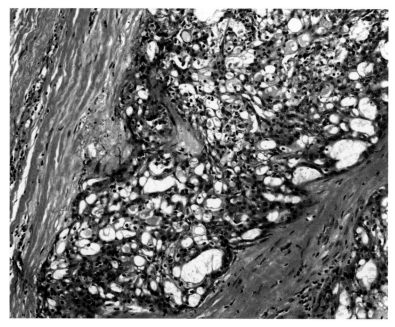

Fig. 20.41 Secretory-type DCIS. Note that the tumor cells form numerous small microglandular lumina and have a vacuolated cytoplasm. Secretory material is seen in the small glandular lumina.

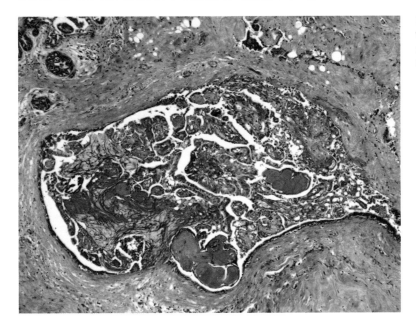

Fig. 20.42 Mucinous DCIS. Papillary lesion with predominantly clinging-type carcinoma with production of extracellular mucin.

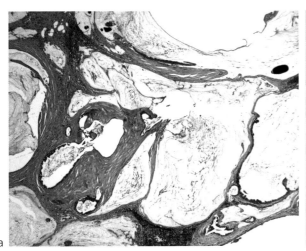

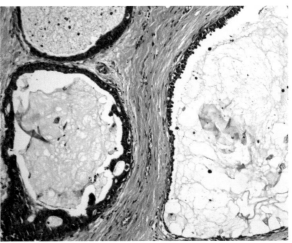

a   b

Fig. 20.43a–b Mucocele-like DCIS.
20.43a Low power view showing large amounts of extracellular mucin in cystically dilated TDLUs. There is spilling of mucin into the fibrous background eliciting an inflammatory reaction. Many cysts lack an epithelial lining.
20.43b Higher magnification showing cysts with a malignant clinging/micropapillary epithelium in the left field combined with bland flat to cuboidal epithelium with apocrine snouts in the right field.

this lesion with an invasive component [207–209]. Malignant mucocele-like lesions furthermore are usually combined with areas of their benign counterpart showing only bland flat to cuboidal epithelium [207–210]. Rupture of cysts with spilling of mucin into surrounding tissue may exacerbate difficulties in distinguishing these lesions from invasive mucinous carcinoma. The presence of benign mucocele-like areas and of DCIS helps in recognizing their true nature. Furthermore, the mucin in mucinous carcinoma is interspersed with blood vessels, in contrast to the mucinous lakes of mucocele-like lesions. In core biopsies these lesions are classified as B3 or B4, usually requiring an excisional biopsy for a definite diagnosis.

SIGNET-RING CELL DCIS

Two types of signet-ring cell carcinomas are described in the most recent WHO classification. One is characterized by intracytoplasmic lumina and usually related to lobular carcinoma, while the other is characterized by an accumulation of cytoplasmic mucosubstances [211]. Signet-ring cell DCIS [212] is characterized by abundant intracellular production of mucin, which stains positively with diastase-PAS or alcian blue and which is immunoreactive for E-cadherin (Fig. 20.44). A second type of signet-ring change is caused by intracytoplasmic lumina that displace the nucleus to one side. This type may be found in lobular neoplasia

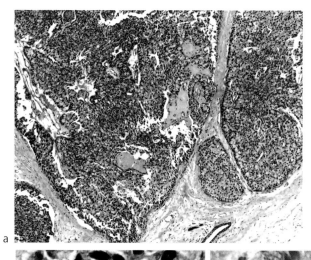

Fig. 20.44a–e Signet-ring cell DCIS.
20.44a Low power view with distended 'ductal structures' containing a papillary proliferation with typical signet-ring cells.

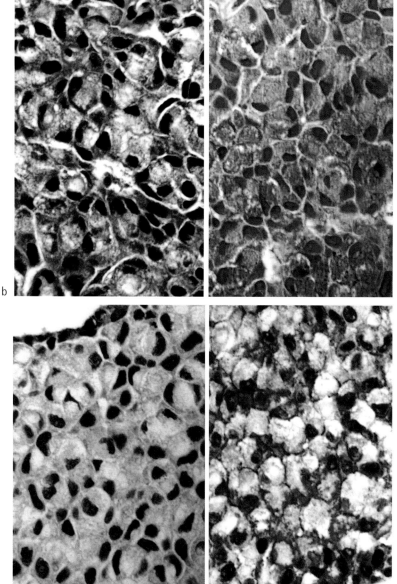

20.44b High power view demonstrating the signet-ring cell appearance.
20.44c Accumulation of mucin with the formation of vacuolated cytoplasm stained with alcian blue.
20.44d Immunostaining for Ck5/6 demonstrates some original normal cells at the luminal border.
20.44e Immunostaining for E-cadherin. Intense reaction for E-cadherin indicating the ductal phenotype.

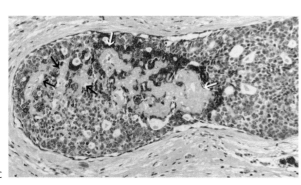
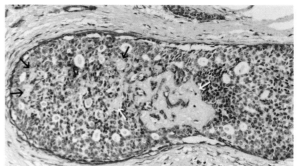

c   d

Fig. 20.48a–d DCIS associated with a classic-type adenoid cystic carcinoma.
20.48c Ck5/6 staining of the same lesion showing mainly Ck5/6+ cells, which surround the hyaline spherules, with basement membrane material (arrows). The latter immunostains for collagen IV and laminin.
20.48d Sm-actin staining at higher magnification to show the myoepithelial cells surrounding the spherules (arrows).

DIFFERENTIAL DIAGNOSIS

In most cases, diagnosis of DCIS is straightforward and can be reached by morphological assessment alone. Some lesions, however, may present diagnostic difficulties, and in such cases, immunohistochemical studies usually help to solve the problem.

CONVENTIONAL DCIS (LOW, HIGH AND INTERMEDIATE GRADE DCIS)

LOW GRADE DCIS MUST BE DISTINGUISHED FROM UDH (SEE CHAPTER 8)

The distinguishing features between these lesions are summarized in Table 8.2 in Chapter 8. To render a diagnosis of UDH the lesion must consist of a heterogeneous cell population with variability in cellular and nuclear shape, in size and placement, with streaming of cells and the formation of irregular secondary lumina. In Ck5/14 immunohistochemistry, a mosaicism of Ck5/14+ and Ck5/14– cells is characteristic. This is in contrast to the homogeneous clonal proliferation of Ck8/18+ and Ck5/14– cells in ADH and in low grade DCIS with its typical 'rigid' and geometric growth pattern. Recently established molecular data showing differences between UDH and ADH/low grade DCIS support this view, but are of no practical importance in daily routine diagnosis.

It should further be borne in mind that residual normal cells that stain for cytokeratin 5 and 14 may persist in ADH/DCIS. These can easily be distinguished from the Ck5/14– neoplastic cells, and their presence should not, therefore, lead to an erroneous diagnosis of UDH.

DISTINGUISHING ADH FROM LIMITED EXAMPLES OF LOW GRADE DCIS REMAINS A MAJOR PROBLEM (SEE CHAPTER 19)

It has been shown in several studies that the current qualitative and quantitative criteria proposed to define ADH still lead to unacceptably low levels of inter-observer agreement even among experienced breast pathologists, with kappa statistics as low as 0.25 [243–245]. The major problem appears to be determining a threshold above which a given lesion is diagnosed as low grade DCIS. The WHO working group was unable to reach a consensus on a size threshold that should be applied in differential diagnosis. As is discussed in more detail in Chapter 19, the fact that ADH is usually confined to one or a few separate lobules, whereas low grade DCIS is characterized by its segmental ductal extension may be helpful. This is in line with the quantitative approach of Page et al. [246] and Tavassoli et al. [247], defining ADH as a predominantly small lesion (about 2 mm or less than two basement-bound spaces) restricted to a single or separate ductal lobular structure(s).

DIFFERENTIAL DIAGNOSIS OF LOW GRADE DCIS ALSO INCLUDES CLASSIC ALH/LCIS

This is especially true if the lesion forms more solid growth patterns. Difficulties may be caused by similarities in cell type with small monomorphic cells and round, usually hyperchromatic nuclei, and the overlap in lobular/ductal extension, with ductal involvement by ALH/LCIS and lobular involvement by DCIS. Finally, some lesions consist of coexisting DCIS/LCIS in the same breast and even in the same ductal lobular unit. In rare cases the cytological features are sufficiently indeterminate to preclude a definitive diagnosis. Poor cellular cohesion and the presence of intracytoplasmic lumina favor ALH/LCIS, whereas cohesive growth, lack of cytoplasmic lumina, polarization of cells at the periphery of the involved spaces and microacinar formation favor a diagnosis of low grade DCIS [192]. In problematical cases, immunostaining for E-cadherin may be of value, since ALH/LCIS are usually E-cadherin-negative whereas the cells of DCIS are E-cadherin-positive.

DIAGNOSING HIGH GRADE DCIS IS USUALLY FAIRLY EASY

These lesions are composed of large cells with enlarged pleomorphic nuclei, often prominent nucleoli, and numerous, sometimes atypical mitoses. In evaluating the nuclear grade it may be helpful to compare the nuclear size of the tumor cells with adjacent red blood cells. The nuclear size of high grade DCIS usually exceeds three red blood cells in diameter. Often there is associated periductal fibrosis and inflammatory reaction. This may cause irregularities of the contours of the involved spaces and thus lead to an erroneous diagnosis of microinvasion (see above). Less than 3% of high grade DCIS cases express Ck5/6 and Ck8/18. Coexpression of these cytokeratins in this histological context should not lead to an erroneous diagnosis of UDH.

DISTINGUISHING INTERMEDIATE GRADE DCIS FROM UDH MAY BE A PROBLEM (SEE CHAPTER 19)

This problem may arise because the cellular/nuclear features and the growth patterns of intermediate grade DCIS and some cases of UDH may overlap. Even with the use of standardized histological criteria, it may not be possible to reach a definite diagnosis based on H&E sections alone. In this context the use of cytokeratin 5 and 14 immunostaining is very helpful, in as much as UDH displays the typical Ck5/14 mosaicism in contrast to the Ck8/18+, Ck5/14− tumor cells of DCIS.

Pitfalls of Ck5/14+ clonal proliferations with monotonous cells and nuclei are discussed in Chapter 19.

SPECIAL TYPES OF DCIS

PAPILLARY TYPE DCIS VS. PAPILLOMA (SEE CHAPTER 10)

A variety of benign and malignant lesions exhibit papillae, so that the presence of papillae alone is insufficient for reaching a definite diagnosis. In papillary lesions the absence of myoepithelial cells may be helpful in making a diagnosis of papillary carcinoma. However, the presence of myoepithelial cells does not exclude a diagnosis of papillary malignancy [168]. From our own experience, we fully support this view. Smaller lesions, in particular, may show both distinct, clearly malignant epithelium and a distinct myoepithelial lining. Thus, the presence of malignant cells with usually hyperchromatic nuclei and a characteristic

growth pattern is the true indicator of DCIS, in striking contrast to the bland appearing nuclei in papillomas. In most of these lesions DCIS in the surrounding breast tissue can be recognized. In solid papillary DCIS, the spindling of the cells may cause problems in differential diagnosis with papilloma associated with UDH. In this context Ck5 and 14 immunostaining nearly always leads to the right diagnosis, as the tumor cells of papillary carcinomas are Ck5/14− in contrast to the Ck5/14 mosaicism of the epithelium of a papilloma with UDH (see Chapters 8 and 11).

MALIGNANT APOCRINE LESIONS (SEE CHAPTER 19)

These lesions must be distinguished from benign apocrine metaplasia and hyperplasia. As apocrine cells represent metaplasias of differentiated glandular cells it follows that Ck5/14 immunostains are of no help in this differential diagnostic context. Rather, it is the type of proliferating cell and its architectural features that allow malignant apocrine proliferation to be distinguished from benign apocrine cells. This is discussed in more detail above and in Chapter 19.

DCIS WITH DIFFERENT TYPES OF 'SECRETORY FEATURES'

Such DCIS poses special problems in differential diagnosis from benign 'counterparts'. Mucocele-like lesions seem to represent a continuum from benign to malignant invasive mucinous carcinoma [210]. The distinguishing feature between mucocele-like DCIS and benign mucocele-like lesions is the presence of highly atypical cells with clinging or micropapillary growth. Cystic hypersecretory DCIS on the other hand combines a typical colloid-like, eosinophilic secretion with the features of a malignant epithelium. Benign counterparts again have a bland, benign epithelium. A careful search for malignancy in both types of lesions by investigating multiple blocks is necessary.

Special types of DCIS such as those associated with adenoid cystic carcinoma and adenosquamous carcinoma are not described as pure in-situ malignancy. The question as to whether collagenous spherulosis is a precursor of adenoid cystic carcinoma is theoretically interesting, but has no practical and clinical implications as these lesions are not known to be associated or followed by breast carcinoma (Chapter 3).

PURE SQUAMOUS CELL DCIS (SEE CHAPTER 3)

This type of lesion is exceptionally rare. It is easily recognized by its prickle cell appearance and its horn pearls. These tumors express both Ck5/6 and Ck10 and are thus easily distinguished from grade 3 DCIS, which expresses Ck8/18 and, in a small number of cases, coexpresses Ck5/6.

REFERENCES

1. Holland R, Faverley D. The local distribution of ductal carcinoma in-situ of the breast: whole-organ studies. In: Silverstein MJ, Recht A, Lagios MD, editors. Ductal Carcinoma In-Situ of the Breast. 2nd ed. Philadelphia: Lippincott Williams & Wilkins; 2003. p.240–8.
2. Betsill WL, Jr., Rosen PP, Lieberman PH, Robbins GF. Intraductal carcinoma. Long-term follow-up after treatment by biopsy alone. JAMA 1978;239:1863–7.
3. Page DL, Dupont WD, Rogers LW, Landenberger M. Intraductal carcinoma of the breast: follow-up after biopsy only. Cancer 1982;49:751–8.
4. Page DL, Dupont WD, Rogers LW, Jensen RA, Schuyler PA. Continued local recurrence of carcinoma 15–25 years after a diagnosis of low grade ductal carcinoma in-situ of the breast treated only by biopsy. Cancer 1995;76:1197–200.
5. Silverstein MJ, Lagios MD, Groshen S, et al. The influence of margin width on local control of ductal carcinoma in-situ of the breast. N Engl J Med 1999; 340:1455–61.
6. Lagios MD. Heterogeneity of ductal carcinoma in-situ of the breast. J Cell Biochem Suppl 1993;17G:49–52.
7. Lagios MD, Margolin FR, Westdahl PR, Rose MR. Mammographically detected duct carcinoma in-situ. Frequency of local recurrence following tylectomy and prognostic effect of nuclear grade on local recurrence. Cancer 1989;63:618–24.
8. Holland R, Hendriks JH, Vebeek AL, Mravunac M, Schuurmans Stekhoven JH. Extent, distribution, and mammographic/histological correlations of breast ductal carcinoma in-situ. Lancet 1990;335:519–22.
9. Lagios MD, Westdahl PR, Margolin FR, Rose MR. Duct carcinoma in-situ. Relationship of extent of noninvasive disease to the frequency of occult invasion, multicentricity, lymph node metastases, and short-term treatment failures. Cancer 1982;50:1309–14.
10. Bijker N, Peterse JL, Duchateau L, et al. Histological type and marker expression of the primary tumour compared with its local recurrence after breast-conserving therapy for ductal carcinoma in-situ. Br J Cancer 2001;84:539–44.
11. Goldstein NS, Murphy T. Intraductal carcinoma associated with invasive carcinoma of the breast. A comparison of the two lesions with implications for intraductal carcinoma classification systems. Am J Clin Pathol 1996;106:312–8.
12. Buerger H, Otterbach F, Simon R, et al. Comparative genomic hybridization of ductal carcinoma in-situ of the breast-evidence of multiple genetic pathways. J Pathol 1999;187:396–402.
13. Buerger H, Simon R, Schafer KL, et al. Genetic relation of lobular carcinoma in-situ, ductal carcinoma in-situ, and associated invasive carcinoma of the breast. Mol Pathol 2000;53:118–21.
14. Lagios MD. Duct carcinoma in-situ. Pathology and treatment. Surg Clin North Am 1990;70:853–71.
15. Tavassoli FA. Ductal intraepithelial neoplasia. In: Pathology of the Breast. 2nd ed. Stanford, Connecticut: Appleton & Lange; 1999. p.260–323.
16. Buerger H, Schmidt H, Beckmann A, et al. Genetic characterisation of invasive breast cancer: a comparison of CGH and PCR based multiplex microsatellite analysis. J Clin Pathol 2001;54:836–40.
17. Boecker W, Moll R, Dervan P, et al. Usual ductal hyperplasia of the breast is a committed stem (progenitor) cell lesion distinct from atypical ductal hyperplasia and ductal carcinoma in-situ. J Pathol 2002;198:458–67.
18. Vos CB, ter Haar NT, Rosenberg C, et al. Genetic alterations on chromosome 16 and 17 are important features of ductal carcinoma in-situ of the breast and are associated with histologic type. Br J Cancer 1999;81:1410–8.
19. Kuukasjärvi T, Tanner M, Pennanen S, et al. Genetic changes in intraductal breast cancer detected by comparative genomic hybridization. Am J Pathol 1997; 150:1465–71.
20. Tavassoli FA. Ductal intraepithelial neoplasia of the breast. Virchows Arch 2001;438:221–7.
21. Cleton-Jansen AM, Buerger H, Haar N, et al. Different mechanisms of chromosome 16 loss of heterozygosity in well- versus poorly differentiated ductal breast cancer. Genes Chromosomes Cancer 2004;41:109–16.
22. Otterbach F, Bankfalvi A, Bergner S, et al. Cytokeratin 5/6 immunohistochemistry assists the differential diagnosis of atypical proliferations of the breast. Histopathol 2000;37:232–40.
23. Korsching E, Packeisen J, Agelopoulos K, et al. Cytogenetic alterations and cytokeratin expression patterns in breast cancer: integrating a new model of breast differentiation into cytogenetic pathways of breast carcinogenesis. Lab Invest 2002;82:1525–33.
24. Perou CM, Sorlie T, Eisen MB, et al. Molecular portraits of human breast tumours. Nature 2000;406:747–52.
25. Sorlie T, Perou CM, Tibshirani R, et al. Gene expression patterns of breast carcinomas distinguish tumor subclasses with clinical implications. Proc Natl Acad Sci U S A 2001;98:10869–74.
26. Siziopikou KP, Schnitt SJ. MIB-1 Proliferation Index in Ductal Carcinoma In-Situ of the Breast: Relationship to the Expression of the Apoptosis-Regulating Proteins bcl-2 and p53. Breast J 2000;6:400–6.
27. Dooley WC, Ljung BM, Veronesi U, et al. Ductal lavage for detection of cellular atypia in women at high risk for breast cancer. J Natl Cancer Inst 2001;93:1624–32.
28. Stomper PC, Margolin FR. Ductal carcinoma in-situ: the mammographer's perspective. AJR Am J Roentgenol 1994;162:585–91.
29. Leborgne RA. The breast in roentgen diagnosis. Montevideo: 1953.
30. Tabár L, Dean PB, Tot T. Teaching Atlas of Mammography. 3rd ed. Stuttgart, New York: Thieme; 2001.
31. Black JW, YOUNG B. A radiological and pathological study of the incidence of calcification in diseases of the breast and neoplasms of other tissues. Br J Radiol 1965;38:596–8.
32. Citoler P. Microcalcifications of the breast. In: Grundmann B, editor. Early diagnosis of breast cancer. New York: Fischer,G.; 1978. p.113–8.
33. Egan RL, McSweeney MB, Sewell CW. Intramammary calcifications without an associated mass in benign and malignant diseases. Radiology 1980;137:1–7.

34. Gershon-Cohen J. Atlas of mammography. Berlin: Springer; 1970.
35. Holland R, Hendriks JH. Microcalcifications associated with ductal carcinoma in-situ: mammographic-pathologic correlation. Semin Diagn Pathol 1994;11:181–92.
36. Millis RR, Davis R, Stacey AJ. The detection and significance of calcifications in the breast: a radiological and pathological study. Br J Radiol 1976;49:12–26.
37. Wellings SR, Jensen HM, Marcum RG. An atlas of subgross pathology of the human breast with special reference to possible precancerous lesions. J Natl Cancer Inst 1975;55:231–73.
38. Azzopardi JG. Problems in Breast Pathology. 1st ed. London: W.B. Saunders; 1979.
39. Ohtake T, Abe R, Kimijima I, et al. Intraductal extension of primary invasive breast carcinoma treated by breast-conservative surgery. Computer graphic three-dimensional reconstruction of the mammary duct-lobular systems [see comments]. Cancer 1995;76:32–45.
40. Schwartz GF, Patchefsky AS, Finklestein SD, et al. Nonpalpable in-situ ductal carcinoma of the breast. Predictors of multicentricity and microinvasion and implications for treatment. Arch Surg 1989;124:29–32.
41. Ottesen GL, Graversen HP, Blichert-Toft M, Zedeler K, Andersen JA. Ductal Carcinoma in-Situ of the Female Breast. Short-Term Results of a Prospective Nationwide Study. Am J Surg Pathol 1992;16:1183–96.
42. Page DL. Breast disease in the 1990s: patchwork quilt or growth industry. Am J Clin Pathol 1993;99:225–6.
43. Johnson JE, Dutt PL, Page DL. Extent and multicentricity of in-situ and invasive carcinoma. In: Bland KI, Copeland EM, editors. The Breast: Comprehensive Management of Benign and Malignant Diseases. 2nd ed. Philadelphia: W.B. Saunders; 1998. p.296–306.
44. Page DL, Rogers LW, Schuyler PA, Dupont WD, Jensen RA. The natural history of ductal carcinoma in-situ of the breast. In: Silverstein MJ, Recht A, Lagios MD, editors. Ductal carcinoma in-situ of the breast. 2nd ed. Philadelphia: Lippincott Williams & Wilkins; 2002. p.17–21.
45. Faverly DR, Burgers L, Bult P, Holland R. Three dimensional imaging of mammary ductal carcinoma in-situ: clinical implications. Semin Diagn Pathol 1994;11:193–8.
46. Millis RR. Classification of ductal carcinoma in-situ. Adv Anat Pathol 1996;3:114–29.
47. Douglas-Jones AG, Gupta SK, Attanoos RL, Morgan JM, Mansel RE. A critical appraisal of six modern classifications of ductal carcinoma in-situ of the breast (DCIS): correlation with grade of associated invasive carcinoma. Histopathol 1996;29:397–409.
48. Bethwaite PB, Smith N, Delahunt B, Kenwright D. Reproducibility of new classification schemes for the pathology of ductal carcinoma in-situ of the breast. J Clin Pathol 1998;51:450–4.
49. Poller DN, Silverstein MJ, Galea M, et al. Ductal Carcinoma in-Situ of the Breast: A Proposal for a New Simplified Histological Classification Association Between Cellular Proliferation and c-erbB2 Protein Expression. Mod Pathol 1994;7:257–62.
50. Silverstein MJ, Poller DN, Waisman JR, et al. Prognostic classification of breast ductal carcinoma-in-situ. Lancet 1995;345:1154–7.
51. Holland R, Peterse JL, Millis RR, et al. Ductal Carcinoma in-Situ: A Proposal for a New Classification. Semin Diagn Pathol 1994;11:167–80.
52. Bellamy CO, McDonald C, Salter DM, Chetty U, Anderson TJ. Noninvasive ductal carcinoma of the breast: the relevance of histologic categorization. Hum Pathol 1993;24:16–23.
53. Schnitt SJ, Connolly JL. Classification of ductal carcinoma in-situ: striving for clinical relevance in the era of breast conserving therapy. Hum Pathol 1997;28:877–80.
54. Consensus conference on the classification of ductal carcinoma in-situ. Hum Pathol 1997;28:1221–5.
55. Schnitt SJ, Harris JR, Smith BL. Developing a prognostic index for ductal carcinoma in-situ of the breast. Are we there yet? Cancer 1996;77:2189–92.
56. Bijker N, Peterse JL, Duchateau L, et al. Risk factors for recurrence and metastasis after breast-conserving therapy for ductal carcinoma-in-situ: analysis of European Organization for Research and Treatment of Cancer Trial 10853. J Clin Oncol 2001;19:2263–71.
57. Allred DC, Bryant J, Land S, et al. Estrogen receptor expression as a predictive marker of the effectiveness of tamoxifen in the treatment of DCIS: Findings from NSABP Protocol B-24. Breast Cancer Res Treat 2002;76:36.
58. Shoker BS, Sloane JP. DCIS grading schemes and clinical implications. Histopathol 1999;35:393–400.
59. Scott MA, Lagios MD, Axelsson K, et al. Ductal carcinoma in-situ of the breast: reproducibility of histological subtype analysis. Hum Pathol 1997;28:967–73.
60. Tavassoli FA. Pathology of the Breast. 1st ed. Norwalk: 1992.
61. Sloane JP, Amendoeira I, Apostolikas N, et al. Consistency achieved by 23 European pathologists in categorizing ductal carcinoma in-situ of the breast using five classifications. European Commission Working Group on Breast Screening Pathology. Hum Pathol 1998;29:1056–62.
62. Anderson TJ, Battersby S. Radial scars of benign and malignant breasts: comparative features and significance. J Pathol 1985;147:23–32.
63. The Consensus Conference Committee. Consensus Conference on the classification of ductal carcinoma in-situ. Cancer 1987;80:1798–802.
64. Recht A, Rutgers EJ, Fentiman IS, et al. The fourth EORTC DCIS Consensus meeting (Chateau Marquette, Heemskerk, The Netherlands, 23–24 January 1998) – conference report. Eur J Cancer 1998;34:1664–9.
65. Tabár L, Dean PB. Basic principles of mammographic diagnosis. Diagn Imaging Clin Med 1985;54:146–57.
66. Eusebi V, Mai KT, Taranger-Charpin A. Tumours of the nipple. In: Tavassoli FA, Devilee P, editors. Tumours of the Breast and Female Genital Organs. Lyon: IARC-Press; 2003. p.104–6.
67. De Potter CR, Foschini MP, Schelfhout AM, Schroeter CA, Eusebi V. Immunohistochemical study of neu protein overexpression in clinging in-situ duct carcinoma of the breast. Virchows Arch A Pathol Anat Histopathol 1993;422:375–80.

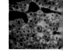

68. Schelfhout VR, Coene ED, Delaey B, et al. Pathogenesis of Paget's disease: epidermal heregulin-alpha, motility factor, and the HER receptor family. J Natl Cancer Inst 2000;92:622–8.

69. Inaji H, Koyama H, Motomura K, Noguchi S. Differential distribution of ErbB2 and pS2 proteins in ductal carcinoma in-situ of the breast. Breast Cancer Res Treat 1996;37:89–92.

70. Quinn CM, Ostrowski JL, Harkins L, Rice AJ, Loney DP. Loss of bcl-2 expression in ductal carcinoma in-situ of the breast relates to poor histological differentiation and to expression of p53 and c-erbB2 proteins. Histopathol 1998;33:531–6.

71. Albonico G, Querzoli P, Ferretti S, Rinaldi R, Nenci I. Biological profile of in-situ breast cancer investigated by immunohistochemical technique. Cancer Detect Prev 1998;22:313–8.

72. Bobrow LG, Happerfield LC, Gregory WM, Millis RR. Ductal carcinoma in-situ: assessment of necrosis and nuclear morphology and their association with biological markers. J Pathol 1995;176:333–41.

73. Naidu R, Yadav M, Nair S, Kutty MK. Expression of c-erbB3 protein in primary breast carcinomas. Br J Cancer 1998;78:1385–90.

74. Done SJ, Arneson NC, Ozcelik H, Redston M, Andrulis IL. p53 mutations in mammary ductal carcinoma in situ but not in epithelial hyperplasias. Cancer Res 1998;58:785–9.

75. Wilbur DC, Barrows GH. Estrogen and progesterone receptor and c-erbB2 oncoprotein analysis in pure in-situ breast carcinoma: an immunohistochemical study. Mod Pathol 1993;6:114–20.

76. van de Vijver MJ, van de BR, Devilee P, et al. Amplification of the neu (c-erbB2) oncogene in human mammmary tumors is relatively frequent and is often accompanied by amplification of the linked c-erbA oncogene. Mol Cell Biol 1987;7:2019–23.

77. Rudas M, Neumayer R, Gnant MF, et al. p53 protein expression, cell proliferation and steroid hormone receptors in ductal and lobular in-situ carcinomas of the breast. Eur J Cancer 1997;33:39–44.

78. Tsuda H, Iwaya K, Fukutomi T, Hirohashi S. p53 mutations and c-erbB2 amplification in intraductal and invasive breast carcinomas of high histologic grade. Jpn J Cancer Res 1993;84:394–401.

79. O'Malley FP, Vnencak JC, Dupont WD, et al. p53 mutations are confined to the comedo type ductal carcinoma in-situ of the breast. Immunohistochemical and sequencing data. Lab Invest 1994;71:67–72.

80. Poller DN, Snead DR, Roberts EC, et al. Oestrogen receptor expression in ductal carcinoma in-situ of the breast: relationship to flow cytometric analysis of DNA and expression of the c-erbB2 oncoprotein. Br J Cancer 1993;68:156–61.

81. Gandhi A, Holland PA, Knox WF, Potten CS, Bundred NJ. Evidence of significant apoptosis in poorly differentiated ductal carcinoma in-situ of the breast. Br J Cancer 1998;78:788–94.

82. Shen KL, Harn HJ, Ho LI, et al. The extent of proliferative and apoptotic activity in intraductal and invasive ductal breast carcinomas detected by Ki-67 labeling and terminal deoxynucleotidyl transferase-mediated digoxigenin-11-dUTP nick end labeling. Cancer 1998;82:2373–81.

83. Kapucuoglu N, Losi L, Eusebi V. Immunohistochemical localization of Bcl-2 and Bax proteins in in-situ and invasive duct breast carcinomas. Virchows Arch 1997; 430:17–22.

84. Leal CB, Schmitt FC, Bento MJ, Maia NC, Lopes CS. Ductal carcinoma in-situ of the breast. Histologic categorization and its relationship to ploidy and immunohistochemical expression of hormone receptors, p53, and c-erbB2 protein. Cancer 1995;75:2123–31.

85. Mourad WA, Setrakian S, Hales ML, Abdulla M, Trucco G. The argyrophilic nucleolar organizer regions in ductal carcinoma in-situ of the breast. The significance of ploidy and proliferative activity analysis using this silver staining technique. Cancer 1994;74:1739–45.

86. Killeen JL, Namiki H. DNA analysis of ductal carcinoma in-situ of the breast. A comparison with histologic features. Cancer 1991;68:2602–7.

87. Radford DM, Fair KL, Phillips NJ, et al. Allelotyping of Ductal Carcinoma in-Situ of the Breast: Deletion of Loci on 8p, 13q, 16q, 17p and 17q. Cancer Research 1995;55:3399–405.

88. O'Connell P, Pekkel V, Fuqua SA, et al. Analysis of loss of heterozygosity in 399 premalignant breast lesions at 15 genetic loci. J Natl Cancer Inst 1998;90:697–703.

89. Fujii H, Marsh C, Cairns P, Sidransky D, Gabrielson E. Genetic divergence in the clonal evolution of breast cancer. Cancer Res 1996;56:1493–7.

90. Stratton MR, Collins N, Lakhani SR, Sloane JP. Loss of heterozygosity in ductal carcinoma in-situ of the breast. J Pathol 1995;175:195–201.

91. Lininger RA, Park WS, Man YG, et al. LOH at 16p13 is a novel chromosomal alteration detected in benign and malignant microdissected papillary neoplasms of the breast. Hum Pathol 1998;29:1113–8.

92. Tsuda H, Fukutomi T, Hirohashi S. Pattern of gene alterations in intraductal breast neoplasms associated with histological type and grade. Clin Cancer Res 1995;1: 261–7.

93. Tsuda H, Takarabe T, Susumu N, et al. Detection of numerical and structural alterations and fusion of chromosomes 16 and 1 in low grade papillary breast carcinoma by fluorescence in-situ hybridization. Am J Pathol 1997;151:1027–34.

94. Tsuda H, Callen DF, Fukutomi T, Nakamura Y, Hirohashi S. Allele loss on chromosome 16q24.2-qter occurs frequently in breast cancers irrespectively of differences in phenotype and extent of spread. Cancer Res 1994; 54:513–7.

95. Radford DM, Fair K, Thompson AM, et al. Allelic loss on a chromosome 17 in ductal carcinoma in-situ of the breast. Cancer Res 1993;53:2947–9.

96. Anbazhagan R, Fujii H, Gabrielson E. Allelic loss of chromosomal arm 8p in breast cancer progression. Am J Pathol 1998;152:815–9.

97. Yaremko ML, Recant WM, Westbrook CA. Loss of heterozygosity from the short arm of chromosome 8 is an early event in breast cancers. Genes Chromosomes Cancer 1995;13:186–91.

98. Yaremko ML, Kutza C, Lyzak J, et al. Loss of heterozygosity from the short arm of chromosome 8 is associated with invasive behavior in breast cancer. Genes Chromosomes Cancer 1996;16:189–95.

99. Coene ED, Schelfhout V, Winkler RA, et al. Amplification units and translocation at chromosome 17q and c-erbB2 overexpression in the pathogenesis of breast cancer. Virchows Arch 1997;430:365–72.

100. Munn KE, Walker RA, Varley JM. Frequent alterations of chromosome 1 in ductal carcinoma in-situ of the breast. Oncogene 1995;10:1653–7.

101. Chappell SA, Walsh T, Walker RA, Shaw JA. Loss of heterozygosity at chromosome 6q in preinvasive and early invasive breast carcinomas. British Journal of Cancer 1997;75:1324–9.

102. Chappell SA, Walsh T, Walker RA, Shaw JA. Loss of heterozygosity at the mannose 6-phosphate insulin-like growth factor 2 receptor gene correlates with poor differentiation in early breast carcinomas. Br J Cancer 1997;76:1558–61.

103. Marsh KL, Varley JM. Loss of heterozygosity at chromosome 9p in ductal carcinoma in-situ and invasive carcinoma of the breast. Br J Cancer 1998;77:1439–47.

104. Chuaqui RF, Zhuang Z, Emmert-Buck MR, Liotta LA, Merino MJ. Analysis of loss of heterozygosity on chromosome 11q13 in atypical ductal hyperplasia and in-situ carcinoma of the breast. Am J Pathol 1997;150:297–303.

105. James LA, Mitchell EL, Menasce L, Varley JM. Comparative genomic hybridisation of ductal carcinoma in-situ of the breast: identification of regions of DNA amplification and deletion in common with invasive breast carcinoma. Oncogene 1997;14:1059–65.

106. Fleming ID, American Joint Committee on Cancer, American Cancer Society. AJCC cancer staging manual. 5th ed. Philadelphia: Lippincott-Raven; 1997.

107. Sloane JP. Quality assurance guidelines for pathology in mammography screening. In: Perry N, Broeders W, de Wolf C, Törnberg S, editors. European guidelines for quality assurance in mammography screening. 3rd ed. 2001. p.159–72.

108. Schuh ME, Nemoto T, Penetrante RB, Rosner D, Dao TL. Intraductal carcinoma. Analysis of presentation, pathologic findings, and outcome of disease. Arch Surg 1986;121:1303–7.

109. Rosner D, Lane WW, Penetrante R. Ductal carcinoma in-situ with microinvasion. A curable entity using surgery alone without need for adjuvant therapy. Cancer 1991;67:1498–503.

110. Wong JH, Kopald KH, Morton DL. The impact of microinvasion on axillary node metastases and survival in patients with intraductal breast cancer. Arch Surg 1990;125:1298–301.

111. Solin LJ, Fowble BL, Yeh IT, et al. Microinvasive ductal carcinoma of the breast treated with breast-conserving surgery and definitive irradiation. Int J Radiat Oncol Biol Phys 1992;23:961–8.

112. Patchefsky AS, Schwartz GF, Finkelstein SD, et al. Heterogeneity of intraductal carcinoma of the breast. Cancer 1989;63:731–41.

113. Silver SA, Tavassoli FA. Mammary ductal carcinoma in-situ with microinvasion. Cancer 1998;82:2382–90.

114. Fisher ER. Pathobiological considerations relating to the treatment of intraductal carcinoma (ductal carcinoma in-situ) of the breast. CA Cancer J Clin 1997;47:52–64.

115. Kerner H, Lichtig C. Lobular cancerization: incidence and differential diagnosis with lobular carcinoma in-situ of breast. Histopathol 1986;10:621–9.

116. Eusebi V, Collina G, Bussolati G. Carcinoma in-situ in sclerosing adenosis of the breast: an immunocytochemical study. Semin Diagn Pathol 1989;6:146–52.

117. Oberman HA, Markey BA. Noninvasive carcinoma of the breast presenting in adenosis. Mod Pathol 1991;4:31–5.

118. Youngson BJ, Cranor M, Rosen PP. Epithelial displacement in surgical breast specimens following needling procedures. Am J Surg Pathol 1994;18:896–903.

119. Youngson BJ, Liberman L, Rosen PP. Displacement of carcinomatous epithelium in surgical breast specimens following stereotaxic core biopsy. Am J Clin Pathol 1995;103:598–602.

120. Lagios MD. Microinvasion in ductal carcinoma in-situ. In: Silverstein MJ, editor. Ductal Carcinoma in-Situ of the Breast. 1st ed. Baltimore: Williams and Wilkins; 1997. p.241–6.

121. Barsky SH, Siegal GP, Jannotta F, Liotta LA. Loss of basement membrane components by invasive tumors but not by their benign counterparts. Lab Invest 1983;49:140–7.

122. Sakr WA, Crissman JD. Immunohistologic distribution of basement membrane in breast neoplasia. Surg Pathol 1988;1:3–12.

123. Gottlieb C, Raju U, Greenwald KA. Myoepithelial cells in the differential diagnosis of complex benign and malignant breast lesions: an immunohistochemical study. Mod Pathol 1990;3:135–40.

124. Hijazi YM, Weiss MA. Use of anti-actin and S-100 protein antibodies in differentiating benign and malignant sclerosing breast lesions. Surg Pathol 1989;2:125–35.

125. Yaziji H, Gown AM, Sneige N. Detection of stromal invasion in breast cancer: the myoepithelial markers. Adv Anat Pathol 2000;7:100–9.

126. Lele SM, Graves K, Gatalica Z. Immunohistochemical detection of maspin is a useful adjunct in distinguishing radial sclerosing lesion from tubular carcinoma of the breast. Appl Immunohistochem Mol Morphol 2000;8:32–6.

127. Barbareschi M, Pecciarini L, Cangi MG, et al. p63, a p53 homologue, is a selective nuclear marker of myoepithelial cells of the human breast. Am J Surg Pathol 2001;25:1054–60.

128. Moritani S, Kushima R, Sugihara H, et al. Availability of CD10 immunohistochemistry as a marker of breast myoepithelial cells on paraffin sections. Mod Pathol 2002;15:397–405.

129. Silverstein MJ. Ductal carcinoma in-situ with microinvasion. In: Silverstein MJ, editor. Ductal Carcinoma in-Situ of the Breast. 1st ed. Baltimore: Williams and Wilkins; 1997. p.557–62.

130. Akhtar S, Michaelson RA, Hutter RV, Leitner SP. Predictors of axillary lymph node mestastases in small (one centimeter or less) T1a,b primary breast cancer. J Clin Oncol 1998;17:120a.

131. Penault-Llorca F, Pomel C, Feillel V, Dauplat J, de Latour M. Microinvasive carcinoma of the breast: Is axillary lymph node dissection indicated? Lab Invest 1998;78:25a.

132. Prasad ML, Osborne MP, Giri DD, Hoda SA. Micro-invasive carcinoma (T1mic) of the breast: clinicopathologic profile of 21 cases. Am J Surg Pathol 2000;24:422–8.

133. Zavotsky J, Hansen N, Brennan MB, Turner RR, Giuliano AE. Lymph node metastasis from ductal carcinoma in-situ with microinvasion. Cancer 1999;85:2439–43.

134. Padmore RF, Fowble B, Hoffman J, et al. Microinvasive breast carcinoma: clinicopathologic analysis of a single institution experience. Cancer 2000;88:1403–9.

135. Mann GB, Port ER, Rizza C, et al. Six-year follow-up of patients with microinvasive, T1a, and T1b breast carcinoma. Ann Surg Oncol 1999;6:591–8.

136. Klauber-DeMore N, Tan LK, Liberman L, et al. Sentinel lymph node biopsy: is it indicated in patients with high-risk ductal carcinoma-in-situ and ductal carcinoma-in-situ with microinvasion? Ann Surg Oncol 2000;7:636–42.

137. De Mascarel I, MacGrogan G, Picot V, Mathoulin-Pelissier S. Prognostic significance of immunohisto-chemically detected breast cancer node metastases in 218 patients. Br J Cancer 2002;87:70–4.

138. Sneige N, Lagios MD, Schwarting R, et al. Interobserver reproducibility of the Lagios nuclear grading system for ductal carcinoma in-situ. Hum Pathol 1999;30:257–62.

139. Wells WA, Carney PA, Eliassen MS, Grove MR, Tosteson AN. Pathologists' agreement with experts and reproducibility of breast ductal carcinoma-in-situ classification schemes. Am J Surg Pathol 2000;24:651–9.

140. Boyages J, Delaney G, Taylor R. Predictors of local recurrence after treatment of ductal carcinoma in-situ: a meta-analysis. Cancer 1999;85:616–28.

141. Harris EE, Solin LJ. The Diagnosis and Treatment of Ductal Carcinoma In-Situ of the Breast. Breast J 2000;6:78–95.

142. Silverstein MJ, Lagios MD, Craig PH, et al. A prognostic index for ductal carcinoma in-situ of the breast. Cancer 1996;77:2267–74.

143. Silverstein MJ. The University of Southern California/Van Nuys prognostic index for ductal carcinoma in-situ of the breast. Am J Surg 2003;186:337–43.

144. Allred DC. Biologic characteristics of ductal carcinoma in-situ. In: Silverstein MJ, editor. Ductal Carcinoma in-Situ of the Breast. Philadelphia: Lippincott Williams & Wilkins; 2002. p.37–48.

145. Vicini FA, Recht A. Age at diagnosis and outcome for women with ductal carcinoma-in-situ of the breast: a critical review of the literature. J Clin Oncol 2002;20:2736–44.

146. Cardenosa G, Eklund GW. Benign papillary neoplasms of the breast: mammographic findings. Radiology 1991;181:751–5.

147. Carter DJ. Intraductal Papillary Tumors of the Breast. A Study of 78 Cases. Cancer 1977;39:1689–92.

148. Fisher ER, Costantino J, Fisher B, et al. Pathologic findings from the National Surgical Adjuvant Breast Project (NSABP) Protocol B-17. Five-year observations concerning lobular carcinoma in-situ. Cancer 1996;78:1403–16.

149. Haagensen CD. Diseases of the Breast. 3rd ed. Philadelphia: W.B. Saunders; 1986.

150. Lefkowitz M, Lefkowitz W, Wargotz ES. Intraductal (intracystic) papillary carcinoma of the breast and its variants: a clinicopathological study of 77 cases. Hum Pathol 1994;25:802–9.

151. Schaefer G, Rosen PP, Lesser ML, Kinne DW, Beattie EJ, Jr. Breast carcinoma in elderly women: pathology, prognosis, and survival. Pathol Annu 1984;19 Pt 1:195–219.

152. Flint A, Oberman HA. Infarction and squamous metaplasia of intraductal papilloma: a benign breast lesion that may simulate carcinoma. Human Pathology 1984;15:764–7.

153. Soo MS, Williford ME, Walsh R, Bentley RC, Kornguth PJ. Papillary carcinoma of the breast: imaging findings. AJR Am J Roentgenol 1995;164:321–6.

154. Carter D, Orr SL, Merino MJ. Intracystic papillary carcinoma of the breast. After mastectomy, radio-therapy or excisional biopsy alone. Cancer 1983;52:14–9.

155. Ciatto S, Andreoli C, Cirillo A, et al. The risk of breast cancer subsequent to histologic diagnosis of benign intraductal papilloma follow-up study of 339 cases. Tumori 1991;77:41–3.

156. Murad TM, Contesso G, Mouriesse H. Papillary tumors of large lactiferous ducts. Cancer 1981;48:122–33.

157. Kraus FT, Neubecker RB. The differential diagnosis of papillary tumors of the breast. Cancer 1962;15:444–55.

158. Tavassoli FA. Pathology of the Breast. 2nd ed. Norwalk: Appleton and Lange; 1999.

159. Rosen PP. Rosen's Breast Pathology. 2nd ed. Philadelphia: Lippincott Williams & Wilkins; 2001.

160. Maluf HM, Koerner FC. Solid papillary carcinoma of the breast. A form of intraductal carcinoma with endocrine differentiation frequently associated with mucinous carcinoma. Am J Surg Pathol 1995;19:1237–44.

161. Dickersin GR, Maluf HM, Koerner FC. Solid papillary carcinoma of breast: an ultrastructural study. Ultrastruct Pathol 1997;21:153–61.

162. Tsang WY, Chan JK. Endocrine ductal carcinoma in-situ (E-DCIS) of the breast: a form of low grade DCIS with distinctive clinicopathologic and biologic characteristics. Am J Surg Pathol 1996;20:921–43.

163. Sapino A, Righi L, Cassoni P, et al. Expression of apocrine differentiation markers in neuroendocrine breast carcinomas of aged women. Mod Pathol 2001;14:768–76.

164. Raju U, Vertes D. Breast papillomas with atypical ductal hyperplasia: a clinicopathologic study. Hum Pathol 1996;27:1231–8.

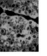

165. Papotti M, Gugliotta P, Ghiringhello B, Bussolati G. Association of breast carcinoma and multiple intra-ductal papillomas: A histological and immunohisto-chemical investigation. Histopathol 1984;8:963–75.

166. Murad TM, Swaid S, Pritchett P. Malignant and benign papillary lesions of the breast. Hum Pathol 1977;8: 379–90.

167. Azzopardi JG. Papilloma and papillary carcinoma. In: Problems in Breast Pathology. 1st ed. Philadelphia: WB Saunders; 1979. p.150–66.

168. Raju UB, Lee MW, Zarbo RJ, Crissman JD. Papillary neoplasia of the breast: immunohistochemically defined myoepithelial cells in the diagnosis of benign and malignant papillary breast neoplasms. Mod Pathol 1989;2:569–76.

169. Chan JK, Saw D. One or two cell types in papillary carcinoma of the breast? Pathology 1986;18: 479–80.

170. McDivitt RW, Holleb AI, Foote F-WJ. Prior breast disease in patients treated for papillary carcinoma. Arch Pathol 1968;85:117–24.

171. Carlo VP, Hwang H, Barry T, Gown AM, Schnitt SJ. Cystic Papillary Carcinoma and Solid Papillary Carcinomas of the Breast: In-Situ or Invasive Lesions? [abstract]. Mod Pathol 2004;17:25A.

172. MacGrogan G, Moinfar F, Raju U. Intraductal papillary neoplasms. In: Tavassoli FA, Devilee P, editors. Tumours of the Breast and Female Genital Organs. Lyon: IARC Press; 2003. p.76–80.

173. Moinfar F, Man YG, Lininger RA, Bodian C, Tavassoli FA. Use of keratin 35betaE12 as an adjunct in the diagnosis of mammary intraepithelial neoplasia-ductal-type – benign and malignant intraductal proliferations. Am J Surg Pathol 1999;23:1048–58.

174. Abati AD, Kimmel M, Rosen PP. Apocrine mammary carcinoma. A clinicopathologic study of 72 cases. Am J Clin Pathol 1990;94:371–7.

175. Leal C, Henrique R, Monteiro P, et al. Apocrine ductal carcinoma in-situ of the breast: histologic classification and expression of biologic markers. Hum Pathol 2001;32:487–93.

176. Tavassoli FA, Norris HJ. Intraductal apocrine carcinoma: a clinicopathologic study of 37 cases. Mod Pathol 1994;7:813–8.

177. Azzopardi JG. Apocrine carcinoma. In: Problems in Breast Pathology. London: W.B. Saunders; 1979. p.341–5.

178. Frable WJ, Kay S. Carcinoma of the breast. Histologic and clinical features of apocrine tumours. Cancer 1968;21:756–63.

179. Damiani S, Eusebi V, Losi L, D'Adda T, Rosai J. Onco-cytic carcinoma (malignant oncocytoma) of the breast. Am J Surg Pathol 1998;22:221–30.

180. Eusebi V, Millis RR, Cattani MG, Bussolati G, Azzopardi JG. Apocrine carcinoma of the breast. A morphologic and immunocytochemical study. Am J Pathol 1986;123:532–41.

181. O'Malley FP, Page DL, Nelson EH, Dupont WD. Ductal Carcinoma In-Situ of the Breast With Apocrine Cytology. Definition of a Borderline Category. Hum Pathol 1994;25:164–8.

182. Ellis IO, Elston CW, Poller DN. Ductal carcinoma in-situ. In: Elston CW, Ellis IO, editors. The Breast. Edinburgh, London, New York: Churchill Livingstone; 1998. p.249–81.

183. Raju U, Zarbo RJ, Kubus J, Schultz DS. The Histologic Spectrum of Apocrine Breast Proliferations: A Comparative Study of Morphology and DNA Content by Image Analysis. Hum Pathol 1993;24:173–81.

184. Jensen RA, Page DL. Cystic hypersecretory carcinoma: what's in a name? [letter]. Arch Pathol Lab Med 1988;112:1179–50.

185. Selim AG, Wells CA. Immunohistochemical localisation of androgen receptor in apocrine metaplasia and apocrine adenosis of the breast: relation to oestrogen and progesterone receptors. J Clin Pathol 1999;52: 838–41.

186. Mazoujian G, Bodian C, Haagensen DE, Jr., Haagensen CD. Expression of GCDFP-15 in breast carcinomas. Relationship to pathologic and clinical factors. Cancer 1989;63:2156–61.

187. Mazoujian G, Pinkus GS, Davis S, Haagensen DE, Jr. Immunohistochemistry of a gross cystic disease fluid protein (GCDFP-15) of the breast. A marker of apocrine epithelium and breast carcinomas with apocrine features. Am J Pathol 1983;110:105–12.

188. Kumar S, Mansel RE, Jasani B. Presence and possible significance of immunohistochemically demonstrable prolactin in breast apocrine metaplasia. Br J Cancer 1987;55:307–9.

189. Tavassoli FA, Purcell CL, Bratthauer GL. Androgen receptor positivity along with loss of bcl-2, ER and PR expression in benign and malignant apocrine lesions of the breast. Implications for therapy. Breast 1996;2: 1–10.

190. Costa MJ, Silverberg SG. Oncocytic carcinoma of the male breast. Arch Pathol Lab Med 1989;113: 1396–9.

191. McDivitt R, Stewart FW, Berg JW. Atlas of Tumour Pathology. 2nd series ed. Washington: 1968.

192. Sloane JP. Biopsy Pathology of the Breast. Vol. 24, 2nd edition ed. London: Arnold; 2001.

193. Guerry P, Erlandson RA, Rosen PP. Cystic hyper-secretory hyperplasia and cystic hypersecretory duct carcinoma of the breast. Pathology, therapy, and follow-up of 39 patients. Cancer 1988;61:1611–20.

194. Page DL, Dupont WD, Jensen RA. Papillary apocrine change of the breast: associations with atypical hyper-plasia and risk of breast cancer. Cancer Epidemiol Biomarkers Prev 1996;5:29–32.

195. Yildirim E, Turhan N, Pak I, Berberoglu U. Secretory breast carcinoma in a boy. Eur J Surg Oncol 1999;25: 98–9.

196. Akhtar M, Robinson C, Ali MA, Godwin JT. Secretory carcinoma of the breast in adults. Light and electron microscopic study of three cases with review of the literature. Cancer 1983;51:2245–54.

197. Hartman AW, Magrish P. Carcinoma of breast in children. Ann Surg 1955;141:792–7.

198. Lamovec J, Bracko M. Secretory carcinoma of the breast: light microscopical, immunohistochemical and flow cytometric study. Mod Pathol 1994;7:475–9.

199. Nguyen GK, Neifer R. Aspiration biopsy cytology of secretory carcinoma of the breast. Diagn Cytopathol 1987;3:234–7.

200. Capella C, Usellini L, Papotti M, et al. Ultrastructural features of neuroendocrine differentiated carcinomas of the breast. Ultrastruct Pathol 1990;14:321–34.

201. Capella C, Eusebi V, Mann B, Azzopardi JG. Endocrine differentiation in mucoid carcinoma of the breast. Histopathol 1980;4:613–30.

202. Koenig C, Tavassoli FA. Nodular hyperplasia, adenoma, and adenomyoma of Bartholin's gland. Int J Gynecol Pathol 1998;17:289–94.

203. Scopsi L, Andreola S, Pilotti S, et al. Mucinous carcinoma of the breast. A clinicopathologic, histochemical, and immunocytochemical study with special reference to neuroendocrine differentiation. Am J Surg Pathol 1994;18:702–11.

204. Komaki K, Sakamoto G, Sugano H, Morimoto T, Monden Y. Mucinous carcinoma of the breast in Japan. A prognostic analysis based on morphologic features. Cancer 1988;61:989–96.

205. Kim Y, Takatsuka Y, Morino H. Mucocele-like Tumor of the Breast: A Case Report and Assessment of Aspirated Cytological Specimens. Breast Cancer 1998; 5:317–20.

206. Yeoh GP, Cheung PS, Chan KW. Fine-needle aspiration cytology of mucocelelike tumors of the breast. Am J Surg Pathol 1999;23:552–9.

207. Ro JY, Sneige N, Sahin AA, et al. Mucocelelike tumor of the breast associated with atypical ductal hyperplasia or mucinous carcinoma. A clinicopathologic study of seven cases. Arch Pathol Lab Med 1991;115:137–40.

208. Kulka J, Davies JD. Mucocele-like tumours: more associations and possibly ductal carcinoma in-situ? Histopathol 1993;22:511–2.

209. Fisher CJ, Millis RR. A mucocele-like tumour of the breast associated with both atypical ductal hyperplasia and mucoid carcinoma. Histopathol 1992;21:69–71.

210. Weaver MG, Abdul-Karim FW, al Kaisi N. Mucinous lesions of the breast. A pathological continuum. Pathol Res Pract 1993;189:873–6.

211. Ellis IO, Schnitt SJ, Sastre-Garau X, et al. Invasive breast carcinoma. In: Tavassoli FA, Devilee P, editors. Tumours of the Breast and Female Genital Organs. Lyon: IARC-Press; 2003. p.13–62.

212. Harris M, Wells S, Vasudev KS. Primary signet ring cell carcinoma of the breast. Histopathol 1978;2: 171–6.

213. Merino MJ, LiVolsi VA. Signet ring carcinoma of the female breast: a clinicopathologic analysis of 24 cases. Cancer 1981;48:1830–7.

214. Fukunaga M, Ushigome S. Small cell (oat cell) carcinoma of the breast. Pathol Int 1998;48:744–8.

215. Sebenik M, Nair SG, Hamati HF. Primary small cell anaplastic carcinoma of the breast diagnosed by fine needle aspiration cytology: a case report. Acta Cytol 1998;42:1199–203.

216. Papotti M, Gherardi G, Eusebi V, Pagani A, Bussolati G. Primary oat cell (neuroendocrine) carcinoma of the breast. Report of four cases. Virchows Arch A Pathol Anat Histopathol 1992;420:103–8.

217. Wade PM, Jr., Mills SE, Read M, et al. Small cell neuroendocrine (oat cell) carcinoma of the breast. Cancer 1983;52:121–5.

218. Francois A, Chatikhine VA, Chevallier B, et al. Neuroendocrine primary small cell carcinoma of the breast. Report of a case and review of the literature. Am J Clin Oncol 1995;18:133–8.

219. Wolff M, Reimis MS. Breast cancer in the male: clinicopathological study of 40 patients and review of the literature. In: Fenoglio C, Wolff M, editors. Progress in surgical pathology. New York: Mason Publishing; 1981. p.77–109.

220. Samli B, Celik S, Evrensel T, Orhan B, Tasdelen I. Primary neuroendocrine small cell carcinoma of the breast. Arch Pathol Lab Med 2000;124:296–8.

221. Deeley TJ. Secondary deposits in the breast. Br J Cancer 1965;19:738–43.

222. Hadju SI, Urban JA. Cancers metastatic to the breast. Cancer 1972;29:1691–6.

223. Shin SJ, Delellis RA, Rosen PP. Small cell carcinoma of the breast – additional immunohistochemical studies. Am J Surg Pathol 2001;25:831–2.

224. Fisher ER, Palekar AS, Gregorio RM, Paulson JD. Mucoepidermoid and squamous cell carcinomas of breast with reference to squamous metaplasia and giant cell tumors. Am J Surg Pathol 1983;7:15–27.

225. Kaufman MW, Marti JR, Gallager HS, Hoehn JL. Carcinoma of the breast with pseudosarcomatous metaplasia. Cancer 1984;53:1908–17.

226. Wargotz ES, Norris HJ. Metaplastic carcinomas of the breast: V. Metaplastic carcinoma with osteoclastic giant cells. Hum Pathol 1990;21:1142–50.

227. Wargotz ES, Norris HJ. Metaplastic carcinomas of the breast. III. Carcinosarcoma. Cancer 1989;64:1490–9.

228. Raju GC. The histological and immunohistochemical evidence of squamous metaplasia from the myoepithelial cells in the breast. Histopathol 1990;17:272–5.

229. Palmer JO, Ghiselli RW, McDivitt RW. Immunohistochemistry in the differential diagnosis of breast diseases. Pathol Annu 1990;25 Pt 2:287–315.

230. Foote FW, Becker WF, Stewart FW. Muco-epidermoid tumours of the salivary glands. Ann Surg 1945;122: 820–44.

231. Foschini MP, Marucci G, Eusebi V. Low grade mucoepidermoid carcinoma of salivary glands: characteristic immunohistochemical profile and evidence of striated duct differentiation. Virchows Arch 2002; 440:536–42.

232. Lamovec J, Us-Krasovec M, Zidar A, Kljun A. Adenoid cystic carcinoma of the breast: a histologic, cytologic, and immunohistochemical study. Semin Diagn Pathol 1989;6:153–64.

233. Eusebi V. Lipid-rich carcinoma. In: World Health Organization, editor. Tumours of the Breast and Female Genital Organs, Chapter 1: Tumours of the Breast. 2000. p.47–8.

234. Azzopardi JG, Smith OD. Salivary gland tumours and their mucins. J Path Bacteriol 1959;77:131–40.

235. Zaloudek C, Oertel YC, Orenstein JM. Adenoid cystic carcinoma of the breast. Am J Clin Pathol 1984;81: 297–307.

236. Foschini MP, Eusebi V. Carcinomas of the breast showing myoepithelial cell differentiation. A review of the literature. Virchows Arch 1998;432:303–10.
237. Koss LG, Brannan CD, Ashikari R. Histologic and ultrastructural features of adenoid cystic carcinoma of the breast. Cancer 1970;26:1271–9.
238. Tavassoli FA, Norris HJ. Mammary adenoid cystic carcinoma with sebaceous differentiation. A morphologic study of the cell types. Arch Pathol Lab Med 1986;110:1045–53.
239. Caselitz J, Becker J, Seifert G, Weber K, Osborn M. Coexpression of keratin and vimentin filaments in adenoid cystic carcinomas of salivary glands. Virchows Arch A Pathol Anat Histopathol 1984;403:337–44.
240. Kasami M, Olson SJ, Simpson JF, Page DL. Maintenance of polarity and a dual cell population in adenoid cystic carcinoma of the breast: an immunohistochemical study. Histopathol 1998;32:232–8.
241. Ro JY, Silva EG, Gallager HS. Adenoid cystic carcinoma of the breast. Hum Pathol 1987;18:1276–81.
242. Trendell-Smith NJ, Peston D, Shousha S. Adenoid cystic carcinoma of the breast: a tumour commonly devoid of oestrogen receptors and related proteins. Histopathol 1999;35:241–8.
243. Swanson Beck J, members of the Medical Research Council Breast Tumour Pathology Panel. Observer variability in reporting of breast lesions. J Clin Pathol 1985;38:1358–65.
244. Sloane JP, Ellman R, Anderson TJ, et al. Consistency of histopathological reporting of breast lesions detected by screening: findings of the U.K. National External Quality Assessment (EQA) Scheme. U. K. National Coordinating Group for Breast Screening Pathology. Eur J Cancer 1994;30A:1414–9.
245. Wells WA, Carney PA, Eliassen MS, Tosteson AN, Greenberg ER. Statewide study of diagnostic agreement in breast pathology. J Natl Cancer Inst 1998;90:142–5.
246. Page DL, Dupont WD, Rogers LW, Rados AM. Atypical Hyperplastic Lesions of the Female Breast. A Long-Term Follow-Up Study. Cancer 1985;55:2698–708.
247. Tavassoli FA. Ductal intraepithelial neoplasia (IDH, AIDH and DCIS). Breast Cancer 2000;7:315–20.

Content

21

LOBULAR NEOPLASIA

RAJENDRA S. RAMPAUL, SARAH E. PINDER, JOHN F.R. ROBERTSON AND IAN O. ELLIS

The terms 'lobular carcinoma in-situ' (LCIS) and atypical lobular hyperplasia (ALH) are used to describe the histological features of a characteristic proliferation of monomorphic atypical cells within breast lobules. The generic term lobular neoplasia (LN) was recently introduced and refers to the entire spectrum of noninvasive atypical epithelial proliferations of lobular-type. LN is multicentric and often lobulated. The diagnosis of LN indicates an increased relative risk of developing invasive carcinoma in either breast. Molecular studies suggest that LN may be a direct precursor of invasive lobular carcinoma.

Lobular neoplasia

■ DEFINITION

Synonyms: carcinoma lobulare in-situ (CLIS), lobular carcinoma in-situ (LCIS), atypical lobular hyperplasia (ALH), lobular neoplasia (LN), lobular intraepithelial neoplasia (LIN)

WHO: Lobular neoplasia
ICD-O code: 8520/2

The term 'lobular carcinoma in-situ' (LCIS) was first used in 1941 by Foote and Stewart to describe the histological features of a characteristic proliferation of monomorphic atypical cells within breast lobules [1]. Their description was limited to well-developed examples and, as such, LCIS is a firmly established histopathological entity (Fig. 21.1). Histologically similar but less well-developed examples, such as atypical lobular hyperplasia were not specifically reported on in earlier studies. Recently, strict histological criteria for its diagnosis have been formulated [2, 3]. This is particularly important as some aspects of the biology of these lesions have a different natural course to ductal carcinoma in-situ. Haagensen suggested the term 'lobular neoplasia' for these lesions [4]. This term was also adopted as a designation to refer to all noninvasive atypical proliferative lesions of lobular-type. Although the term 'lobular neoplasia' is more appealing than the word 'carcinoma', we prefer the terms LCIS and ADH as these terms are well-established in the literature and imply different risks of developing carcinoma.

■ CONCEPTUAL APPROACH

The relationship between LCIS and invasive cancer is unresolved and remains controversial. However, some recent advances have led us to a greater understanding of the biology of this entity. Loss of heterozygosity studies in primary tumors have identified deletions at chromosomal region 16q22.1 in half of the informative breast cancer cases, suggesting a possible tumor suppressor gene [22–25]. E-cadherin, a transmembrane protein responsible

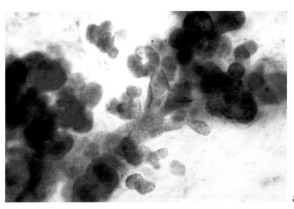

a

Fig. 21.1a–b Lobular carcinoma in-situ, classic variant.
21.1a Submacroscopic view of an LCIS showing distension of all acini and the terminal duct.

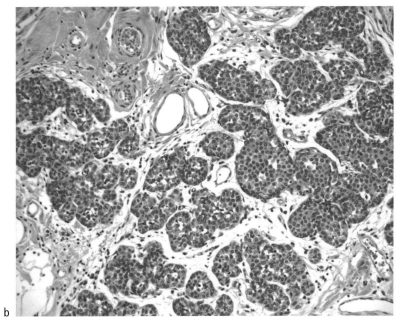

b

21.1b The acini of the lobule in the right field are distended and filled with monotonous, small tumor cells characteristic of lobular neoplasia. The left field shows a lobule with incompletely filled acini which, in addition to neoplastic cells, contain interspersed benign cells.

for cell-cell adhesion, is localized in this region and has been implicated. In support of this, reduced E-cadherin expression has been recorded in 50% of infiltrating ductal carcinomas, and complete loss of E-cadherin has been shown in most infiltrating lobular carcinomas [26–30]. Berx et al. demonstrated truncation mutations in four of seven invasive lobular breast cancers in which there was a loss of the wild-type E-cadherin allele [31]. Interestingly, no mutations in 42 infiltrative ductal and medullary carcinomas were detected in this study. Comparative genomic hybridization analyses of LCIS and invasive cancer have shown some similarities at the chromosomal level, but significant differences also exist [32].

Early age of onset and multicentricity of neoplasms is suggestive of heritable cancer predisposition syndromes, which suggests LCIS may be the result of an inherited susceptibility. Indeed, Lakani et al. have provided support for this hypothesis by showing that foci of LCIS are likely to be clonal [33]. A priori evidence suggests that E-cadherin may be a candidate for an LCIS predisposition gene. This hypothesis has recently been tested, building on the identification of constitutional E-cadherin mutations that predispose to familial diffuse gastric cancer [34]. Rahman et al. examined lymphocytic DNA from 65 individuals with LCIS for germline alterations in E-cadherin: none were found. Recently however, an inherited frameshift mutation in exon 3 of E-cadherin was reported in a patient with LCIS who had a strong family history of gastric cancer [35].

These studies suggest a molecular pathway from LCIS to invasive disease. Further studies are eagerly awaited as they may provide clues on chemotherapeutic/preventative strategies.

■ CLINICAL FEATURES, EPIDEMIOLOGY AND ▪ TREATMENT

CLINICAL FEATURES AND EPIDEMIOLOGY

LCIS and ALH both possess similar clinical features (Table 21.1). The incidence is greatest before the menopause, with a decrease thereafter (less than 10% of patients with LCIS are postmenopausal) [5]. Lobular neoplasia characteristically affects both breasts in a multifocal, multicentric pattern. If LCIS is present in a breast biopsy, more than half of cases will contain residual LCIS in the ipsilateral breast. If the contralateral breast is biopsied extensively, more than a third will contain LCIS [6]. At Nottingham City Hospital, following a review of 3822 core biopsies, 13 (0.3%) were classified as B3 with lobular neoplasia, 5 were an incidental finding and 8 underwent diagnostic excision (4 invasive, 2 DCIS, 1 benign and 1 lobular neoplasia). Liberman [7] has recently reported findings on 1315 consecutive lesions; of these 16 (1.2%) were LCIS. Elsheikh and Silverman [8] described a series of 22 patients with pleomorphic calcification; 7 had LCIS in core biopsies. Tarjan et al. [9] found a 3.6% incidence of lobular neoplasia in 2280 sequential core biopsies.

Involvement is often greatest in areas containing the most breast parenchyma, for instance beneath the nipple and the upper, outer quadrant [10]. Discovery of LCIS or ALH is almost always an incidental finding in a biopsy performed for other reasons. No specific mammographic features of lobular neoplasia have been described [12]. Nonetheless, it is important to appreciate that adjacent breast tissue will sometimes contain microcalcifications [11, 13].

Accurately assessing the incidence of lobular neoplasia within the general population is difficult as most diagnoses represent an incidental discovery at breast biopsy. Only about a quarter of patients with LCIS subsequently develop invasive carcinoma, which suggests that most lesions must remain clinically silent [14]. It is also likely that, as the vast majority of diagnoses of LCIS or ALH occur in premenopausal women, lobular neoplasia probably regresses after the menopause. Since no clinical or mammographic signs are associated with LCIS, we may assume that the incidence of lobular neoplasia within the general population is equivalent to the incidence in breast biopsies. It is estimated that if 1–2% of otherwise benign breast biopsies contain lobular neoplasia, the general population may be assumed to have a similar incidence [15]. However, its incidence appears to have increased over the last 30 years for several reasons:

1. mammographic detection of calcifications, which have a slight association with adjacent LCIS;
2. a lower threshold of suspicion leading to more biopsies i. e., a lower threshold for intervention; and
3. more thorough histological sectioning and examination of specimens by pathologists.

Tab. 21.1 Features of LCIS and ALH

Multifocal, multicentric, bilateral.
Decreasing incidence after the menopause.
Nonpalpable, macroscopically not visible.
Incidental finding even at mammography.
Slight association with adjacent calcification.
Risk indicators of developing invasive carcinoma.
At molecular level also a precursor lesion of invasive lobular carcinoma.

469

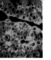

LOBULAR NEOPLASIA AS A RISK INDICATOR

Lobular neoplasia encompasses a histological spectrum with LCIS at one extreme. It is now widely accepted that such a spectrum of risk is also present and parallels histological extent of involvement. It was only in 1978 that Haagensen and Rosen independently reported on the clinical implications of LCIS when they described their experience with patients who were diagnosed with LCIS at biopsy, but who were given no further treatment [4, 5]. These patients were subsequently shown to have an increased risk of developing a subsequent invasive carcinoma upon long-term follow-up. ALH as a term was later instituted in order to place diagnostic boundaries within the spectrum of lobular neoplasia. This approach has helped to separate lesser examples of lobular neoplasia and resulted in more clinical implications [2, 3].

Several studies of lobular neoplasia and its risk implications now exist. One group, however, has also stratified cancer risk by separating marked examples (LCIS) from lesser examples (ALH) [3]. Frykberg, in compiling 12 reported studies involving 874 women with LCIS who underwent long-term follow-up, showed an overall rate of developing invasive carcinoma of 18–37% over a follow-up of to 24–47 years [47]. However, the design, selection bias, differences in length and completeness of follow-up and accuracy of histological diagnosis has caused some doubt as to the validity of these figures [48]. The National Surgical Adjuvant Breast and Bowel Project (NSAPB) P-1 prevention trial provides data on breast cancer risk in women with LCIS and atypical hyperplasia [49]. From this study, a 100% greater incidence of invasive breast carcinoma occurred in the control group of women with a history of LCIS over a median 55 month follow-up. Tamoxifen prevention studies in the US have demonstrated a reduction in risk greatest in women with a history of LCIS (56% relative risk reduction) and atypical hyperplasia (86% reduction). In contrast, European studies using different risk evaluation models and entry criteria have found no benefit.

Irrespective of the differences in terminology used and the number of cases, there are significant similarities among these studies. One such example is the average age at biopsy and the relative risk of subsequent development of an invasive carcinoma. An obvious difference, in contrast, is the incidence of lobular neoplasia in otherwise benign breast biopsies, ranging from 0.5% to 3.8%. Haagensen's series in 1978 had a higher incidence of lobular neoplasia with a concomitant lower percentage of patients developing an invasive carcinoma [4]. Both these observations could be explained by the inclusion of what we would recognize as ALH. What is more, if all patients in the Nashville series were analyzed as two separate groups (ALH and LCIS), the incidence of lobular neoplasia would be equal to 2.1% of the 223 biopsies [3, 14], with only 15% of patients later developing an invasive carcinoma.

Time to development of invasive carcinoma is another important difference in these studies of lobular neoplasia. In Page's study [14] two thirds of those who developed a carcinoma did so within 15 years following biopsy. However, in Rosen's series [5, 6] more than half the invasive lesions developed after 15 years. Nonetheless the relative risk figures are not dissimilar. Ottesen et al., with a median follow-up of 5 years, cited an 11% incidence of invasive carcinoma developing after LCIS alone. This supports the idea that the risk is greatest within the first 10–15 years after discovery [50].

There has also been controversy about the time interval after which risk of subsequent carcinoma decreases following diagnosis of lobular neoplasia. Uzieblo et al. recently addressed this in 92 patients with LCIS alone. The mean follow-up was 21 years, 26 patients developed subsequent carcinoma, the mean interval to carcinoma was 14 years (45% of which developed carcinoma after 15 years) and 5 developed carcinoma 20 years or more after LCIS diagnosis [51].

ALH also has important implications in risk assessments. Indeed it has been questioned whether risk assessments have been 'diluted' by the inclusions of these lesser examples. It must be borne in mind that, by recognizing and diagnosing ALH, we are assigning a moderately increased risk of subsequent carcinoma 4–5 times that of the general population [2, 3]. Using strict histological criteria, Page et al. [3] were able to demonstrate that the risk implications of ALH are approximately half that of LCIS. Another aspect that must be considered in these ALH cases is the influence of a positive family history, in particular a first-degree relative with breast carcinoma. Patients with ALH but no family history have an 8–10% risk of developing an invasive carcinoma within 10–15 years. In those with a first-degree relative, the risk increases to 20% for the same time frame, equivalent to that associated with LCIS [2, 3]. Interestingly, a positive family history does not further affect risk in LCIS [14].

In any analysis of data for risk assessment, two aspects must be considered: relative risk and absolute risk. Relative risk statements are used to compare groups and must be interpreted in terms of a carefully pre-established denominator. Absolute risk is the likelihood of an individual patient or group of patients developing a disease within a given period of time, expressed as a percentage [52]. Thus for a patient with ALH, the absolute risk is 8% (invasive carcinoma within 10–15 years) and 17–20% in LCIS. These ranges are most relevant to women in their fifth decade.

Clinically, LCIS is becoming accepted as a risk indicator. However, how this information is being used to manage patients remains varied [11].

Several studies have shown that in LCIS the risk of developing an invasive carcinoma applies to both breasts, with a slight preponderance of subsequent carcinomas on the ipsilateral side [14], but some now argue this risk is equal [47]. For example, in Page's 1991 series, five patients developed carcinomas in the ipsilateral breast, three in the opposite and one developed bilateral cancers [14]. These were predominantly invasive lobular or a variant thereof. In other series, the majorities were ductal [15] or lobular [4, 45].

Recently, Page et al. examined the laterality and risk implications of invasive breast cancer in women with ALH [46]. They followed 252 women diagnosed with ALH from 1950–1985. Fifty (20%) patients developed invasive breast cancer. The relative risk (RR) was 3.1 (95% CI 2.3–4.3, p < 0.001). Sixty-eight percent developed ipsilateral cancer. This data suggests that in ALH invasive cancer is about three times more likely to arise in the ipsilateral breast, and therefore challenges previous data that risk is equal in both breasts.

TREATMENT

A greater understanding of LCIS only started to emerge with the advent of screening mammography. Anecdotal observation of a high rate of multicentricity and bilaterality, coexistence with invasive disease and reports of further development of breast cancer in the future caused many surgeons to believe an aggressive therapeutic approach was the only option to effectively manage these patients. Thus until the 1970s ipsilateral mastectomy was the standard treatment for LCIS [1, 54, 55].

We now understand much more about the biology and epidemiology of LCIS and have a better idea of its long-term outcome [53]. As a result, major changes in treatment have been adopted.

Haagensen was the first to suggest nonoperative observation with lifelong surveillance for LCIS [4]. Recent studies have now shown that the risk of such an approach is very low [56–59]. Most importantly, mastectomy has never been shown to reduce mortality compared to observation alone. Thus nonoperative observation is now the most widely accepted and rational option for LCIS. Recent studies of cancer-related mortality that strictly excluded invasive disease and that more accurately distinguished LCIS from DCIS and hyperplasia, report a less than 7.2% or even absent mortality in these women over long-term follow-up. These figures are the result of women with LCIS undergoing strict clinical and mammographic surveillance due to their known risk,

leading to an earlier detection, smaller size [19] and thus better prognosis.

Although LCIS is widely disseminated throughout the breast, there is no evidence to date that all biopsy specimens need re-excision with 'clear' excision margins. It has never been shown that such a course of action reduces subsequent risk of invasive breast cancer.

A few indications for diagnostic excision following lobular neoplasia on core biopsy do however exist:
1. overlapping features with DCIS,
2. the presence of an additional high-risk lesion,
3. radiological/histological discordance,
4. extensive lobular neoplasia with comedonecrosis.

In 1988, only 54% of respondents to a survey of the Society of Surgical Oncology and the American Society of Breast Surgeons agreed with observation alone. This increased to 87% in 1996 [20]. With the accumulating evidence that nonoperative management is acceptable, the necessity or validity of a rigid distinction between LCIS and ALH [2, 54, 5] is now being increasingly challenged.

The real challenge with LCIS however, is to accurately determine which women will subsequently develop carcinoma. Being able to identify a high-risk subgroup is highly desirable, as it will allow for selective application of more aggressive approaches such as definitive surgery. The grade and extent of lobular involvement have been suggested by Page as indicators of poor outcome [14]. Frykberg [59] has suggested additional risk factors such as family history, nulliparity and atypical hyperplasia.

The NSABP P-1 prevention trial has addressed the issue of LCIS and tamoxifen [49]. In the recent analysis 13 175 women were randomized to either tamoxifen or placebo. In 826 women with LCIS, a 56% reduction in the incidence of invasive breast carcinoma among women taking tamoxifen was found. For those with ALH (n = 1193) this reduction was approximately 86% for the tamoxifen group. The use of tamoxifen is now approved for use in these women. Although this data provides an exciting avenue for chemotherapeutic strategies, several unanswered questions remain, such as the appropriate duration of tamoxifen administration, the extent of its risks and, naturally, the further identification of other prognostic factors.

In conclusion, an observational approach to patients with LCIS is appropriate and evidence-based [47]. Tamoxifen appears to provide an advantage in risk reduction, but it requires further research to address several issues. Bilateral mastectomy should be reserved only for those at exceptionally high risk. Accurate identification of this group remains our chief challenge.

■ PATHOLOGY

MACROSCOPY

Macroscopically no characteristic features of lobular neoplasia exist.

MICROSCOPY

The characteristic features of lobular neoplasia are summarized in Table 21.2 [38]. In lobular neoplasia the defining atypical cell type is round, cuboidal, or polygonal with clear or light cytoplasm. Nuclei are round-to-oval, cytologically bland, with an occasional small nucleolus. Mitotic figures and hyperchromatism are not features of lobular neoplasia but may occasionally be seen. Within the involved spaces there is an even, discohesive distribution of cells, and cellular monotony is the rule (Fig. 21.2). Intracytoplasmic lumina are often present and, though helpful, are not required for diagnosis [16]. These lumina are clear when stained with H&E and are accentuated with alcian blue and/or PAS stains [17]. Ultrastructural analysis reveals these lumina are lined by microvilli [17]. The presence of cells containing intracytoplasmic lumina in a fine-needle aspirate strongly suggests a diagnosis of lobular neoplasia [18]. The morphology of the type of LCIS described above is referred to as type A to distinguish it from a variant type B that contains slightly larger cells with larger monomorphous nuclei and usually visible nucleoli (Fig. 21.3). The histological description holds true for both LCIS and ALH; it is the degree of involvement of breast lobules that distinguishes one from the other. The anatomical distribution of LCIS in lobules and terminal ducts, and changes in the morphology of these structures, influences the histopathological appearances of LCIS in any given case. In the postmenopausal atrophic breast, Foote and Stewart observed that LCIS arises from the terminal ducts, whereas it appears to do so in the TDLUs of the premenopausal breast [19].

The point of reference for determining any type of lobular neoplasia is the normal acinus. Given the fact that a total of two cells layers normally line an acinus, the presence of three or more cells of characteristic morphology above the basement membrane implies ALH. In typical lobular neoplasia the normal glandular epithelium of the acini and intralobular ductules is replaced by neoplastic cells. These cells may cause expansion of the normal lobular-ductal architecture, as well as enlargement of the lobule in relation to uninvolved lobules in the adjacent breast. Although lobular enlargement is not an absolute diagnostic criterion, the diagnosis of LCIS does require that:

1. the involved acini be populated exclusively by the characteristic cells; and
2. these cells fill, distend, and distort at least one half of the acini within the lobular unit (Figs 21.1 and 21.2).

ALH is diagnosed when:
1. fewer than half of the acini are expanded and distorted (Fig. 21.4);
2. filling is incomplete i.e., interspersed intercellular spaces remain; or
3. other cell types are intermixed (Fig. 21.4b–c).

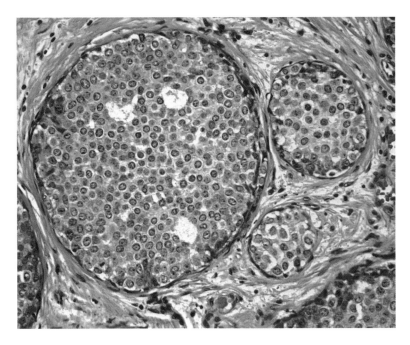

Fig. 21.2 Lobular carcinoma in-situ. Higher magnification showing distended acini filled with monotonous small cells (type A) with an even, discohesive distribution. Note the rounded cytoplasmic compartment of the atypical cells, which are completely discohesive due to a lack of the adhesion molecule E-cadherin.

It is important to note however that, although quantitative factors have been included among the diagnostic criteria, the extent of lobular involvement for such a diagnosis remains unanswered.

Diagnosis rests on finding characteristic neoplastic cells within lobules. Not infrequently, cytologically identical cells may focally involve the ducts; a condition called 'pagetoid' involvement (Fig. 21.5a–b) [1]. This involves a proliferation of neoplastic cells just above the basement membrane, tending to undermine the normal lining epithelial cells (Fig. 21.5a–b). When only pagetoid involvement can be identified without

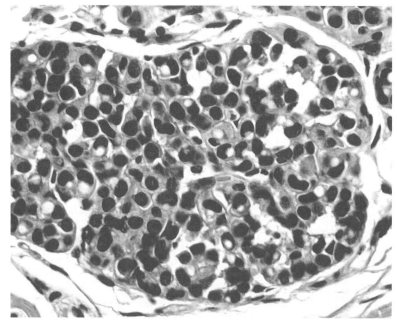

Fig. 21.3 Lobular carcinoma in-situ. This distended acinus contains larger cells (type B), some of which display intracytoplasmic lumina.

Tab. 21.2 Distinguishing features of lobular neoplasia, FEA/ADH and low grade DCIS

Lesion	Lobular neoplasia	FEA/ADH and DCIS, low grade
Definition	Proliferation of atypical, discohesive monotonous cells in TDLUs.	Proliferation of uniform atypical, cohesive cells, low grade.
Cellular composition	Proliferation of cells with round, cuboidal, or polygonal shape and light cytoplasm. Nuclei monotonous, round-to-oval, slightly enlarged with an occasional small nucleolus. Intracytoplasmic lumina common.	Proliferation of atypical cells with a cuboidal to polygonal shape. Even spacing of cells. Nuclei slightly enlarged, round-to-oval with occasional nucleoli. Flat growth or more complex cohesive patterns with trabecular bars, Roman bridges, micropapillae of cribriform growth. Intracytoplasmic lumina rare.
Immunohistochemistry	Ck8/18+, Ck5/14–, ER+, E-cadherin–.	Ck8/18+, Ck5/14–, ER+, E-cadherin+.
Lobular architecture	Lobular architecture usually preserved. Rare exceptions.	In early stages lobular architecture preserved with dilated ductules (FEA/ADH). Later unfolding of lobules and extension into the ductal system (DCIS).
Spread	Discohesive infiltration and finally replacement of original epithelium within lobules (ducts often involved). Pagetoid spread usually present.	Cohesive growth with destruction and replacement of original cells within TDLUs (FEA/ADH) or within the ductal-lobular tree (DCIS). Pagetoid spread usually absent.
Subtypes	Polymorphous, signet-ring cell, apocrine, extensive LCIS with comedonecrosis.	Apocrine.
B-classification	B3 or B5a.	B3 or B5a according to stage.

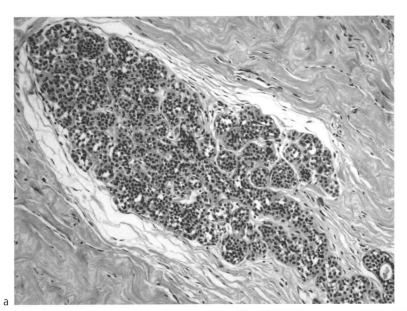

a

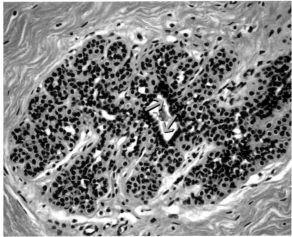

b

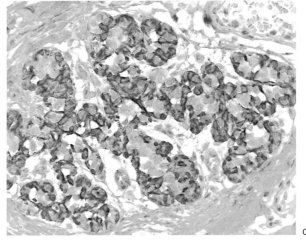

c

Fig. 21.4a−c Atypical lobular hyperplasia.
21.4a This lobule shows acini incompletely filled by cells characteristic of lobular neoplasia. Note the presence of residual lumina in some acini. Only few acini are distended. This lesion would classify as ALH.

21.4b Another lobule in the same slide. Monotonous, round, atypical cells replace the normal cells of the lobular acini without expansion or distortion of the acini. In the center the normal luminal epithelium is retained (arrows). Furthermore other cell types are intermixed in acinar structures with the neoplastic cells.

21.4c Ck5/6-immunostaining of a lobule showing the characteristic Ck5/6− atypical cells, which are interspersed with compressed glandular and myoepithelial cells heavily staining for Ck5/6. Sm-actin staining may show a similar result.

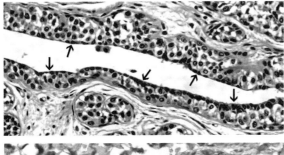

a

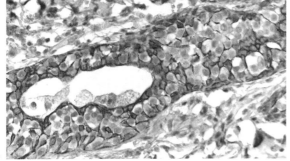

b

Fig. 21.5a−b Lobular carcinoma in-situ with pagetoid spread of neoplastic cells in adjacent ducts.

21.5a This example shows the proliferation of neoplastic cells just above the basement membrane undermining the residual glandular cells at the luminal border (arrows). Furthermore there are residual displaced and distorted glandular and myoepithelial cells between the tumor cells.

21.5b Ck5/14-immunostaining highlights the luminal and myoepithelial cells. The neoplastic cells characteristically do not express basal cytokeratins 5 and 14. Note also the compressed Ck5/14+ cells between the proliferating atypical cells. These also stain for sm-actin, being in part myoepithelial cells (not shown here).

the more characteristic cellular changes of lobular neoplasia, diagnosis is frequently more difficult to achieve. In this instance, a careful search within the breast for lobular involvement by LCIS or ALH is indicated. Pagetoid involvement is more common and its presence more extensive in LCIS than ALH. This association with LCIS does not affect risk implications. However, ductal involvement in association with ALH increases the subsequent cancer risk to a level intermediate between ALH and LCIS [21].

Using the above guidelines, diagnosis of LCIS relies on the presence of a single population of characteristic cells filling the acini of a lobular unit, with over half of the acini being distended and distorted. In practice, a diagnosis of LCIS requires full distension of acini, which is equivalent to eight or more cells across the diameter of an acinus. If these diagnostic guidelines are followed, most examples of LCIS are not difficult to recognize.

Several electron microscopic studies have described the origin of LCIS to be lobular epithelial cells. Ultrastructurally, the typical case reveals intracytoplasmic lumina lined by microvilli. The basement membrane in LCIS has been studied in detail by Anderson who demonstrated discontinuity and noted that such gaps could be detected in both LCIS and normal lobules.

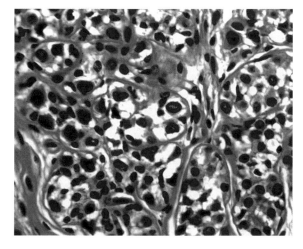

Fig. 21.6 Lobular carcinoma in-situ, pleomorphic variant. This lesion shows a proliferation of tumor cells with polygonal disheveled cytoplasmic bodies and many more polymorphic and hyperchromatic nuclei. It would classify as polymorphic-type LCIS.

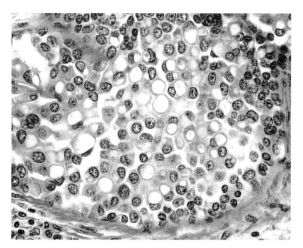

Fig. 21.8 Lobular carcinoma in-situ, signet-ring cell type, with typical large intracytoplasmic lumina, which displace the nucleus towards the periphery. Note that the neoplastic cells display a discohesive cell growth.

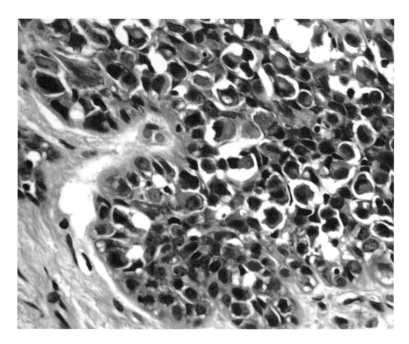

Fig. 21.7 Lobular carcinoma in-situ, apocrine variant. The tumor cells show abundant eosinophilic, finely granular cytoplasm characteristic of apocrine metaplasia. Some of the cells contain intracytoplasmic lumina.

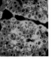

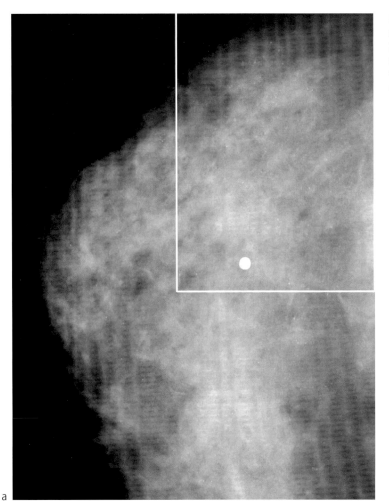

Fig. 21.9a – c Extensive lobular carcinoma in-situ with comedonecrosis.
21.9a Mammography of the right breast showing a homogeneously dense background with widely spread, coarse microcalcifications (courtesy of C. Grellmann).

a

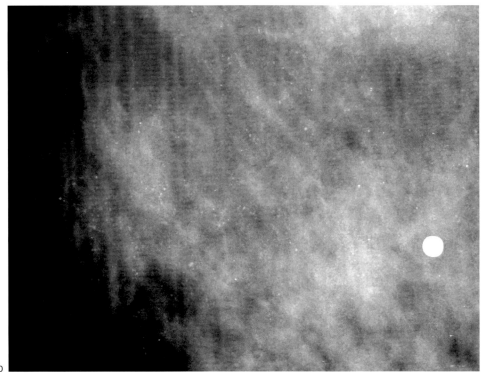

21.9b Higher magnification reveals polymorphic clustered and linear microcalcifications.

Continuation

b

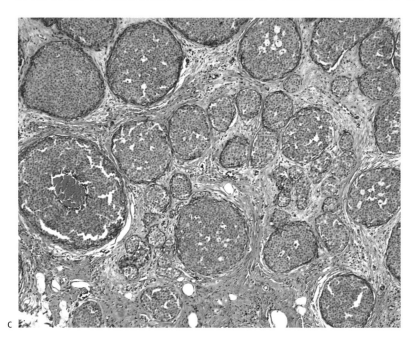

c

Fig. 21.9a–c Extensive lobular carcinoma in-situ with comedonecrosis.
21.9c Low power view displaying distension of the ductal-lobular tree due to proliferation of neoplastic discohesive cells characteristic of lobular neoplasia with comedonecrosis. This growth pattern is unusual for lobular neoplasia and requires therapeutic excision of the lesion, similar to DCIS. The comedonecrosis leads to polymorphic calcification similar to comedo DCIS. Note that this type of LCIS also shows the same ductal-lobular spread as comedo-type DCIS. Many of these patients require wide excision or simple mastectomy.

Variants of lobular neoplasia include pleomorphic (Fig. 21.6), apocrine (Fig. 21.7) and signet-ring cell type types (Fig. 21.8), as well as extensive LCIS with comedonecrosis (Fig. 21.9a–c).

INTERPRETATION OF CORE AND VACUUM-ASSISTED BIOPSIES

Classic LN (ALH and LCIS) should be classified as B3. It is usually a coincidental finding in a core biopsy from a screen-detected lesion. Therefore, a multidisciplinary discussion is essential to determine whether an abnormality that has been radiologically identified is also represented at microscopy. These cases must be managed cautiously.

On occasions a small cell epithelial proliferation in lobules and/or ducts may not be clearly classified as lobular neoplasia or low grade DCIS, and in these circumstances a numerically higher category (B4 or B5) is prudent and should be considered. Sometimes E-cadherin may help in the differential diagnosis. Pleomorphic LCIS and LCIS with comedonecrosis must be classified as B5.

IMMUNOHISTOCHEMISTRY

E-cadherin is lost in the neoplastic cells of lobular neoplasia (Fig. 21.10). Estrogen (Fig. 21.11) and progesterone are usually strongly positive in 60–90% of cases, while erbB2 and p53 are usually negative. The tumor cells express glandular cytokeratins 8/18 but not high molecular weight Ck5 and 14 (Fig. 21.12). Sometimes tumor cells infiltrating the ductal epithelium are seen in clusters between normal or even hyperplastic cells, the latter usually being Ck5/14+ and also sometimes sm-actin+ (Fig. 21.5).

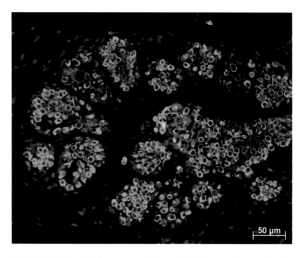

Fig. 21.10 Double immunostaining of lobular carcinoma in-situ for E-cadherin (red signal) and Ck8/18 (green signal). Note the complete absence of E-cadherin in the neoplastic cells, contrasting with the residual E-cadherin+ normal cells and myoepithelial cells.

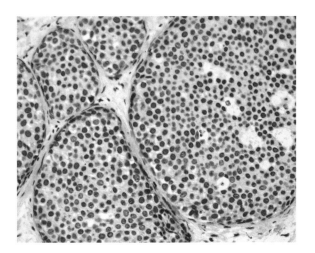

Fig. 21.11 Immunostaining for estrogen showing a moderate to intensive reaction in most of the tumor cells.

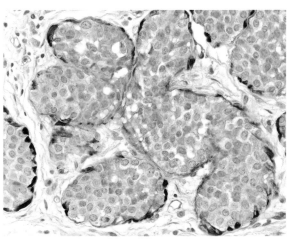

Fig. 21.12 Fully developed LCIS. Ck5/6 immunostaining highlights the myoepithelial cells. The tumor cells do not react for Ck5/6.

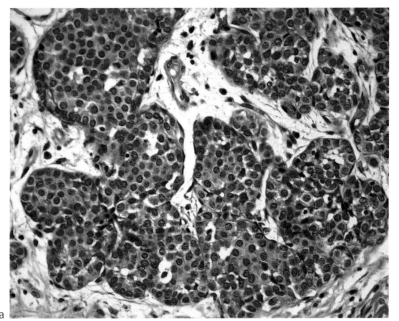

a

Fig. 21.13a–d Differential diagnosis of LCIS and DCIS.
21.13a LCIS of more solid growth with some irregular spaces. Note the discohesive cell pattern.

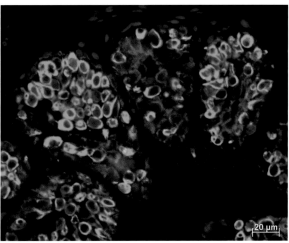

b

21.13b Immunostaining for E-cadherin (red signal) and Ck8/18 (green signal) highlights the loss of this adhesion molecule in the tumor cells, contrasting with residual normal cells.

Continuation

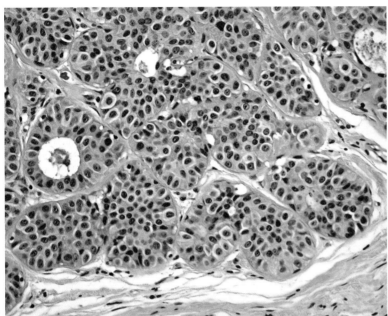

c

Fig. 21.13a – d Differential diagnosis of LCIS and DCIS.

21.13c Low grade DCIS. The neoplastic cells have a round to polygonal shape. The tumor cells show a solid growth pattern with formation of glandular spaces indicative of ductal-type neoplasia.

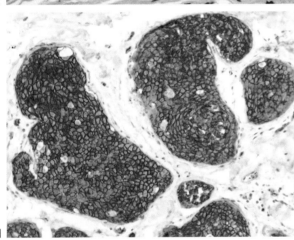

d

21.13d Immunostaining for E-cadherin of the lesion in Fig. 21.13c showing a strong membranous reaction.

MOLECULAR GENETICS

See 'conceptual approach' and Chapter 17.

DIFFERENTIAL DIAGNOSIS

The differential diagnosis of LCIS/ALH includes several conditions with proliferative changes affecting the terminal ducts and lobules, including 'pseudolactational hyperplasia', clear cell change, and apocrine metaplasia. It can be difficult in rare cases to distinguish some types of DCIS from LCIS. The presence of a diagnostic category of 'low nuclear grade, solid pattern (noncomedo) DCIS' clearly demonstrates that such patterns can overlap or closely approximate those seen in LCIS (Fig. 21.13a – d). This is due to the presence in both conditions of filling of distended,

basement membrane-bound spaces by cells, without defining intercellular spaces, to form cribriform or papillary formations. Having similar, or even overlapping, histological and cytological criteria gives rise to situations where both diagnoses must be made in order to explain the patterns present [36]. Small secondary glandular-like spaces within the solid masses of cells may be present, even if only a suggestion of a ductal pattern can be seen. These may be rosette-like and are a feature of many so-called 'solid noncomedo DCIS' (Fig. 21.13c – d). The placement of cells and their relation with each other at the plasma membrane is a subtle, but defining and important feature. The cells of lobular neoplasia are considered to be somewhat 'disheveled' in appearance. The sharp definition of cell membranes usually seen in DCIS is absent, and cells appear to be arranged as several linear segments, whereas in LCIS it almost seems like the rounded cytoplasmic compartment defined by each cell has no relationship to adjacent cells. The cytoplasm is clear in both solid DCIS and LCIS and so presents no helpful discerning criterion, except in the case of the intracytoplasmic lumina or vesicles so characteristic of lobular neoplasia. However, these intracytoplasmic lumina may be present even when a completely ductal pattern is present [37]. One final criterion helpful in making this difficult histological differential diagnosis is the appearance of these lesions at low power: LCIS is characteristically lobulocentric due to the regular dilatation of the acini within the lobular units.

DCIS extending into individual acini without destruction of lobular architecture also poses a difficult differential challenge (Fig. 21.14). This growth pattern has been termed 'cancerization of lobules' by Azzopardi [38]. Careful attention to cytological features and architectural patterns will facilitate the distinction from lobular neoplasia. Lobular neoplasia may also be found within lobular alterations of the breast that commonly produce a mass.

Fibroadenoma [40–42] and sclerosing adenosis (Fig. 21.15) [39, 40] may occasionally contain foci of otherwise characteristic lobular neoplasia. Lobular

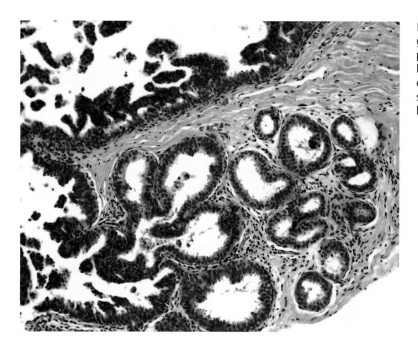

Fig. 21.14 Lobular cancerization of low grade DCIS. The lobular structures are preserved, and the acinar structures are lined by monotonous cohesive neoplastic cells with a clinging growth pattern. This should not lead to a misdiagnosis of lobular neoplasia.

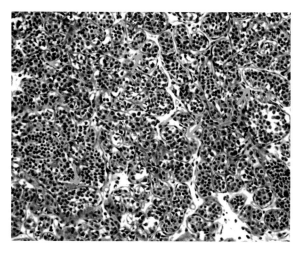

Fig. 21.15 Lobular neoplasia in a sclerosing adenosis. The tubular structures are slightly distended by the characteristic neoplastic cells. Note that the basal membranes around the tubules are preserved (arrows). This lesion should not lead to a misdiagnosis of invasive carcinoma.

neoplasia within sclerosing adenosis can be a potential source of confusion with invasive carcinoma [39]. Jensen et al. showed a threefold increase in the incidence of ALH in biopsy specimens with sclerosing adenosis compared to those without. However, only 1 in 21 such specimens had ALH within the sclerosed lobular units [43]. This tendency for ALH and sclerosing adenosis to be associated in the same biopsy specimen should prompt pathologists to look carefully for ALH in cases of sclerosing adenosis. The relative risk for such patients may be greater than for either of these entities individually (6–7 times that of the general population), as shown in a single study [43]. Risk implications associated with lobular neoplasia within a fibroadenoma remain unknown, but are probably greater than lobular neoplasia alone [44].

There are occasions when features of both DCIS and LCIS cannot be denied, and in such instances both diagnoses should be made (Fig. 21.16a–b).

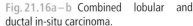

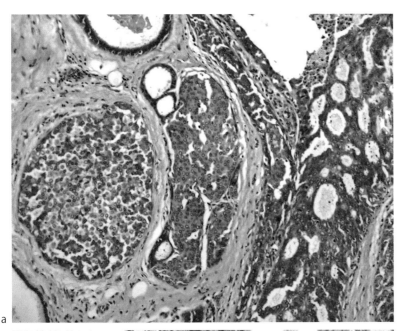

Fig. 21.16a–b Combined lobular and ductal in-situ carcinoma.
21.16a H&E staining showing low grade DCIS with a cribriform growth pattern in the right field and LCIS with a discohesive cell growth in the left field.

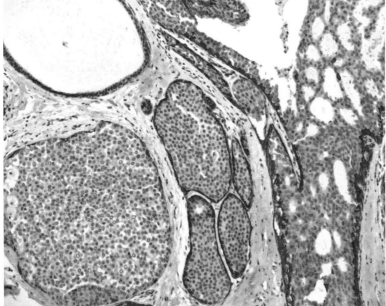

21.16b Ck5/6 staining highlights the strong reactivity of the myoepithelial cells. The neoplastic cells of both the ductal and lobular-type do not react.

REFERENCES

1. Foote F, Stewart F. Lobular carcinoma in-situ: a rare form of mammary carcinoma. Am J Pathol 1941; 17: 491–496.
2. Dupont WD, Page DL. Risk factors for breast cancer in women with proliferative disease. N Engl J Med 1985; 312: 146–151.
3. Page DL, Dupont WD, Rogers LW, Rados MS. Atypical hyperplastic lesions of the female breast. A long-term follow-up study. Cancer 1985; 55: 2698–2708.
4. Haagensen CD, Lane N, Lattes R, Bodian C. Lobular neoplasia (so-called lobular carcinoma in-situ) of the breast. Cancer 1978; 42: 737–769
5. Rosen PP, Lieberman PH, Braun DW Jr, et al. Lobular carcinoma in-situ of the breast: detailed analysis of 99 patients with average follow-up of 24 years. Am J Surg Pathol 1978; 2: 224–251.
6. Rosen PP, Braun DW Jr, Lyngholm B, et al. Lobular carcinoma in-situ of the breast: preliminary results of treatment by ipsilateral mastectomy and contralateral breast biopsy. Cancer 1981; 47: 813–819
7. Liberman L et al. Am J Roentgenology. 1999; 173; 291–299
8. Elsheikh E et al. USCAP 2001; Abs 127
9. Tarjan et al. USCAP 2001; Abs 205

10. Lambird PA, Shelley WM. The spatial distribution of lobular in-situ mammary carcinoma. JAMA 1969; 210: 689–693.
11. Shack RB, Page DL. The patient at risk for breast cancer: pathologic and surgical considerations. Prospectives in Plastic Surgery 1988; 2: 43–59.
12. Sonnenfeld MR, Frenna TH, Weidner N, Meyer JE. Lobular carcinoma in-situ: mammographic-pathologic correlation of results of needle-directed biopsy. Radiol 1991; 181: 363–367.
13. Pope T, Fechner R, Wilhelm M, et al. Lobular carcinoma in-situ of the breast: mammographic features. Radiol 1988; 168: 63–66.
14. Page DL, Kidd TE Jr, Dupont WD, et al. Lobular neoplasia of the breast: higher risk for subsequent invasive cancer predicted by more extensive disease. Hum Pathol 1991; 22: 1232–1239.
15. Bartow SA, Pathak DR, Black WC, et al. Prevalence of benign, atypical, and malignant breast lesions in populations at different risk for breast cancer. Cancer 1987; 60: 2751–2760.
16. Quincey C, Raitt N, Bell J, Ellis IO. Intracytoplasmic lumina – a useful diagnostic feature of adenocarcinomas. Histopathol 1991; 19: 83–87.
17. Battifora H. Intracytoplasmic lumina in breast carcinoma, a helpful histopathologic feature. Arch Pathol 1975; 99: 614–617.
18. Salhany KE, Page DL. Fine-needle aspiration of mammary lobular carcinoma in-situ and atypical lobular hyperplasia. Am J Clin Pathol 1989; 92: 22–26.
19. McDivitt RW, Hutter RVP, Foote FW, Stewart F. In-situ lobular carcinoma: a prospective follow-up study indicating cumulative patient risks. JAMA 1967; 201: 96–100.
20. Gump FE. Implications and management of lobular carcinoma in-situ of the breast (LCIS). Breast J 1997; 3: 196–99.
21. Page DL, Dupont WD, Rogers LW. Ductal involvement by cells of atypical lobular hyperplasia in the breast: a long-term follow-up study of cancer risk. Hum Pathol 1988; 19: 201–207.
22. Cleton-Jansen AM et al. At least two different regions are involved in allecic imbalance on chromosome arm 16q in breast cancer. Genes Chromosomes Cancer 1994; 9: 1010–107.
23. Devilee P et al. Somatic genetic changes in human breast cancer. Bichem Biophy Acta. 1994; 1198:113–0.
24. Rodriguez E et al. Genetic changes in epithelial solid neoplasia. Cancer Res. 1994; 54:3398–406.
25. Tsuda H et al. Alleic loss on chromosome 16q24.2 qter occurs frequently in breast cancers irrespectively of differences in phenotype and extent of spread. Cancer Res. 1994;54:513–17.
26. Rimm D et al. Reduced a-catenin and E-cadherin expression in breast cancer. Lab Invest. 1995; 5: 506–12.
27. Berg J et al. Breast Cancer. Cancer; 1995; 75: 257–69.
28. Gamallo C et al Correlation of E-Cadherin expression with differentiation grade and histologic type in breast cancer. Am J Pathol. 1993; 142: 987–93.
29. Moll R et al. Differential loss of E-Cadherin expression in infiltrating ductal and lobular breast carcinomas. Am J Pathol 1993; 143: 1731–42.
30. Rasbridge S et al. Epithelial and placental cadherin cell adhesion molecule expression in breast carcinoma. J Path. 1993; 169: 245–50.
31. Berx G et al. Cadherin is a tumour supressor gene mutated in human lobular breast cancers. EMBO J 1995; 14: 6107–115.
32. Lu Y et al. Comparative genomic hybridization analysisof lobular carcinoma in-situ and atypical lobular hyperplasia and potential role for gains and losses of genetic material in breast neoplasia. Cancer Res. 1998; 58:4721–7.
33. Rahman N et al . Lobular carcinoma in-situ of the breast is not caused by cotitutional mutations in the E-cadherin gene. BJC 2000; 82: 568–570.
34. Gayther SA et al. Identification of germ-line E-cadherin mutations in gastric cancer families of European origin. Cancer Res. 1998; 58: 4086–4089.
35. Keller G et al. Diffuse type gastric and lobular breast carcinoma in a familial gastric patient with an E-cadherin germline mutation. Am J Pathol. 1999; 155: 337–342.
36. Page DL, Anderson TJ, Rogers LW. Carcinoma in-situ. In: Diagnostic Histopathology of the Breast. Page DL, Anderson TJ eds. Edinburgh: Churchill Livingstone, 1987; 181.
37. Fisher ER, Brown R. Intraductal signet ring carcinoma: a hitherto undescribed form of intraductal carcinoma of the breast. Cancer 1985; 55: 2533–2537.
38. Azzopardi JG. Problems in breast pathology. London: W.B. Saunders, 1979; 203.
39. Fechner RE. Lobular carcinoma in-situ in sclerosing adenosis. Am J Surg Pathol 1981; 5: 233–239.
40. Haagensen CD, Lane N, Lattes R. Neoplastic proliferation of the epithelium of the mammary lobules: adenosis, lobular neoplasia, and small cell carcinoma. Surg Clin North Am 1972; 52: 497–524.
41. Pick PW, Iossifides IA. Occurrence of breast carcinoma within a fibroadenoma, a review. Arch Pathol Lab Med 1984; 108: 590–594.
42. Diaz NM, Palmer JO, McDivitt RW. Carcinoma arising within fibroadenomas of the breast, a clinicopathologic study of 105 patients. Am J Clin Pathol 1991; 95: 614–622.
43. Jensen RA, Page DL, Dupont WD, Rogers LW. Invasive breast cancer risk in women with sclerosing adenosis. Cancer 1989; 64: 1977–1983.
44. Dupont WD, Page DL, Parl FF. Breast cancer risk associated with fibroadenomas. Lab Invest 1990; 62: 28A.
45. Page DL, Kidd TE Jr, Dupont WD, et al. Lobular neoplasia of the breast: higher risk for subsequent invasive cancer predicted by more extensive disease. Hum Pathol 1991; 22: 1232–1239.
46. Page DL, Schuyler PA et al. Atypical lobular hyperplasia as a unilateral predictor of breast cancer risk: a retrospective cohort study. Lancet. 2003; (361): 125–9.
47. Frykberg ER. Lobular Carcinoma of the Breast. The Breast. 1999; 5 (5):296–302.
48. Gump FE. Lobular carcinoma in-situ: pathology and treatment. Surg Clin N Am 1990; 70: 873–83.
49. Fisher B et al. Tamoxifen for prevention of breast cancer:

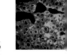
report of the National Surgical Adjuvant Breast and Bowel Project P-1 study. J Natl Cancer Inst 1998; 90: 1371–88.

50. Ottesen GL, Graversen HP, Blichert-Toft M, et al. Lobular carcinoma in-situ of the female breast: short-term results of a prospective nationwide study. Am J Surg Pathol 1993; 17: 14–21.

51. Uzieblo and Goldstein. USCAP 2001; Ab 211.

52. Dupont WD, Page DL. Relative risk of breast cancer varies with time since diagnosis of atypical hyperplasia. Hum Pathol 1989: 20: 723–725.

53. Andersen JA. Lobular carcinoma in-situ: a long-term follow-up in 52 cases. Acta Pathol Microbiol Scand 1974; 82: 519–533.

54. Hutter RVP. The management of patients with lobular carcinoma of the breast. Cancer 1984; 53: 798–802.

55. Page DL, Kidd TE, Dupont WD, et al. Lobular neoplasia of the breast: higher risk for subsequent invasive cancer predicted by more extensive disease. Hum Pathol. 1991; 22: 1232–39.

56. Carson W, Sanchez-Forgach E, Stomper P, et al. Lobular carcinoma in-situ: observation without surgery as an appropriate therapy. Ann Surg Oncol 1994; 1: 141–46.

57. Zurrida S, Bartoli C, Galimberti V, et al. Interpretation of risk associated with the unexpected finding of lobular carcinoma in-situ. Ann Surg Oncol 1996; 3: 57–61.

58. Bodian CA, Perzin KH, Lattes R. Lobular neoplasia: long term risk of breast cancer and relation to other factors. Cancer 1996; 78: 1024–34.

59. Frykberg ER, Santiago F, Betstill WL, O' Brien PH, Lobular carcinoma in-situ of the breast. Surg Gynaecol Obstet 1987; 164: 285–301.

Content

22

THE CYTOLOGY OF PRENEOPLASTIC DISEASE

CLIVE WELLS

Preneoplasia within the breast is histologically one of the most difficult areas for breast pathologists, and hence it is no surprise that assessment of these lesions can be fraught with problems. **This is especially true for cytologists due to the relative lack of architectural features** available to them compared to those that can be obtained from histological sections. **The main premalignant lesions that will be discussed here are atypical ductal and atypical lobular hyperplasia, atypical apocrine hyperplasia and apocrine adenosis, radial scars, mucocele-like lesions and multiple papilloma syndrome.**

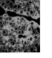
The cytology of preneoplastic disease

■ DEFINITION

As in cervical cytology, which was originally intended to detect early invasive carcinoma, mammographic screening for small invasive cancers has led to the recognition of premalignant lesions and carcinoma in-situ with much greater frequency than in the prescreening era. Just as the recognition of the cytological appearances of preneoplastic lesions and carcinoma in-situ in cervical cytology followed from the introduction of screening, breast cytology has also been forced to deal with these problems. This has, in particular, led to small areas of atypical ductal hyperplasia with calcification being aspirated by stereotaxis. These lesions present new challenges and pitfalls for the breast pathologist.

■ ATYPICAL DUCTAL HYPERPLASIA (ADH)

Aspiration of areas of atypical ductal hyperplasia can occur by chance in a palpable area of fibrocystic change without clinical or radiological signs relating to the atypia, but, as ADH is a rare lesion, this is very uncommon. The more likely scenarios are either where the area of ADH has undergone microcalcification and has been detected at mammographic screening or where ADH is a component of another lesion, such as a radial scar or papilloma. As ADH essentially represents a stage before the development of low grade ductal carcinoma in-situ (DCIS), interpretation of its cytological appearance may be extremely difficult and can easily be misinterpreted. In addition, its appearance varies somewhat when an underlying lesion is also present.

Smears from ADH not associated with another lesion are generally poorly cellular. Similar to low grade DCIS, compact clusters of cells can usually be seen, which are relatively monomorphic but may have occasional benign cells mixed in with the mildly atypical cells. Dissociation is not a common feature and bare nuclei are common, so these smears may easily be interpreted as totally benign (C2). This is especially true if other features of a benign condition such as fibrocystic change are present. The smears are, however, often recognized as atypical (C3) or suspicious (C4) due to the presence of abnormal chromatin and nuclear enlargement within the clusters. Cases in which nuclear abnormalities are pronounced are at risk of being overdiagnosed as malignant (C5) [1].

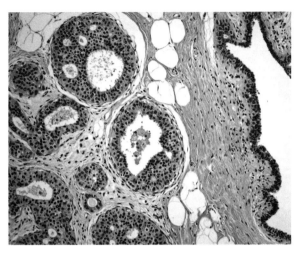

Fig. 22.1 Part of a lobule showing a group of dilated ductules with proliferation of monomorphic atypical cells and normal epithelium in the interlobular duct in the right field. H&E.

ADH associated with a radial scar is a particularly difficult scenario for the cytologist. Mayers and Sloane showed that about a third of all clinically relevant radial scars are associated either with malignancy or ADH [2]. Larger radial scars were more prone to such change. Smears from these lesions can show the difficult combination of atypical clusters of cells with small tubules and can be easily overdiagnosed as malignant.

Diagnosis of ADH is essentially histological, ADH being originally defined as a hyperplastic lesion that has some but not all of the features of low grade DCIS [3]. As the full histological architecture and extent of lesions are not apparent in cytological smears, many of the features used in making this diagnosis histologically are not seen. It is, therefore, not surprising that this is an extremely difficult lesion for cytopathologists.

ADH is cytologically rather variable in appearance, mainly depending on whether it is associated with another lesion such as a papilloma or radial scar. Isolated ADH not associated with another lesion (Fig. 22.1) often gives a cytological picture similar to usual ductal hyperplasia (UDH): three-dimensional clusters of cells (Figs 22.2 and 22.3) without papillary cores but with some minor dissociation of atypical cells from the edges of the clusters (Figs 22.4 and 22.5). The clusters of cells are, however, more monomorphic than in regular hyperplasia [4] and show less attempt at streaming than in usual ductal hyper-

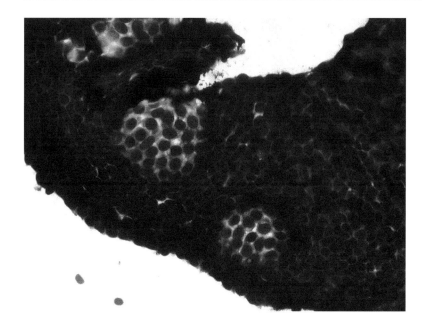

plasia (Fig. 22.6). Nucleoli are more prominent than in regular hyperplasia. Sometimes the clusters of cells do not take the form of three-dimensional spheres but of monolayers [5]. In this situation, their architecture is helpful, and straight edges and round holes from the cribriform center of the lesion may be seen (Fig. 22.6). Cells with atypical nuclear features may merge with areas where the chromatin pattern is more regular, and there are more obviously two cell types, as seen in usual ductal hyperplasia (Fig. 22.7). The cytological features are therefore difficult to differentiate on one hand from usual ductal hyperplasia, and on the other, from low grade cribriform or micropapillary carcinoma in-situ [6]. Assessment of the architectural pattern of the clusters is necessary when attempting to differentiate between these lesions. Bibbo has devised a scoring system in a scenario of intraductal epithelial proliferations to attempt to give the cytologist aid in deciding whether significant atypia are sufficiently present in a cytological smear to warrant further investigation [7]. This is based on four criteria (Table 22.1).

A score of 4–8 is not considered significant, while a score of 9–12 is considered worrying and worthy of further investigation. It should also be recognized that these lesions are extremely difficult on standard core biopsy [8] due to the limited extent of sampling which can be performed. These difficult lesions may be better assessed by the mammotome technique or by localization biopsy.

Tab. 22.1 Four criteria used in deciding whether further investigation of intraductal hyperplasia is warranted (Bibbo et al. [7])

Criterion	Score
Myoepithelial cells (bare nuclei)	
Many	1
Moderate	2
Few	3
Cellular arrangement	
Monolayer	1
Overlapping	2
Clustering	3
Cellular composition of cell groups	
Heterogeneous	1
Variable	2
Homogeneous	3
Chromatin pattern	
Regular, fine	1
Regular, coarse	2
Irregular, coarse	3

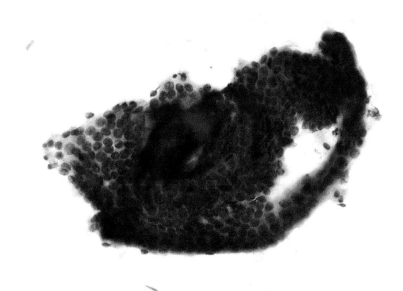

Fig. 22.3 A Papanicolaou stained slide of a group of cells showing calcification and a relatively monotonous group of cells.

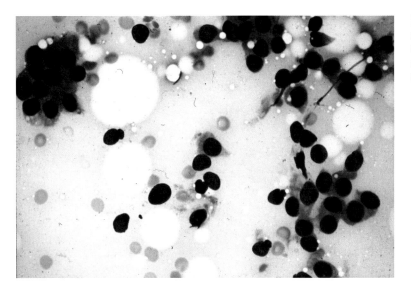

Fig. 22.4 Another case of ADH on cytology showing some dissociation of columnar cells from the edge of the duct. Some bare nuclei can also be seen, however, in the same field. May-Grunewald Giemsa.

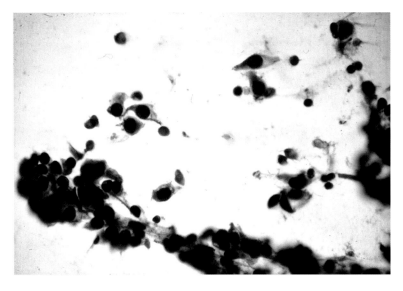

Fig. 22.5 The same case as Fig. 22.4 showing similar dissociation of columnar cells in the Papanicolaou stain.

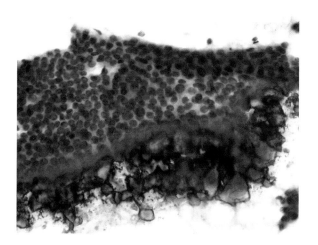

Fig. 22.6 A cluster of cells with calcification, showing a monotonous cell composition and little attempt at streaming of cells, as is often seen in usual ductal hyperplasia. Papanicolaou.

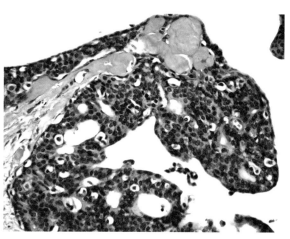

Fig. 22.9 Higher power view of the area of ADH within a papilloma. H&E.

Fig. 22.7 The same case as Fig. 22.6 showing apocrine cells and calcification as well as a more monotonous cluster with well-defined edges similar to the previous figure. May-Grunewald Giemsa.

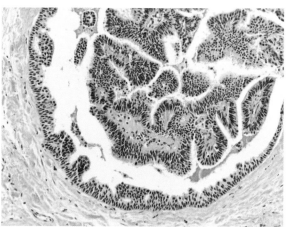

Fig. 22.8 A papillary lesion with extensive flat and micro-papillary epithelial atypia. H&E.

ADH associated with other lesions such as radial scars, complex sclerosing lesions and papillary lesions (Figs 22.8–22.11) can also be aspirated and may cause confusion, as the fundamental clinical or radiological features are those of the underlying lesion rather than the fine punctate calcification associated with isolated ADH.

It should be remembered that distinguishing ADH from ductal carcinoma in-situ is only difficult in cases of low grade DCIS. An accurate fine needle aspiration (FNA) from high grade DCIS will show obvious malignant cells and necrosis, neither of which are features of ADH. The difficulty in distinguishing low grade DCIS from ADH in breast screening has been cited as a reason for adoption of core biopsy on areas of microcalcification. However, as the majority of DCIS detected in breast screening are high grade, there is no a priori reason, despite opinions to the contrary, why FNA should not be used as a first line method of investigation.

ATYPICAL LOBULAR HYPERPLASIA (ALH)

Atypical lobular hyperplasia is a lesion defined as partial filling or involvement of a lobule or number of lobules with neoplastic lobular cells resembling those of lobular carcinoma in-situ. The distinction is really one of extent and is partially subjective. Lobular carcinoma in-situ (LCIS) is diagnosed when greater than 50% of a lobule has its acini filled and expanded by a uniform population of neoplastic lobular cells. ALH, in contrast, is diagnosed when less than 50% of the acini show these features. Accordingly, a proliferation that fills but does not expand the acini, that is still a mixed proliferation but includes cells recognizable as lobular neoplasia, or that does not completely fill the

acini is designated as ALH (Fig. 22.13). Thus defined, the lesion has a relative risk of subsequent invasive carcinoma of approximately 4.5-times [3]. Recognizing the difficulty of assigning a lesion to one or other of these categories, some authors have advocated the term 'lobular neoplasia' for these lesions. ALH may extend into terminal ducts, increasing its relative risk of subsequent invasive malignancy approximately 9-times, a level comparable to fully developed LCIS [9].

ALH and LCIS do not have a distinctive mammographic or clinical appearance and are likely to be aspirated only by chance in association with another lesion such as fibrocystic change or radial scar. Very occasionally, LCIS may calcify and produce appearances similar to low grade DCIS of solid type, but this is the exception rather than the rule.

The cytological appearances of ALH (Figs 22.13–22.15) are those of small clusters of atypical cells with round or lens-shaped nuclei with some dissocia-

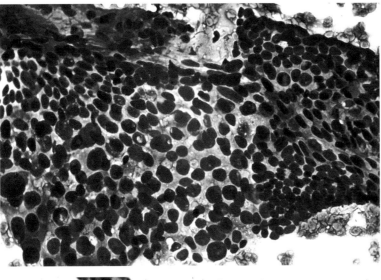

Fig. 22.10 Highly atypical cells on cytology. These cells appear cytologically malignant but merge with more monomorphous cells within the same group, which obviously contains two cell types. May-Grunewald Giemsa.

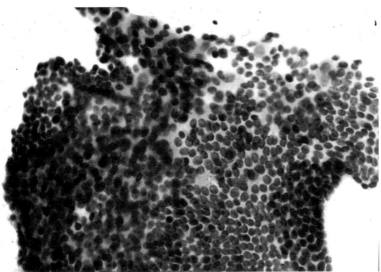

Fig. 22.11 The same case on Papanicolaou staining showing a similar cluster composed of two cell types, with atypical cells and more regular cells merging in the same cluster. Care should be taken not to overinterpret these changes as unequivocal malignancy.

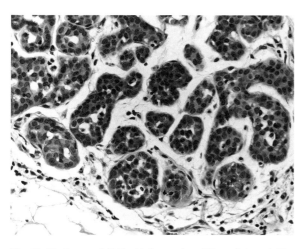

Fig. 22.12 A case of ALH with incomplete filling of the acini by neoplastic lobular cells. H&E.

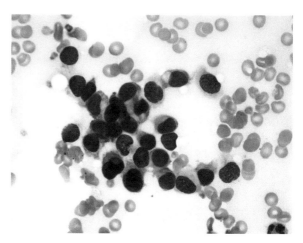

Fig. 22.15 A cluster of atypical neoplastic lobular cells in another case of ALH. May-Grunewald Giemsa.

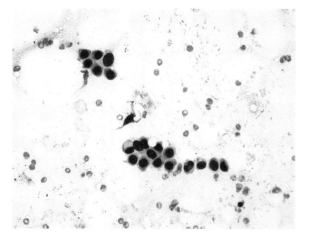

Fig. 22.13 Small atypical neoplastic lobular cells in a cytological aspirate from the same case as Fig. 22.12. These neoplastic lobular cells are rarely a major feature of smears from cases of ALH. They can, however, be mistaken for lobular carcinoma cells. May-Grunewald Giemsa.

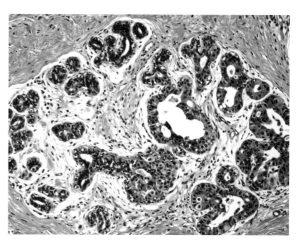

Fig. 22.16 A case of atypical apocrine hyperplasia. The patient developed an invasive apocrine carcinoma seven years later. Despite this, the features in this case are not sufficient for a diagnosis of apocrine DCIS. H&E.

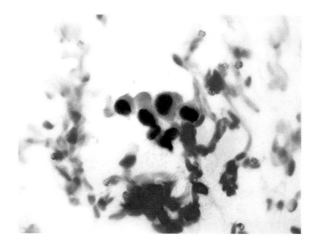

Fig. 22.14 A similar small group of atypical lobular cells from the same case. Papanicolaou.

tion [10]. Smears are usually poorly cellular and generally have the features of the underlying lesion associated with the atypical cells, unlike smears from invasive lobular carcinoma. For example, fibrocystic change with associated ALH will show the general features of fibrocystic change: apocrine cells, benign ductal epithelial cells and foamy macrophages with occasional small groups of atypical cells showing some dissociation. This is in contrast to the cytological picture of a poorly cellular smear with a monotonous population of neoplastic lobular cells, which would be suggestive of invasive lobular carcinoma. The atypical cells from ALH are small and have a high nuclear cytoplasmic ratio and an abnormal chromatin pattern. Some of the cells may contain intracytoplasmic mucin droplets, which stain with alcian blue/periodic acid Schiff (AB/PAS) staining. Although these droplets are

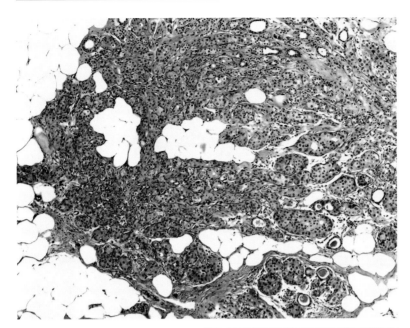

Fig. 22.17 A low power view of atypical apocrine change within sclerosing adenosis. The low power view still has a lobular configuration. H&E.

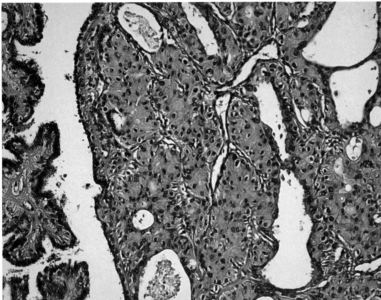

Fig. 22.18 An area of atypical apocrine change within a papilloma. Note the normal epithelium of the papilloma in the left field. H&E.

also highly characteristic of lobular carcinoma their presence in ALH means they are not necessarily indicative of malignancy.

■ ATYPICAL APOCRINE HYPERPLASIA (AAH) ■ AND ATYPICAL APOCRINE ADENOSIS (AAA)

These lesions have been described as premalignant by Seidman et al. with a 5.5-times increased relative risk of subsequent malignancy [11]. AAH is defined as an intraluminal proliferation of atypical apocrine cells with a greater than three-fold variation in nuclear size and a complex growth pattern with micropapillae and bridges akin to low grade nonapocrine DCIS

(Fig. 22.16). AAA is defined as atypical apocrine cells with a greater than three-fold variation in nuclear size associated with sclerosing adenosis [12] (Fig. 22.17).

AAH is an intraductal lesion or intra-acinar proliferation, which is sometimes associated with cyst formation. This can lead to difficulties in cytological diagnosis [13]. AAA is also problematic for cytologists as it also often coexists with radial scars or complex sclerosing lesions [14, 15].

Atypical apocrine hyperplasia within a papilloma is also problematic (Fig. 22.18).

Histologically, both of these conditions are usually identified due to the marked nuclear atypia within the apocrine cells, and therefore it is not so surprising that they can cause problems in cytological interpretation.

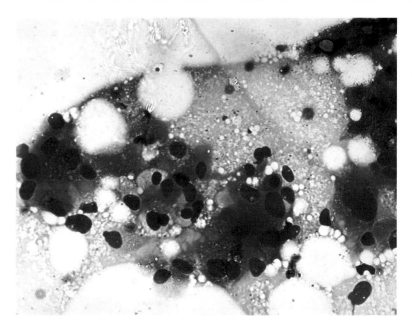

Fig. 22.19 Atypical apocrine cells on cytology. Care must be taken when interpreting such cytological changes, as they can easily be misdiagnosed as malignant. The presence of spindle cells from the sclerosing adenosis in conjunction with the apocrine cells can be a helpful feature. May-Grunewald Giemsa.

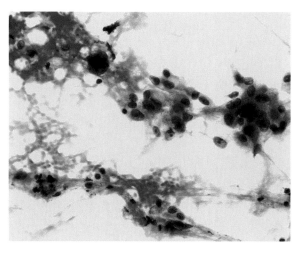

Fig. 22.20 Atypical apocrine cells on Papanicolaou staining from the same case.

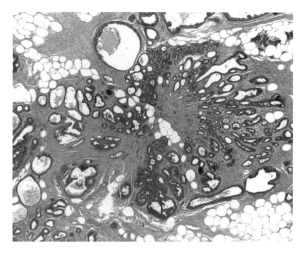

Fig. 22.21 A typical radial scar on histology with a central hyaline elastotic scar. H&E.

Aspiration from apocrine adenosis can produce bizarre apocrine cells in clusters with some dissociation of cells at the edge of the clusters (Figs 22.19 and 22.20). The clusters, unlike those of apocrine carcinomas, do however show a mixture of two distinct cell types, with spindle cells from the sclerosing component intermingling with the atypical apocrine cells. Necrosis and mitotic figures are not features of these conditions, and their presence should alert the reader to the likelihood of carcinoma. Conversely, in their absence, smears containing recognizable apocrine cells, even if bizarre, should not be unequivocally diagnosed as malignant. In cases of AAH associated with papillary lesions, recognizable nonapocrine papillary structures and foamy macrophages are usually present in addition to the atypical apocrine cells.

RADIAL SCAR

Radial scars are characterized histologically by pseudoinfiltrative epithelial structures with a variable degree of hyperplasia radiating outwards from a central core of elastotic fibrous tissue (Fig. 22.21). Their possible relationship to subsequent malignancy is unproven, and their inclusion in a chapter on preneoplastic lesions may be controversial. Nonetheless they do appear to be frequently associated with hyperplasia and atypia, as detailed above and illustrated in a number of publications [2]. This makes their cytological features variable. They bear a resemblance mammographically to low grade carcinoma, especially tubular carcinoma. Cytologically, differentiating these

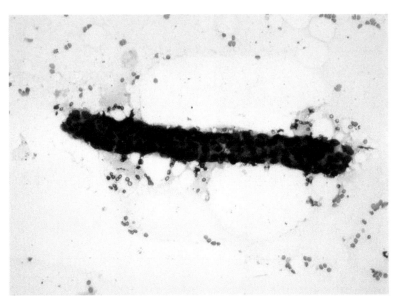

Fig. 22.22 An elongated tubule from the radial scar in Fig. 22.21. May-Grunewald Giemsa.

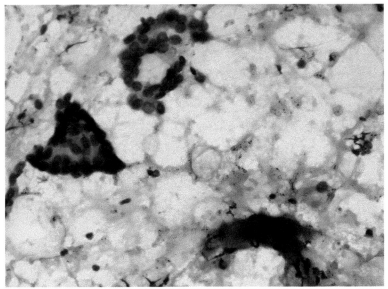

Fig. 22.23 Angular tubule formation also from the same radial scar. Note however the myoepithelial layer and bare nuclei. Hematoxylin.

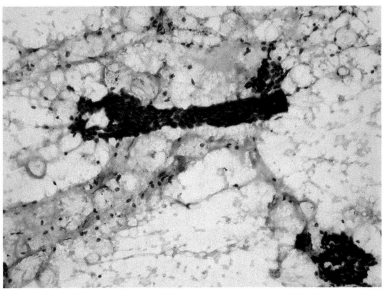

Fig. 22.24 Similar tubule formation with bare nuclei in a hematoxylin stained cytology smear.

lesions from low grade invasive carcinoma is difficult. Both may show tubular profiles on cytology (Figs 22.22 and 22.23), and smears from both may also contain bare nuclei (Fig. 22.24). Elastosis may be seen on cytological smears, if the aspiration technique is sufficiently good and hits the center of the lesion, but elastic tissue may also be obtained from the center of low grade carcinomas, especially tubular carcinoma. These lesions are responsible for a significant number of false results, if the cytologist is not aware of their radiological appearance.

MUCOCELE-LIKE LESIONS

Mucin secretion within the ducts of fibrocystic change is not uncommon, but the condition of mucocele-like lesions associated with ADH and DCIS of mucin secreting type is less commonly recognized, despite this being a significant cause of microcalcification of unusual morphology [16, 17] (Fig. 22.25). Cytologically, these lesions can resemble mucinous carcinoma, although generally without the ramifying vessels and the malignant cells within the mucous seen in that condition (Figs 22.25 and 22.26). In most other respects mucocele-like lesions can simulate mucinous carcinoma cytologically, especially if associated with atypical hyperplasia or mucinous DCIS [18, 19]. The clue to diagnosis is the absence of the characteristic mass-like lesion of a mucinous carcinoma on mammography and the presence of microcalcification only.

MULTIPLE PAPILLOMAS

The cytological features of multiple papilloma syndrome (multiple peripheral papillomas) are only poorly described in the literature, and cytology is not a

Fig. 22.26 Mucin and some benign appearing cells from the same case as Fig. 22.26. This should not be confused with mucinous carcinoma. The cells are usually relatively benign in appearance, even if there is concomitant atypia. May-Grunwald Giemsa.

particularly good test in investigating this condition. The lesion is defined by the presence of multiple peripheral papillomas, as opposed to the solitary papillomas occurring in major nipple ducts (Fig. 22.27). The condition should also not be confused with juvenile papillomatosis, which is generally not regarded as premalignant and is not associated with papilloma formation. It is also distinct from papillary duct hyperplasia of adolescence, where the papillary projections into the ducts are hyperplastic, in other words have multiple connections to the duct wall in contrast to true papillomas [20]. Multiple peripheral papillomas may develop ADH and low grade DCIS, eventually leading to low grade invasive carcinoma in approximately 25% of cases [21]. It is therefore fortu-

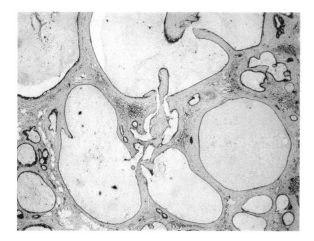

Fig. 22.25 A mucocele-like lesion that presented as microcalcification at mammographic screening. H&E.

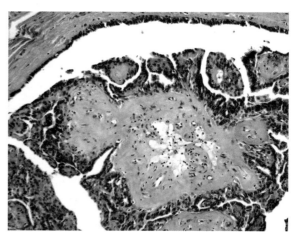

Fig. 22.27 A sclerosed papilloma from a case of multiple peripheral papillomas. H&E.

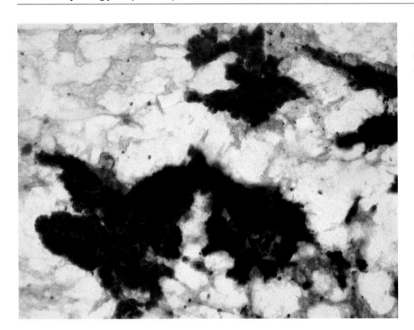

Fig. 22.28 Cytology from the same case showing papillary groups of cells with stromal cores. It is very difficult to exclude coexisting low grade DCIS in these cases. Papanicolaou.

nate that this lesion is rare. The papillomas in this condition have a myoepithelial layer, and low grade cribriform DCIS develops around the edge of the dilated duct preferentially. The cytological features [22] are those of a papilloma, with papillary cores within three-dimensional clusters of cells (Fig. 22.28). These are seen on Giemsa staining as metachromatic stroma within the clumps. On Papanicolaou staining, the clusters are seen to have a myoepithelial cell layer, but excluding in-situ disease in these circumstances is not possible. Indeed with smears from papillomas in general, it is often difficult to definitively exclude a diagnosis of intracystic papillary carcinoma.

JUVENILE PAPILLOMATOSIS

Juvenile papillomatosis (Swiss cheese disease) is a benign breast condition that is usually unilateral and is characterized by multiple apocrine-lined cysts with coexisting usual ductal hyperplasia, foamy macrophages and often sclerosing adenosis. Recurrent bilateral lesions with a positive family history have been suggested to have an increased incidence of malignancy, whereby unilateral nonrecurrent lesions do not appear to carry any increased risk [23]. In the absence of clinical features, cytological features are nonspecific, consisting of sheets of hyperplastic breast epithelium with areas resembling fibroadenoma, macrophages, and apocrine cells [24].

REFERENCES

1. Sneige N, Fornage BD, Saleh G. Ultrasound-guided fine-needle aspiration of nonpalpable breast lesions. Cytologic and histologic findings. American Journal of Clinical Pathology 1994;102;98–101.

2. Sloane JP, Mayers MM. Carcinoma and atypical hyperplasia in radial scars and complex sclerosing lesions: importance of lesion size and patient age [see comments]. Histopathology 1993;23;225–231.

3. Page DL, Dupont WD. Anatomic indicators (histologic and cytologic) of increased breast cancer risk. [Review]. Breast Cancer Research & Treatment 1993;28;157–166.

4. Marshall CJ, Schumann GB, Ward JH, Riding JM, Cannon-Albright L, Skolnick M. Cytologic identification of clinically occult proliferative breast disease in women with a family history of breast cancer [see comments]. American Journal of Clinical Pathology 1991;95;157–165.

5. Abendroth CS, Wang HH, Ducatman BS. Comparative features of carcinoma in-situ and atypical ductal hyperplasia of the breast on fine-needle aspiration biopsy specimens. American Journal of Clinical Pathology 1991;96;654–659.

6. Sneige N, Staerkel GA. Fine-needle aspiration cytology of ductal hyperplasia with and without atypia and ductal carcinoma in-situ. Human Pathology 1994;25;485–492.

7. Bibbo M, Scheiber M, Cajulis R, Keebler CM, Wied GL, Dowlatshahi K. Stereotaxic fine needle aspiration cytology of clinically occult malignant and premalignant breast lesions [published erratum appears in Acta Cytol 1992 May-Jun;36(3):460]. Acta Cytologica 1988;32;193–201.

8. Bellocq JP, Zafrani B, Chenard MP. – [Diagnostic difficulties and limits in breast histopathology in core biopsies (breast microbiopsies)]. [French]. – Archives d Anatomie et de Cytologie Pathologiques 1998;46(4): 257–60257–600.

9. Page DL, Kidd TE, Jr., Dupont WD, Simpson JF, Rogers LW. Lobular neoplasia of the breast: higher risk for subsequent invasive cancer predicted by more extensive disease. Human Pathology 1991;22;1232–1239.

10. Salhany KE, Page DL. Fine-needle aspiration of mammary lobular carcinoma in-situ and atypical lobular hyperplasia. American Journal of Clinical Pathology 1989;92;22–26.

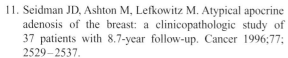
11. Seidman JD, Ashton M, Lefkowitz M. Atypical apocrine adenosis of the breast: a clinicopathologic study of 37 patients with 8.7-year follow-up. Cancer 1996;77; 2529 – 2537.

12. Tavassoli FA. Atypical hyperplasia: a morphologic risk factor for subsequent development of invasive breast carcinoma. [Review]. Cancer Investigation 1992;10; 433 – 441.

13. Sneige N. Fine-needle aspiration of the breast: a review of 1,995 cases with emphasis on diagnostic pitfalls. Diagnostic Cytopathology 1993;9;106 – 112.

14. Makunura CN, Curling OM, Yeomans P, Perry N, Wells CA. Apocrine adenosis within a radial scar: a case of false positive breast cytodiagnosis. Cytopathology 1994; 5;123 – 128.

15. Bonzanini M, Gilioli E, Brancato B, Pellegrini M, Mauri MF, Dalla PP. Cytologic features of 22 radial scar/complex sclerosing lesions of the breast, three of which associated with carcinoma: clinical, mammographic, and histologic correlation. – Diagnostic Cytopathology 1997 Nov;17(5):353 – 62 1997;353 – 622.

16. Chinyama CN, Davies JD. Mammary mucinous lesions: congeners, prevalence and important pathological associations. Histopathology 1996;Dec;29(6);533 – 539.

17. Hamele-Bena D, Cranor ML, Rosen PP. Mammary mucocele-like lesions. Benign and malignant. Am J Surg Pathol 1996;Sep;20(9):1081 – 1085.

18. Wong NL, Wan SK. Comparative cytology of mucocele-like lesion and mucinous carcinoma of the breast in fine needle aspiration. Acta Cytologica 2000;Sep-Oct;44(5); 765 – 770.

19. Yeoh GP, Cheung PS, Chan KW. Fine-needle aspiration cytology of mucocelelike tumors of the breast. Am J Surg Pathol 1999;May;23(5);552 – 559.

20. Wilson M, Cranor ML, Rosen PP. Papillary duct hyperplasia of the breast in children and young women. Mod Pathol 1993;Sep;6(5);570 – 574.

21. Papotti M, Gugliotta P, Ghiringhello B, Bussolati G. Association of breast carcinoma and multiple intraductal papillomas: an histological and immunohistochemical investigation. Histopathology 1984;Nov;8(6);963 – 975.

22. Jeffrey PB, Ljung BM. Benign and malignant papillary lesions of the breast. A cytomorphologic study. Am J Clin Pathol 1994;Apr;101(4);500 – 507.

23. Rosen PP, Kimmel M. Juvenile papillomatosis of the breast. A follow-up study of 41 patients having biopsies before 1979. Am J Clin Pathol 1990;May;93(5); 599 – 603.

24. Ostrzega N. Fine-needle aspiration cytology of juvenile papillomatosis of breast: a case report. Diagn Cytopathol 1993;Aug;9(4);457 – 460.

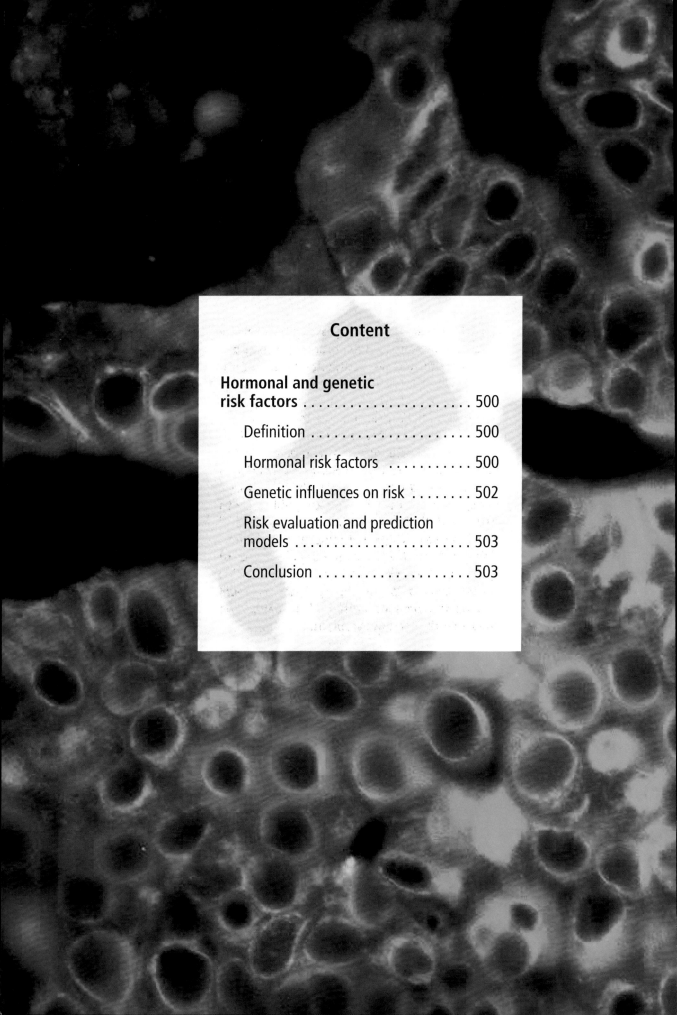

Content

HORMONAL AND GENETIC RISK FACTORS

RAJENDRA S. RAMPAUL, SARAH E. PINDER, DOUGLAS R. MACMILLAN AND IAN O. ELLIS

Breast cancer is a complex, multifactorial disease involving numerous interrelations with genetic and environmental factors. Each year, over one million new cases are diagnosed, making it the commonest malignancy in women (18% of all female cancers). In the United Kingdom, the age-standardized incidence and mortality are the highest in the world and in the United States over 180,000 women are diagnosed annually [1]. Worldwide, breast cancer is a major public health issue, and thus efforts to better understand the disease are of paramount importance. **Epidemiological studies have attempted to quantify the risk associated with invasive breast carcinoma. In this chapter we will discuss the data of hormonal influences on breast carcinoma development.**

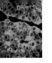

Hormonal and genetic risk factors

■ Definition

A risk factor is defined as the characteristic of individual patients that increase their chances of developing breast cancer to about the level of risk in the general population.

Risk factors can be classified as genetic (family history), hormonal, nutritional, morphologic (previous benign disease), and radiation-related. It is important to remember however that absence of risk factors does not exclude the development of cancer.

One of the main results arising from the recognition of breast cancer risk has been the use of age to determine recommendations for mammographic screening programs. There is now a growing impetus for physicians to become versed in evaluating breast cancer risk and in counseling women on medical decisions.

The last decade has witnessed a great thrust in breast cancer research, and there is now good data on various etiologic factors in the development of breast cancer. For example, two major susceptibility genes (BRCA1 and BRCA2) have been identified and isolated, the human genome project has demonstrated regions that have revealed as yet unidentified breast cancer-related genes, and some somatically altered genes have been characterized.

Up to 10% of all breast cancers can be accounted for by the inheritance of BRCA1 or BRCA2 mutations [2]. However, it is important to appreciate that non-genetic factors also play a role in familial clustering. Very little is known about the interaction of genes with environmental pressures, and much work must therefore be done to better understand the factors involved in the development of breast cancer.

■ Hormonal risk factors

It is now known that estrogen exposure is associated with the risk of developing breast cancer. Increased or prolonged exposure is associated with an increased risk [3, 4], whereas reducing exposure is considered to provide a protective effect [5]. Female sex, and menstrual and reproductive history all strongly implicate steroid sex hormones in the development of mammary cancer.

Reproductive steroid hormones are thought to exert an influence on carcinogenesis by affecting prolifera-

tion kinetics, differentiation and stem cell atrophy – all of which can result in an increase in susceptible cells. Factors associated with a greater number of menstrual cycles such as early age of menarche, nulliparity, and late onset menopause [6–8] increase the likelihood of breast cancer.

Pike et al. [4] demonstrated from a case-control study of women aged 32 or less that oral contraception use before full term pregnancy was associated with an elevated risk of breast cancer (p < 0.01). It was also observed that a first trimester abortion before a first full term pregnancy was associated with a 2.4-fold risk increase (p < 0.005). Thus women who start menstruating early in life have a twofold increase in relative risk (RR).

The same holds true for those with a late menopause. Women with a natural menopause after the age of 55 possess a breast cancer RR twice that of women undergoing the menopause before the age of 45 [9]. Oophorectomy provides protection inversely related to age at oophorectomy.

Nulliparity and late age at first birth both increase the lifetime risk of breast cancer. Nulliparous women have an RR of 1 compared with 0.5 for those who have their first child before the age of 20. Women who choose to have their first child after the age of 37 are at highest risk (1.4).

Not surprisingly, evidence shows that decreasing the number of ovulatory cycles caused by moderate exercise [10, 11] and a longer lactation period [12] can be protective.

Oral contraceptive hormones

To date, studies on the relationship between the use of the oral contraceptive pill (OCP) and the risk of breast cancer have arrived at differing conclusions. Several early studies [13–15] were unable to demonstrate a relationship between the two, whereas later studies in long-term users of the OCP and also in women on estrogen-progestogen replacement therapy do seem to indicate a link.

Data from the *Cancer and Steroid Hormone Study* (CASH) were used to assess whether OCP use had different effects on the risk of breast cancer at different ages of diagnosis [16]. This hypothesis followed on from the observation of age-specific differences in breast cancer risk factors and age-specific differences in the cancer-parity relationship. Women in the 20 to

34 age group using the OCP were found to have a slightly increased risk (odds ratio [OR], 1.4; 95% CI, 1.0–2.1) when compared to those who had never used the OCP. No association between OCP use and the development of breast carcinoma was seen in women in the 35 to 44 age range. OCP use actually decreased the risk of breast cancer (OR, 0.9; 95% CI, 0.8–1.0) in women between 45 and 54 years of age. The authors concluded that, even though the slightly increased risk estimates for the youngest women were compatible with findings by other investigators, the data provide no reasons for changing prescribing practices or for altering OCP use associated with a risk of breast cancer.

The Collaborative Group on Hormonal Factors in Breast Cancer performed a reanalysis of data on 53,297 women with and 100,239 women without breast cancer from 54 epidemiologic studies. This showed that women taking the combined OCP have a slightly increased risk of developing breast carcinoma, with the effect persisting for ten years after termination of use [16, 17].

The cancers that did develop in this study population were generally confined to the breast. Those in the group taking the OCP had clinically less advanced cancers than those who did not.

Miller et al. examined the relation between risk of breast cancer before 45 years of age and OCP use in a case-control study of 407 patients with breast cancer and 424 controls [14]. From their data the authors concluded that, for less than ten years of exogenous steroid use, the RR estimate was 2.0, while for women with more than ten years use this rose to 4.1 (95% CI, 1.8–9.3). These finding suggest that length of exposure may influence risk of development of breast cancer in very long-term users.

Hormone replacement therapy (HRT)

Evidence suggests that hormone replacement therapy reduces the risk of coronary heart disease and osteoporosis by about 50% but increases the risk of breast cancer by 30–40% [18–20]. The fact that the reduction in coronary disease and osteoporosis is larger than the increase in breast cancer, and that women have a greater probability of dying of coronary events than breast cancer, have led some experts to consider that the benefits of HRT outweigh the risks [21, 22]. This approach must, however, be taken cautiously, as the balance between risks and benefits are quite different for women at increased risks. The relative risk associated with HRT in women with a family history of breast cancer does not appear to be any higher than those without a family history. However, data based on decision analyses suggest that the absolute benefit of HRT falls as the risk of breast cancer increases [22–24].

In current users of HRT and those who have used HRT in the previous one to four years, RR increases by 1.023 (1.011–1.036) for each year of use. The risk of breast cancer also appears higher with combined estrogen and progesterone preparations.

HRT formulation and pattern of positive use have varied quite considerably over the years. This has of course posed a limitation to the interpretation of data examining the relationship between HRT and breast cancer.

Findings of six meta-analyses [25, 26] and a large pooled analysis [27] of epidemiologic studies investigating the possible relationship between postmenopausal estrogen use and risk of breast cancer show RR estimates across studies range from 1.01–1.07. In the pooled analysis the RR was 1.14 [27]. However, women who have used HRT have, overall, little or no risk compared to women who have never used these hormones. The criterion 'ever use' is a poor measure of exposure as it can neither distinguish between short- and long-term use nor between recent and past users.

Data from the meta-analyses show a significant increase in risk of 30–40% in patients using HRT for longer than five years. However, when compared to results from several case control studies [28, 29], a significant positive association was not observed. The elevated RR seen in the meta-analysis was also encompassed in the 95% confidence interval of these case-controlled studies. Case control studies do possess limitations such as the non-participation of controls. This must be borne in mind when interpreting data from such work.

Assessment of risk based on recent use is difficult, as many studies have not clearly delineated this from current usage. Some studies quote a RR for current use of 1.63 for those with a natural menopause and 1.48 for a surgical menopause [30]. The *Breast Cancer Detection Demonstration Project* (BCDDP) showed a positive association with invasive breast cancer among current users with 5–15 years of use (RR 1.0–1.4) [31].

The effect of current or recent use of HRT on breast cancer risk was evaluated in detail in the pooled analysis [27]. A statistically significant association was observed between current/recent use and risk of breast cancer. The strongest positive association was seen with longest duration of use. In those using postmenopausal hormones within the previous five years the RR were 1.08 (1–4 years use), 1.31 (5–9 years of use), 1.24 (10–14 years of use) and 1.56 (more than 15 years of use). No significant increase in breast cancer risk was seen in women who had stopped using post menopausal hormones for five or more years.

Interestingly, it has been suggested that increased surveillance among women taking hormones may

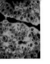

account for the increased risk seen in several studies. Support for this comes from the observation that a higher RR is associated with in-situ disease rather invasive disease [29, 30].

GENETIC INFLUENCES ON RISK

It is now well established that a positive family history carries an increased risk of developing breast cancer [31]. Farrell et al. [31] have shown from pooled data that the RR conferred by a first-degree relative is 2.0, and up to 10% of breast cancers are known to develop from germ line mutations in susceptibility genes which are inherited as autosomal dominant.

Two breast cancer susceptibility genes, BRCA1 and BRCA2, have been isolated and characterized in the last ten years. These have been shown to be responsible for up to 80% of large breast cancer kindreds.

BRCA1 GENE

Using segregation analysis Williams and Anderson [32] evaluated all genetic models that could explain the aggregation of breast cancer in families and rejected all but the inheritance of a highly penetrative autosomal susceptibility allele. This approach was vindicated with the isolation of the BRCA1 gene on chromosome 17q [32, 33].

Between 15–45% of hereditary breast cancers are now known to be associated with a BRCA1 germ line mutation [34, 35]. The lifetime risk of breast cancer among female mutation carriers is 60–80% [36, 37], with a 20–40% risk of developing ovarian cancers [40, 41].

Cancers arising from BRCA1 germ line mutations possess several characteristic clinical features: an earlier age of onset compared to sporadic cases, a higher prevalence of bilateral cancer and the presence of associated tumors (in particular ovarian but also colon and prostatic cancers) [36, 40].

BRCA1 consists of 24 exons, 22 of which code for a protein composed of 1,863 amino acids. The gene contains a C3HC4 zinc-binding RING finger in the domain at the amino terminal and has a simian virus 40-type nuclear localization sequence in exon 11 [35]. The gene also has a conserved acidic carboxyl terminus [35] called the BRCT domain [41–45]. BRCT motives have been described in several proteins involved in cell cycle control and DNA damage repair pathways [44, 45], providing support for the role of BRCA1 in cellular responses to DNA damage. The most common founder mutations in BRCA1 are 185 del AG and 5382 ins C [46, 47] and may account for up to 10% of all mutations in BRCA1. These mutations also occur at a tenfold higher frequency in

Ashkenazi Jews [48, 49]. When combined, these two mutations account for almost all BRCA1 mutations in this population. The 185 del AG mutation has also been reported in Moroccan, Spanish and non-Jewish families [50–53], suggesting that the short tandem repeat at this locus may be prone to mutations. Approximately 20% of Jewish women with early onset breast cancer (less than 40 years old) carry the 185 del AG mutation [54].

There are a few reports of mutations in other European populations. The 5382 ins C and the 4153 del AA mutations have been detected in studies of Russian populations [55]. The 2802 del AA mutation has been seen in the Netherlands [56, 57], and 1675 del A and 1135 ins A [58] have been described in Norwegian populations. Llede et al. have recently described a new founder mutation among people of Scottish ancestry [59].

Large or partial genomic deletions are also an important source of mutation in BRCA1. The high frequency of the Alu repeat element in intronic regions of BRCA1 has been postulated as a cause [32]. Studies on Dutch and Belgian populations reveal three large genomic deletions which accounted for 30% of all BRCA1 mutations in these families.

BRCA2 GENE

Wooster et al. have demonstrated the existence of a second dominant breast cancer susceptibility gene using linkage analysis from 22 families. These families possessed early onset female breast cancer and included one case of male breast cancer. Polymorphic markers in these families enabled the BRCA2 locus to be linked to chromosome 13q. For BRCA2 mutation carriers, lifetime risk of breast cancer has been estimated at 60–85%, and lifetime risk of ovarian cancer at 10–20%. Patients may also be associated with an increase in colon, prostatic, pancreatic, bowel duct and stomach cancers.

BRCA2 cDNA is approximately 11.5 kb long and is composed of 26 exons in the coding region. The BRCA2 protein consists of 3,418 amino acids and has a molecular mass of 384 kDa. Code mutation on sporadic BRCA2 is not well established. Current research is progressing at a rapid rate, and at present over 250 mutations have been found. A number of founder mutations have been identified in BRCA2. In Ashkenazi Jews there is a prevalence of 1.2% for the 6174 del T mutation. The 999 del 5 mutation has been observed in Icelandic and Finnish populations. It is thought that this mutation has been shared by both these populations. A common haplotype covering the regions spanning the BRCA2 gene was found and suggests that this mutation was carried by individuals who migrated during ancient times. BRCA2, similar to

BRCA1, is postulated to play a role in DNA damage response pathways.

LOW PENETRANCE BREAST CANCER SUSCEPTIBILITY GENES

Susceptibility alleles of low penetrance are defined in this instance as genes in which subtle sequence variance or polymorphisms may be associated with an altered risk of breast cancer. Such variance in these genes is common in the general population. It is currently thought that each variant may be associated with a much higher attributable risk of cancer than high penetrance genes, and may therefore be responsible for more breast cancers than the highly penetrant BRCA1 and BRCA2 genes. Modifier genes operate on the basis of biologic causality and as such can be found in a number of pathways such as steroid metabolism, DNA damage response and immunomodulatory pathways. One such gene is the mutated ataxia-telangiectasia (ATM) gene. Epidemiological studies have suggested that around 1% of the female population carries a mutated ATM gene, significantly increasing their RR of breast cancer (3.9–6.4). This may account for up to five percent of all breast cancers [32]. Other candidate genes include p53 (Li Fraumeni syndrome), CYP1A1, CYP17 and several protooncogenes.

RISK EVALUATION AND PREDICTION MODELS

In the United Kingdom average individual risk is approximately one in ten and in the United States this figure is closer to one in eight for the female population [37]. This risk naturally decreases with increasing age (assuming no development of cancer).

Currently there are four models available to assess risk. Of these the Gail model is most popular. It estimates the breast cancer risk in white women screened annually with mammography [60] and predicts the cumulative risk according to decade up to the age of 90. Variables include current age, age at menarche, age at first live birth, number of breast biopsies, presence of atypical hyperplasia and number of first degree relatives with breast cancers. In the United States the Gail model is also employed to guide patient cohort selection for clinical breast cancer prevention trials. While it provides a good estimate in selected populations, the model does possess limitations. It over-predicts for the younger women, women younger than 20 at first birth and those that do not participate in annual screening programs. It may also overestimate the risk for women whose mother or sisters developed late onset breast cancer as well as under-estimate the risk for those with multiple second, or third degree relatives affected by breast cancer.

Claus et al. using data from the CASH study developed another commonly used model [2]. The Claus model is based on the assumption of high penetrant genes due to a rare autosomal dominant mutation. The model incorporates more information about family history but is not useful in very high-risk pedigree and does not take environmental, behavioral or reproductive factors into account.

Genetic testing for BRCA1/2 mutations can be assessed using the BRCAPRO software, which is available online at **www.jhsph.edu/biostats/brcapro**.

CONCLUSION

Clinicians involved in the care of breast cancer patients are often asked: 'What are my chances of developing breast cancer?' And: 'Will my children develop breast cancer?'

Thus physicians must become adept in evaluating breast cancer risk using the most up-to-date risk assessment tools and knowledge of the literature supporting its use. Risk assessment can be used directly to guide HRT, mammography, use of Tamoxifen for prevention, counseling, use of prophylactic mastectomy and genetic testing for BRCA1/2 mutations.

One of the first steps in this process for a woman with a risk factor for BRCA1 or BRCA2 mutation is to determine if she is interested in pursuing genetic testing before testing actually is undertaken. She should be provided with information on the probability of her carrying a mutation and on the benefits, risks and limitations of available testing. It is imperative that an informed decision about BRCA1 testing is made.

Because BRCA1 mutations are rare in non-Ashkenazi Jews, genetic testing is unlikely to provide useful information for women from families with no risk factors for BRCA mutation [61].

As discussed earlier, there are several methods and factors available for stratifying risk and predicting a woman's individual risk of breast cancer. Each method has its own merits and may be appropriate in completely different settings. Qualitative assessment of breast cancer risk may be sufficient for a woman in her fourth or fifth decade to make a decision about screening mammography, but making a decision on whether to undergo prophylactic mastectomy would involve genetic susceptibility testing.

For women with risk factors for carrying a BRCA1 or BRCA2 mutation, but who subsequently test negative or do not choose to undergo testing, the Claus model offers the most comprehensive assessment of their family history. In the UK there are now guidelines developed to help physicians provide care and counseling for such patients who require genetic counseling and screening mammography [62].

REFERENCES

1. Kelsey, J. and P. Horn-Ross, Breast cancer: magnitude of the problem and escriptive epidemiology. Epidemiologic Reviews, 1993. 15: p. 7–16.
2. Claus, E., et al., The genetic attributable risk of breast and ovarian cancer. Cancer, 1996. 77: p. 2318–2324.
3. Begg, L., et al., Endogenous sex hormone levels and breast cancer risk. Genetic Epidemiology, 1987. 4: p. 233–247.
4. Pike, M., et al., The hormonal basis of breast cancer. National Cancer Institute Monograph, 1979. 53: p. 187–193.
5. Hulka, B., Epidemiologic analysis of breast and gynecologic cancers. Progress in Clinical & Biological Research, 1997. 396: p. 17–29.
6. Trichopoulos, D., B. MacMahon, and P. Cole, Menopause and breast cancer risk. Journal of the National Cancer Institute, 1972. 48: p. 605–613.
7. Kampert, J., A. Whittemore, and R.J. Paffenbarger, Combined effect of childbearing, menstrual events, and body size on age-specific breast cancer risk. American Journal of Epidemiology, 1988. 128: p. 962–979.
8. White, E., Projected changes in breast cancer incidence due to the trend toward delayed childbearing. American Journal of Public Health, 1987. 77: p. 495–497.
9. Henderson, B., Endogenous and exogenous endocrine factors. Hematol Oncol Clin North Am, 1989. 3: p. 577–598.
10. Berg, J. and R. Hutter, Breast Cancer. Cancer, 1995. 75: p. 257–269.
11. Yuan, J., et al., Risk factors for breast cancer in Chinese women in Shanghai. Cancer Research, 1988. 48: p. 1949–1953.
12. Bergkvist, L., et al., The risk of breast cancer after estrogen and estrogen-progestin replacement. New England Journal of Medicine, 1989. 321: p. 293–297.
13. McPherson, K., A. Neil, and M.e.a. Vessey, Oral contraceptives and breast cancer. Lancet, 1983. 17: p. 1414–1415.
14. Miller, A., G. How, and G.e.a. Sherman, Mortality from breast cancer afer irradiation during fluoroscopic examinations in patients being treated for tuberculosis. New England Journal of Medicine, 1989. 321: p. 1285–1289.
15. Pike, M., B. Henderson, and J. Calagrande, Oral Contraceptive use and early abortion risk as factors for breast cancer in young women. British Journal of Cancer, 1981. 43: p. 72–76.
16. Collaborative Group on Hormonal Factors in Breast Cancer, Breast cancer and hormonal contraceptives: Collaborative re-analysis of individual data on 53,297 women with breast cancer and 100,239 women without breast cancer from 54 epidemiologic studies. Lancet, 1996. 347: p. 1713–1727.
17. Grodstein, F., M. Stampfer, and G.e.a. Colditz, Post-menopausal hormone therapy and mortality. New England Journal of Medicine, 1997. 336: p. 1769–1775.
18. Folsom, A., et al., Hormonal replacement therapy and morbidity and mortality in a prospective study of post-menopausal women. American Journal of Public Health, 1995. 85: p. 1128–1132.
19. Colditz, G., S. Hankinson, and D.e.a. Hunter, The use of estrogens and progestins and the risk of breast cancer in postmenopausal women. New England Journal of Medicine, 1995. 332: p. 1589–1593.
20. Grady, D., S. Rubin, and D.e.a. Petitti, Hormone therapy to prevent disease and prolong life in postmenopausal women. Ann Intern Med, 1992. 117: p. 1016–1037.
21. Col, N., M. Eckman, and R.e.a. Karas, Patient-specific decisions about hormone replacement therapy in post-menopausal women. JAMA, 1997. 277: p. 1140–1147.
22. Col, N., S. Pauker, and R.e.a. Goldberg, Individualizing therapy to prevent long-term consequences of estrogen deficiency in postmenopausal women. Arch Intern Med, 1999. 159: p. 1458–1466.
23. Colditz, G., B. Rosner, and F. Speizer, Risk factors for breast cancer according to family history of breast cancer. J Natl Cancer Inst, 1996. 88: p. 365–371.
24. Dupont, W. and D. Page, Menopausal estrogen replacement therapy and breast cancer. Arch Intern Med, 1991. 151: p. 67–72.
25. Grady, D., S. Rubin, and D.e.a. Petitti, Hormone therapy to prevent disease and prolong life in postmenopausal women. Ann Intern Med, 1992. 117: p. 1016–1036.
26. Collaborative Group on Hormonal Factors in Breast Cancer, Breast Cancer and hormone replacement therapy: collaborative reanalysis of data from 51 epidemiologic studies of 52,705 women with breast cancer and 108,411 women without breast cancer. Lancet, 1997. 1997(350).
27. Newcomb, P., M. Longnecker, and B.e.a. Storer, Long-term hormone replacement therapy and risk of breast cancer in postmenopausal women. American Journal of Epidemiology, 1995. 332: p. 1589–1593.
28. Stanford, J., et al., Combined estrogen and progestin hormone replacement therapy in relation to risk of breast cancer in middle-aged women. JAMA, 1995. 274 (137–142).
29. Schairer, C., et al., Menopausal estrogen and estrogen-progestin replacement therapy and risk of breast cancer (United States). Cancer Causes Control, 1994. 5: p. 491–500.
30. Martin, A.-M. and L. Weber, Genetic and Hormonal Risk Factors in Breast Cancer. Journal of the National Cancer Institute, 2000. 92(14): p. 1126–1135.
31. Pharoah, P., N. Day, and S.e.a. Duffy, Family history and the risk of breast cancer: a systematic review and meta-analysis. International Journal of Cancer, 1997. 71: p. 800–809.
32. Williams, W. and D. Anderson, Genetic epidemiology of breast cancer: segregation analysis of 200 Danish pedigrees. Genet Epidemiol, 1984. 1: p. 7–20.
33. Miki, Y., et al., A strong candidate for the breast and ovarian cancer susceptibility gene GRCA1. Science, 1994. 266: p. 66–71.
34. Narod, S., et al., An evluation of genetic heterogeneity in 145 breast-ovarian cancer families. Breast Cancer Linkage Consortium. American Journal of Hum Genet, 1995. 56: p. 254–264.
35. Easton, D., D. Ford, and J. Peto, Inherited susceptibility to breast cancer. Cancer Survey, 1993. 18: p. 95–113.

36. Couch, F., et al., BRCA 1 mutations in women attending clinics that evaluate the risk of breast cancer. New England Journal of Medicine, 1997. 336: p. 1409–1415.

37. Easton, D., et al., Genetic linkage analysis in familial breast and ovarian cancer: results from 214 families. The Breast Cancer Linkage Consortium. American Journal of Hum Genet, 1993. 52: p. 678–701.

38. Struewing, J., et al., BRCA1 mutations in young women with breast cancer [letter]. Lancet, 1996. 347: p. 1493.

39. Easton, D., D. Ford, and D. Bishop, Breast and ovarian cancer incidence in BRCA 1-mutation carriers. Breast Cancer Linkage Consortium. American Journal of Hum Genet, 1995. 56: p. 265–271.

40. Nelson, C., et al., Familial clustering of colon, breast, uterine and ovarian cancers as assessed by family history. Genet Epidemiol, 1993. 10: p. 235–244.

41. Anderson, D. and M. Badzioch, Familial breast cancer risks. Effects of prostate and other cancers. Cancer, 1993. 72: p. 114–119.

42. Arason, A., R. Barkardottir, and V. Egilsson, Linkage analysis of chromosome 17q markers and breast-ovarian cancer in Icelandic families, and possible relationship to prostatic cancer. American Journal of Hum Genet, 1993. 52: p. 711–717.

43. Koonin, E., S. Altschul, and P. Bork, BRCA 1 protein products: functional motifs. Nat Genet, 1996. 13: p. 266–268.

44. Callebaut, I. and J. Mornon, From BRCA1 to RAP1: a widespread BRCT module closely associated with DNA repair. FEBS Lett, 1997. 400: p. 25–30.

45. Abel, J., et al., Mouse Brca1: localization sequence analysis and identification of evolutionarily conserved domains. Hum Mol Genet, 1995. 4: p. 2265–2273.

46. Bork, P., et al., A supervamily of conserved domains in DNA damage-responsive cell cycle checkpoint proteins. FASEB J, 1997. 11(68–76).

47. Couch, F. and B. Weber, Mutations and polymorphisms in the familial early-onset breast cancer (BRCA1) gene. Breast Cancer Information Core. Hum Mutat, 1996. 8: p. 8–18.

48. Tonin, P., et al., BRCA1 mutations in Ashkenazi Jewish women [letter]. American Journal of Hum Genet, 1995. 57: p. 189.

49. Struewing, J., et al., The risk of cancer associated with specific mutations of BRCA1 and BRCA2 among Ashkenazi jews. New England Journal of Medicine, 1997. 336: p. 1401–1408.

50. Berman, D., et al., Two distinct origins of a common BRCA1 mutation in breast-ovarian cancer families: a genetic study of 15,185 delAG-mutation kindreds. American Journal of Hum Genet, 1996. 58: p. 1166–1176.

51. Bar-Sade, R., et al., The 185delAG BRCA1 mutation originated before the dispersion of Jews in the diaspora and is not limited to Askhenazim. Hum Mol Genet, 1998. 7: p. 801–805.

52. Diez, O., et al., Prevalence of BRCA1 and BRCA2 Jewish mutations in Spanish breast cancer patients. British Journal of Cancer, 1999. 79: p. 1302–1303.

53. FitzGerald, M., et al., Germ-line BRCA1 mutations in Jewish and non-Jewish women with early-onset breast cancer. New England Journal of Medicine, 1996. 334: p. 143–149.

54. Offit, K., et al., Germline BRCA1 185delAG mutationsin Jewish women with breast cancer. Lancet, 1996. 347: p. 1643–1645.

55. Szabo, C. and M. King, Population genetics of BRCA1 and BRCA2 [editorial]. American Journal of Hum Genet, 1997. 60: p. 1013–1020.

56. Petrij-Bosch, A., et al., BRCA1 genomic deletions are major founder mutations in Dutch breast cancer patients [published erratum appears in Nat Genet 1997;17:503]. Nat Genet, 1997. 17: p. 341–345.

57. Abbott, D., et al., BRCA1 expression restores radiation resistance in BRCA1-defective cancer cells through enhancement of transcription-coupled DNA repair. J Biol Chem, 1999. 274: p. 18808–1812.

58. Andersen, T., A. Borresden, and P. Moller, A common BRCA1 mutation in Norwegian breast and ovarian cancer families? [letter]. American Journal of Hum Genet, 1996. 59: p. 486–487.

59. Leide, A., et al., A breast cancer patient of Scottish descent with germ-line mutations in BRCA1 and BRCA2 [letter]. American Journal of Hum Genet, 1998. 62: p. 1543–1544.

60. Gail, M., et al., Projecting individualized probabilities of developing breast cancer for white females who are being examined annually. Journal of the National Cancer Institute, 1989. 81: p. 1879–1886.

61. Parmigiani, G., D. Berry, and O. Aguilar, Determining carrier probabilities for breast cancer-susceptibility genes BRCA1 and BRCA2. American Journal of Human Genetics, 1998. 62: p. 145–158.

62. Eccles, D., D. Evans, and J. Mackay, Guidelines for a genetic risk based approach to advising women with a family history of breast cancer. UK Cancer Family Study Group. Journal for Medical Genetics, 2000. 37: p. 203–207.

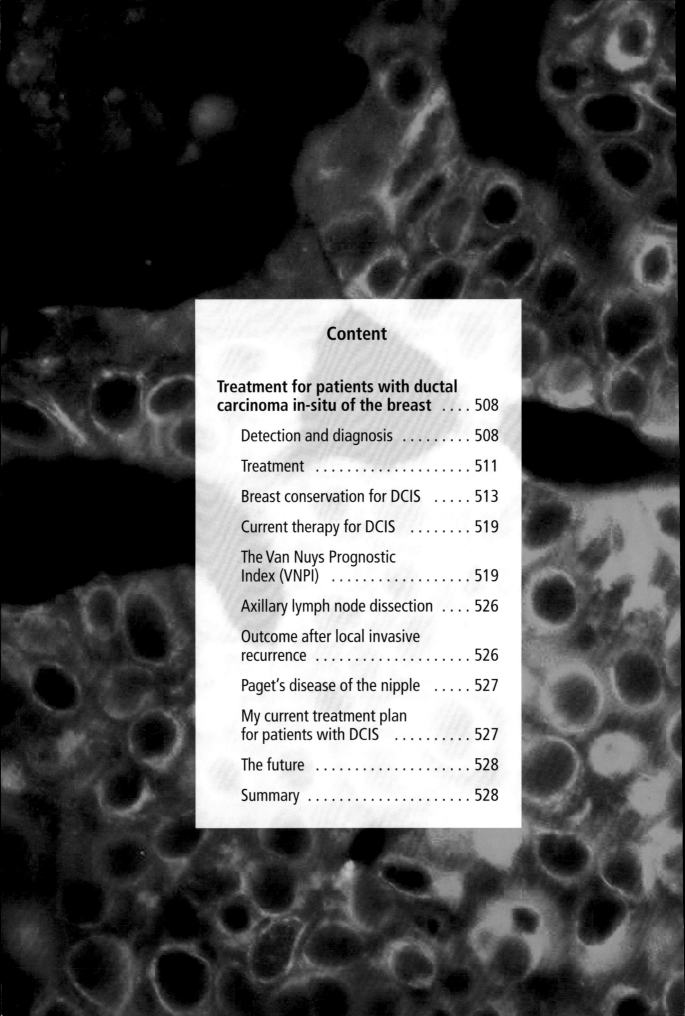

Content

TREATMENT FOR PATIENTS WITH DUCTAL CARCINOMA IN-SITU OF THE BREAST

MELVIN J. SILVERSTEIN

Prior to 1980, DCIS was a rare disease, representing about 1% of all breast cancer [46] and generally presenting as a palpable mass, nipple discharge, or Paget's disease [2]. The treatment for most patients with DCIS at that time was mastectomy. Since 1980, with the acceptance, improved technology and increased use of mammography, the clinical presentation of DCIS has changed dramatically. Today, **most DCIS is nonpalpable and discovered mammographically**. It is a completely different disease from that seen two decades ago. **Currently, DCIS represents at least 15–20%** [10, 11] of all newly diagnosed cases of breast cancer and as much as 20–40% of cases diagnosed by mammography [10, 11]. During the year 2004, there were more than 57,000 new cases of DCIS in the United States [26]. It is not entirely clear whether the increase in breast cancer incidence can be explained by increased and improved mammography or whether there is also a true increase in the incidence of breast cancer.

Today, **most patients with DCIS can be successfully treated with breast preservation**, with or without radiation therapy. In this chapter, I will demonstrate how easily available data can be used to help in the complex treatment selection process.

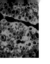
Treatment for patients with ductal carcinoma in-situ of the breast

■ DETECTION AND DIAGNOSIS

MAMMOGRAPHY

During the last five years, 91% of the DCIS patients in my personal series presented with nonpalpable lesions. A few percent were detected as random findings during a biopsy for a breast thickening or some other benign fibrocystic change; the vast majority, however, were detected by mammography. The most common mammographic findings were microcalcifications, frequently clustered and generally without an associated soft tissue abnormality. With this said, I will add that ultrasound is performed on all patients with suspicious nonpalpable mammographic findings. In a small percentage, an associated mass can be detected.

Overall, 80% of our DCIS patients exhibited microcalcifications on preoperative mammography. The patterns of these microcalcifications may be focal, diffuse, or ductal with variable size and shape. Comedo DCIS tends to have 'casting calcifications' which are linear, branching, or bizarre and are almost pathognomonic for comedo DCIS [83]. Almost all comedo lesions – more than 90% in our series – have calcifications that can be visualized on mammography.

In our series, 50% of noncomedo lesions did not have mammographic calcifications, making them more difficult to find and the patients more difficult to follow, if treated conservatively. When noncomedo lesions are calcified, they tend to have fine granular punctate calcifications.

A major problem confronting surgeons relates to the fact that calcifications do not always map out the entire DCIS lesion, particularly those of the noncomedo subtype. Even though all the calcifications are removed, the surgeon may be leaving significant amounts of DCIS behind. Sometimes, the majority of the calcifications are benign. In other words, the DCIS lesion may be smaller, larger, or the same size as the calcifications that lead to its identification. Calcifications more accurately approximate the size of comedo lesions than noncomedo lesions [30]. Despite these difficulties, the mammographic detection of suspicious microcalcifications in an asymptomatic patient has become extremely important in understanding the natural history of DCIS.

Before mammography was common or of good quality, most DCIS was clinically apparent and could be diagnosed by palpation or inspection; it was gross disease. Gump et al. [27] divided DCIS by method of diagnosis into gross and microscopic disease. Similarly, Schwartz et al. [57] divided DCIS into two groups: clinical and subclinical. Both groups felt patients presenting with a palpable mass, a nipple discharge, or Paget's disease of the nipple required more aggressive treatment. Schwartz stated that palpable DCIS should be treated as though it were an invasive lesion. He suggested that the pathologist simply had not found the area of invasion. While it makes perfect sense to believe that the change from nonpalpable to palpable disease is a poor prognostic sign, our group has not been able to demonstrate this for DCIS. In our series, when equivalent patients with palpable and nonpalpable DCIS are compared, they do not differ in the rate of local recurrence or mortality. In other words, palpability is not a significant predictor of local recurrence in patients with DCIS. We have, however, demonstrated a poorer prognosis for palpable invasive breast cancer when compared with similarly sized nonpalpable invasive breast cancer [69].

BIOPSY

Should breast biopsy be required, four types are available: fine needle aspiration (FNA), stereotactic biopsy, ultrasound-guided (a more comfortable alternative to stereotactic biopsy if the lesion is discernible on ultrasound), and needle-directed open (surgical) biopsy. FNA is generally of little help for nonpalpable DCIS. With FNA, it is possible to obtain cancer cells, but as there is no tissue, no architecture exists. So while the cytopathologist can say that malignant cells are present, they generally cannot say whether or not the lesion is invasive [43].

The importance of stereotactic core biopsy has increased dramatically over the last few years. Dedicated prone digital tables make this a precise tool in experienced hands. For DCIS, stereotactic 14 gauge core biopsy presents some problems. Since the biopsy sample is small, one cannot always rule out invasion or may not even be able to make the diagnosis. Decisions that require knowledge as to whether or not invasion is present, such as when deciding on sentinel node biopsy, may need to be based on excision of the entire lesion rather than core biopsy. If multiple core biopsies have been performed and the lesion is subsequently surgically removed, the area of the core biopsies –

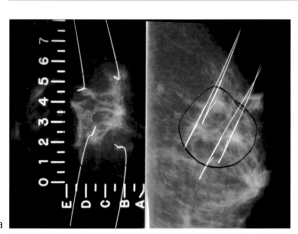

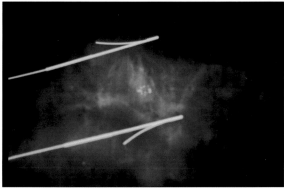

Fig. 24.1a – b
24.1a Craniocaudal and mediolateral mammograms taken after insertion of four bracketing wires around an area of architectural distortion.
24.1b Specimen radiograph of a double wire directed breast biopsy showing a cluster of microcalcifications excised with clear margins.

done with a 14 gauge needle – might be disrupted, making it difficult to tell whether there is true invasion.

This problem was largely remedied in the mid 1990s with the development of a number of new larger core vacuum-assisted tissue acquisition systems for percutaneous minimally invasive breast biopsy. These tools take significantly larger cores of tissue compared with the 14 gauge needle and allow tissue samples to be taken contiguously. Consequently, upgrading or changing the diagnosis at the time of definitive surgery is far less frequent: only about 11 – 13 % [8].

Vacuum biopsy devices must be used judiciously, as small clusters of microcalcifications may be removed in their entirety, leaving no landmarks for a subsequent surgical excision. A small microclip should always be placed at the time of biopsy to facilitate localization procedures as well as future mammographic evaluation. Because these devices use a 7 – 11 gauge needle, the risk of post-procedure hematoma formation is higher, and thus adequate compression of the biopsy cavity should be performed post-procedure. I prefer a bias pressure wrap technique.

If the diagnosis cannot be made with a minimally invasive technique (this should occur very infrequently, less than 5 % of the time), needle-directed breast biopsy is the next step. I believe that the first attempt to remove the lesion is the most important. The first excision is the best chance to remove the entire lesion and to achieve the best possible cosmetic result. Currently, I prefer two to four wires to bracket the lesion [61, 62, 67] (Fig. 24.1). This technique makes complete removal during the initial biopsy more likely. I never remove a possible DCIS using a single wire, since it may lead to incomplete removal of the abnormality, calcifications at the edge of the specimen, positive histologic margins, and the need to re-excise the lesion (Fig. 24.2). If a single wire is used,

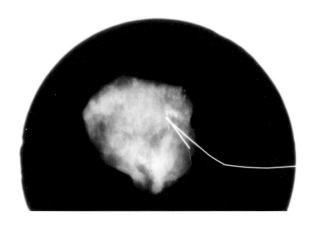

Fig. 24.2 Specimen radiograph of a single wire directed breast biopsy showing microcalcifications at the edge of the specimen.

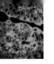

the surgeon should make certain that the excision is adequate by personally reviewing the intraoperative specimen radiography with the radiologist and inspecting the gross margins with the pathologist. The bigger problem, however, is that the distribution of microcalcifications does not always accurately map out the extent of disease. Multiple wires do not help with this problem.

Needle localization, intraoperative specimen radiography, and correlation with the preoperative mammogram should be performed in every nonpalpable case. Margins should be inked or dyed, and specimens should be serially sectioned at 2–3 mm intervals. The tissue sections should be arranged and processed in sequence. Pathologic evaluation should include a description of all architectural subtypes, nuclear grade, polarization, an assessment of necrosis, the measured or estimated size or extent of the lesion, and the margin status with measurement of the closest margin.

Tumor size should be determined by direct measurement or ocular micrometry from stained slides for smaller lesions. For larger lesions, a combination of direct measurement and estimation, based on the distribution of the lesion in a sequential series of slides, should be used. The proximity of DCIS to an inked margin should be determined by direct measurement or ocular micrometry. The closest single distance between any involved duct containing DCIS and an inked margin should be reported.

If the lesion is large and the diagnosis unproven, I would suggest stereotactic vacuum-assisted biopsy as a first step to prove that malignant cells are present and to obtain enough tissue to make a definitive histologic diagnosis. If the patient is motivated for breast conservation, an MRI should be performed to make certain the wide local excision is feasible. Following this, a multiple wire directed excision can be planned. This will give the patient her best chance at two opposing goals: clear margins and good cosmesis. Our best

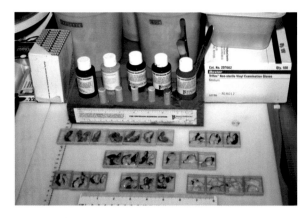

Fig. 24.4 The specimen has been color coded with dyes and serially sectioned.

chance at completely removing a large lesion is with a large initial excision. Our best chance at good cosmesis is with a small biopsy. It is the surgeon's job to optimize these opposing goals. A large quadrant resection should not be performed unless there is cytologic or histologic proof of malignancy. This type of resection may lead to breast deformity, and, should the diagnosis prove to be benign, the patient will be quite unhappy.

Removal of nonpalpable lesions is best performed with an integrated team consisting of a surgeon, a radiologist, and a pathologist. The radiologist who places the wires must be experienced, as must the surgeon who removes the lesion and the pathologist who processes the tissue.

At Van Nuys Breast Center, a facility that I directed from 1979–1998, the team developed an optimal setup for needle-directed breast biopsy. A pathologist was always with us in the operating room to receive the specimen and to be oriented as to its exact position in the patient. Our pathologist then took the specimen to our radiology department, only 25 meters away and on the same floor, where specimen radiology was carried out under the direction of the radiologist who placed the wires. I believe it is a mistake for the pathologist to perform the specimen radiology in the pathology department, particularly if the mammographic abnormality is a subtle mass or an architectural distortion. The pathologist should not be responsible for determining whether or not the surgeon has properly removed an area that was initially identified by another physician, the radiologist. Ideally, the radiologist who identified the lesion initially should place the wires, read the specimen radiogram, and inform the surgeon and the pathologist that the proper area has been removed and that the margins appear adequate by specimen radiography. When multiple physicians are involved, passing the case from one to another, there is a greater risk of error.

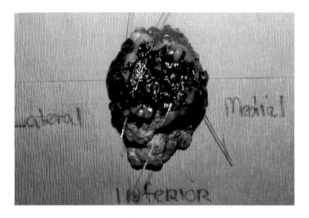

Fig. 24.3 The color-coded excision specimen with multiple wires in place.

Once our radiologist confirms that the proper area has been removed, our pathologist returns to the pathology laboratory and dyes the specimen, using a different color for each surface (Fig. 24.3). Should the red surface show involved margins on final histopathologic evaluation, we know it is the superior surface of the biopsy specimen, and it will be relatively easy to re-excise. The entire specimen should be serially sectioned and sequentially submitted for histologic evaluation (Fig. 24.4). No tissue should be discarded. No frozen sections should be performed on nonpalpable lesions. Hormone receptors, DNA analysis, HER2/neu etc., can be determined on the formalin fixed and paraffin embedded blocks.

Once the surgeon has been told that the proper area has been removed, the biopsy cavity should be marked with metallic clips (Fig. 24.5). This will identify the area of the biopsy if radiation therapy is elected or if there is a local recurrence. It will also help if re-excision has to be performed.

COUNSELING THE PATIENT WITH BIOPSY-PROVEN DCIS

It is never easy to tell a patient that she has breast cancer. But is DCIS really cancer? When we think of cancer, we generally think of a disease that, if untreated, runs an inexorable course toward death. That is certainly not the case with DCIS. We must emphasize to the patient that she has a borderline cancerous lesion – a 'pre-invasive' lesion – which, at this time, is not a threat to her life. In my series of 911 patients with DCIS, the mortality rate is less than 0.6%. Numerous other DCIS series [2, 13, 15, 17, 42] confirm an extremely low mortality rate. One of the most frequent concerns expressed by patients once a diagnosis of cancer has been made is the fear that the cancer has 'spread throughout her body.' We are able to assure patients with DCIS that no invasion was seen microscopically and that the likelihood of systemic spread is minimal.

The patient needs to be educated that the term breast cancer encompasses a multitude of lesions of varying degrees of aggressiveness and lethal potential. The patient with DCIS needs to be reassured that she has a minimal lesion and that she is likely to need some additional treatment, which may include surgery, radiation therapy or possibly hormonal therapy. She needs reassurance that she will not need chemotherapy, that her hair will not fall out and that in all likelihood she is not going to die from this lesion. She will, of course, need careful clinical follow-up for the rest of her life.

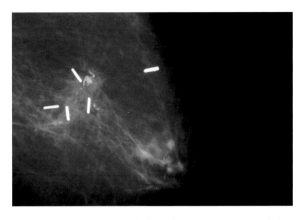

Fig. 24.5 Postoperative mediolateral mammogram. Metal clips mark biopsy cavity.

TREATMENT

Let us start by saying that for most patients there will be no single correct treatment. Right or wrong, a choice of treatment generally exists. As the choices increase and become more complicated, frustration will increase for both the patient and her physician [60]. As treatments vary, the local recurrence rate is affected. But, at the present time and regardless of which treatment is chosen, no study has shown a significant benefit in terms of breast cancer specific survival, the single most important endpoint.

MULTICENTRICITY AND MULTIFOCALITY

Multicentricity is defined as DCIS in a quadrant other than the quadrant in which the original DCIS (index quadrant) was diagnosed. There must be normal breast tissue separating the two foci. However, definitions of multicentricity vary from author to author. Hence, the reported incidence of multicentricity also varies. Rates from 0 to 78% [21, 41, 55, 58], averaging about 30% have been reported.

Holland [29, 30] evaluated 119 mastectomy specimens by taking a whole organ section every five millimeters. Each section was radiographed, and paraffin blocks were made from every radiographically suspicious spot. In addition, 25 blocks on average were taken from the quadrant containing the index cancer, and random samples were taken from all other quadrants, the central subareolar area and the nipple. The microscopic extension of each lesion was verified on the radiographs. This technique permitted a three-dimensional reconstruction of each lesion. This elegant study demonstrated that most DCIS lesions were larger than expected (50% greater than 50 mm), they involved more than one quadrant by continuous extension (23%), but, most importantly, they were

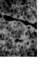
unifocal (99%). Only 1 of 119 mastectomy specimens (0.8%) had 'true' multicentric distribution, with a separate lesion in a different quadrant and in a different ductal system. From this, it is clear that complete excision of a DCIS lesion is possible due to unifocality but may be extremely difficult due to larger than expected size. This information, when combined with the fact that most local recurrences are at or near the original DCIS (91% in my series), suggests that the concept of multicentricity per se is not important in the treatment decision-making process.

Multifocality is defined as separate foci of DCIS within the same quadrant. The studies of Holland et al. [29, 30] and Noguchi et al. [47], suggest that multifocality may be artifactual: resulting from looking at a three-dimensional arborizing entity in two dimensions on a glass slide. It would be analogous to saying that the branches of a tree were not connected if the branches were cut through one plane, placed separately on a slide, and viewed in cross-section.

In essence then, most DCIS are unicentric but commonly multifocal. This means that complete excision, while often difficult, is theoretically possible in most patients.

MASTECTOMY

Until the 1980s, most breast cancer, including DCIS, was treated with mastectomy. As clinicians began using breast conservation (excision of the tumor, axillary dissection, and whole breast irradiation) for small invasive lesions, the treatment of DCIS lagged behind. Surgeons continued to perform mastectomies for DCIS while recommending breast conservation for more aggressive invasive lesions. Because of this, there is a large amount of data available regarding outcome after mastectomy for DCIS, although most mastectomy studies reflect lesions that were palpable and generally larger than those routinely discovered today.

Swain [82], in a review of 12 series of DCIS patients, with a total of 723 patients treated with mastectomy noted a local recurrence rate of 5% (range 0–10%). The mortality rate was 1.3% (range 0–8%). Most of these patients had palpable DCIS. Fowble [22], in her review of 14 studies, containing 1061 patients treated with mastectomy, noted a local recurrence rate of only 1%. The mortality rate was 1.7%. Barth et al. [4], in their review of 15 studies with 1342 patients, found the local recurrence rate to be 1.1%. The mortality rate was 1.3%. There is some patient overlap in these three reviews.

In our series, there are 319 patients treated with mastectomy: two of these (0.06%) have recurred locally (both with invasive lesions), but neither (0%) has died from breast cancer. Mastectomy clearly works

for DCIS. For many patients, however, it represents too much treatment. Mastectomy is deforming and may be psychologically mutilating even with breast reconstruction. Our challenge is to select only those patients for mastectomy who genuinely require it: those cases where a lesser procedure would lead to an unacceptably high local recurrence rate.

Mastectomy is indicated for large diffuse lesions, for patients with documented multicentric disease (biopsy proof of DCIS in multiple quadrants), for patients unwilling to take even the slightest increased risk of death due to an invasive recurrence, for patients who have no interest in breast conservation or who are medically unsuited for breast conservation, and for patients who are unwilling and/or unable to undergo careful clinical follow-up. In a subsequent section, entitled 'The Van Nuys Prognostic Index', our guidelines and patient selection process will become clearer.

When mastectomy is required and reconstruction desired, I generally perform a procedure that our group calls glandular replacement therapy (GRT) [32]. Glandular replacement therapy is a combination of skin-sparing mastectomy and autologous tissue reconstruction. Since DCIS does not invade the skin, there is no reason to discard large amounts of skin as when a mastectomy is performed for a large invasive breast cancer close to or involving overlying skin (Fig. 24.6). By saving most of the skin, the original skin envelope is preserved. When this is filled with autologous tissue, it generally yields a breast of similar size, shape, and consistency when compared with the remaining contralateral breast (Fig. 24.7a–c). I do not save the nipple. Our usual choice for autologous tissue is a TRAM (transrectus abdominus myocutaneous) flap; either free with microvascular anastomoses or pedical. Reconstruction with latissimus dorsi flaps or implants should be considered for appropriate patients.

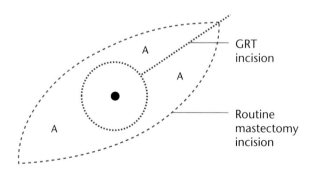

Fig. 24.6 Skin incision for glandular replacement therapy (skin-sparing mastectomy and immediate reconstruction).

THE DANGER OF LOCAL RECURRENCE

A few words are required about the dangers of local recurrence. If all local recurrences were noninvasive, there would be little indication for mastectomy as the initial procedure. In our own series and in most other reported series, approximately half of all local recurrences are invasive [38, 42, 80]. Local recurrences are therefore extremely important. When they occur in patients who have struggled to save their breasts, they are both demoralizing and, theoretically, a threat to life. By avoiding mastectomy, we gain both psychological and physical advantages but when there is an invasive recurrence, we have allowed an almost totally curable noninvasive lesion to advance to a potentially less curable form. Ultimately, this may translate to a higher mortality rate for patients treated conservatively.

■ BREAST CONSERVATION FOR DCIS

Today, we live in an era where breast conservation therapy for small invasive tumors is being used with ever increasing frequency. With this in mind, it becomes extremely difficult to justify the continued use of mastectomy for less aggressive noninvasive disease.

Breast conservation for DCIS is performed differently from breast conservation for invasive lesions. An invasive breast cancer requires excision of the primary lesion with clear margins, axillary node dissection or sentinel node biopsy, and some form of radiation therapy. It also requires chemotherapy, if nodes are positive or if the primary tumor has poor prognostic features. Breast conservation for DCIS is different. It requires, at a minimum, excision of the primary tumor, generally with clear histologic margins. Radiation therapy may or may not be added. There is no need for chemotherapy or formal axillary dissection. A small percentage of ER-positive patients may take tamoxifen.

Because of the serial subgross work of Holland et al. [29, 30] previously described in the section on multi-centricity and multifocality, we now know that, theoretically, many DCIS lesions can be completely excised. Unfortunately, in 23% of cases from this work, the lesion occupied more than a full quadrant of the breast. Nevertheless, in a large percentage of cases, it is potentially possible to remove the entire lesion while achieving acceptable cosmetic results. High-quality mammography and an aggressive biopsy policy utilizing stereotactic cores and multiple hooked-wires will yield a higher percentage of smaller lesions that can be completely excised with excellent cosmetic results.

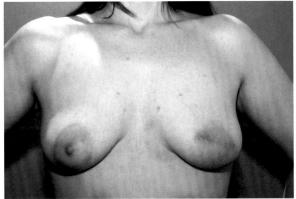

a

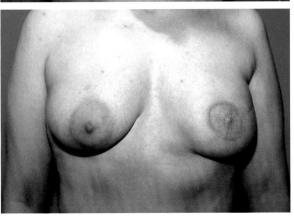

c

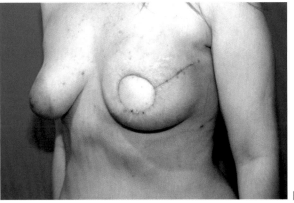

b

Fig. 24.7a–c Cosmetic results of glandular replacement therapy.
24.7a Preoperative photograph of a 34-year-old female. The left nipple had been removed two years earlier for Paget's disease. She presented with an 8 cm recurrence of high grade comedo DCIS.
24.7b A reconstructed breast after skin-sparing mastectomy and TRAM flap reconstruction (GRT). The island of skin that has been replaced is circular and exactly the same size as the nipple/areolar complex that has been removed.

24.7c The nipple/areolar complex has been reconstructed.

WHAT CONSTITUTES A CLEAR MARGIN?

I have already talked about how tissues should be processed and how important it is to mark (ink or dye) all margins. When this has been done and the pathologist tells us that the margins are free of disease, what does that mean? Does it really mean that we have excised the entire lesion? A first step is to define what we mean by a 'clear margin'. Our initial problem is that there is no consensus on what this term constitutes; different researchers use different criteria. In the past, our group had used one millimeter. I will shortly show, however, that one millimeter is inadequate. Solin et al. have used two millimeters [80]. The National Surgical Adjuvant Breast and Bowel Project (NSABP) [21] and the European Organization for Research and Treatment of Cancer (EORTC) require that the tumor

has not been transected: only a few fibrous or adipose cells between the tumor and the inked margin are needed to call the margin clear. Holland and associates [31]) require normal breast structures between the tumor and the margin. The Nottingham group has required 10 mm in all directions [59]. The work of Faverly et al. [12] suggests that 10 mm would be an excellent choice for clear margins. Using the serial subgross technique, they showed that only about 10% of DCIS lesions have gaps (skip lesions) greater than 10 mm.

I have looked at the importance of margins in our series. Figure 24.8 compares the actuarial local recurrence rates when one millimeter or more is used as the definition of a clear margin. Figure 24.9 compares the local recurrence rates when 10 mm or more is used as the definition of a clear margin. The local recurrence

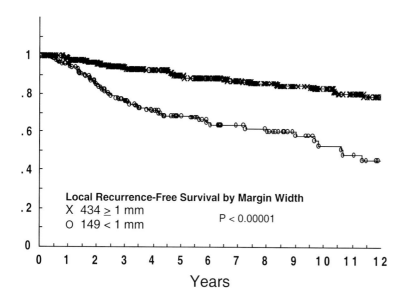

Fig. 24.8 Probability of local recurrence-free survival comparing margins ≥ 1 mm with margins < 1 mm for 583 breast conservation patients.

Local Recurrence-Free Survival by Margin Width
X 434 ≥ 1 mm
O 149 < 1 mm   P < 0.00001

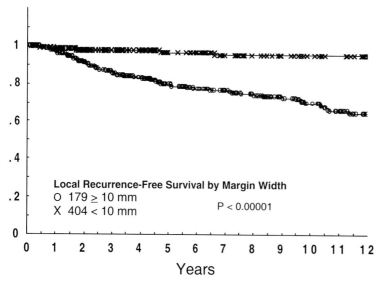

Local Recurrence-Free Survival by Margin Width
O 179 ≥ 10 mm
X 404 < 10 mm   P < 0.00001

Fig. 24.9 Probability of local recurrence-free survival, comparing margins ≥ 10 mm with margins < 10 mm for 583 breast conservation patients.

rate drops dramatically when 10 mm is required in every direction. As mentioned above, the three-dimensional work of Faverly and associates [12] suggests that skip areas are generally less than 10 mm and that 10 mm margins may be the gold standard.

I must, however, acknowledge that 10 mm in every direction is difficult to achieve while obtaining good cosmesis. In the operating room, the surgeon is faced with a difficult problem: DCIS is a lesion that generally can neither be seen nor felt. The surgeon's best chance for a complete excision with widely clear margins comes only with the placement of multiple hooked-wires in a lesion whose extent is well marked by calcifications. If the lesion extends significantly beyond the calcifications, complete excision is far less likely and will only occur if the surgeon is not only highly competent but also lucky.

CAN DCIS BE COMPLETELY REMOVED USING A COSMETIC WIDE EXCISION [68]?

Do clear margins mean that no residual DCIS has been left behind? Do involved margins mean that we are certain to find residual DCIS if we perform a mastectomy? No matter how exhaustive the evaluation of the margins, it is not perfect. Thousand of slides could be made from a 50 mm biopsy specimen. Generally, our group will submit about 20–30 cassettes from a 50 mm excision; this is a mere sampling. The evaluation of margins is, at best, a scientific approximation.

I have unpublished data on 568 patients with DCIS in whom an initial excision was performed and who subsequently underwent mastectomy or re-excision of the initial biopsy site. This allowed us to histologically evaluate how much DCIS was left behind and to correlate whether or not the initial margin status was a good predictor of residual DCIS. As expected, 71% (327/459) of patients with involved margins had residual DCIS; surprisingly, 38% (41/109) of patients with 'clear' margins of one millimeter or more also had residual DCIS. Similar data is available from the NSABP Protocol B-06. In this study, 22 patients with negative margins underwent mastectomy. Residual DCIS was found in 41% [21].

From this, we can conclude that DCIS is difficult to excise completely using a cosmetic wide local excision. If the object is to completely excise DCIS while preserving the breast, a true quadrantectomy may be required in many cases. This is best achieved using modern oncoplastic procedures. We also can conclude that our evaluation of the initial biopsy margins leaves something to be desired. In spite of a thorough evaluation, with color coding of all margins, 38% of patients with what we thought were clear margins (using one millimeter or more as the definition of clear margins) had residual disease. While I

believe factors like nuclear grade and comedo-type necrosis are important, inadequate excision of the primary lesion is probably the most important cause of local failure after conservative treatment for ductal carcinoma in-situ of the breast.

When re-excision of the entire biopsy cavity is required because of positive histologic margins, I generally wait two to four months for the induration and inflammatory response to subside since there is no biologic urgency with DCIS. Immediate re-excision often yields an inferior cosmetic result when compared with delayed re-excision. However, if one re-excises immediately, it is easier to define the biopsy cavity, and it may be possible to re-excise only the involved or close margins.

WIDE EXCISION ONLY

Lagios and associates [39, 41, 42] have been leaders in breast conservation without radiation therapy for more than a decade. In the 1970s, they began treating selected patients with DCIS by excision only. Their strict criteria for eligibility required that all lesions be nonpalpable, discovered mammographically, 25 mm or less in maximum size, and free of microcalcifications on postoperative mammography. Lagios [38] reported a 12% actuarial local recurrence rate at five years and 16% at ten years. There were no breast cancer related deaths, and no patients have developed distant metastases. These are among the lowest local recurrence rates reported to date for DCIS treated by excision only.

A number of other investigators [15, 48, 57] have reported similar but slightly higher rates of local recurrence for DCIS treated by excision only. The NSABP has reported an actuarial local recurrence rate of 20.9% at five years [15]. Schwartz et al. [57] have reported a 15.3% (absolute rate) at four years. On an actuarial basis this is likely to be about 20% at five years, similar to the NSABP.

The average size of Lagios' tumors was only seven millimeters. In addition, Lagios' protocol used the strictest inclusion criteria, which may explain why his local recurrence rate is lower, in spite of a longer follow-up period.

I believe that excision only is an acceptable form of treatment for carefully selected patients with DCIS. I will elaborate on our selection process in the section entitled 'The Van Nuys Prognostic Index'.

WIDE EXCISION PLUS RADIATION THERAPY

Numerous retrospective analyses of patients with DCIS treated with breast conserving surgery and radiation therapy have been published [6, 14, 37, 44, 52, 54, 57, 65, 77, 79, 80, 86]. Follow-up is relatively

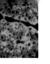

short. Local recurrence rates average about 8–10% at 5 years. The largest of these retrospective radiation analyses is that of Solin et al. [77, 79, 80] which combined the data of nine institutions in the United States and Europe. 261 DCIS lesions were treated with excision plus breast irradiation. The 15-year actuarial local recurrence rate was 19%. Half of the recurrences were DCIS, and half were invasive. The 15-year breast cancer specific survival rate was 96% [77].

In 1985, the NSABP began a prospective randomized study to evaluate the value of postoperative breast irradiation after excision of the DCIS lesion. After excision of the lesion with clear margins (NSABP nontransection definition), patients were randomized to receive ipsilateral breast irradiation or no further therapy. Axillary node dissection was required until June 1987, but was optional thereafter (at the surgeon's discretion). If an axillary dissection was performed, the nodes had to be negative for the patient to be included in the study.

In 1993, the first NSABP report was published [15]. A total of 790 patients were evaluable: 391 treated by excision only and 399 treated by excision plus breast irradiation. The five-year actuarial local recurrence rate was 10.4% for excision plus irradiation and 20.9% for excision only. The difference was highly significant. There were a total of 64 recurrences in the excision-only group, exactly half of which were invasive. There were 28 recurrences in the excision plus irradiation group, only eight of which were invasive (29%). The NSABP concluded that excision plus breast irradiation was more appropriate than excision alone for patients with localized DCIS, and if there were a local recurrence, radiation statistically decreased the likelihood that it would be invasive. After years of retrospective analyses, this was the first prospective randomized clinical trial for patients with DCIS, and it is of profound importance.

The NSABP recommended excision of the lesion and irradiation for all conservatively treated patients with localized DCIS and clear margins (by their definition of nontransection), regardless of histologic subtype, nuclear grade, or size of the DCIS lesion. In other words, they concluded that excision alone for DCIS was inappropriate. While I give great credit to the NSABP for organizing and conducting an outstanding study, it is difficult for clinicians to use global recommendations in an age of sophisticated consumer medicine.

The initial NSABP report gave no recurrence analysis by subset. Readers were told that almost 50% of the patients had comedo-type necrosis, that more than 85% of the patients had lesions 20 mm or smaller and that 81% of the lesions were nonpalpable. However, physicians were not told how any of these parameters affected outcome. Because there was no

subset analysis, there was no way to determine whether the outcome was different for a three millimeter low grade micropapillary lesion with widely clear margins compared with a 20 mm high grade comedo DCIS with minimally clear margins. The NSABP did not state whether patients with palpable DCIS recurred at a higher rate than patients with nonpalpable lesions. Due to these shortcomings, some reviewers were critical [40, 50].

In 1995, the NSABP published a second report, from a pathological perspective [19]; these data were updated in 1999 [20]. Approximately three fourths of the patients had microscopic slides available for central pathology review. In the 1995 analysis, both comedo-type necrosis and margin status (close/involved) were found to be significant predictors of an increased likelihood of local recurrence. In the 1999 update, only comedo-type necrosis was significant as an independent predictor of local recurrence. The NSABP continued to recommend that all patients with DCIS electing breast conservation receive radiation therapy, in addition to excision with clear margins.

The outcome results of B-17 were updated in 1998 [17]. At eight years, 27% of patients treated with excision alone had recurred locally, whereas, only 12% of those treated with excision plus irradiation had recurred. There was a significant decrease in local recurrence of both DCIS and invasive breast cancer among the irradiated patients. The eight-year data led the NSABP to reconfirm their 1993 position and to continue to recommend postoperative radiation therapy for all patients with DCIS who chose to save their breasts. Perhaps, more importantly, there was no significant difference in breast cancer mortality, regardless of which treatment was used. In fact, there were more breast cancer deaths in those patients who received radiation therapy, but the difference was not statistically significant.

The favorable results of B-17, in support of radiation therapy for patients with DCIS, led the NSABP to perform Protocol B-24 [16]. In this trial, 1804 patients with DCIS were treated with excision and radiation therapy, and then randomized to receive either tamoxifen or a placebo. At five years of actuarial follow-up, 9% of patients treated with placebo had recurred locally, compared with 6% of those treated with tamoxifen. When all breast cancer events were analyzed, including new contralateral breast cancers as well as regional and distant recurrences, the cumulative rate was 8.2% for those who received tamoxifen and 13.4% for those who received placebo (p = 0.0009). The results of B-17, B-24 and P-1 (the NSABP chemoprevention study) [16] led the NSABP to recommend both radiation therapy and tamoxifen for all patients with DCIS treated with breast preservation [85].

In 2000, the EORTC published the results of its prospective randomized DCIS study [33], a trial with a similar randomization to B-17. This trial included 1010 patients: at four years, 9% of patients treated with excision plus radiation therapy had recurred locally compared with 16% of patients treated with excision alone. These results are almost identical when compared with the NSABP's at four years.

A CLOSER LOOK AT NSABP PROTOCOL B-17 AND EORTC PROTOCOL 10853

The initial 1993 NSABP study [15] was criticized for a number of reasons, including the NSAPB's definition of clear margins, no requirement for specimen radiography, no requirement for postbiopsy/preradiation therapy mammography to exclude residual disease, no requirement for the inking or marking of margins, no requirement for size estimation, and most importantly, no requirement for complete tissue processing, without which invasive foci and margin involvement cannot be excluded [40, 50]. While the NSABP Protocol B-17 study was a prospective randomized trial of two different treatments, its histopathologic data published in 1995 [19] and updated in 1999 [20], were not prospectively acquired. The analysis of nine pathologic factors, including grade, size, and margins, was retrospective and based upon central review after the trial had been concluded. Two factors, margins and size, require more detailed comment.

MARGINS

The NSABP considered a margin 'clear' if the tumor was not transected. In other words, only a fat cell or a collagen fiber between the DCIS and the inked margin was required to consider that margin clear. Many margins were obviously significantly wider than that. NSABP surgeons certainly did not set out to achieve the smallest possible margins. Rather, Protocol B-17 was designed for simplicity and reproducibility. The margin was either clear or not clear: the DCIS was either transected or not transected. No color coding or inking had to be performed, meaning no time-consuming margin measurements by ocular micrometry had to be made or could be made. There was no requirement for the number of slides that had to be submitted per centimeter of resected tissue. The fewer blocks that were processed, the less likely one was to find a transected duct with DCIS at the margin or an unsuspected area of invasion. Moreover, 23% of the cases were not available for review by the central pathologist in the 1999 update [20].

Clearly, the NSABP patients designated as having clear margins had a wide range of margin widths. It is likely that many NSABP patients alleged to have clear margins, in reality, had extremely close margins and significant residual disease. Therefore, on average, patients in the untreated arm were likely to have high local recurrence rates. This in fact turned out to be the case: 27% at eight years [17].

In the Van Nuys series, at eight years, patients with margins less than 1 mm had a 58% local recurrence rate, those with margins 1 mm to less than 10 mm had a 20% local recurrence rate, and for those with 10 mm or greater margins, the local recurrence rate was only 3% [70]. Margin width is a continuum: the wider the margin width, the less likely there is to be a local recurrence [64].

SIZE

There was no requirement in NSABP Protocol B-17 for estimating and reporting tumor size. In the initial NSABP report, more than 40% of patients had no size recorded. In this group of patients, the size was inadvertently listed as being less than 1 mm [15]. It was only later, after a retrospective central review [19, 20] that approximately 90% of the tumors were reported to be 10 mm or smaller. The retrospective size analysis measured the largest dimension on a single slide.

In the Van Nuys series, lesions were three-dimensionally reconstructed. In general, the largest diameter on a single slide was smaller than the size recorded. With almost 90% of NSABP tumors measuring 10 mm or smaller, the average size must have been only 8–9 mm. With tumors this small, the NSABP reported a 12% recurrence rate at eight years after radiation therapy and a 27% recurrence rate when radiation therapy was not given [17]. If the analysis of the Van Nuys series is limited to tumors 20 mm or smaller (twice the size of the NSABP), the local recurrence rate at eight years after radiation therapy was 13% (essentially the same as the NSABP) and 18% when radiation therapy was not given (9% less than the NSABP), in spite of the fact that the Van Nuys tumors were twice the size (unpublished data). Clearly, the two groups are measuring lesions differently. Using the method employed in the Van Nuys series, the NSABP tumors would be larger. Using the NSABP method, the Van Nuys tumors would be smaller.

The EORTC trial corroborated the main conclusion of the B-17 study: radiation therapy decreases local recurrence rates of both invasive and noninvasive disease in conservatively treated patients with DCIS [33]. The EORTC study, unfortunately, is subject to the same criticism that was leveled at the initial B-17 publication: these include a lack of a subset analysis that would permit physicians to estimate local recurrence rates for various subgroups of patients, for example high grade (nuclear grade 3) versus low grade lesions; wide excision margins versus narrow margins; and those with comedo-type necrosis versus those without. Currently there are too few recurrences in the EORTC trial for such a subset analysis, but a subsequent central pathology review is forthcoming.

A singular finding in the B-17 trial was the 3.5-fold reduction in invasive local recurrences following radiation therapy [15, 17], an observation not seen in the EORTC trial or any other study of breast conservation employing radiation therapy [33, 70, 72, 77]. While DCIS recurrences were reduced by 47% in the NSABP trial if radiation therapy was given, invasive recurrences were reduced by 71% [17]. In contrast, the EORTC demonstrated an essentially equal reduction for both in-situ and invasive local recurrences following radiation therapy. The NSABP has used the marked decrease in invasive local recurrence as the principal rationale for their recommendation that all conservatively treated patients with DCIS receive postoperative breast irradiation.

The EORTC trial, like the NSABP trial, showed that, regardless of which of the two treatments was used, excision alone or excision plus radiation therapy, the most important endpoints, the distant recurrence rate and the mortality rate, were essentially identical. The authors point out that, with increased follow-up, there is a greater potential for distant disease in patients who recur with invasive breast cancer. Consequently, the most important reason to give radiation therapy would be to prevent invasive local recurrence. Of some concern is the fact that after only 4.25 years of follow-up, there are 24 patients with metastatic breast cancer in the EORTC trial compared with only 15 in the NSABP trial after eight years of follow-up.

Both the NSABP and EORTC trials did exactly what they were designed to do: they proved that, overall, radiation therapy was effective for patients with DCIS. Neither protocol, however, was designed to answer the compelling questions that sophisticated patients and their physicians ask today. Namely, exactly which subgroups will benefit from irradiation and by exactly how much?

Why not give radiation therapy to all conservatively treated patients with DCIS?

Radiation therapy is expensive, time consuming, and accompanied by side effects in a small percentage of patients [53]. Radiation fibrosis of the breast is a somewhat more common side effect. New technologies with more uniform dose distribution may reduce this. Radiation fibrosis, when it occurs, changes the texture of the breast and skin, may make mammographic follow-up more difficult, and may result in delayed diagnosis, if there is a local recurrence. Should there be an invasive recurrence at a later date, radiation therapy cannot be used again (although some

have tried this). Should there be significant skin and vascular changes following radiation therapy, skin-sparing mastectomy, if needed in the future, is clearly more difficult to perform. Finally, the most compelling reason not to use radiation therapy for all patients with DCIS is that no benefit has been shown in the single most important endpoint, breast cancer-specific survival, regardless of treatment. The NSABP's 1999 update reported four breast cancer deaths among the excision-only group and seven among the excision plus radiation therapy group [20]. The EORTC study also failed to show a difference in breast cancer mortality between the two treatment arms.

Recently, the Early Breast Cancer Trialists' Collaborative Group published a meta-analysis of the 10- and 20-year results from 40 unconfounded randomized trials of radiotherapy for early breast cancer [9]. Radiotherapy regimens routinely produced a reduction in local recurrence along with a reduction, in the range of 2–4%, in 20-year breast cancer mortality. However, cardiovascular mortality was increased in those who received radiotherapy. Because of this the absolute survival gain with radiotherapy was only 1.2% [36]. The studies reported in the meta-analysis were conducted between 1961 and 1990. More modern radiotherapy techniques are designed to minimize cardiopulmonary exposure but long-term cardiovascular mortality data do not exist. Physicians must be secure that the benefits of radiation therapy significantly outweigh the potential side effects, complications, inconvenience and costs for a given subgroup of patients, particularly those with relatively nonlethal malignancies such as DCIS.

Should all conservatively treated patients with DCIS receive postoperative radiation therapy?

I believe that the answer to this question is no. I agree it is clear that breast irradiation reduces the local recurrence rate by about 50% at five years (from around 20% to around 10%). Series with longer follow-up [77, 79], however, suggest that, as time passes, recurrences will continue to accrue in the patients treated with radiation. This raises the speculation, that at least in some patients, radiation merely delays, rather than prevents an inevitable recurrence. I believe that there is now sufficient, easily available information that can aid clinicians in differentiating patients who require radiation therapy after excision from those who do not. These same data can delineate patients who are better served by mastectomy because of unacceptably high recurrence rates with or without radiation therapy.

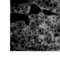

CURRENT THERAPY FOR DCIS

Currently, there is a wide range of acceptable treatments for the patient with DCIS. Treatment varies from simple excision to numerous forms of wider excision (segmental resection, quadrant resection, etc.), all of which may or may not be followed by radiation therapy. If the patient is a poor candidate for breast preservation, then mastectomy – with or without immediate reconstruction – is recommended. Since DCIS is a biologically heterogeneous group of lesions rather than a single entity and because patients have a wide variety of personal needs and agendas that must be considered throughout the treatment selection process, it is clear that no single approach is appropriate for all forms of the disease or for all patients.

The most benign appearing forms of DCIS (for example, low nuclear grade, small celled without necrosis, estrogen and progesterone receptor positive, HER2/neu-negative, etc.), if untreated, may never progress to invasive disease. Long-term actuarial analyses reveal that approximately 40% of untreated low grade lesions develop into invasive breast cancer after 25–30 years of follow-up [49]. About half of these patients go on to die of breast cancer. In other words, only one patient in five with untreated low grade DCIS goes on to die from breast cancer. This finding again raises an issue discussed earlier regarding whether or not DCIS, and in particular low grade DCIS, should be considered breast cancer. Alternatively, the most aggressive appearing forms of DCIS (high nuclear grade, large celled with comedo-type necrosis, HER2/neu-positive, etc.), if left untreated, are much more likely to develop into invasive carcinomas in significantly shorter periods of time.

The most important questions today are: Which lesions, if untreated, are going to become invasive breast cancer? How long will it take for this to happen? Are there biologic or genetic markers that can be used to predict ultimate invasion? Which DCIS lesions, if treated conservatively, have such high rates of local recurrence, regardless of radiation therapy, that mastectomy should be the preferred initial treatment? In patients who do not require mastectomy, which lesions can be treated with excision alone and which lesions need postoperative breast irradiation? These are simple questions whose answers, however, are both difficult and complex.

A histologic, biologically based classification by itself does not yield enough information to determine proper treatment. Two additional factors, tumor size and margin width, have also been shown to be independent predictors of local recurrence in conservatively treated patients with DCIS [5, 39, 56, 64, 72, 73, 80]. It may be possible, by using a combination of these factors, to select subgroups of patients who do not require irradiation, if breast conservation is elected, or conversely to select patients whose recurrence rate is so high, even with breast irradiation, that mastectomy is preferable.

THE VAN NUYS PROGNOSTIC INDEX (VNPI)

There are numerous clinical, pathologic, and laboratory factors that might aid clinicians and patients wrestling with the difficult treatment decision-making process. Our research [65, 73] and the research of others have shown that various combinations of nuclear grade, the presence of comedo-type necrosis, tumor size, age, and margin status are all important factors in predicting local recurrence in patients with DCIS who elect breast conservation [5, 19, 39, 41, 42, 48, 51, 57, 80, 87]. By using a combination of these factors, it may be possible to select subgroups of patients who do not require irradiation or to select patients whose recurrence rate is potentially so high, even with breast irradiation, that mastectomy is preferable.

We used the first two of these prognostic factors (nuclear grade and necrosis) to develop the histopathologic classification [73] described earlier in this chapter. But nuclear grade and comedo-type necrosis are inadequate as the sole guidelines in the treatment selection process. Tumor size and margin status are also important.

The Van Nuys Prognostic Index (VNPI) [72] was devised by combining three statistically significant predictors (by multivariate analysis) of local tumor recurrence in patients with DCIS: tumor size, margin status, and pathologic classification [73]. A score of 1 (best prognosis) to 3 (worst prognosis) was given for each of the three predictors. The objective of all three predictors was to create three statistically different subgroups for each predictor, using local recurrence as a marker of treatment failure. Cut-off points were determined by statistical analyses, using the log rank test with an optimum p-value approach.

SIZE SCORE

A score of 1 was given for a small tumors 15 mm or less, 2 was given for intermediate size tumors 16–40 mm, and 3 was given for large tumors 41 mm or more in diameter.

MARGIN SCORE

A score of 1 was given for widely clear tumor-free margins of 10 mm or more. This was most commonly achieved by re-excision with the finding of no residual DCIS or only focal residual DCIS at the biopsy cavity. A score of 2 was given for intermediate margins of 1–9 mm and 3 for margins less than 1 mm.

PATHOLOGIC CLASSIFICATION SCORE

A score of 3 was given for tumors classified as group 3 (all high nuclear grade lesions), 2 for tumors classified as group 2 (non-high nuclear grade lesion with comedo-type necrosis), and 1 for tumors classified as group 1 (non-high nuclear grade lesion without comedo-type necrosis).

DETERMINING THE VAN NUYS PROGNOSTIC INDEX

The initial VNPI formula was determined using the beta values obtained from the multivariate analysis, which show the relative contribution of each factor in the estimation of the likelihood of local recurrence [63, 72]. Additional analyses revealed that the formula could be simplified, without compromising validity, by omitting the beta weighting suggested by the multivariate analysis, and by readjusting the numerical range for each of the three subgroups. The final formula for the Van Nuys Prognostic Index became:

VNPI = pathologic classification score + margin score + size score

This formula yielded seven groups with whole number scores ranging from 3 to 9. The best possible VNPI score was 3, a score of 1 for each predictor (e.g. a 5 mm low grade lesion, with widely clear margins by re-excision would earn a score of 3). The worst possible score was 9, a score of 3 for each predictor (e.g. a 50 mm high grade lesion with involved margins would earn a score of 9). Table 24.1 summarizes the scoring for the VNPI.

RESULTS OF ANALYSIS USING THE VNPI

The VNPI was initially evaluated on 254 breast conservation patients from The Van Nuys Breast Center (mastectomy patients were omitted from the analysis since they no longer had their ipsilateral breast at risk for local recurrence – the endpoint of this study). Following this, the VNPI was independently validated by analyzing Lagios' series of 79 patients. Both groups use similar tissue processing and have consulted one another for more than 15 years. The disease-free survival curves for comparable patients in each group were almost identical with no statistical differences found in any subgroup tested. The two groups of patients were therefore combined to yield a total of 333 patients with DCIS treated with breast preservation. These results were published in 1996 [72]. For this chapter, I have updated the results through the year 2000 to include 583 breast conservation patients.

Treatment for these patients was highly selective. However, selection (treatment bias) is not an important bias in this series since we are testing a prognostic index rather than analyzing treatment. Although the patient and her clinician control treatment selection, they cannot control final margins, tumor size, or pathologic classification. The fact that some patients opted for suboptimal treatments that were not recommended (e.g. 66 patients with VNPI scores of 8 or 9 who selected BCT were all advised to undergo mastectomy) was actually helpful in developing and evaluating the VNPI.

The disease-free survival for all 583 patients is shown by tumor size in Figure 24.10, by margin width in Figure 24.11, and by pathologic classification in Figure 24.12. The differences between every survival

Tab. 24.1 The University of Southern California/Van Nuys Prognostic Index Scoring System

	Score		
	1	2	3
Size (mm)	≤ 15	16–40	≥ 41
Margin width (mm)	≥ 10	1–9	< 1
Pathologic classification	Non-high grade without necrosis (grade 1 or 2)	Non-high grade with necrosis (grade 1 or 2)	High grade with or without necrosis (grade 3)
Age (yrs)	> 60	40–60	< 40

One to three points are awarded from each of four different predictors of local breast recurrence (size, margin width, pathologic classification, and age). Scores for each of the predictors are totaled to yield a Van Nuys Prognostic Index score ranging from a low of 4 to a high of 12

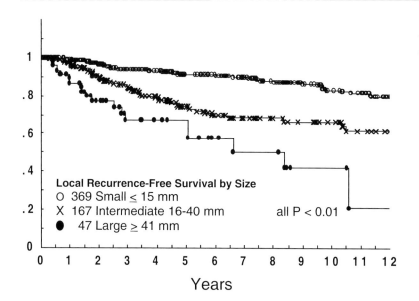

Local Recurrence-Free Survival by Size
O 369 Small ≤ 15 mm
X 167 Intermediate 16-40 mm   all P < 0.01
● 47 Large ≥ 41 mm

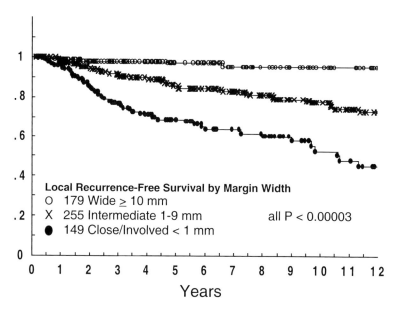

Local Recurrence-Free Survival by Margin Width
O 179 Wide ≥ 10 mm
X 255 Intermediate 1-9 mm   all P < 0.00003
● 149 Close/Involved < 1 mm

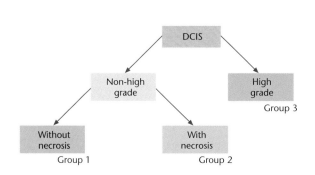

Fig. 24.12a Van Nuys DCIS pathologic classification.

curve for each of the three predictors that make up the VNPI are statistically significant.

Figure 24.13 groups patients with low (VNPI = 3 or 4), intermediate (VNPI = 5, 6, or 7), or high (VNPI = 8 or 9) recurrence rates together. Each of these three groups are statistically different from one another.

Patients with VNPI scores of 3 or 4 do not show a disease-free survival (DFS) benefit from breast irradiation (Fig. 24.14) (p = 0.43). Patients with an intermediate rate of local recurrence, VNPI 5, 6, or 7, are benefited by irradiation (Fig. 24.15). There is a statistically significant average 15% decrease in local recurrence rate in irradiated breasts compared to those treated by excision alone (p = 0.02). Figure 24.16

divides patients with a VNPI of 8 or 9 into those treated by excision plus irradiation and those treated by excision alone. Although, the difference between the two groups is significant (p = 0.03), conservatively treated DCIS patients with a VNPI of 8 or 9 recur at an extremely high rate with or without radiation therapy.

Although mastectomy is curative for approximately 98–99% of patients with DCIS [2, 7, 65], mastectomy represents significant overtreatment for the majority of cases detected by current methods. When breast conservation is elected rather than mastectomy, radiation therapy statistically decreases the likelihood of local recurrence when compared with excision alone [15]; but radiation therapy, like mastectomy, may also represent overtreatment for a significant number patients who elect breast preservation.

Subsets of patients who are not likely to receive any significant benefit from radiation therapy can be identified, such as those with VNPI scores of 3 or 4 in the series presented here, low grade lesions in the series of Lagios et al. [38, 39, 42], small noncomedo lesions with uninvolved margins in the series of Schwartz et al. [57] or the well-differentiated lesions of Zafrani et al. [87]. Such patients may account for more than 30% of the total DCIS group [38, 39, 57, 73, 87].

The broad recommendation by the NSABP, that radiation therapy is appropriate for all patients with DCIS who are treated with breast preservation, while clearly correct based on their 1993 data, does not consider the histologic heterogeneity of DCIS nor the differences in subsets demonstrated by our data

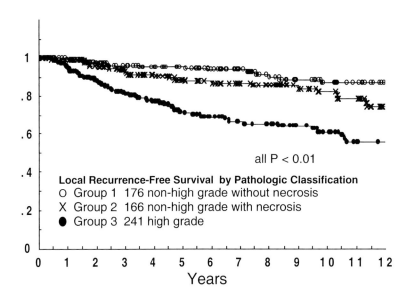

Fig. 24.12b Probability of local recurrence-free survival using Van Nuys DCIS pathologic classification for 583 breast conservation patients.

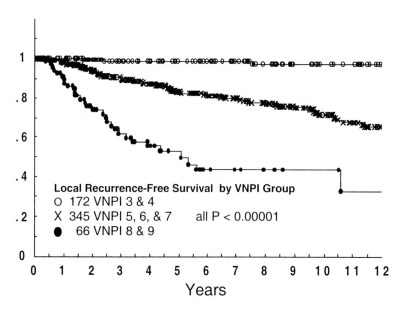

Fig. 24.13 Probability of local recurrence-free survival grouped by VNPI score for 583 breast conservation patients.

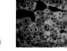

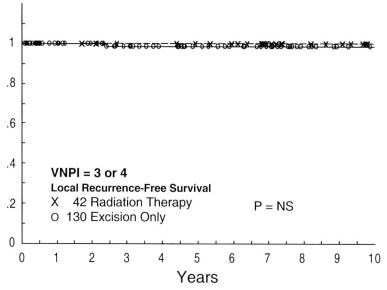

Fig. 24.14 Probability of local recurrence-free survival by treatment for 172 breast conservation patients with VNPI scores of 3 or 4.

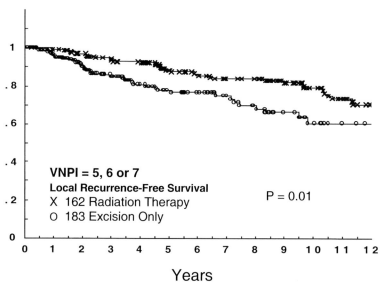

Fig. 24.15 Probability of local recurrence-free survival by treatment for 345 breast conservation patients with VNPI scores of 5, 6, or 7.

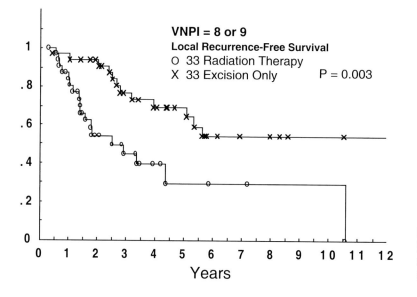

Fig. 24.16 Probability of local recurrence-free survival by treatment for 66 breast conservation patients with VNPI scores of 8 or 9.

[65, 73], their 1995 data [19], and the data of others [5, 39, 41, 42, 48, 51, 57, 73, 87].

Radiation therapy is not without side effects. It changes the texture of the breast, makes subsequent mammography more difficult to interpret, and, perhaps most importantly, its use precludes additional radiation therapy and breast conservation should a meta-chronous invasive breast cancer develop. For these reasons, radiation therapy should only be offered to those patients with DCIS likely to obtain a benefit.

Patients in this series with VNPI scores of 8 or 9 present a different problem. While these patients show the greatest relative benefit from postexcisional radiation therapy, their local recurrence rate continues to be unacceptably high, and a recommendation for mastectomy should be seriously considered.

Treatment recommendations for the intermediate group (patients with scores of 5, 6, or 7) are the most difficult. For patients with intermediate VNPI scores and margin scores of 2 or 3, re-excision may improve DFS. If the score remains intermediate after re-excision, radiation therapy should be considered. However, some patients with scores of 7 may be better treated with mastectomy (e.g. a patient with a large nuclear grade 2 lesion without necrosis and with less than 1 mm margins after re-excision), while some patients with scores of 5 (e.g. a patient with widely clear margins, small tumor size, but high nuclear grade) may elect no further treatment. These are independent judgments that must be made by the patient and her physician. I would hope that the VNPI would be a helpful adjunct to these difficult decisions.

Our work demonstrates that DCIS patients can be stratified into specific subsets based on the pathologic classification (using nuclear grade and necrosis), the size of the lesion, and the adequacy of surgical treatment as determined by pathologic margin assessment. If appropriate criteria are provided, pathologists should have little trouble making these determinations.

Counseling patients with DCIS in a rational manner can be extremely difficult when the range of treatment options is extreme. The VNPI allows a scientifically based discussion with the patient, using the parameters of the lesion obtained after an initial excision. Thus, in some cases, a patient can choose a re-excision, in an effort to 'downscore' her lesion. Successful downscoring of a patient with a VNPI of 8 or 9 could result in substantial reduction in the risk of local recurrence, perhaps changing a recommendation from mastectomy to radiation therapy. Similarly, patients with close or involved margins, with VNPI scores of 5 or 6 after initial excision could opt for re-excision. Successful downscoring by achieving widely clear margins could result in a final VNPI score sufficiently low to avoid breast irradiation.

Downscoring can be achieved only by re-excising

patients with margins scores of 2 or 3. Re-excision will not lower the pathologic classification score nor will it reduce the size of the tumor. In some cases, re-excision will 'upscore' the tumor, increasing the VNPI score by revealing a larger tumor size, a higher nuclear grade, the presence of previously undetected comedo necrosis, or an involved margin.

The proposed VNPI may be useful to clinicians because it divides DCIS into three groups with different risks for local recurrence after breast conservation therapy. Although there is an obvious treatment choice for each group (excision only for patients with scores of 3 or 4, excision plus radiation therapy for patients with scores of 5, 6, or 7, and mastectomy for patients with scores of 8 or 9), the VNPI is offered only as a guideline, a starting place in the discussions with patients.

The VNPI was the first attempt to quantify known important prognostic factors in DCIS, making them clinically useful in the treatment decision-making process. Clearly, the validity of the VNPI must be independently confirmed by other groups with large series of DCIS patients and sufficient data to complete the subset analysis as outlined here.

CASE PRESENTATIONS USING THE VNPI TO AID IN TREATMENT

CASE 1

A 47-year-old woman with microcalcifications detected on screening mammography. Wire-directed excision yielded a 10 mm non-high grade (cribriform) DCIS with comedo-type necrosis. The closest margin was less than 1 mm. VNPI score = 6 (size score = 1, pathologic classification score = 2, and margin score = 3). Re-excision was performed and no residual DCIS was found. This procedure downscored the lesion by converting her margin score to 1. The patient now has a VNPI of 4 and can be considered for careful clinical follow-up without additional radiation therapy.

CASE 2

A 54-year-old woman with microcalcifications detected on screening mammography. Wire-directed biopsy revealed a 10 mm, (solid) DCIS of intermediate grade with focal comedo-type necrosis. The margins were involved. VNPI score = 6 (size score = 1, pathologic classification score = 2, and margin score = 3). This score, of course, is inaccurate since the lesion was transected, and the true size was not known. Re-excision was performed and extensive residual disease measuring 42 mm was found. In addition, foci of high grade comedo DCIS were found. The closest margin was now 1 mm. VNPI score = 8 (size score = 3, pathologic classification score = 3, and margin score = 2). This procedure upscored the lesion by converting her size score to 3, her pathologic classification score to 3 and her margin score to 2. The patient now has a VNPI of 8 and would be best treated with mastectomy. An alternative would be to re-excise one more time in the hope of obtaining widely clear margins. If this were to happen, her margin score would become 1 and her VNPI would equal 7 and at that point, radiation therapy would be an alternative to mastectomy.

CASE 3

A 6 mm low grade (micropapillary) DCIS without necrosis was found inadvertently within a breast reduction specimen in a 44-year-old woman. Because this was a reduction, tissue margins were not marked and tissue was not serially sectioned. All additional, previously unprocessed, formalin fixed tissue was then processed but no additional DCIS was found. Microscopically, the margins of the initial DCIS appeared widely clear, but we cannot be certain. Prereduction mammography was negative. VNPI score = 3 or 4 (size score = 1, pathologic classification score = 1, and margin score = 1 or 2). A VNPI score of 3 or 4 is our best guess in this case. In light of this, I would not treat this patient with radiation therapy. However, reduction mammoplasty causes scarring, and this patient's future mammographic follow-up will not be optimal.

CASE 4

A 74-year-old woman with a 5 mm area of microcalcifications detected on screening mammography. Wire-directed breast biopsy revealed a 5 mm high grade (comedo) DCIS. The margins were widely clear (> 10 mm in all directions). VNPI score = 5 (size score = 1, pathologic classification score = 3, and margin score = 1). Patients in the intermediate group (5, 6, or 7) generally require more thought and discussion. Some patients with scores of 5 may be better served by omitting radiation. Some patients with scores of 7 may be better served by mastectomy. In this particular case, I would not irradiate for the following reasons. The lesion was well marked by calcifications. It measured 5 mm on mammography and 5 mm on the microscopic slide – a good mammographic/pathologic correlation. Postoperative mammography showed no residual calcifications. The margins were widely clear. I prefer to omit radiation therapy in a patient of this age whenever possible. I would have no quarrel with the physician who elected to give radiation to this patient.

CASE 5

A 47-year-old women with a palpable upper outer quadrant thickening. Mammography showed a non-diagnostic architectural distortion. FNA revealed highly atypical cells. Core biopsy revealed a low grade (micropapillary) DCIS without necrosis. The patient was strongly motivated for breast conservation. A 4-wire bracketed upper outer quadrant segmental resection was done. A 6 cm DCIS identical to the core biopsy, extending tenuously close to three margins, was found. VNPI = 7 (size score = 3, pathologic classification score = 1, and margin score = 3). In this particular case, I would prefer skin-sparing mastectomy with immediate free TRAM reconstruction. I would choose this because the lesion is large and extends to three margins. Because it is not calcified, it is more difficult to excise completely, and it will be more difficult to follow if this patient selects breast preservation. As an alternative, the wound could be allowed to heal for 3–6 months, and a formal quadrantectomy performed. With a low grade lesion, there is little risk in delaying definitive treatment for 6 months. If the margins were widely clear (> 10 mm) after quadrantectomy the VNPI score would now be 5 (size score = 3, pathologic classification score = 1, and margin score = 1), and consideration could be given to adding radiation therapy, However, data is weak regarding the benefits of radiation therapy for low grade lesions, and I would like to follow this patient closely without adding radiation therapy.

MARGIN WIDTH AS A PREDICTOR OF LOCAL RECURRENCE

Margin width is the distance between DCIS and the closest inked margin and reflects the completeness of excision. Although the multivariate analysis used to derive the VNPI suggests approximately equal importance for the three significant factors (margin width, tumor size and biologic classification), the fact that DCIS can be thought of in Halstedian terms (it is a local disease and complete excision should cure the patient) suggests that margin width should be the single most important factor in terms of local recurrence.

Serial subgross evaluation of more than 100 breasts after mastectomy for DCIS suggests that when margin widths exceed 10 mm the likelihood of residual disease is relatively small, in the range of 10–15% [12, 29]. In 1999, we published data suggesting that there is little to be gained from postoperative breast irradiation when all margins are greater than 10 mm, regardless of nuclear grade, tumor size, or the presence of comedo-type necrosis [70].

I have been asked by colleagues whether publication of these data in the New England Journal of Medicine [70] meant that we were abandoning the VNPI. My answer was absolutely not. The VNPI is a superior tool because it takes into account not only margin width but tumor size and biologic classification. To score best (lowest) using the VNPI, one needs a small, well excised, low grade lesion. This type of lesion is not likely to recur, with or without radiation therapy. Through June, 2000, there were 162 patients who scored 3 or 4 on the VNPI, only two of whom had recurred locally. In the recently published series using only margin width, there were three recurrences among 133 patients with margins of 10 mm or more; updated through June 2000, there were five recurrences among 170 such patients. The VNPI is a slightly better predictor of local recurrence (and it should be), but it requires more data and is clearly more difficult to use and reproduce from laboratory to laboratory.

AGE AS A PREDICTOR OF LOCAL RECURRENCE

Early in the year 2000, a series of papers from William Beaumont Hospital in Royal Oak, Michigan, USA, called attention to young age as a poor prognostic factor [84], and in 2001, it was added to the VNPI.

◼ AXILLARY LYMPH NODE DISSECTION

In 1986, our group suggested that axillary lymph node dissection be abandoned for DCIS [74, 75]. In 1987, the NSABP made axillary node dissection for patients with DCIS optional, at the discretion of the surgeon. Since that time, we have published a series of papers which continue to show that axillary node dissection is not indicated for patients with DCIS [65, 66, 68, 76]. To date, our group had performed a total of 417 node dissections (301 level I and II dissections and 116 samplings of less than 10 nodes). In two patients, a single positive node was found by hematoxylin and eosin staining and routine sectioning without evidence of invasion or microinvasion in the primary. Frykberg et al. [24] compiled in their review of the management of DCIS data from nine studies with a total of 754 patients. The incidence of axillary lymph node metastasis for patients with DCIS was 1.7%. In spite of these numbers, some authors continue to advocate removal of the axillary nodes in patients with palpable extensive DCIS, who have a higher risk of occult invasion [3, 27, 57].

Our current policy is as follows. In any patient with DCIS who is undergoing breast preservation, I do not remove any axillary nodes. In patients being treated with mastectomy, a thorough dissection of the axillary tail often yields 1–10 nodes [18]. In addition, most of our current patients who undergo mastectomy are reconstructed with a free TRAM flap. This procedure requires dissection of the subscapular vessels. It is not uncommon to remove a few nodes during the dissection as the vessels are exposed. The final point revolves around the fact that most patients undergoing mastectomy have larger tumors, creating a greater

possibility for occult invasion missed during routine histologic evaluation. In light of this, most patients are generally happy to have a few lower axillary nodes examined pathologically. Uncovering a few negative nodes buys additional peace of mind for many patients.

There is now uniform agreement that, for patients with DCIS, the axilla does not need treatment [58, 106, 110]. For patients with DCIS undergoing breast conservation, the axilla should not be irradiated, and no form of axillary sampling or dissection needs to be performed. For patients treated with excision plus postoperative radiation therapy, the lower axilla is included by the tangential fields to the breast.

For patients with DCIS lesions large enough to merit mastectomy, a sentinel node biopsy [1, 25, 28, 35] using a vital blue dye, radioactive tracer or both can be performed at the time of mastectomy. This is done in the event that permanent sections of the mastectomy specimen reveal one or more foci of invasion. If invasion is documented, no matter how small, the lesion is no longer considered to be DCIS but, rather, an invasive breast cancer. The sentinel node or nodes are evaluated by hematoxylin and eosin (H&E) staining followed by immunohistochemistry for cytokeratin when routine H&E stains are negative.

Preliminary data are now available on the results of sentinel node biopsy in patients with DCIS. Nodal positivity ranges from 5–13% by immunohistochemistry for patients with high-risk DCIS [34]. High-risk DCIS is generally defined as lesions with high nuclear grade, large size, palpability, or those requiring mastectomy. In our own series, I have performed 145 sentinel node biopsies on patients with DCIS undergoing mastectomy; eight patients (6%) have had a single node with cytokeratin positive cells. I have elected not to treat these patients as stage 2, although others do. There have been no recurrences in this small group, with only 30 months of median follow-up.

◼ OUTCOME AFTER LOCAL INVASIVE RECURRENCE

Local recurrence after treatment for DCIS is demoralizing, and if invasive it is a threat to life [71]. Approximately 50% of all local recurrences are invasive [38, 66, 76, 78]. For the last decade, local recurrence (both invasive and noninvasive) has been used as the marker of treatment failure for patients with DCIS.

Updated outcome charts after local recurrence through mid 2000 for 911 patients in the Van Nuys series revealed a total of 112 local recurrences: 45 (44%) invasive and 57 (56%) noninvasive. No patient with a noninvasive recurrence developed distant metastases, and none died of breast cancer. For the 50 patients with invasive recurrences, 52% presented with stage 2A or more disease at the time of local recurrence, eight developed distant metastases and five died of breast cancer. The breast cancer mortality rate at 12 years for the subgroup of patients with invasive local recurrences was 11%, and the distant disease rate for this subgroup was 20% (rates similar to those reported by other groups). Invasive recurrence after treatment for DCIS is a significant event, converting a patient with previous stage 0 disease to a patient, on average, with stage 1 to 2A breast cancer (ranging from stage 1 to stage 4). Treatment for a patient with an invasive recurrence should be based on the stage of the recurrent disease. In spite of these five mortalities, one should bear in mind that, overall, DCIS is an extremely favorable disease. When the entire Van Nuys series of 911 patients is considered, the actuarial probability of an invasive recurrence at eight years is 7% and the probability of a breast cancer specific mortality is only 1.1%. It is, however, a tragedy, when a patient with DCIS recurs with invasive breast cancer and then goes on to die of metastatic disease.

DCIS is an extremely favorable disease and the likelihood of dying from breast cancer is small, regardless of what type of treatment is received [71]. No study to date, including the prospectively randomized NSABP studies [17] or the EORTC study [33], has shown a significant difference in breast cancer specific mortality, regardless of treatment.

PAGET'S DISEASE OF THE NIPPLE

Paget's disease presents with eczematoid changes of the nipple. In many cases, there is an underlying lesion that may or may not be palpable. The underlying lesion may be invasive or noninvasive. After a complete mammographic work-up, I biopsy the nipple using local anesthesia and, if present, the underlying lesion. Treatment depends on many factors. If the underlying lesion is invasive, I excise it, along with the nipple areolar complex, perform a sentinel node biopsy and treat the whole breast with radiation therapy. The cosmetic results for central lesions are generally quite good (Fig. 24.7c). Modified radical mastectomy can be performed if the patient chooses so.

If the underlying lesion is DCIS, I generally excise the nipple areolar complex with a generous wedge of breast tissue which includes the underlying lesion. If the underlying lesion is marked with microcalcifications, I use wires to direct the wedge resection; if it is not calcified, the excision is done blindly. All edges of the resected specimen are color coded, and the tissue is serially sectioned. If no underlying lesion is found, I do nothing further. If an underlying DCIS is found, I use the VNPI as a guideline for suggesting treatment. If histologic margins are involved, I either re-excise or perform a mastectomy with immediate reconstruction, depending on the size of the breast and the degree of margin involvement. I generally do not irradiate patients after complete excision with widely clear margins. Selected cases of Paget's disease can be treated with nipple preservation and radiation [81]. Nipple areolar reconstruction should be delayed until permanent sections are available which reveal clear histologic margins and a decision has been made whether or not radiation therapy is going to be used.

MY CURRENT TREATMENT PLAN FOR PATIENTS WITH DCIS

With the development of high-quality screening mammography, it has become common to see an asymptomatic patient in whom routine mammography has revealed an area of microcalcifications. During the 1980s, this patient would have had a wire or dye-directed breast biopsy to make a diagnosis. During this time period, approximately 70–75% of biopsies for microcalcifications yielded benign lesions. In addition, surgeons did not fully appreciate the radial segmental distribution of most DCIS lesions nor the profound importance of clear margins. During the early and mid 1980s, we were irradiating all conservatively treated patients. We were not anxious to perform a wide segmental-type resection initially when the majority of lesions were benign, and we often accepted close or focally involved margins without suggesting re-excision. We assumed that radiation therapy would deal with any residual cancer cells.

Our approach changed in the late 1980s as we developed a greater appreciation for the extent and distribution of DCIS. We became much more concerned with clear margins, and our enthusiasm for radiation therapy for DCIS decreased. The development of stereotactic core biopsy went hand in hand with this new approach. By the early 1990s, it was now possible, using a specially designed table with the patient in the prone position, to make a preoperative diagnosis with a 14 gauge core biopsy. This allowed preoperative consultation and planning, and for most patients it meant only one trip to the operating room for definitive treatment. The main problem with the 14 gauge core biopsy was that, because of the relatively small sample size, the final diagnosis was upstaged about 20–25% of the time following definitive surgery. In other words, one patient in five diagnosed with DCIS as a result of 14 gauge core biopsy actually had invasive breast cancer. This generally forced us back to the operating room on

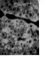

another day to dissect the axilla or perform a sentinel node biopsy. We had the same problem with a 14 gauge stereotactic biopsy that yielded a diagnosis of atypical ductal hyperplasia (ADH). Again, about 20% of the time, at definitive surgery these lesions turned out to be DCIS. Because of this, we routinely recommend open biopsy following 14 gauge core biopsy with a diagnosis of atypical hyperplasia.

By the late 1990s, this problem was remedied, to a major extent, with the development of a number of new larger core vacuum assisted tissue acquisition systems for percutaneous minimally invasive breast biopsy. The 7–11 gauge vacuum assisted probes take significantly larger cores of tissue when compared with the 14 gauge needle and afford the ability to sample tissue contiguously. Consequently, upgrading or changing the diagnosis at the time of definitive surgery is far less frequent, only about 10% in large series [8].

With this and everything else previously said in this chapter as a basis, I currently manage patients with suspicious nonpalpable mammographic lesions in the following manner. Our first step is to get an 11 gauge vacuum-assisted biopsy. If the diagnosis of DCIS is made, I counsel the patient thoroughly about the nature of the disease, paying particular attention to the size and distribution of her disease as seen mammographically. If she is a good candidate for breast preservation (an area of DCIS that I think can be removed completely and with clear margins without dramatically deforming the breast) and she is anxious to preserve her breast, I generally perform a 4-wire-directed segmental resection, and I commonly use a radial incision to take advantage of the radial distribution of DCIS. I often remove a small amount of skin and dissect the entire segment down to and including the pectoralis major muscle fascia. This generally guarantees that the anterior and posterior margins will be clear. If widely clear margins are obtained – 10 mm or more in the other four directions (superior, inferior, medial, and lateral) – I generally do not recommend postoperative radiation therapy. If the margins are 1–9 mm, I may re-excise or consider adding radiation therapy.

In patients whose lesions are too large mammographically to yield clear margins and an acceptable cosmetic result, I prefer to go directly to skin-sparing mastectomy and autologous reconstruction, generally with a TRAM flap. Having performed only a percutaneous minimally invasive breast biopsy in these patients, I am seldom faced with a skin incision in the wrong place or a biopsy scar that needs re-excision.

Some DCIS lesions extend well beyond their mammographic signs and may be extremely difficult to excise completely. These patients are probably better served with mastectomy and reconstruction.

Patients with DCIS treated with breast preservation should be followed closely. At the Lee Breast Center within the Norris Comprehensive Cancer Center of the University of Southern California, they are examined physically every six months for the rest of their life. Mammography is performed every six months on the ipsilateral breast and yearly on the contralateral breast. MRI is performed yearly.

THE FUTURE

Our current treatment approach to noninvasive breast cancer is phenotypic rather than genotypic. It is based on morphology rather than etiology. Genetic changes routinely precede morphologic evidence of malignant transformation. Using basic science, medicine must learn how to recognize these genetic changes, exploit them and, ultimately, prevent them. DCIS is a group of lesions in which the complete malignant phenotype of unlimited growth, angiogenesis, genomic elasticity, invasion, and metastasis has not been fully expressed. With sufficient time, most DCIS lesions will learn how to invade and metastasize. We must learn how to prevent this.

SUMMARY

DCIS is now relatively common, and its frequency is increasing. Most of this is due to better mammographic detection. We are not sure whether there is a true increase in incidence. Not all microscopic DCIS will progress to clinical cancer, but if a patient has DCIS and is not treated with a mastectomy, she is more likely to develop an ipsilateral invasive breast cancer than a woman without DCIS.

The comedo subtype of DCIS is more aggressive and malignant in its histologic appearance and is more likely to be associated with subsequent invasive cancer than the noncomedo subtypes. Comedo DCIS is more likely to have a high S-phase, overexpress HER2/neu and show increased thymidine labeling when compared to noncomedo DCIS. Comedo DCIS treated conservatively is also more likely to recur locally than noncomedo DCIS. However, separation of DCIS into two groups by architecture is an oversimplification and does not reflect the biologic complexity of the lesion. Because many DCIS lesions are admixtures of multiple architectural types of DCIS, our group no longer stratifies DCIS by comedo versus noncomedo subtypes. Rather, we use nuclear grade and the presence or absence of comedo-type necrosis to classify lesions.

Most DCIS detected today will be nonpalpable. They will most likely be detected by mammographic

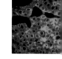
calcifications. It is not uncommon for DCIS to be larger than expected by mammography, to involve more than one quadrant of the breast and to be unicentric in its distribution.

Preoperative evaluation should include film-screen mammography with compression magnification. The surgeon and the radiologist should plan the excision procedure carefully. The first attempt at excision is the best chance to get a complete excision with a good cosmetic result. Re-excisions may yield poor cosmetic results. In patients with lesions that look like DCIS, consideration should be given to stereotactically directed vacuum assisted biopsy to make a definitive diagnosis.

Following the establishment of the diagnosis, the patient can be counseled. If she is motivated for breast conservation, the surgeon and radiologist should plan the procedure carefully, using multiple wires to map out the extent of the lesion. Once the multiple-wire-directed excisional biopsy has been done, two factors can be evaluated: cosmesis and histopathology. If the cosmetic result is acceptable and the margins are clear, the patient can proceed with breast conservation. The published prospective randomized trials run by the NSABP and the EORTC have proven that, overall, conservatively treated patients have a lower local recurrence rate if postoperative radiation therapy is given. However, these studies show no benefit in breast cancer survival, regardless of which treatment is given. Because of this, many physicians and patients prefer not to use radiation therapy if prognostic factors suggest a low local recurrence rate.

If a patient has a VNPI score or 3 or 4, or a margin with of 10 mm or more, she may be considered for careful clinical follow-up. If her score is 5 or above and initial margins are close or involved, re-excision can be considered, but this may yield a poor cosmetic result if the breast is small. In addition, the margins may continue to be involved.

At this point, patients with intermediate VNPI scores of 5, 6 or 7 or intermediate margin widths (1–9 mm) should be considered for breast irradiation. Patients with high VNPI scores of 8 or 9, should be considered for mastectomy with or without immediate reconstruction. Skin-sparing mastectomy is appropriate for patients with DCIS since this lesion does not involve the skin.

Reconstruction can be accomplished with a variety of techniques, including expander, implant, and TRAM flap. In general, immediate reconstruction is preferred. It eliminates at least one surgical procedure in the future, and it usually results in a happier patient with a better cosmetic result.

The most controversial point in DCIS treatment is whether or not to additionally administer radiation therapy to a patient who has a, seemingly, complete excision of her DCIS. Much more information needs to be gathered on this subject. At the current time, I do not irradiate any patients with DCIS with a VNPI score of 3 or 4. For patients with scores of 5, 6 or 7, with margin scores of 2 or 3, re-excision is considered. If the score remains in the mid-range, radiation therapy is generally added to the patient's treatment plan. For patients with scores of 8 or 9, a mastectomy with immediate reconstruction is usually recommended.

For women with larger lesions (relative to breast size) that cannot be totally excised, mastectomy remains the treatment of choice. All patients with DCIS are counseled regarding tamoxifen therapy.

REFERENCES

1. Albertini J, Lyman G, Cox C, al e (1996) Lymphatic mapping and sentinel node biopsy in the patient with breast cancer. JAMA 276: 1818–1822
2. Ashikari R, Hadju S, Robbins G (1971) Intraductal carcinoma of the breast. Cancer 28: 1182–1187
3. Balch C, Singletary E, Bland K (1993) Clinical decision-making in early breast cancer. Ann Surg 217: 207–222
4. Barth A, Brenner J, Giuliano A (1995) Current management of ductal carcinoma in-situ. Western J Med 163: 360–366
5. Bellamy C, McDonald C, Salter D, Chetty U, Anderson T (1993) Noninvasive ductal carcinoma of the breast: the relevance of histologic categorization. Human Pathology 24: 16–23
6. Bornstein B, Recht A, Connolly J, al e (1991) Results of treating ductal carcinoma in-situ of the breast with conservative surgery and radiation therapy. Cancer 67: 7–13
7. Bradley S, Weaver D, Bouwman D (1990) Alternative in the surgical management of in-situ breast cancer. Am Surg 56: 428–432
8. Burak W, Owens K, Tighe M, Kemp L, Dinges S, Hitchcock C, Olsen J (2000) Vacuum-Assisted Stereotactic Breast Biopsy: Histologic Underestimation of Malignant Lesions. Arch Surg 135: 700–703
9. Early Breast Cancer Trialists' Collaborative Group (2000) Favorable and unfavorable effects on long-term survival of radiotherapy for early breast cancer. Lancet 355: 1757–1770
10. Ernster V, Barclay J, Kerlikowske G, Henderson I (1996) Incidence of and treatment for ductal carcinoma in-situ of the breast. JAMA 275: 913–918
11. Ernster V, J B, Kerlikowske K, Wilkie H, Ballard-Barbash R (2000) Mortality among women with ductal carcinoma in-situ of the breast in population-based surveillance, epidemiology and end results program. Arch Intern Med 160: 953–958
12. Faverly D, Burgers L, Bult P, Holland R (1994) Faverly DRG, Burgers L, Bult P & Holland R 1994 Three dimensional imaging of mammary ductal carcinoma is situ: Clinical implications. Semin in Diag Pathol 11: 193–198

13. Fentiman I, Fagg N, Millis R, Haywood J (1986) In-situ ductal carcinoma of the breast: Implications of disease pattern and treatment. Eur J Surg Oncol 12: 261–266

14. Findlay P, Goodman R (1983) Radiation therapy for treatment of intraductal carcinoma of the breast. Am J Clin Oncol 6: 281–285

15. Fisher B, Costantino J, Redmond C, Fisher E, Margolese R, Dimitrov N, Wolmark N, Wickerham D, Deutsch M, Ore L, Mamounas E, Poller W, Kavanah M (1993) Lumpectomy compared with lumpectomy and radiation therapy for the treatment of intraductal breast cancer. N Engl J Med 328: 1581–1586

16. Fisher B, Dignam J, Wolmark N, al e (1999) Tamoxifen in treatment of intraductal breast cancer: National Surgical Adjuvant Breast and Bowel Project B-24 randomized controlled trial. Lancet 353: 1993–2000

17. Fisher B, Dignam J, Wolmark N, Mamounas E, Castantino J, Poller W, Fisher E, Wickerham D, Deutsch M, Margolese R, Dimitrov N, Kavanah M (1998) Findings from National Surgical Adjuvant Breast and Bowel Project B-17. J Clin Oncol 16: 441–452

18. Fisher B, Montague E, Redmond C, al e (1977) Comparison of radical mastectomy with alternative treatments for primary breast cancer. Cancer 39: 2827–2839

19. Fisher E, Constantino J, Fisher B, al e (1995) Pathologic findings from the National Surgical Adjuvant Breast Project (NSABP) Protocol B-17. Cancer 75: 1310–1319

20. Fisher E, Dignam J, Tan-Chiu E, al e (1999) Pathologic findings from the National Surgical Adjuvant Breast Project (NSABP) eight-year update of Protocol B-17: Intraductal Carcinoma. Cancer 86: 429–438

21. Fisher E, Sass R, Fisher B, al e (1986) Pathologic findings from the National surgical Adjuvant Breast Project (Protocol 6) i. Intraductal carcinoma (DCIS). Cancer 57: 197–208

22. Fowble B, Hanlon A, Fein D (1997) Results of conservative surgery and radiation for mammographically detected ductal carcinoma in-situ (DCIS). Int J Radiat Oncol Biol Phys 38: 949–957

23. Fraass B, Roberson P, Lichter A (1985) Dose to the contralateral breast due to primary breast irradiation. Int J Radiol Oncol Phys 11: 485–497

24. Frykberg E, Masood S, Copeland E, Bland K (1993) Duct carcinoma in-situ of the breast. Surg Gynecol Obstet 177: 425–440

25. Giuliano A, Dale P, Turner R, al e (1995) Improved axillary staging of breast cancer with sentinel lymphadenectomy. Ann Surg 222: 394–401

26. Jemal A, Tirari R, Murray T, et al. (2004) Cancer Statistics, 2004. CA, A Cancer Journal for Clinicians 54: 8–29.

27. Gump F, Jicha D, Ozzello L (1987) Ductal carcinoma in-situ (DCIS): A revised concept. Surgery 102: 190–195

28. Hansen N, Giuliano A (1997) Axillary dissection for ductal carcinoma in-situ. Williams and Wilkins, Baltimore

29. Holland R, Faverly D (1997) Whole Organ Studies. Williams and Wilkins, Baltimore

30. Holland R, Hendriks J, Verbeek A, Mravunac M, Schuurmans S (1990) Extent, distribution, and mammographic/histologic correlations of breast ductal carcinoma in-situ. Lancet 335: 519–522

31. Holland R, Veling S, Mravunac M, Hendriks J (1985) Histologic multifocality of Tis, T1–2 Breast carcinomas. Implications for clinical trials of breast conserving surgery. Cancer 56: 979–990

32. Jensen J, Handel N, Silverstein M, al e (1995) Glandular replacement therapy (GRT) for intraductal breast carcinoma (DCIS). Proc Am Soc Clin Oncol 14: 138

33. Julien J, Bijker N, Fentiman I, Peterse J, Delledonne V, Rouanet PA, A, Sylvester R, Mignolet F, Bartelink H, Van Dongen J (2000) Radiotherapy in breast conserving treatment for ductal carcinoma in-situ: First results of EORTC randomized phase III trial 10853. Lancet 355: 528–533

34. Klauber-DeMore N, Tan L, Liberman L, Kaptain S, Fey J, Borgen PH, A (2000) Sentinel lymph node biopsy: Is it indicated in patients with high-risk ductal carcinoma in-situ of ductal carcinoma in-situ with microinvasion? Ann Surg Oncol 7: 636–642

35. Krag D, Weaver D, Alex J, al e (1993) Surgical resection and radiolocalization of sentinel lymph node in breast cancer using a gamma probe. Ann Surg Oncol 2: 335–340

36. Kurtz J (2000) Radiotherapy for early breast cancer: was a comprehensive overview of trials needed? Lancet 355: 1739–1740

37. Kuske R, Bean J, Garcia D, al e (1993) Breast conservation therapy for intraductal carcinoma of the breast. Int J Radiat Oncol Biol Phys 26: 391–396

38. Lagios M (1995) Controversies in diagnosis, biology, and treatment. Breast J 1: 68–78

39. Lagios M, Margolin F, Westdahl P, Rose N (1989) Mammographically detected duct carcinoma in-situ. Frequency of local recurrence following tylectomy and prognostic effect of nuclear grade on local recurrence. Cancer 63: 619–624

40. Lagios M, Page D (1993) Radiation therapy for in-situ or localized breast cancer (letter). N Engl J Med 321: 1577–1578

41. Lagios M, Westdahl P, Margolin F, Rose M (1982) Duct Carcinoma in-situ: Relationship of extent of noninvasive disease to the frequency of occult invasion, multicentricity, lymph node metastases, and short-term treatment failures. Cancer 50: 1309–1314

42. Lagios MD (1990) Duct carcinoma in-situ: pathology and treatment. Surgical Clinics of North America 70: 853–871

43. Lee C, Carter D, Philpotts L, Couce M, Horvath L, Lange R, Tocino I (2000) Ductal carcinoma in-situ diagnosed with stereotactic core needle biopsy: Can invasion be predicted? Radiology 217: 466–470

44. McCormick B, Rosen P, Kinne D, Cox L, Yahalom J (1991) Duct carcinoma in-situ of the breast: An analysis of local control after conservation surgery and radiotherapy. Int J Radiat Oncol Biol Phys 21: 289–292

45. Muller-Runkel R, Kalokhe G (1990) Scatter dose from tangential breast irradiation to the uninvolved breast. Radiology 175: 873–876

46. Nemoto T, Vana J, Bedwani R, Baker H, McGregor F, Murphy G (1980) Management and survival of female breast cancer: Results of a national survey by The American College of Surgeons. Cancer 45: 2917–2924

47. Noguchi S, Aihara T, Koyama H, Motomura K, Inaji H, Imaoka S (1994) Discrimination between multicentric and multifocal carcinomas of breast through clonal analysis. Cancer 74: 872–877

48. Ottesen G, Graversen H, Blichert-Toft M, Zedeler K, Andersen J (1992) Ductal carcinoma in-situ of the female breast. Short-term results of a prospective nationwide study. Am J Surg Pathol 16: 1183–1196

49. Page D, Dupont W, Rogers L, Jensen R, Schuyler P (1995) Continued local recurrence of carcinoma 15–25 years after a diagnosis of low grade ductal carcinoma in-situ of the breast treated only by biopsy. Cancer 76: 1197–1200

50. Page D, Lagios M (1995) Pathologic analysis of the NSABP-B17 Trial. Cancer 75: 1219–1222

51. Poller D, Silverstein M, Galea M, al e (1994) Ductal carcinoma in-situ of the breast: a proposal for a new simplified histological classification association between cellular proliferation and c-erbB2 protein expression. Modern Pathology 7: 257–262

52. Ray G, Adelson J, Hayhurst E, Marzoni A, Gregg D, Bronk M, McClenathan J, Bitar N, Macio I (1993) Ductal carcinoma in-situ of the breast: Results of treatment by conservative surgery and definitive radiation. Int J Radiat Oncol Biol Phys 28: 105–111

53. Recht A (1997) Side Effects of Radiation Therapy. In: Silverstein M (ed) Ductal Carcinoma in-Situ of the Breast. Williams and Wilkins, Baltimore, pp 347–352

54. Recht A, Danoff B, Solin L, Schnitt S, Connolly J, Botnick L, Goldberg I, Goodman R, Harris J (1985) Intraductal carcinoma of the breast: Results of treatment with excisional biopsy and irradiation. J Clin Oncol 3: 1339–1343

55. Rosen P, Senie R, Schottenfeld D, Ashikari R (1979) Noninvasive breast carcinoma: Frequency of unsuspected invasion and implications for treatment. Ann Surg 1989: 377–382

56. Schwartz G (1994) The role of excision and surveillance alone in subclinical DCIS of the breast. Oncology 8: 21–26

57. Schwartz G, Finkel G, Carcia J, Patchefsky A (1992) Subclinical ductal carcinoma in-situ of the breast: treatment by local excision and surveillance alone. Cancer 70: 2468–2474

58. Schwartz G, Patchefsky A, Finkelstein S, al e (1989) Nonpalpable in-situ ductal carcinoma of the breast. Arch Surg 124: 29–32

59. Sibbering D, Blamey R (1997) Nottingham Experience. In: Silverstein M (ed) Ductal Carcinoma In-Situ of the Breast. Williams and Wilkins, Baltimore, pp 367–372

60. Silverstein M (1991) Intraductal breast carcinoma: Two decades of progress? Am J Clin Oncol 14: 534–537

61. Silverstein M (1994) Noninvasive breast cancer: The dilemma of the 1990s. Obstet Gynecol Clinics N Amer 21: 639–658

62. Silverstein M (1995) The first chance is the best chance. J Surg Oncol 58: 229–230

63. Silverstein M (1997) Van Nuys Prognostic Index for DCIS. In: Silverstein M (ed) Ductal Carcinoma In-Situ of the Breast. Williams and Wilkins, Baltimore, pp 491–504

64. Silverstein M (1998) Prognostic factors and local recurrence in patient with ductal carcinoma in-situ of the Breast. Breast J 4: 349–362

65. Silverstein M, Barth A, Poller D, Gierson E, Colburn W, Waisman J, Gamagami P (1995) Ten-year results comparing mastectomy to excision and radiation therapy for ductal carcinoma in-situ of the breast. Eur J Cancer 31A: 1425–1427

66. Silverstein M, Cohlan B, Gierson E, al e (1992) Duct carcinoma in-situ: 227 cases without microinvasion. Eur J. Cancer 28: 630–634

67. Silverstein M, Gamagami P, Colburn W, al e (1989) Nonpalpable breast lesions: Diagnosis with slightly overpenetrated screen-film mammography and hook wire-directed breast biopsy in 1014 cases. Radiology 171: 633–638

68. Silverstein M, Gierson E, Colburn W, al e (1994) Can intraductal breast carcinoma be excised completely by local excision? Clinical and pathologic predictors. Cancer 73: 2985–2989

69. Silverstein M, Gierson E, Waisman J, Colburn W, Gamagami P, al e (1995) Predicting axillary node positivity in patients with invasive carcinoma of the breast by using a combination of T category and palpability. J Am Coll Surg 180: 700–704

70. Silverstein M, Lagios M, Groshen S, Waisman J, Lewinsky B, Martino S, Gamagami P, Colburn W (1999) The influence of margin width on local control in patients with ductal carcinoma in-situ (DCIS) of the breast. New Engl J Med 340: 1455–1461

71. Silverstein M, Lagios M, Martino S, Lewinsky B, Craig P, Beron P, Gamagami P, Waisman J (1998) Outcome after local recurrence in patients with ductal carcinoma in-situ of the breast. J Clin Oncol 16: 1367–1373

72. Silverstein M, Poller D, Craig P, al e (1996) A prognostic index for ductal carcinoma in-situ of the breast. Cancer 77: 2267–2274

73. Silverstein M, Poller D, Waisman J, Colburn W, Barth A, Gierson E, Lewinsky B, Gamagami P, Slamon D (1995) Prognostic classification of breast ductal carcinoma-in-situ. Lancet 345: 1154–1157

74. Silverstein M, Rosser R, Gierson E, al e (1986) Axillary Lymph node dissection for intraductal carcinoma – is it indicated? Proc Am Soc Clin Oncol . 5: 265

75. Silverstein M, Rosser R, Gierson E, Waisman J, Gamagami P, Hoffman R, Colburn W, Lewinsky B, Fingerhut A (1987) Axillary Lymph node dissection for intraductal carcinoma – is it indicated? Cancer 59: 1819–1824

76. Silverstein M, Waisman J, Gierson E, al e (1991) Radiation therapy for intraductal carcinoma: Is it an equal alternative? Arch Surg 126: 424–428

77. Solin L, Kurtz J, Fourquet A, Amalric R, Recht A, Kuske R, Taylor M, Barrett W, Fowble B, Haffty B, Schultz D, McCormick B, McNeese M (1996) Fifteen year results of breast conserving surgery and definitive breast irradiation for treatment of ductal carcinoma in-situ of the breast. J Clin Oncol 14: 754–763

78. Solin L, McCormick B, Recht A, al e (1996) Mammographically detected, clinically occult ductal carcinoma in-situ (intraductal carcinoma) treated with breast

conserving surgery and definitive breast irradiation. Cancer J Sci Am 2: 158–165

79. Solin L, Recht A, Fourquet A, Kurtz J, Kuske R, McNeese M, al e (1991) Ten-year results of breast-conserving surgery and definitive irradiation for intraductal carcinoma of the breast. Cancer 68: 2337–2344

80. Solin L, Yeh I, Kurtz J, al e (1993) Ductal carcinoma in-situ (intraductal carcinoma) of the breast treated with breast-conserving surgery and definitive irradiation. Correlation of pathologic parameters with outcome of treatment. Cancer 71: 2532–2542

81. Stockdale A, Brierley J, Whire W, Folkes A, Rostom A (1989) Radiotherapy for Paget's Disease of the nipple: A Conservative alternative. Lancet II(8664): 664–666

82. Swain S (1989) Ductal carcinoma in-situ – incidence, presentation and guidelines to treatment. Oncology 3: 25–42

83. Tabar L, Dean P (1985) Basic principles of mammographic diagnosis. Diagn Imag Clin Med. 54: 146–157

84. Vicini F, Kestin L, Goldstein N, Chen P, Pettinga J, Frazier R, Martinez A (2000) Impact of Young Age on Outcome in Patients With Ductal Carcinoma-In-Situ Treated With Breast-Conserving Therapy. J Clin Oncol 18: 296–306

85. Wolmark N (1999) Tamoxifen after surgery/RT decreases local recurrence risk in DCIS patients. Oncology News International, vol 8, pp 12

86. Zafrani B, Fourquet A, Vilcoq J, Legal M, Calle R (1986) Conservative management of intraductal breast carcinoma with tumorectomy and radiation therapy. Cancer 57: 1299–1301

87. Zafrani B, Leroyer A, Fourquet A, Laurent M, Trophilme D, Validire P, Sastre-Garau X (1994) Mammographically-detected ductal in-situ carcinoma of the breast anaylyzed with a new classification. A study of 127 cases: correlation with estrogen and progesterone receptors, p53 and c-erbB2 proteins, and proliferative activity. Seminars in Diagnostic Pathology 11: 208–214

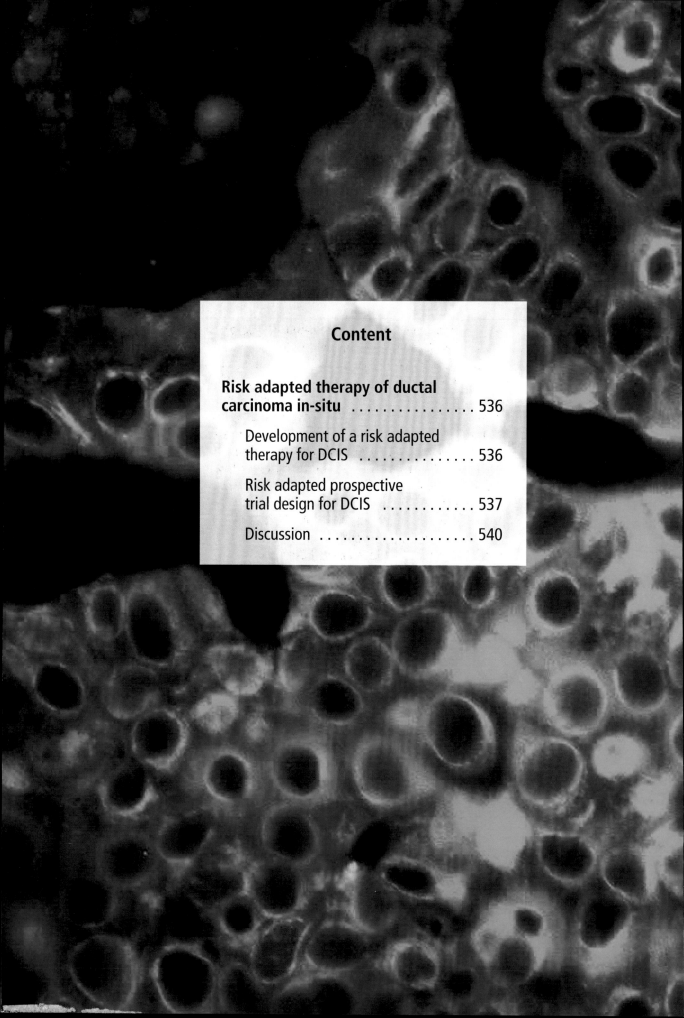

Content

25

RISK ADAPTED THERAPY OF DUCTAL CARCINOMA IN-SITU

AGUSTINUS HARJANTO TULUSAN, MICHAEL BUEHNER, HILDEGARD VOLKHOLZ,
THOMAS HUETTNER AND WOLFGANG SCHULZE

At a time where breast conserving therapy (BCT) for the treatment of invasive breast cancer (IBC) is commonly used, it has become increasingly difficult to further justify the routine use of mastectomy for ductal carcinoma in-situ (DCIS). This seems paradoxical: DCIS is not a single disease but represents a broad heterogeneous group of in-situ breast lesions.

Due to the intensive use of mammography, DCIS diagnosis today is much more frequent and the size of the DCIS lesions much smaller than in the last decades [1]. A DCIS rate of 12.5% in all newly diagnosed breast cancer cases has been calculated based on surveillance, epidemiology, and end results (SEER) data, while in population screening programs for breast cancer the rate of DCIS is approximately 30% [1, 2].

Retrospective studies and prospective trials have shown that BCT due to DCIS is associated with a local relapse rate of 6–45%, depending on the treatment strategies used [3–13]. Of these about 50% will have invasive cancer. After mastectomy the mortality of DCIS patients is only 0–3.7% [3, 7, 14–16]. This makes the optimum choice of DCIS treatment controversial, but DCIS treatment trends from 1983–1992 have shown a 50% reduction in the mastectomy rate [1].

Awareness of DCIS as a heterogeneous disease and the obligatory close cooperation of surgeons, radiologists, pathologists and radiotherapists for treatment of DCIS open up the possibility of more adequate and better tailored therapeutic concepts.

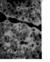

Risk adapted therapy of ductal carcinoma in-situ

■ DEVELOPMENT OF A RISK ADAPTED THERAPY FOR DCIS

EXPERIENCE FROM SURGICAL THERAPY OF DCIS

Varying studies of patients receiving only follow-up after treatment with biopsy for DCIS have shown a 15–30% rate of ipsilateral, invasive or in-situ recurrence within the following 20 years [17].

At the Academic Hospital of the University of Erlangen-Nuremberg in nine patients from the late 1950s DCIS (all noncomedo type) was missed in breast biopsies. In a follow-up for 6–10 years, three of these were diagnosed with invasive cancer in the ipsilateral breast. No in-situ or invasive carcinoma developed in those cases where the DCIS lesions were small and presumably excised with clear margins. It seems therefore that, at least in some circumstances, a wide local excision alone can be entirely adequate for treatment of in-situ disease. On the other hand there is no doubt that breast irradiation could lower the local recurrence rate of patients with invasive or in-situ breast cancer treated with BCT [4, 5].

PATHOLOGICAL CONSIDERATIONS

For a long time classification of DCIS was based only on the histological architecture of lesions. As a result DCIS was classified into comedo and noncomedo (cribriform, micropapillary and papillary, solid, and clinging) subtypes, with Paget's disease representing another special form of DCIS. In the mid 1970s several pathological and radiological studies revealed the importance of the terminal duct lobular unit (TDLU) as the primary site of breast carcinoma development [18–20], with secondary spread into the ductal system [15, 21]. Meticulous serial radial examination of more than 400 mastectomy specimens (Fig. 25.1a–b) in combination with serial specimen radiography of 343 invasive and 75 in-situ breast carcinomas in our institution, disclosed the intraductal spread of DCIS, following the radial segmental anatomical branching of the ductal system.

In 60% of breast carcinoma mastectomies no further tumor is detected outside a simulated segmental resection area. This is especially true for DCIS with an extension of less than 4 cm. DCIS smaller than 1 cm have a less than 4% chance of further in-situ lesions at a distance of more than 1 cm from the primary DCIS.

Larger DCIS (2.5 or more) may show an intraductal spread to the next segment of the ductal tree and may sometimes even occupy the whole breast quadrant or different quadrants of the breast.

From our data we postulate four different patterns of DCIS spread: focal (≤ 1 cm), segmental (> 1–2.5 cm), spread into several segments (> 2.5–4 cm) and spread into different quadrants of the whole breast (> 4 cm; Fig. 25.2a–d).

The most important prognostic parameter of DCIS is the extension at the time of diagnosis [15]. Noncomedo micropapillary DCIS usually has a larger extension than DCIS of comedo type, probably because comedo DCIS tends to be diagnosed earlier as a result of microcalcification.

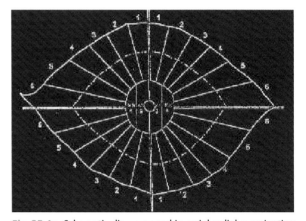

Fig. 25.1a Schematic diagram used in serial radial examination of mastectomy specimens.

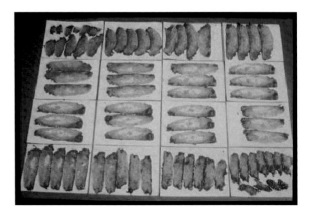

Fig. 25.1b Serial radial examination of one mastectomy specimen in whole slide section.

■ RISK ADAPTED PROSPECTIVE TRIAL DESIGN ■ FOR DCIS

Four patient risk groups were established which were based on two histopathological features: (1) extension of disease and (2) distance of the resection margin in pathological specimens (Table 25.1).

No other morphological features (for instance DCIS histological subtype, malignancy grade or other biological factors such as hormone receptor status or proliferation rate) were employed in this risk group system.

Patients classified as RG I and II were considered to be at low risk, while patients classified as RG III and IV were at a high risk of local recurrence after BCT. Irradiation of the remaining breast after surgery was given only in high risk patients (50 Gy + 10 Gy boost). Once results from the pathological report of the excision biopsy were obtained along with an informed

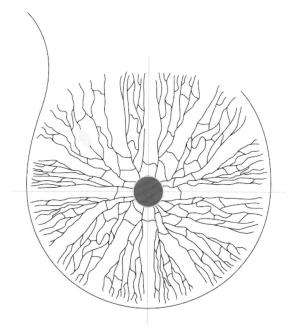

Fig. 25.2a Focal DCIS.

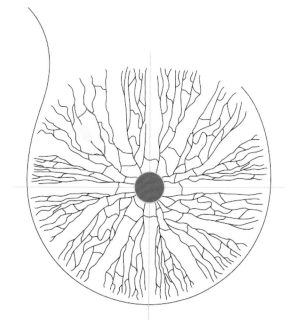

Fig. 25.2b Segmental DCIS.

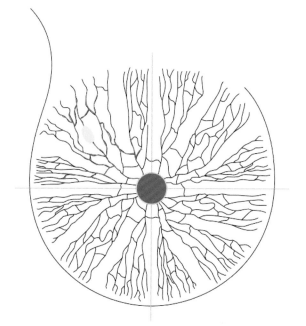

Fig. 25.2c DCIS involving several segments.

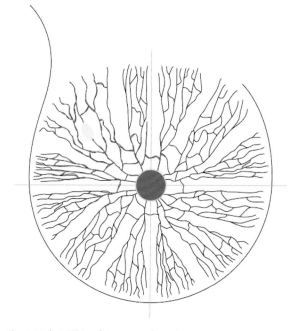

Fig. 25.2d DCIS involving several quadrants

consent to the study, secondary mastectomy could also be chosen as an option for high risk patients.

Mammographic and other imaging technique findings, clinical examination results, inking margins of the surgical specimen, and specimen radiography in comparison with the pathological findings also had to be evaluated before definitively categorizing patients into risk groups. Complete semiserial histological giant sections were used in our lab in processing 90% of surgical specimens, allowing the full extent of DCIS to be easily reconstructed (Fig. 25.3).

Surgery was performed by segmental resection, removing the DCIS within the ductal tree of the involved breast parenchyma in a radial resection with simultaneous reconstruction of the defect using the parenchymal flap technique for good cosmesis (Fig. 25.4).

Other so-called oncoplastic surgical techniques such as the latissimus dorsi myocutaneous flap technique were not utilized for reconstruction of surgical breast defects after segmental resection. For extended DCIS cases, axillary dissection of the lower level was performed, while only a small number of DCIS cases of smaller size also underwent axillary node sampling.

Follow-up was performed by clinical examination and annual or biannual mammography, with the addition of other imaging techniques as necessary. Suspect findings were confirmed histologically by open biopsy or core biopsy.

Recurrences in cases treated without radiotherapy could be re-excised and treated with radiotherapy. Recurrences in cases treated with radiotherapy were mostly treated with mastectomy.

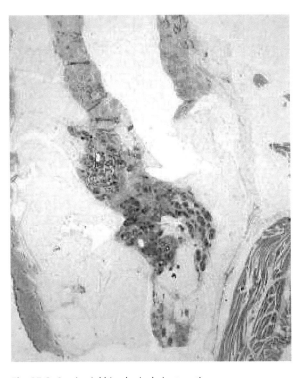

Fig. 25.3 Semiserial histological giant section.

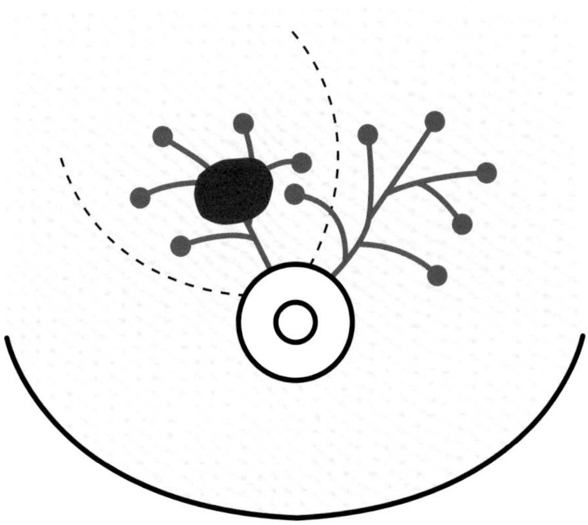

Fig. 25.4 Segmental resection with reconstruction using the parenchymal flap technique.

Tab. 25.1 Risk group classification

Risk group (RG)		Risk of local recurrence	Treatment
RG I	Small disease, < 10 mm size, widely clear tumor-free margins.	Low	BCT without radiotherapy.
RG II	Larger disease, 10–25 mm size, tumor-free margins.	Low	BCT without radiotherapy.
RG III	Extended disease, > 25 mm size, involvement of several segments, close to or not apparently free margins.	High	BCT with radiotherapy or optional mastectomy.
RG IV	Very extended disease, involvement of several quadrants, positive margins – not suited for BCT.		Mastectomy.

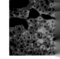

ACCRUAL OF DATA

From 1 January 1985 until mid 1996 122 cases of DCIS for the risk adapted therapy trial were accrued in two centers (Table 25.2). These were cases detected in a non-screening program, usually detected by mammography during annual medical check-up. Acceptance for the study was high. Only four patients (3.3%) were, for a variety of reasons, treated atypically and therefore eliminated from the study. Mean follow-up time was 68 months (12–141 months), and no cases were lost during follow-up.

RESULTS

One hundred and eighteen DCIS cases were treated according to the protocol: 27 DCIS classified as RG I, 44 as RG II, 44 as RG III, and 3 as RG IV.

Twenty-six patients (21.3%; 23 RG III patients and 3 RG IV patients) decided on mastectomy after diagnosis of DCIS. In these mastectomy patients no cases of invasive cancer or of axillary node metastasis at pathological examination of the surgical specimen occurred, with no recurrences or breast cancer deaths.

Ninety-two DCIS cases (76 DCIS and 16 DCIS with LCIS) were treated by BCT with (n = 21) and without (n = 71) radiotherapy (Table 25.3).

All patients in RG I (27) and RG II (44) were treated with segmental resection alone, and 21 in RG III were treated with segmental resection along with local radiotherapy.

Total recurrence was 7.6% (7/92; 4 DCIS and 3 invasive). The median disease-free period was 28 months (6–60 months).

The local recurrence rate correlated closely with the DCIS risk group (Fig. 25.5).

The local recurrence rate for RG I was 0% (0/27), for RG II 9.1% (4/44) and for RG III 14.3% (3/21).

The local recurrence rate for DCIS cases treated by segmental resection alone (RG I and RG II) was therefore 5.6% (4/71) after 6 years of follow-up, and for patients with high risk DCIS treated by segmental resection along with local radiotherapy (RG III) the local recurrence rate was 14.3% (Fig. 25.6).

All seven recurrences were detected within the vicinity of the primary DCIS location. The median disease-free period for nonirradiated patients was 32 months (11–60 months) and 24 months (6–39 months) for irradiated patients. Three of the four recurrences from the non-irradiated patients and two of the three recurrences from the radiated patients were treated once more with breast conserving surgery. The other recurrences were treated with mastectomy.

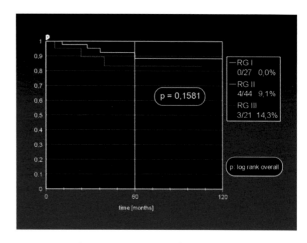

Fig. 25.5 Kaplan-Meier estimates of local recurrence rate for RG I–III.

Tab. 25.2 Patient numbers and tumor characteristics

Period of accrual	1985–1986
Total no. patients	118
▪ Erlangen	▪ 87 (73.7%)
▪ Bayreuth	▪ 31 (26.3%)
Mean age (years)	51.9 (28.2–78.0)
No. bilateral DCIS	4
No. breasts involved	122
No. pure DCIS	103 (84.4%)
No. DCIS + LCIS	19 (15.6%)

Tab. 25.3 Patients treated with BCT and associated tumor characteristics

Period of accrual	1985–1986
Total no. of patients	88
▪ Erlangen	▪ 68 (77.3%)
▪ Bayreuth	▪ 20 (22.7%)
No. bilateral DCIS	4
No. breasts involved	92
No. pure DCIS	76 (82.6%)
No. DCIS + LCIS	16 (17.4%)
Median follow-up (months)	68 (12.1–141.4)

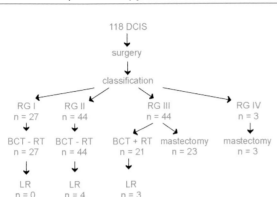

Fig. 25.6 Treatment according to risk group classification and local recurrence rate (RG = risk group, BCT = breast conserving therapy, R = radiotherapy, LR = local recurrence rate).

One patient with invasive recurrence also has a stage 3 ovarian cancer, but she died as a result of the breast disease.

■ Discussion

In contrast to randomized studies, the aim of this prospective DCIS trial was to confirm the possibility of selecting DCIS therapy according to the risk of local recurrence. This approach was deduced from data accrued in various studies. We do not regard any single treatment plan to be optimal for therapy of all DCIS cases. Individualization of therapy, however, needs accurate characterization of DCIS lesions. Disease pattern, extension, surgical resection according to mammographic findings and anatomical branching of the ductal tree, radiographic control of specimens and meticulous workup of the pathological specimen are some of the most important factors for deciding risk in each individual case. Local radiotherapy or further re-excision to reveal clear margins are the most important measures for lowering the risk of recurrence or the risk of side effects of therapy. In our study clear margins and extension of the DCIS were the two factors used in determining risk of local recurrence.

Because DCIS malignancy grades as measured by the Van Nuys Prognostic Index (VNPI) were not primarily used in risk classification in our study, we retrospectively re-evaluated our data and classified cases according to the VNPI criteria (Fig. 25.7).

Fourty-one DCIS cases reclassified as VNPI 3–4 were originally classified as RG I (27) and RG II (14). All cases in this group received no local radiotherapy after surgery, and the local recurrence rate was 4.9%. The 43 DCIS cases that were reclassified as VNPI 5–7

were originally classified as RG II (30) and RG III (13), of which 30.2% were treated with radiotherapy after breast surgery, while the local recurrence rate was 7%. There was no significant difference in the local recurrence rate of the DCIS group reclassified as VNPI 5–7 between cases treated with radiotherapy (7.7%) and those without radiotherapy (6.7%). Of the 8 RG III cases that were reclassified as VNPI 7–9 all received radiotherapy, and the local recurrence rate was 25%.

The analysis of the reevaluation of our study according to the VNPI underlined once more the prognostic significance for local recurrence of marginal status and DCIS disease extension.

VNPI therapy	3-4 (n=41)	5-7 (n=43)	8-9 (n=8)
BCT - RT	4,9 % (2 / 41)	6,7 % (2 / 30)	–
BCT +RT	–	7,7 % (1 / 13)	25,0 % (2 / 8)
total	4,9 % (2 / 41)	7,0 % (3 / 43)	25,0 % (2 / 8)

Fig. 25.7 Local recurrence rate according to van Van Nuys Prognostic Index (VNPI) classification (BRT = breast conserving therapy, RT = radiotherapy).

The VNPI classification system has often been criticized because of its retrospective design. To confirm the significance of VNPI, we thus performed another prospective treatment study. From 1997 to 2003 a new consecutive study, the Bayreuth II prospective therapy trial of DCIS, was performed based on data derived from the VNPI study. This study was aimed at establishing a risk adapted treatment concept for DCIS with regards to surgical therapy, radiotherapy and eventual systemic endocrine therapy.

Sixty-three DCIS cases, detected by microcalcifications (80%), mammographic densities (12%) or pathologic milk duct secretion were treated. Thirty-three DCIS cases of smaller extension could be treated with breast conserving segmental resection (VNPI 3–4) without additional local radiotherapy. Of the 20 DCIS cases with a wider extension 7 could be treated with segmental resection with clear resection margins of more than 1 cm, while in 5 cases a quadrantectomy was performed with reconstruction of the larger tissue defects by oncoplastic surgical techniques (latissimus

DCIS cases (n = 63)	Surgery	Surgery + radiotherapy
VNPI 3–4 (33)	Segmental resection (33)	
VNPI 5–7 (20)	Segmental resection (7) Quadrantectomy + latissimus dorsi (5)	Segmental resection (8)
VNPI 8–9 (10)	Mastectomy (8) Quadrantectomy + latissimus dorsi (1)*	Quadrantectomy + latissimus dorsi (1)

Tab. 25.4 DCIS trial Bayreuth II (1997–2003)

* Local recurrence after 18 months

dorsi myocutaneous flap) to achieve clear resection margins of more than 1 cm. As a result none of these 12 cases required addition local radiotherapy. Segmental resection as well as local radiotherapy were required in the remaining 8 DCIS cases with a wider extent (VNPI 5–7), as clear margins of 1 cm could not be achieved. Mastectomy was necessary in 8 of the 10 cases of very extended DCIS (VNPI 8–9). In 2 of these 10 cases breast conserving surgery – more than the usual quadrantectomy combined with oncoplastic reconstructive measures – was attempted with and without local radiotherapy (Table 25.4).

After a follow-up of 6–70 months (a mean of 48 months) only 1 local recurrence (DCIS) occurred in the VNPI 8–9 group with breast conserving surgery and reconstruction by latissimus dorsi muscle flap without radiotherapy. This patient was treated by skin sparing mastectomy and immediate breast reconstruction with a silicone implant and is now, 40 months after this second course of treatment, free of disease.

Based on the risk adapted treatment concept of DCIS, BCT could be performed in 87% of the 63 DCIS cases in this prospective study: in 12% using oncoplastic reconstructive techniques and in 15% with additional local radiotherapy. Mastectomy was necessary in 13% of these 63 DCIS cases, and after a mean follow-up of 48 months only 1 local recurrence occurred.

This Bayreuth II DCIS trial confirms and underlines that the application of VNPI is feasible, reasonable and associated with low local recurrence rates with a very high rate of BCT for DCIS. This risk adapted treatment concept is only possible under strict interdisciplinary collaboration and linked to a very high complexity of pathologic tissue processing. In the future the use of digital 'postprocessing' of digital mammography images could gain greatly in importance in preoperative planning of the resection area to avoid multiple surgical procedures (Fig. 25.8).

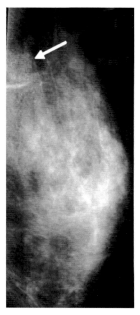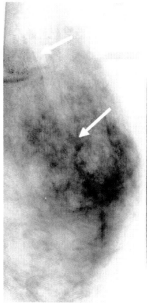

Fig. 25.8 Mammography before and after digital 'postprocessing' shows clearly better identification of the extent of microcalcifications (arrows) and therefore better possibility of preoperative planning of the resection area.

In the future more attention should also be paid to the role of oncoplastic surgery for BCT of larger DCIS, as it makes removal of more tissue possible without cosmetic defects. Local radiotherapy can be given in cases with a high risk of recurrence due to disease malignancy grade or in cases where a definite classification of DCIS according to the risk group classification as used in this study (RG I–IV) or the VNPI classification cannot be made. The high local recurrence rate in our study of 14% in RG III (25% in the reevaluated VNPI 7–9 cases) showed that radiotherapy does not compensate for inadequate surgical clearance of DCIS. This has also been confirmed in other recent studies [22].

REFERENCES

1. Ernster VL: Epidemiology and Natural History of Ductal Carcinoma in-Situ. In: Ductal carcinoma in-situ of the breast. Ed.: Silverstein MJ. Baltimore: Williams & Wilkins, (1997) 23–33

2. Ernster VL, Barclay J, Kerlikowske K, Grady D, Henderson C (1996). Incidence of and treatment for ductal carcinoma in-situ of the breast. JAMA 275: 913–918

3. Fisher ER, Leeming R, Anderson S, Redmond C, Fisher B (1991). Conservative management of intraductal carcinoma (DCIS) of the breast. J Surg Oncol 47:139–147

4. Fisher B, Costantino J, Redmond C, et al. (1993). Lumpectomy compared with lumpectomy and radiation therapy for the treatment of intraductal breast cancer. N Engl J Med 328:1581–1586

5. Fisher B, Dignam J, Wolmark N, et al. (1998). Lumpectomy and radiation therapy for the treatment of intraductal breast cancer: findings from National Surgical Adjuvant Breast and Bowel Project B-17. J Clin Oncol 16:441–452

6. Fisher B, Dignam J, Wolmark N, et al. (1999). Tamoxifen in treatment of intraductal breast cancer: National Surgical Adjuvant Breast and Bowel Project B-24 randomised controlled trial. Lancet 353:1993–2000

7. Fisher ER, Dignam J, Tan-Chiu E, et al. (1999). Pathologic findings from the National Surgical Adjuvant Breast Project (NSABP) eight-year update of Protocol B-17: intraductal carcinoma. Cancer 86:429–438

8. Solin LJ, Kurtz J, Fourquet A, et al. (1996). Fifteen-year results of breast-conserving surgery and definitive breast irradiation for the treatment of ductal carcinoma in-situ of the breast. J Clin Oncol 14:754–763

9. Silverstein MJ, Lagios MD, Craig PH, et al. (1996). A prognostic index for ductal carcinoma in-situ of the breast. Cancer 77:2267–2274

10. Schwartz GF, Schwarting R, Cornfield DB, et al. (1996). Subclinical duct carcinoma in-situ of the breast (DCIS): treatment by local excision and surveillance alone. Proc Amer Soc Clin Onc 15:101–101

11. Lagios MD, Margolin FR, Westdahl PR, Rose MR (1989). Mammographically detected duct carcinoma in-situ. Frequency of local recurrence following tylectomy and prognostic effect of nuclear grade on local recurrence. Cancer 63:618–624

12. Lagios MD: Lagios Experience. In: Ductal carcinoma in-situ of the breast. Ed.: Silverstein MJ. Baltimore: Williams & Wilkins, (1997) 23–33

13. Arnesson LG, Olsen K: Linköping Experience. In: Ductal carcinoma in-situ of the breast. Ed.: Silverstein MJ. Baltimore: Williams & Wilkins, (1997) 23–33

14. Silverstein MJ, Cohlan BF, Gierson ED, et al. (1992). Duct carcinoma in-situ: 227 cases without microinvasion. Eur J Cancer 28:630–634

15. Lagios MD, Westdahl PR, Margolin FR, Rose MR (1982). Duct carcinoma in-situ. Relationship of extent of noninvasive disease to the frequency of occult invasion, multicentricity, lymph node metastases, and short-term treatment failures. Cancer 50:1309–1314

16. Bradley SJ, Weaver DW, Bouwman DL (1990). Alternatives in the surgical management of in-situ breast cancer. A meta-analysis of outcome. Am Surg 56:428–432

17. Page DL, Dupont WD, Rogers LW, Landenberger M (1982). Intraductal carcinoma of the breast: follow-up after biopsy only. Cancer 49:751–758

18. Gallager HS, Martin JE. (1969). Early phases in the development of breast cancer 243:1170–1178.

19. Wellings SR, Jensen HM (1973). On the origin and progression of ductal carcinoma in the human breast. J Natl Cancer Inst 50:1111–1118

20. Wellings SR, Jensen HM, Marcum RG (1975). An atlas of subgross pathology of the human breast with special reference to possible precancerous lesions. J Natl Cancer Inst 55:231–273

21. Evans A, Pinder S, Wilson R, et al. (1994). Ductal carcinoma in-situ of the breast: correlation between mammographic and pathologic findings. AJR Am J Roentgenol 162:1307–1311

22. Chan KC, Knox WF, Sinha G et al. (2001). Extent of Excisison Margin Width Required in Breast Conserving Surgery for Ductal Carcinoma In-Situ. Cancer 91:9–16.

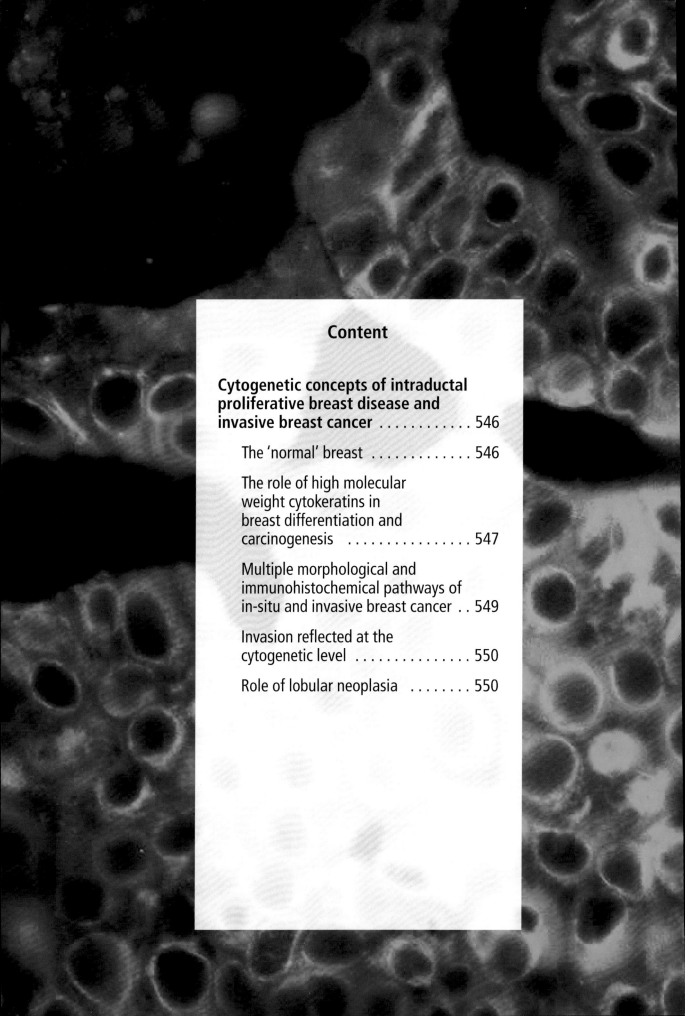

Content

CYTOGENETIC CONCEPTS OF INTRADUCTAL PROLIFERATIVE BREAST DISEASE AND INVASIVE BREAST CANCER

HORST BUERGER AND WERNER BOECKER

The molecular and formal pathogenesis of invasive breast cancer is still a matter of intense debate. Different models of breast cancer evolution and progression may give rise to different diagnostic and clinical approaches. Therefore a clear understanding of the pathogenetic mechanisms involved in breast cancer evolution – associated with morphologically detectable distinct phenotypes – is both of fundamental interest and high clinical value.

After the outstanding work of Page and coworkers in the early 1980s [1], the morphological steps within a linear progression model of breast carcinogenesis appeared clarified and were treated almost as dogma, even though other models of breast cancer evolution were also discussed [2]. The definition of different morphological forms of proliferative breast lesions, each associated with an increased risk of developing breast cancer in the future, remains the major achievement of this work. The epidemiological observation of a stepwise increase in breast cancer risk associated with usual ductal hyperplasia (UDH) through to atypical ductal hyperplasia (ADH) and ductal carcinoma in-situ (DCIS) was thought to justify an equally stepwise, linear, model of progression. It was assumed this was mirrored by changes on a genetic level, as had already been described in various other epithelial neoplasms. Nevertheless, in a multitude of recent morphological, immunohistochemical and genetic studies on normal and malignant breast proliferations data has emerged, that has led to new interpretations of previous findings.

It is the aim of this chapter to provide a comprehensive overview of such developments as well as of the theoretical and possible practical consequences for our changing understanding of breast carcinogenesis.

Cytogenetic concepts of intraductal proliferative breast disease and invasive breast cancer

THE 'NORMAL' BREAST

It is now widely accepted that cancer is a 'genetic' disease: various kinds of mutations affecting a multitude of different oncogenes and tumor suppressor genes drive a normal resting breast cell towards malignant behavior [3]. Breast cancer finally occurs when sufficient numbers of such alterations have accumulated. In breast cancer research the presence of genetic alteration was therefore automatically regarded as a sign of a clonal proliferation [4] and was, in consequence, assumed to be both a hallmark of an initial neoplasia and of malignancy. The 'normality' of morphologically unaltered breast tissue is nowadays a matter of intense debate. With the findings of a 'loss of heterozygosity' (LOH) in normal breast tissue adjacent to invasive breast cancer, the interpretation of previous molecular data has been challenged and even seems questionable [5, 6]. Even though only a small minority of patients were shown to possess such mutations, it became clear that, rather than affecting the whole breast, the mutations were restricted to small areas or 'fields', which were not automatically connected to each other. Since the extension of these fields could not be reliably defined, the authors of one study suggested the existence of a hypothetical 'field defect' or 'genetic field' [7], as in other epithelia. The definition of 'adjacent' in the context of this study, however, remained unclear; due to the tree-like organization of the breast and the invasive growth properties of breast cancer, the impression of 'adjacent' cancer and tumor-free tissue may be of secondary importance, not reflecting the true nature of the tissue. It has since been shown that the distribution of these genetically altered cells is more widespread than previously believed, with the finding of genetic alterations 'distant' to synchronous human breast cancer. The distribution of LOH in normal breast tissue seems to be fairly random for most genetic loci so far analyzed.

At our present state of knowledge, the wide distribution of genetically altered TDLUs in human breast tissue, with or without associated breast cancer, opens up the possibility of different biological mechanisms. The tree-like, anatomic organization of the human breast with multiple patches of per se monoclonal cells [8, 9] might lend weight to the hypothesis that alterations take place during pubertal development of the breast, with a random distribution over several TDLUs. Another plausible, but nevertheless highly speculative, model to explain such findings could be that of modified breast-specific 'field cancerization', requiring a horizontal motility of non-neoplastic cells along preformed anatomic structures such as might be seen after postlactational breast reconstruction.

Despite this problem it has become obvious that the frequency of genetic alterations varies significantly. Whereas only a small minority of breast lobules obtained from reduction mammoplasties for cosmetic reasons showed these alterations, the frequency of genetic alterations within breast tissue of normal appearance was significantly higher in patients undergoing therapeutic breast surgery due to a diagnosis of atypical hyperplasia or invasive breast carcinoma [10]. To what extent so-called 'malignancy associated changes' described by means of very elaborated morphometric techniques mirror these genetic changes remains an open question for further research [11].

In addition to the fact that the distribution of these altered cell patches remains poorly understood, varying mechanisms underlying the acquisition of such genetic changes have now been discussed. Thus, an overall, and so far undefined, breast-specific genetic instability at a chromosomal level cannot be excluded. In particular such a mechanism [12] is suggested by the identification of similar unbalanced chromosomal translocations in bilateral lobular carcinoma in-situ (LCIS).

Normal epithelial breast cells undergo cyclic, periodical proliferative and apoptotic changes as well as variations in their functional parameters [13], principally as a result of hormonal influences and to a lesser, but nevertheless probably underestimated, extent due to the effects of endogenous and exogenous carcinogens. On the one hand this might seem an advantage as it guarantees a constant and finally balanced cell renewal, providing a mechanism for the elimination of genetically altered cells. On the other hand, a periodically increased rate of proliferation represents a phase of increased vulnerability, since somatic mutations are mainly due to DNA replication errors. Little is known about the basic somatic mutation rate in human tissues in general, and in breast tissue in particular. In T-cells derived from human lymphocytes a somatic mutation rate of 0.5% has been described in contrast to 1.2% in normal appearing, nontumorous breast tissue – almost double the basic somatic mutation rate [10]. An increased basic somatic mutation rate in normal breast tissue – the suggested

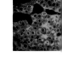

role for BRCA1 and 2 [14] – would provide a fascinating model for breast carcinogenesis. It should, however, be borne in mind that this definition of an increased mutation rate against the background of cyclical breast proliferation may merely reflect an increased opportunity for the acquisition of genetic alterations. Despite these drawbacks, further research in this field has provided fascinating new insights into breast carcinogenesis, in particular the demonstration of the prognostic relevance of such alterations in terms of breast cancer recurrence and their cell biological background.

What are the consequences of these advances for conventional models of breast cancer progression [15]? The synchronous presence of distinct genetic alterations, for example both in a UDH lesion and an associated invasive breast carcinoma, was interpreted as a proof of a clonal relationship of both lesions [16]. Given that genetic alterations are also present in normal breast tissue however, it does not automatically hold true that a relationship between both lesions must necessarily exist. Rather, it seems equally logical and intriguing to regard UDH as one of several different morphological reflections of genetic alterations that

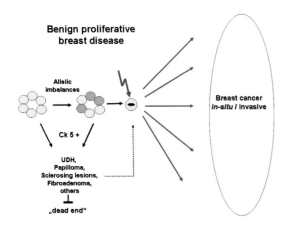

Fig. 26.1 With the repeated findings of molecular changes in benign, morphologically unaltered breast tissue, the understanding and interpretation of ductal hyperplasia as an obligate precursor lesion of breast cancer is under question. As identical alterations had also been demonstrated in DCIS and/or invasive breast carcinoma, allelic imbalances were regarded in the past as a sign of a neoplastic, clonal proliferation, indicating the first steps towards malignancy. However, the presence of allelic imbalances in UDH and morphologically unaltered breast tissue instead suggests that they should now be regarded as an indicator for an increased risk rather than as obligate factor. Since there is considerable difference between cytokeratin expression patterns in UDH and (pre)malignant breast disease, the overwhelming majority of UDH must be regarded as 'dead-end' lesions. However, the force which drives a genetically altered, but morphologically unaltered, cell towards malignancy remains to be elucidated.

have already taken place in normal breast tissue (Fig. 26.1), whereby a coexisting DCIS or an invasive breast cancer might be the result of additional and different genetic alterations [7]. Thus, UDH cannot automatically be interpreted as a precursor lesion of invasive breast cancer. The putative existence and definition of a 'genetic field' with different benign and malignant morphologies therefore substantially improves our understanding of the pathogenesis of multifocal breast cancers [17] or unrelated tumor clones in DCIS [18] and invasive breast cancer [19, 20]. At the present state of investigation, it is unclear which intracellular forces or changes are able to drive a genetically altered breast cell towards malignancy, or vice versa which mechanisms take place to prevent the malignant state. Starting points for further, clarifying research have been provided by the demonstration that at least some of these alterations have a functional and clinical consequence, with an increased recurrence rate in patients undergoing breast conserving surgery [6, 21, 22]. Further studies have also been able to show that even distinct gene amplifications of sequences regulating the transcription of the epidermal growth factor receptor gene (EGFR) occur in morphologically unaltered breast tissue, with a correlation to tumor recurrence [6]. Studies of Lakhani and coworkers clearly demonstrated that genetic alterations occur in myoepithelial as well as in luminal cells, one interpretation being that they take place in common precursor or progenitor cells [23].

■ THE ROLE OF HIGH MOLECULAR WEIGHT CYTOKERATINS IN BREAST DIFFERENTIATION AND CARCINOGENESIS

In Chapter 1 the existence of different cellular compartments within the resting female breast, mainly differentiated by their cytokeratin expression patterns, is extensively described. In what way does this knowledge alter our understanding of intraductal proliferative breast disease?

Which cells within a complex tissue give rise to the development of cancer has long been a matter of debate. A satisfactory answer is still forthcoming. Evidence exists that some tumor entities may arise from early, stem cell-like compartments [24]. During carcinogenesis they may show features of cellular differentiation explaining bilinear differentiation. Nevertheless, different cellular subgroups within a complex, more mature tissue might equally function as starting points for carcinogenesis [25]. The various morphological differentiation grades with their distinct protein and (probably) RNA expression patterns might

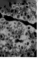
in this regard be interpreted as rudimentary, caricature-like remnants of their more or less differentiated cells of origin [26].

Recent immunohistochemical and cell biological studies in murine and human cells have provided evidence for an important role of high molecular weight cytokeratins for these putative progenitor cells [27, 28]. As outlined in detail above, the interpretation of these findings may represent clear evidence of a hierarchical order of these cellular compartments. In brief, cells with predominant expression of Ck5, a high molecular weight cytokeratin, give rise to the development of glandular and myoepithelial cell lineages [29]. According to these results, development leads either to the pure glandular subtype with a predominant expression of Ck8/18 or, in contrast, to the intermediate myoepithelial cell type characterized by coexpression of Ck5 and sm-actin, some of which will finally develop a pure monoexpression of sm-actin. These findings indicate that varying cellular compartments may function as different progenitors of invasive breast cancer and its proposed precursor lesions [30].

High molecular weight cytokeratins are rarely expressed in invasive breast cancer or in DCIS, in sharp contrast to benign lesions such as UDH, and this represents an accepted and reproducible feature of the proposed precursor lesions of invasive breast cancer [31]. Since cytokeratin expression patterns are highly preserved during carcinogenesis and tumor progression [32], a close direct relationship between these lesions seems doubtful. In addition, the fact that different cellular compartments exist in the female breast further weakens the case for such a relationship. Immunophenotypically, UDH resembles a progenitor cell lesion, in contrast to DCIS, which displays a mature glandular phenotype. Nevertheless, further evidence for the existence of progenitor cell-derived lesions is mounting. Sorlie and Perou [33, 34] clearly demonstrated the existence of a subgroup of invasive breast cancer cases characterized by expression of basal, high molecular weight cytokeratins, including Ck5 [35]. This and previous studies were able to demonstrate that these rather rare tumors are associated with a worse prognosis [36] and more frequently

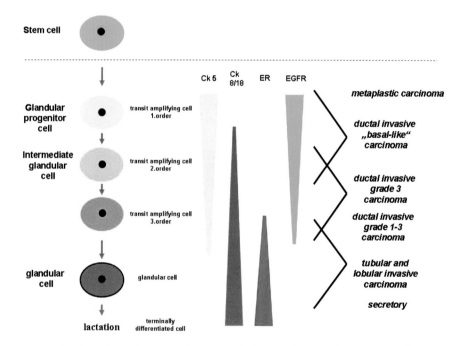

Fig. 26.2 Recent advances in determining tissue specific stem cells have pointed to the existence of primary stem cells and so-called first-, second- and n-order 'transit amplifying cells'. As discussed in previous chapters, it seems that early progenitor, intermediately differentiated and glandular cells are the morphological hallmarks of these cell populations within the breast. Combining existing, experimental data on stem/progenitor cells within the breast, a distinct immunohistochemical pattern becomes obvious.

Early progenitor cells are typically Ck5+, Ck8/18− (or weakly Ck8/18+) and ER-negative, are highly proliferative and EGFR-dependent. As breast cells differentiate, these factors change their expression patterns. Comparing this data from physiological breast cells with the different subgroups of invasive breast carcinomas, significant parallel findings are evident. One might therefore speculate that the different types of carcinomas arise from different target cells and that the original expression patterns are partially maintained during carcinogenesis. A dedifferentiation of invasive carcinomas is nevertheless possible. However, cytogenetic findings make this event rather unlikely.

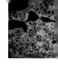

carry BRCA1 mutations [37, 38]. Further cytogenetic and immunohistochemical analyses of a large series of invasive breast cancer cases correlated cytokeratin expression with protein and cytogenetic alteration patterns. In particular, frequent losses of chromosomal 16q characterize these carcinomas as a separate, independent subgroup, rather than as the end stage of a dedifferentiation [39, 40]. In consequence, the transfer of our knowledge about physiological breast differentiation onto the level of breast carcinogenesis enables a feasible explanation for the large heterogeneity of invasive breast cancer, comprising well-differentiated glandular tumors on one end of the morphological and immunohistochemical spectrum through to poorly-differentiated carcinomas on the other (Fig. 26.2). These results are clear evidence for an important role of cellular subpopulations within the normal breast functioning as cytogenetic pathway-specific precursor cells of breast cancer [26, 41]. Whereas a carcinogenic hit of 'early progenitor cells' may cause a poorly-differentiated breast cancer to evolve, tumor associated dedifferentiation of a glandular cell seems to be associated with a better differentiated, low grade tumor.

■ MULTIPLE MORPHOLOGICAL AND IMMUNOHISTOCHEMICAL PATHWAYS OF IN-SITU AND INVASIVE BREAST CANCER

Even though classification systems of preinvasive breast disease still favor a stepwise dedifferentiation of in-situ and invasive breast cancer, the introduction of new technologies has given us important insights into the genetic mechanisms and pathways of breast carcinogenesis over the last decades.

The introduction of 'comparative genomic hybridization' (CGH) has facilitated a much improved classification of breast disease. It enables a global overview of all unbalanced chromosomal alterations within a tumor and is not biased by prior selection of markers, as is the case in microsatellite analysis [42]. It has become obvious that DCIS is the morphological reflection of at least two different, parallel genetic pathways. Well-differentiated as well as intermediately-differentiated DCIS are characterized by a loss of 16q chromosomal material [43–46]. In contrast, this chromosomal alteration is rather uncommon in poorly-differentiated DCIS (Fig. 26.3). Poorly-differentiated DCIS instead reveals a multitude of genetic alterations, for example gains of 20q and 17q as well as losses of 13q and 17p, resulting in a significantly higher degree of cytogenetic instability. An obligate cytogenetic and morphological progression from well to poorly-differentiated DCIS in the sense of a

16q-losses and differentiation

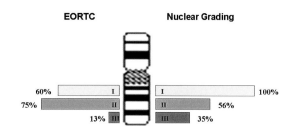

Genetic progression seems not to be the rule

Fig. 26.3 In a series of more than 50 DCIS of varying grade it became obvious that the presence of chromosomal 16q losses, revealed by CGH, is rather common in well-differentiated DCIS compared to intermediately and poorly-differentiated DCIS. This finding was independent of the classification scheme used. The variation of the relative numbers of 16q losses in the respective DCIS subgroups reflects the uncertainties associated with classification, especially of the intermediate subgroup.

morphological dedifferentiation is not the rule [47]. In consequence, it now seems obvious that multiple parallel pathways in DCIS must exist, irrespective of the pathological classification system used (Fig. 26.4). Since all the existing data about DCIS characterizes this lesion as the ultimate precursor of invasive breast cancer, it also follows that other similar pathways might be delineated leading to invasive breast cancer. A number of cytogenetic studies of invasive breast cancer support the hypothesis of multiple, predominantly parallel progression pathways in breast cancer (Fig. 26.5). Further data has accumulated to indicate

Clonal proliferation

-16q

+11q13
+17q12
+20q13

DCIS
Low grade

DCIS
High grade

Fig. 26.4 From the distribution of 16q losses in DCIS, it is evident that several cytogenetic pathways in invasive breast cancer exist. Losses of 16q define one pathway, whereas changes such as gains or even high-level amplifications of 11q13, 17q and 20q are hallmarks of other lines of breast cancer evolution.

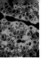

that these pathways are associated with specific phenotypic and prognostic parameters, especially the pathway involving a loss of 16q. Recent studies have also given first hints of the existence of different genetic mechanisms, resulting in 16q losses in well and poorly-differentiated invasive breast cancers as measured by microsatellite analysis [48]. Nevertheless, a stepwise dedifferentiation in breast carcinogenesis could not be ruled out by any of these studies. Recent studies have now been able to define patterns of chromosomal alteration associated with a putative progression from well to poorly-differentiated breast cancer, including gains of 7p and 5p combined with losses of 9q [49]. Again, these alteration patterns seem to define a particular prognostic subgroup [50, 51]. They represent a backbone of the current morphological systems of classification [7].

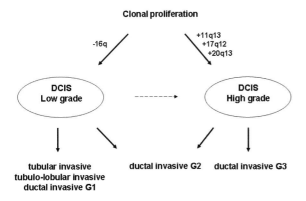

Fig. 26.5 Genetic and morphological evolution is continuous from DCIS through to invasive carcinoma. Tubular, tubulolobular and ductal invasive grade 1 carcinomas display an almost identical alteration pattern to well-differentiated DCIS. The same relationship is found between poorly-differentiated DCIS and ductal invasive grade 3 carcinomas. Ductal invasive grade 2 carcinomas are in this regard a morphological mixture, comprising tumors originating in the well-differentiated pathway as well as in the poorly-differentiated pathway.

INVASION REFLECTED AT THE CYTOGENETIC LEVEL

Tumor progression can be defined from various perspectives, whereby a change in tumor grade is only one parameter. From a clinical point of view it is of course of much higher importance to define genetic events associated with the acquisition of invasive growth properties. In a model based on multiple pathways of progression, such a definition may be

hampered by the fact that a multitude of different, alternative mechanism are likely to exist. It is therefore not surprising that various markers have been associated with the gain of invasiveness. The loss of chromosomal 14q material nevertheless seems to be a protective event for tumor invasion in DCIS. Likewise, gain of 6q material has been detected at a greater frequency in LCIS than lobular invasive breast cancer [43, 12]. The importance of 14q losses has further been strengthened by studies in invasive breast cancer: LOH on 14q was significantly associated with a lower incidence of lymph node metastasis in invasive breast cancer [52]. In contrast, gains of 11q13 and 8q were associated with tumor invasion in DCIS [53, 54]. The characteristic changes in protein expression have not yet been described in detail.

ROLE OF LOBULAR NEOPLASIA

Lobular neoplasia has long been regarded as a mere risk indicator for invasive breast cancer rather than as a true carcinoma. Various cytogenetic and molecular investigations comparing ductal and lobular breast tumors directly and/or indirectly point to an alternative interpretation and clinical role of LN. It could be shown that LN shares a high degree of homology with well-differentiated DCIS in quantitative and qualitative cytogenetic alteration patterns – again with losses of 16q and gains of 1q as the most frequent, recurrent alterations. Based on these findings we consider DCIS and LN different morphological phenotypes of a partly similar, shared genotype. This would explain the clinical observation that patients with a diagnosed LN have a 20% likelihood of developing invasive breast cancer of ductal subtype and that the same frequency could be observed in patients with DCIS who consequently suffered from lobular invasive breast cancer. Such a genetic relationship could also explain the existence of invasive breast cancer with mixed ductal and lobular differentiation. Why LN seems to progress towards overt malignancy at a much lower rate than DCIS remains an issue for further investigation.

This hypothesis has, however, received support from a comparison of different tumors in the same patient. Rare cases of DCIS with adjacent lobular invasive carcinomas shared a large number of identical cytogenetic alterations, again pointing to the genotype-phenotype relationship described above [45]. The major difference – probably explaining the different morphology of these tumors – was the staining pattern for E-cadherin, whose gene is located on 16q. Since all these DCIS cases displayed an intermediate differentiation grade and 16q losses, we suggest that a point mutation of E-cadherin is the second hit, according to

Knudson's two-hit theory [55–57]. We consider these results to be the foundation of a unifying concept of lobular and ductal breast tumors (Fig. 26.6).

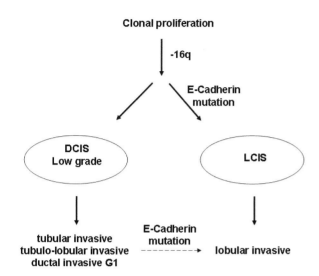

Fig. 26.6 Cytogenetic studies revealed that chromosomal 16q losses were the predominant and, sometimes, the only findings in well-differentiated DCIS and LCIS. In contrast to DCIS, E-cadherin mutations are almost exclusively found in LCIS. One might therefore interpret LCIS and well-differentiated DCIS as two morphologically different phenotypes of a shared, cytogenetic genotype. Inactivating point mutations within the E-cadherin gene might also occur at the level of invasive breast cancer, explaining the possibility of a mixed ductal and lobular differentiation.

REFERENCES

1. Dupont, W. D. and Page, D. L. Risk factors for breast cancer in women with proliferative breast disease. J Natl Cancer Inst 1981; 312: 146–151.
2. Allred, D. C., O'Connell, P., Fuqua, S. A., and Osborne, C. K. Immunohistochemical studies of early breast cancer evolution. Breast Cancer Res Treat 1994; 32: 13–18.
3. Hanahan, D. and Weinberg, R. A. The hallmarks of cancer. Cell 2000; 100: 57–70.
4. Lakhani, S. R., Slack, D. N., Hamoudi, R. A., Collins, N., Stratton, M. R., and Sloane, J. P. Detection of allelic imbalance indicates that a proportion of mammary hyperplasia of usual type are clonal, neoplastic proliferations. Lab Invest 1996; 74: 129–135.
5. Deng, G., Lu, Y., Zlotnikov, G., Thor, A. D., and Smith, H. S. Loss of heterozygosity in normal tissue adjacent to breast carcinomas. Science 1996; 274: 2057–2059.
6. Tidow, N., Boecker, A., Schmidt, H., Agelopoulos, K., Boecker, W., Buerger, H., and Brandt, B. Distinct Amplification of an Untranslated Regulatory Sequence in the egfr Gene Contributes to Early Steps in Breast Cancer Development. Cancer Res 2003; 63: 1172–1178.
7. Boecker, W., Buerger, H., Schmitz, K., Ellis, I. O., van Diest, PJ., Sinn, HP., Geradts, J., Poremba, C., and Herbst, H. Ductal epithelial proliferations of the breast: a biological continuum? Comparative genomic hybridization and high-molecular-weight cytokeratin expression patterns. J Pathol 2001; 195: 415–421.
8. Diallo, R., Schaefer K-L, Poremba, C., Shivazi, N., Willmann, V., Buerger, H., Dockhorn-Dworniczak, B., and Boecker, W. Monoclonality in normal epithelium, hyperplastic and neoplastic lesions of the breast. J Pathol 2001; 193: 27–32.
9. Tsai, Y. C., Lu, Y., Nichols, P. W., Zlotnikov, G., Jones, P. A., and Smith, H. S. Contiguous patches of normal human mammary epithelium derived from a single stem cell: implications for breast carcinogenesis. Cancer Res 1996; 56: 402–404.
10. Larson, P. S., de las Morenas, A., Cupples, L. A., Huang, K., and Rosenberg, C. L. Genetically abnormal clones in histologically normal breast tissue. Am J Pathol 1998; 152: 1591–1598.
11. Mommers, E. C., Poulin, N., Meijer, CLM., Baak, J. P., and van Diest PJ. Malignancy-associated changes in breast tissue detected by image cytometry. Anal Cell Pathol 2000; 20: 187–195.
12. Lu, Y. J., Osin, P., Lakhani, S. R., Di-Palma, S., Gusterson, B. A., and Shipley, J. M. Comparative genomic hybridization analysis of lobular carcinoma in-situ and atypical lobular hyperplasia and potential roles for gains and losses of genetic material in breast neoplasia. Cancer Res 1998; 58: 4721–4727.
13. Potten, C. S., Watson, R. J., Williams, G. T., Roberts, S. A., Harris, M., and Howell, A. The effect of age and menstrual cycle upon proliferative activity of the normal breast. Br J Cancer 1988; 58: 163–170.
14. Venkitaraman, A. R. Functions of BRCA1 and BRCA2 in the biological response to DNA damage. J Cell Sci 2001; 114: 3591–3598.
15. Beckmann, M. W., Niederacher, D., Schnurch, H. G., Gusterson, B. A., and Bender, H. G. Multistep carcinogenesis of breast cancer and tumour heterogeneity. J Mol Med 1997; 75: 429–439.
16. Washington, C., Dalbegue, F., Abreo, F, Taubenberger, J. K., and Lichy, J. H. Loss of heterozygosity in fibrocystiy change of the breast. Genetic relationship between benign proliferative lesions and associated carcinomas. Am J Pathol 2000; 157: 323–329.
17. Dawson P., J., Baekey, P. A., and Clark, R. A. Mechanisms of multifocal breast cancer: an immunocytochemical study. Hum Pathol 1995; 26: 965–969.
18. Fujii, H., Marsh, C., Cairns, P., Sidransky, D., and Gabrielson, E. Genetic divergence in the clonal evolution of breast cancer. Cancer Res 1996; 56: 1493–1497.
19. Teixeira, M. R., Pandis, N., Bardi, G., Andersen, J. A., Mitelman, F., and Heim, S. Clonal heterogeneity in breast cancer: karyotypic comparisons of multiple intra- and extra-tumorous samples from 3 patients. Int J Cancer 1995; 63: 63–68.
20. Going, J. J., Abd El-Monem, H. M., and Craft, J. A. Clonal origins of human breast cancer. J Pathol 2001; 194: 406–412.

21. Li, Z., Moore, D. H., Meng, Z. H., Ljung, B. M., Gray, J., and Dairkee, S. H. Increased risk of local recurrence is asociated with allelic loss in normal lobules of breast cancer patients. Cancer Res 2002; 62: 1000–1003.

22. Li, Z., Meng, Z. H., Chandraserkan, R., Kuo, W. L., Collins, C. C., Gray, J., and Dairkee, S. H. Biallelic inactivation of the thyroid hormone receptor β1 gene in early stage breast cancer. Cancer Res 2002; 62: 1939–1943.

23. Lakhani, S. R., Chaggar, R., Davies, S., Jones, C., Collins, N., Odel, C., Stratton, M. R., and O´Hare, M. Genetic alterations in "normal" luminal and myoepthelial cells of the breast. J Pathol 1999; 189: 496–503.

24. Owens, D. M. and Watt, F. M. Contribution of stem cells and differentiated cells to epidermal tumours. Nat Rev Cancer 2003; 3: 444–451.

25. Sell, S. and Pierce, G. B. Maturation arrest of stem cell differentiation is a common pathway for the cellular origin of teratocarcinomas and epithelial cancers. Lab Invest 1994; 70: 6–22.

26. Olsson, H. Tumour biology of a breast cancer at least partly reflects the biology of the tissue/epithelial cell of origin at the time of initiation – a hypothesis. J Steroid Biochem Mol Biol 2000; 74: 345–350.

27. Dontu, G., Abdallah, W. M., Foley, J. M., Jackson, K. W., Clarke, M. F., Kawamura, M. J., and Wicha, M. S. In vitro propagation and transcriptional profiling of human mammary stem/progenitor cells. Genes Dev 2003; 17: 1253–1270.

28. Deugnier, M. A., Faraldo, M. M., Janji, B., Rousselle, P., Thiery, J. P., and Glukhova, M. A. EGF controls the in vivo developmental potential of a mammary epithelial cell line possessing progenitor properties. J Cell Biol 2002; 159: 453–463.

29. Boecker, W., Moll, R., Poremba, C., Holland, R., van-Diest, P. J., Dervan, P., Buerger, H., Wai, D., Diallo, R., Herbst, H., Schmidt, A., and Buchwallow, I. B. Common adult stem cells in the human breast give rise to glandular and myoepithelial cell lineages: A new cell biological concept. Lab Invest 2002; 82: 737–746.

30. Boecker, W., Moll, R., Dervan, P., Buerger, H., Poremba, C., Diallo, R., Herbst, H., Schmidt, A., and Buchwallow, I. B. Usual ductal hyperplasia of the breast is a committed stem (progenitor) cell lesion distinct from atypical ductal hyperplasia and ductal carcinoma of the breast. J Pathol 2002; in press:

31. Otterbach, F., Bankfalvi, A., Bergner, S., Decker, T., Krech, R., and Boecker, W. Cytokeratin 5/6-immunohistochemistry is helpful in the diagnosis of atypical proliferations of the breast. Histopathology 2000; 37: 232–240.

32. Moll, R., Franke, W. W., Schiller, D. L., Geiger, B., and Krepler, R. The catalog of human cytokeratins: patterns of expression in normal epithelia, tumors and cultured cells. Cell 1982; 31: 11–24.

33. Sorlie, T., Perou, C., Tibshirani, R., Aas, T., Geisler, S., Johnsen, H., Hastie, T., Eisen, M., van de Rijn, M., Jeffrey, S. S., Thorsen, T., Quist, H., Matese, J. C., Brown, P. O., Botstein, D., Lonning, P. E., and Borresen-Dale AL. Gene expression patterns of breast carcinomas distinguish tumor subclasses with clinical implications. Proc Natl Acad Sci U S A 2001; 98: 10869–10874.

34. Sorlie, T., Tibshirani, R., Parker, J., Hastie, T., Marron, J. S., Nobel, A., Deng, S., Johnsen, H., Pesich, R., Geisler, S., Demeter, J., Perou, C. M., Lonning, P. E., Brown, P. O., Borresen-Dale, A. L., and Botstein, D. Repeated observation of breast tumor subtypes in independent gene expression data sets. Proc Natl Acad Sci U S A 2003; 100: 8418–8423.

35. Perou, C., Sorlie, T., Eisen, M., van de Rijn, M., Jeffrey, S. S., Rees, C. A., Pollack, J. R., Ross, D. T., Johnsen, H., Akslen, L. A., Fluge, O., Pergamenschikov, A., Williams, C., Zhu, S., Lonning, P. E., Borresen, Dale AL, Brown, P. O., and Botstein, D. Molecular portraits of human breast tumours. Nature 2000; 406: 747–752.

36. van de, Rijn M., Perou, C. M., Tibshirani, R., Haas, P., Kallioniemi, O., Kononen, J., Torhorst, J., Sauter, G., Zuber, M., Kochli, O. R., Mross, F., Dieterich, H., Seitz, R., Ross, D., Botstein, D., and Brown, P. Expression of cytokeratins 17 and 5 identifies a group of breast carcinomas with poor clinical outcome. Am J Pathol 2002; 161: 1991–1996.

37. Foulkes, W. D., Stefansson, I. M., Chappuis, P. O., Begin, L. R., Goffin, J. R., Wong, N., Trudel, M., and Akslen, L. A. Germline BRCA1 mutations and a basal epithelial phenotype in breast cancer. J Natl Cancer Inst 2003; 95: 1482–1485.

38. van der, Groep P., Bouter, A., van der, Zanden R., Menko, F. H., Buerger, H., Verheijen, R. H., Van Der, Wall E., and van Diest, P. J. Re: Germline BRCA1 mutations and a basal epithelial phenotype in breast cancer. J Natl Cancer Inst 2004; 96: 712–713.

39. Korsching, E., Packeisen, J., Agelopoulos, K., Eisenacher, M., Voss, R., Isola, J., van Diest, PJ., Brandt, B., Boecker, W., and Buerger, H. Cytogenetic alterations and cytokeratin expression patterns in breast cancer – integrating a new model of breast differentiation into cytogenetic pathways of breast carcinogenesis. Lab Invest 2002; 82: 1525–1533.

40. Wang, Z. C., Lin, M., Wei, L. J., Li, C., Miron, A., Lodeiro, G., Harris, L., Ramaswamy, S., Tanenbaum, D. M., Meyerson, M., Iglehart, J. D., and Richardson, A. Loss of heterozygosity and its correlation with expression profiles in subclasses of invasive breast cancers. Cancer Res 2004; 64: 64–71.

41. Li, Y., Welm, B., Podsypanina, K., Huang, S., Chamorro, M., Zhang, X., Rowlands, T., Egeblad, M., Cowin, P., Werb, Z., Tan, L. K., Rosen, J. M., and Varmus, H. E. Evidence that transgenes encoding components of the Wnt signaling pathway preferentially induce mammary cancers from progenitor cells. Proc Natl Acad Sci U S A 2003; 100: 15853–15858.

42. Kallioniemi, A., Kallioniemi, O. P., Piper, J., Tanner, M., Stokke, T., Chen, L., Smith, H. S., Pinkel, D., Gray, J. W., and Waldman, F. M. Detection and mapping of amplified DNA sequences in breast cancer by comparative genomic hybridization. Proc Natl Acad Sci U S A 1994; 91: 2156–2160.

43. Buerger, H., Otterbach, F., Simon, R., Poremba, C., Diallo, R., Decker, T., Riethdorf, L., Brinkschmidt, C., Dockhorn-Dworniczak, B., and Boecker, W. Comparative genomic hybridization of ductal carcinoma in-situ of the breast- evidence of multiple genetic pathways. J Pathol 1999; 187: 396–402.

44. Vos, C. B., ter, Haar NT, Rosenberg, C., Peterse, J. L., Cleton, Jansen AM, Cornelisse, C. J., and van-de, Vijver MJ. Genetic alterations on chromosome 16 and 17 are important features of ductal carcinoma in-situ of the breast and are associated with histologic type. Br J Cancer 2000; 81: 1410–1418.

45. Buerger, H., Simon, R., Schaefer, K. L., Diallo, R., Littmann, R., Poremba, C., van Diest, PJ., Dockhorn-Dworniczak, B., and Boecker, W. Genetic relationship of lobular carcinoma *in-situ*, ductal carcinoma *in-situ* and associated invasive carcinoma of the breast. Mol Pathol 2000; 53: 118–121.

46. Buerger, H., Mommers, E., Littmann, R., Diallo, R., Poremba, C., Brinkschmidt, C., Dockhorn, Dworniczak B., van Diest PJ, and Boecker W. Correlation of morphologic and cytogenetic parameters of genetic instability with chromosomal alterations in in-situ carcinomas of the breast. Am J Clin Pathol 2000; 114: 854–859.

47. Holland, R., Peterse, J. L., Millis, R. R., Eusebi, V., Faverly, D., van-de, Vijver MJ, and Zafrani, B. Ductal carcinoma in-situ: a proposal for a new classification. Semin Diagn Pathol 1994; 11: 167–180.

48. Cleton-Jansen, A. M., Buerger, H., Haar, Nt N., Philippo, K., van de Vijver, M. J., Boecker, W., Smit, V. T., and Cornelisse, C. J. Different mechanisms of chromosome 16 loss of heterozygosity in well- versus poorly differentiated ductal breast cancer. Genes Chromosomes Cancer 2004; 41: 109–116.

49. Korsching, E., Packeisen, J., Helms, M. W., Kersting, C., Voss, R., van Diest, P. J., Brandt, B., Van Der, Wall E., Boecker, W., and Burger, H. Deciphering a subgroup of breast carcinomas with putative progression of grade during carcinogenesis revealed by comparative genomic hybridisation (CGH) and immunohistochemistry. Br J Cancer 2004; 90: 1422–1428.

50. Rennstam, K., Ahlstedt-Soini, M., Baldetorp, B., Bendahl, P. O., Borg, A., Karhu, R., Tanner, M., Tirkkonen, M., and Isola, J. Patterns of chromosomal imbalances defines subgroups of breast cancer with distinct clinical features and prognosis. A study of 305 tumors by comparative genomic hybridization. Cancer Res 2003; 63: 8861–8868.

51. Gray, J. Quantitative analysis of chromosomal CGH in human breast tumours associates copy number abnormalities with p53 status and patient survival. Proc Natl Acad Sci U S A 2001; 98: 7952–7957.

52. O´Connell`, P., Fischbach, K., Hilsenbeck, S. G., Mohsin, S. K., Fuqua, S., Clark, G. C., Osborne, C. K., and Allred, C. Loss of heterozygosity at D14S62 and metastatic potential of breast cancer. J Natl Cancer Inst 1999; 91: 1391–1397.

53. Chuaqui, R. F., Zhuang, Z., Emmert, Buck MR, Liotta, L. A., and Merino, M. J. Analysis of loss of heterozygosity on chromosome 11q13 in atypical ductal hyperplasia and in-situ carcinoma of the breast. Am J Pathol 1997; 150: 297–303.

54. Robanus-Maandag, E. C., Bosch, C. A., Kristel, P. M., Hart, A. A., Faneyte, I. F., Nederlof, P. M., Peterse, J. L., and van de Vijver, M. J. Association of C-MYC amplification with progression from the in-situ to the invasive stage in C-MYC-amplified breast carcinomas. J Pathol 2003; 201: 75–82.

55. Berx, G., Cleton, Jansen AM, Strumane, K., de, Leeuw WJ, Nollet, F., van, Roy F., and Cornelisse, C. E-cadherin is inactivated in a majority of invasive human lobular breast cancers by truncation mutations throughout its extracellular domain. Oncogene 1996; 13: 1919–1925.

56. Berx, G., Cleton, Jansen AM, Nollet, F., de, Leeuw WJ, van-de, Vijver M., Cornelisse, C., and van, Roy F. E-cadherin is a tumour/invasion suppressor gene mutated in human lobular breast cancers. EMBO J 1995; 14: 6107–6115.

57. De-Leeuw, W. J., Berx, G., Vos, C. B., Peterse, J. L., Van, de, V, Litvinov, S., Van-Roy, F., Cornelisse, C. J., and Cleton, Jansen AM. Simultaneous loss of E-cadherin and catenins in invasive lobular breast cancer and lobular carcinoma in-situ. J Pathol 1997; 183: 404–411.

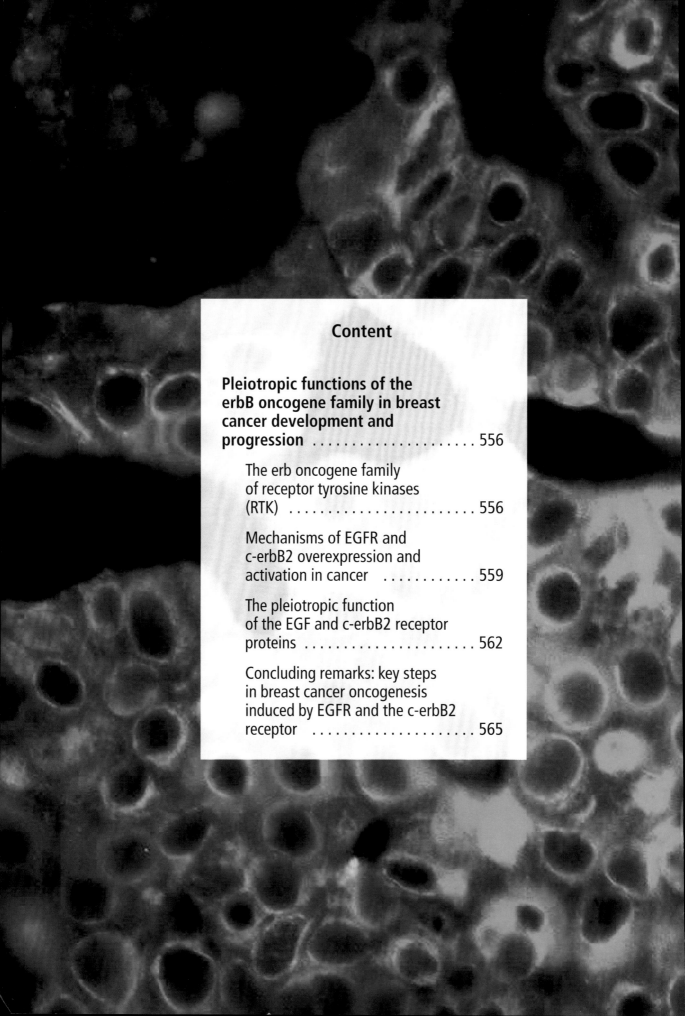

Content

PLEIOTROPIC FUNCTIONS OF THE ERBB ONCOGENE FAMILY IN BREAST CANCER DEVELOPMENT AND PROGRESSION

Burkhard H. Brandt

The database on which the multistep tumor progression model of human breast cancer is founded is still small, and the first genetic molecular hits in the process to breast cancer are still unknown. The concepts of oncogenes, tumor suppressor genes and mutator genes proposed over the last years has given us a deeper insight into the tumor biology of breast cancer. On the basis of these general concepts, first attempts to decipher the fundamental steps in breast cancer development and progression have now been made.

To actively proliferate, normal cells require mitogenic signals involving growth factors. Such stimulation may be endocrine, juxtacrine or paracrine (Fig. 27.1). Oncogenes which confer growth factor self-sufficiency to tumor cells are first order candidates for the initiation and progression of breast cancer development (Fig. 27.1) [2]. In this context, experimental and clinical evidence strongly suggests that upregulated epidermal growth factor receptors (EGFR/c-erbB1) and c-erbB2 receptors are key players [3–7].

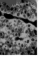

Pleiotropic functions of the erbB oncogene family in breast cancer development and progression

■ THE ERB ONCOGENE FAMILY OF RECEPTOR TYROSINE KINASES (RTK)

STRUCTURE AND FUNCTION

Growth factor receptors of the erbB family are a group of four transmembrane glycoproteins characterized by an extracellular ligand-binding domain, a transmembrane spanning domain and an intracellular domain with tyrosine kinase activity: EGFR (c-erbB1), HER2/neu (c-erbB2), c-erbB3 and c-erbB4. Of these, EGFR, c-erbB3 and c-erbB4 have known extracellular ligands, whereas only EGFR, c-erbB2 and c-erbB4 contain an intracellular tyrosine kinase domain [8–11].

The epidermal growth factor receptor (EGFR/c-erbB1) is a 170 kDa glycoprotein that was first discovered in epidermoid carcinoma [12]. It is expressed in many normal and malignant cell types [13]. The gene is located on chromosome 7p13-p12. It can be activated by its ligands, which include epidermal growth factor (EGF), TGF-α, amphiregulin, betacellulin, epiregulin and heparin-binding EGF. Ligand binding to the extracellular domain of EGFR leads to receptor dimerization, causing downstream activation of signaling pathways and cross-auto-phosphorylation of other transmembrane receptors (Fig. 27.2) [14]. EGFR is also indirectly activated by mechanisms such as binding of certain ligands to other membrane receptors, membrane depolarization, and environmental stressors.

c-erbB2 (HER2/neu) is a gene located on chromosome 17q11.2-q12. It encodes a 185 kDa transmembrane protein that has extensive homology with EGFR. In contrast to EGFR, the c-erbB2 receptor has no direct ligand. Instead, it acts by enhancing signaling of the above-mentioned EGF and EGF-like ligands and the c-erbB3 and c-erbB4 specific neuregulin ligand family (NRG) by the process of receptor heterodimerization with each of the three other erbB family members (Fig. 27.2) [16]. It has also been shown that, of the erbB family members, EGFR is the preferential heterodimerization partner of c-erbB2. Phosphorylated tyrosine residues of the intracellular domain of erbB family RTKs (autophosphorylation sites) act as interaction sites for downstream proteins containing the SH2 (src homology 2) domain, marking the start of complex signaling cascades. SH2 and phosphotyrosine-binding domains containing proteins such as PLCy, PI3K, Src, Shc, Grb2, Grb7 and Nck link RTKs to further downstream signaling pathways that control cell growth, differentiation, and motility. Moreover, the formation of heterodimers with the other erbB receptors brings several effector proteins under the control of c-erbB2 that do not directly bind it [17–20].

Therefore EGFR and the c-erbB2 receptor induce different signal transduction pathways with a variation of secondary messenger responses. The range of intracellular pathways controlled in this way and the respective cell biological responses will be discussed below. The schematic drawing in Figure 27.3 provides an overview of the main signaling pathways of EGFR and the c-erbB2 receptor.

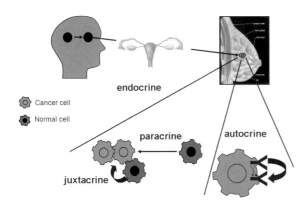

Fig. 27.1 Endocrine, juxtacrine, paracrine, and autocrine mitotic signaling in breast cancer carcinogenesis.

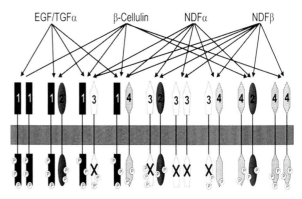

Fig. 27.2 Ligand binding, dimerization, and cross phosphorylation of erbB tyrosine kinase receptors [15].

EGFR AND c-erbB2 AS CLINICAL PROGNOSTICATORS AND THERAPY PREDICTORS

In 1977 Bernard Fisher described breast cancer as a systemic disease [22]. Since then a number of prognostic criteria have been discussed and remain the subject of investigation. In a meta-analysis comprising data from 40 studies the mean percentage of cases classified as EGFR-positive breast cancers amounted to 45% [23]. Nearly all studies disclosed a negative relationship between EGFR and steroid receptors. Most of the studies showed a significant correlation between high EGFR expression and poor differentiation of tumors, but none with tumor size, lymph node metastasis, aneuploidy or proliferation index [24]. There is considerable debate in the literature concerning the prognostic value of EGFR. The majority of follow-up studies showed a significant prognostic value, indicating that patients with EGFR-positive tumors have a poor prognosis [25]. The discriminatory effect of EGFR status with respect to prognosis seems to decrease when the follow-up interval is more than six years.

The c-erbB2 gene is amplified and overexpressed in 20–30% of invasive carcinomas, and in 40–60% of DCIS of the breast [26, 27]. However, data in the literature is conflicting concerning its prognostic significance; a beneficial effect of c-erbB2 amplification and overexpression has even been suggested [28]. This controversy can in part be attributed to a lack of standardization, for example immunohistochemistry, gene dosage determination and Western blot or solid-phase immunoassay techniques. Extensive clinical studies have shown c-erbB2 amplification and overexpression to be inversely correlated with both disease-free and overall survival in node-positive breast cancer patients. Moreover, patients with tumors overexpressing c-erbB2 did not benefit from cyclophosphamide, methotrexate, and 5-fluorouracil adjuvant therapy. However, these patients had a better outcome with more aggressive regimes, including adriamycin [29, 30]. Both EGFR and c-erbB2 have been shown to indicate patients who will not benefit from tamoxifen therapy, even when their tumors were positive for estrogen receptor.

Within prognostically favorable node-negative subpopulations of breast cancer patients, a small cohort of patients who suffered from early hematogenous metastasis could be identified by measuring c-erbB2 amplification and c-erbB2 overexpression [31, 32]. Applying an immunomagnetic separation technique, blood-borne epithelially-derived cell clusters expressing c-erbB2 were discovered [33]. These data suggest that blood-borne clustered cells expressing the c-erbB2 oncogene product may be prime candidates for the metastasis forming unit in breast cancer.

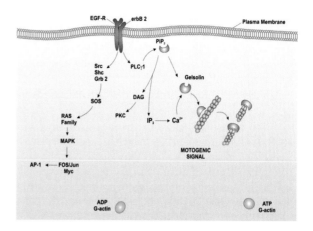

Fig. 27.3 The primary signaling pathways of the EGFR and c-erbB2 receptor tyrosine kinase dimer [21].

THERAPY STUDIES FOR BREAST CANCER TARGETING EGFR AND c-erbB2

Breast cancers that overexpress EGFR and/or c-erbB2 are far more aggressive than those that do not. This conclusion and the observation that the overexpression of these receptors is conserved in metastatic tumors have led to the inauguration of erbB-targeted systemic therapeutic approaches [34–36].

This novel strategy using immune-based therapies has shown promising results. It is based on the assumption that antibodies generated against erbB receptors selectively target those tumor cells. One approach to controlling c-erbB2 using a humanized mouse monoclonal antibody to the c-erbB2 protein (in Europe known as Herceptin®, in USA as trastuzumab) has already been approved by the FDA and launched for clinical application [37, 38]. The antibody inhibits proliferation of cells that overexpress c-erbB2 and induces antibody-dependent cellular cytotoxicity against these cells.

Data from clinical trials indicate that Herceptin® is active in patients with c-erbB2-positive advanced metastatic breast cancer as a single agent and in combination with chemotherapy.

Ongoing clinical trials are extensively testing strategies to target EGFR using monoclonal antibodies against the extracellular domain of the receptor and also inhibitors of its tyrosine kinase [39–41]. The human-to-murine chimeric monoclonal antibody (mAb) C225 and a chimeric human/murine version (IMC-225/Cetuximab) that competes with ligand binding and tyrosine kinase activation has been evaluated, alone and in combination with cisplatin, in phase I clinical trials. The antibody-associated toxicity was minimal, and patients experiencing disease stabilization were seen in all studies. A highly specific and potent inhibitor of the EGFR tyrosine kinase (Gefitinib/ ZD 1839/Iressa) that inhibits the EGF-stimulated proliferation of human carcinoma cells with a 50% inhibitory concentration in the nanomolar range was evaluated in a phase I study.

Another technique targeting c-erbB2 takes advantage of the discovery that E1A, a gene product from the homologous adenovirus gene identified as a suppressor for ras-induced metastasis, also represses c-erbB2 expression via a cis DNA element in the gene promoter [42]. A clinical phase I trial was developed for this E1A gene therapy, targeting breast and ovarian cancer overexpressing c-erbB2 [43]

Many other approaches that have not yet been transferred to clinical trials are also under investigation. Expression of c-erbB2, for example, can be suppressed by antisense oligonucleotides, single chain antibody fragments coupled to toxins, adenovirus-mediated ribozymes and site-directed irreversible inhibitors of the c-erbB2 tyrosine kinase [44].

It may be assumed that cancer chemoprevention trials specifically targeting c-erbB2 will be beneficial for women with c-erbB2-positive precursor lesions, who are at high risk for breast cancer. This is strongly supported by the fact that c-erbB2 is the preferred heterodimerization partner in the erbB receptor family and therefore offers a selective target, including several routes of signal transduction involved in cancer development.

DIAGNOSTIC IMPLICATIONS OF c-erbB2

Overexpression of c-erbB2 has also gained therapeutic implications. The US Food and Drug Administration (FDA) has approved trastuzumab (Herceptin®) – a humanized monoclonal antibody directed against c-erbB2 – and two diagnostic kits – the immunohistochemical DAKO-HercepTest™ and the INFORM-HER-2/neu Gene Detection System (Oncor/Ventana) based on FISH. Several groups have reported excellent sensitivity, reproducibility and high accuracy of the FISH assay in archival breast cancer tissues, and it is currently the method of choice for c-erbB2 gene amplification in histological sections [1, 45]. In contrast, major concerns have been raised concerning a possible oversensitivity of the DAKO-HercepTest™, which potentially indicates a higher frequency of c-erbB2 positive cases than expected in breast cancer patients [46, 47]. Since c-erbB2 overexpression/ amplification is a quantitative rather than a qualitative alteration and dosage changes appear to have a significant clinical impact both on disease outcome and therapeutic response, quantitative assessment of c-erbB2 has become a methodical issue of major importance.

Besides testing for Herceptin® therapy indication required by the FDA, no agreement has been reached on the detection method to be used for c-erbB2 amplification and overexpression in clinical use. In our experience, methods assessing gene dosage alterations provide more reliable and concordant information on c-erbB2 gene status in breast cancer samples than immunohistochemical methods [48]. The degree of c-erbB2 amplification can be determined by FISH and cdPCR, with both procedures showing a high degree of concordance [49]. The novel technique of real-time PCR will further enhance reliability of measurement and reduce turnaround time and costs.

Data on the prognostic and predictive value of c-erbB2 overexpression in breast cancer are primarily derived from immunohistochemical (IHC) studies. In a comparative study we estimated the efficacy of the two clinically most relevant IHC tests for detecting c-erbB2 expression in archival paraffin-embedded breast carcinoma tissues. Using the antibody originally applied in the Clinical Trial Assay for the anti-c-erbB2 studies, a highly significant concordance rate was found between protein overexpression and FISH-detected gene amplification status. In some cases amplification of the c-erbB2 gene as an early event (see 'Amplifications of EGFR and c-erbB2' below) may precede overexpression of the protein. Such cases can readily be detected by the FISH technique in tissue sections, but may be overlooked when IHC is used alone. Low level gene copy signals can also be diluted below detectable limits in extracted tumor DNA required for other gene-based assays.

Conflicting reports exist on whether quantity of c-erbB2 protein expression is an important predictor of outcome and therapy sensitivity in breast cancer. Experimental data have shown that a critical level of c-erbB2 needs to be achieved for tyrosine kinase activation and inappropriate cellular signaling. This can lead, in turn, to acquisition of an invasive phenotype, which determines the metastatic capacity of a tumor even if only small tumor cell clusters are involved. Detection of these 'low-expressor' cases can be directly performed by FISH or by complex methodological techniques, for instance gene dosage estimation by cdPCR or in vivo invasiveness assays, whereas low-level protein expression can be quantified by automated IHC coupled with computer-assisted imaging techniques.

However, it is not only the presence of the c-erbB2 protein on the tumor cell surface, but also the active signaling of the receptor, regulated via reversible phosphorylation events, which is of essential importance for the malignant phenotype. Functional characterization of the overexpressed c-erbB2 receptor using phosphorylation-state-specific antibodies is a new aspect of c-erbB2 studies, potentially enhancing their clinical relevance.

Diagnostic studies of EGFR expression and phosphorylation similar to those on c-erbB2 have still not been performed [50]. Moreover, the genomic rearrangement processes leading to increased EGFR expression levels are more complicated than those associated with c-erbB2 (see 'Modulation of EGFR gene transcription' below). We have now started basic research on the subject. More work is needed before an EGFR DNA-assay can be established in the clinical laboratory [51].

MECHANISMS OF EGFR AND c-erbB2 OVER-EXPRESSION AND ACTIVATION IN CANCER

AMPLIFICATIONS OF EGFR AND c-erbB2

Gene dosage deviations of constitutional genes and oncogenes are frequent events in cancer cells, especially during chemotherapy. Basic research on the mechanisms of gene dosage elevations by amplification have revealed that the most likely mechanism is based on recombination reactions [52]. DNA segments of kb-to-Mb sizes are exchanged in or between chromosomes resulting in gain and loss of genomic material. It is therefore possible to estimate gene dosage by measurement of representative sequences of the target gene by Southern blotting protocols, in-situ hybridization and quantitative PCR [53].

A direct correlation between gene dosage of c-erbB2 and the expression of the membrane receptor has been shown. A relationship between the genotype of distinct loci and a specific phenotype in normal somatic cells is a very rare event, making gene dosage sensitivity rather unlikely. Only specific gene families that are members of a signal transduction system – for instance the erbB receptors – show such sensitivity. Interaction of the gene products in these systems is often the reason for such gene dosage sensitivity. In consequence, it is not only the total number of receptors per cell – for instance the EGFR and c-erbB2 receptors – which leads to proliferation or invasiveness, but the ratio of receptor numbers. Further interaction with other proteins, as has been demonstrated for the erbB oncogenes, leads to modifications of the pathogenic effect of gene dosage and results in a broad variety of phenotypes. Frequent alterations of the erbB oncogenes in breast cancer may therefore be one of the main causes of breast cancer heterogeneity.

Amplifications of EGFR with a gene copy number above 3.0 have been reported at a frequency of $0-20\%$ [54, 55] (Fig. 27.4). Amplifications of c-erbB2 in a range from 3.0 to 50.0 copies as ascertained by

Southern blotting, slot blotting, and quantitative PCR have been observed in $14-15\%$ of patients [56, 57] (Fig. 27.4).

The higher analytical sensitivity of PCR-based methods used in our studies revealed deviations in gene dosage of the erbB oncogenes in the low-level range of $1.6-3.0$. Data from clinical evaluation studies indicate that this range is important in estimating prognosis in primary breast cancer [59, 60].

The c-erbB2 gene dosage (degree of amplification) showed significant correlation with c-erbB2 receptor concentrations in the tumor [61]. These data are in line with results obtained by other techniques, including immunohistochemistry or Western blotting. The c-erbB2 gene dosage is also a prognostic factor for metastasis-free survival. Increased c-erbB2 gene dosages are characteristic features of short-term survival, but the prognostic significance for medium- and long-term survivors is lost. Amplification and overexpression of c-erbB2 associated with EGFR aberrations and EGFR overexpression is a clear cut, clinically relevant prognosticator. Moreover, in patients with node-negative breast cancer, the combination of both parameters was of prognostic value.

Determination of erbB oncogene gene dosage offers an additional method of assessment in primary cancer. Models of how the different erbB protein products (EGFR and c-erbB2) influence tumor progression may seem like putting a complicated puzzle together; the pieces do however fit. The pleiotropic functions of these proteins are discussed below. Such information has aided us in individualizing how breast cancer is monitored and treated.

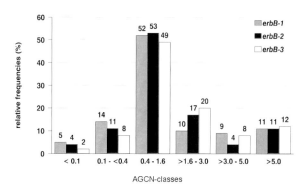

Fig. 27.4 Average gene copy number (AGCN) frequencies of the EGFR and c-erbB2 oncogenes in breast cancer tissues. Distribution of AGCN of erbB oncogenes in primary breast cancer tissue. The relative frequencies of the AGCN class for each erbB oncogene is given above the columns. The data were acquired by the ddPCR method, as described in Brandt et al. 1995 [58].

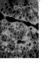

MODULATION OF EGFR AND c-erbB2 GENE TRANSCRIPTION

Up to now, mechanisms regulating the transcription of the EGFR proto-oncogene have been poorly understood. Our knowledge, however, of secondary structures, simple repetitive sequences like CA repeats (CA-SSR) and the function of mutations with regards to negative or positive enhancers is more advanced and will provide new insights into the regulation of gene expression and elucidate the linkage of inherited polymorphisms and cancer.

REGULATION OF EGFR GENE TRANSCRIPTION IN NORMAL TISSUE

Human erbB genes originated from a viral precursor gene, the v-erbB oncogene, carried by retroviruses: the avian leukosis, avian sarcoma and avian erythroblastosis viruses [62]. Unlike v-erbB, EGFR possesses an extracellular domain and is activated after ligand binding. It was initially localized at chromosome 7p13-q22 and later mapped more precisely to p11.2. The EGFR locus covers 193 kbp and 28 exons [63].

Transcription of the EGFR gene results in at least two different mRNA species of 5.8 and 10.5 knt, respectively [64]. These transcripts are detectable in all EGF-expressing tissues and translated to form the 170 kDa EGFR. Another EGFR mRNA of only 1.8 kb has been identified in normal human placenta tissue. It codes for the extracellular domain only and is produced via alternative RNA processing. The ligand-binding protein can form heterodimers with full-length EGF receptors, which may be a way of signal transduction regulation by suppressing the formation of active EGFR homodimers or heterodimers with other members of the erbB family [65].

Production of EGFR mRNA can be stimulated directly or indirectly by treatment of cells with EGF, phorbol, dibutyryl-cAMP, dexamethasone, thyroid hormone, retinoic acids, interferon-α, and wild-type p53. In overexpressing cells the effect can be reversed, causing a suppression of the EGFR promoter [66–68].

The EGFR gene promoter is GC-rich and contains no consensus sequences such as TATA or CAAT boxes [69]. Transcription starts at multiple initiation sites within the promoter region. A further three sequences with enhancer activity have been found within the 5'-region of the gene. Two of them – located upstream of the promoter and downstream in intron 1 close to a polymorphic region – showed cooperative function: the downstream enhancer functioned only in the presence of the upstream element [70]. A large number of experimental studies have shown that expression of the receptor is, in fact, primarily regulated at the level of gene transcription.

MODULATION OF EGFR GENE TRANSCRIPTION BY POLYMORPHIC REPETITIVE SEQUENCES AND MUTATIONS

It has been shown that the first intron of several genes, including EGFR, has an important regulatory function [71]. A polymorphic simple sequence repeat with 14–21 CA dinucleotides (CA-SSR) and a heterozygosity of 72% in a Caucasian reference pedigree [72] has been revealed close to the downstream enhancer element. Differences in the number of repeats in the CA-SSR in EGFR intron 1 indicate different levels of transcription modulation. EGFR transcription activity in vitro declines with increasing length of the CA-SSR (Fig. 27.5).

These results suggest that the polymorphic region has two functions. Firstly, it indirectly regulates transcription in vitro up to fivefold, depending on the number of repeats in the CA-SSR, and, secondly, it blocks RNA elongation independently of the length of the CA-SSR. The observed effect in vitro is also important in vivo at the protein expression level. Allele-dependent modulation of EGFR transcription can be observed in carcinoma cell lines in vivo, but, not surprisingly, there are other regulation mechanisms that can compensate for this [74, 75]. In the case of EGFR, action of a repressor protein that preferentially inhibits transcription of DNA molecules with a longer CA-SSR could explain these results. A loop structure, that brings together the two enhancers

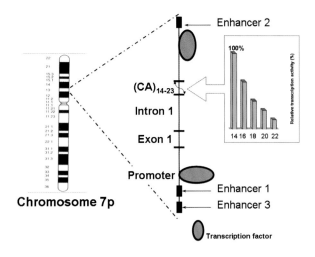

Fig. 27.5 Structure of the 5'-regulatory sequence of the EGFR gene. The insert demonstrates the relationship between length of the CA-SSR and the in vitro transcription activity of the gene [73].

at the 5'-region by the action of one or more DNA-binding proteins may be favored if the polymorphic stretch is prolonged. In this way, a transcriptional repressor protein that binds downstream of the CA-SSR could serve as a mediator of allele-dependent inhibition in EGFR transcription. This is a novel transcriptional regulation mechanism that involves the action of a presumed repressor and is dependent on the length of the CA-SSR and its influence on DNA flexibility.

Using a standardized semiautomated method for microsatellite analysis we identified loss of heterozygosity at this CA-SSR in one third of all primary breast cancer cases [76, 77]. In the cancer tissue a preferred deletion of the longer allele of the CA-SSR was observed. This LOH resulted in an increased EGFR expression in tumor cells. On the basis of this finding it could be hypothesized that mutation of this CA-SSR supports the interaction between enhancer 1 and 2.

In all cases of an EGFR CA-SSR LOH only full-length transcripts could be obtained by RT-PCR analysis of the EGFR mRNA and full-length receptor proteins by Western blotting [78].

Based on these results, microdissected samples of normal, nontumorous breast tissue with known LOH of the EGFR locus in the associated invasive carcinoma were investigated. In 75% of these patients an LOH in the CA-SSR of the EGFR gene in at least two normal, nontumorous breast lobules was detected. This suggests that this genetic alteration is a primary event in breast cancer carcinogenesis. Taking into account the fact that 35% of all informative breast cancer cases displayed this LOH and 75% of these patients also show LOH in normal breast tissue indicates that this alteration is a primary genetic alteration in more than 20% of all sporadic breast cancer cases.

Furthermore, 20% of nontumorous hyperplasias and metaplasias and 80% of atypical ductal hyperplasias presented with an LOH of the CA-SSR. Segregation of LOH was further detected in all cases of associated ductal carcinoma in-situ (DCIS) and also in all lymph node metastases. To our knowledge, no other genomic alteration leading to gene deregulation has so far been reported with such a high frequency in nontumorous breast tissue. In consequence, the enhanced expression of EGFR could contribute to an increased proliferation rate: we were able to detect a highly increased number of MIB-1-positive cells in lobules from these patients displaying LOH in the EGFR CA-SSR.

REGULATION OF c-erbB2 TRANSCRIPTION

As mentioned above, transduction of extracellular signals to the cytoplasm via c-erbB receptors is not solely dependent on ligand binding to the extracellular domain, but is also determined by concentrations of the different receptors on the cell surface. Knowing how the expression levels of c-erbB genes are controlled is therefore crucial. Besides alteration of gene copy numbers (see 'Amplifications of EGFR and c-erbB2' above), modulation of transcription activity of a gene is another way in which expression of an erbB receptor protein can be regulated.

The c-erbB2 gene comprises consensus sequences (TATA, CAAT box) and two palindromic binding sites for basic transcription factors (Sp1, RBPJk) that enhance basal transcription [79]. Mediated by an enhancer element in intron 1, c-erbB2 is down-regulated by estrogen in estrogen-responsive cells [80]. The latter effect explains the observation that there is an inverse relationship between estrogen and c-erbB2 expression in many breast carcinoma cell lines. ESX, a new member of the ETS proto-oncogene family, is another transcription factor upregulating c-erbB2 which, when overexpressed, may be a crucial event in tumorigenic transformation of mammary cells [81]. Transcription of c-erbB2 is indirectly driven by progesterone, cAMP, phorbol, retinoic acid and by cell-cell contact in confluent layers of cultured cells [82].

As mentioned above, overexpression of c-erbB2 is most frequently caused by gene amplification. Overexpression without gene amplification has also been found in a small subset of less than 10% of breast cancers.

TRANSCRIPTION OF c-erbB2 ALTERNATIVE SPLICE VARIANTS

The c-erbB2 gene is transcribed in three different, full length mRNA species of 4.6, 5.8 and 10.5 kb and an alternatively spliced 2.3 kb variant lacking the transmembrane and intracellular portions of the receptor [1]. This truncated c-erbB2 mRNA encodes the extracellular domain (ECD) of the receptor-like tyrosine kinase and diverges 61 nucleotides upstream of the transmembrane domain [83]. Recently, another splice variant deficient in only one exon, slightly upstream of the transmembrane domain, has been found in carcinoma cell lines. It is interesting to note that the point of divergence from full length transcripts is identical in these two splice variants.

The ECD mRNA of the c-erbB2 protein was found to be expressed in tumor cell lines. The resultant 100 kDa protein consisted of the entire ECD except for 20 amino acids. The sequence of the isolated

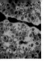

cDNA clone suggested that this region was generated during RNA processing by reading through a splice donor site and an in-frame stop codon upstream of the transmembrane region. The truncated protein has been shown to accumulate in the perinuclear region of a gastric cancer cell line (MKN7) and to double the cell division rate in breast cancer cell lines (BT 474, MDA-468) (Fig. 27.6) [84]. This method of producing truncated c-erbB2 molecules must be distinguished from proteolytic cleavage of full length proteins, where the intracellular domain (ICD) remains within the cell. Unlike soluble receptor ECDs that are shed from the cell surface, translated splice variants may also remain in the cytosol.

In c-erbB2-positive primary breast tumor samples, there was a broad variety of full length to ECD mRNA ratios. Nevertheless, the sample cohort could be divided into two biologic distinct subgroups [88]. The amount of ECD in one subgroup was 4–5-fold that in the other subgroup, with no overlap of the full length to ECD mRNA ratios. Furthermore, most of the lymph node metastases and all bone marrows from patients with metastatic disease presented with a high level of ECD mRNA (Fig. 27.6) [89]. In a further investigation of micrometastatic breast cancer cells, the previous observation that most of the c-erbB2 positive samples expressed elevated levels of truncated c-erbB2 mRNA was supported [87]. In this study with peripheral stem cell collections from breast cancer patients subsequently undergoing high-dose chemotherapy,

c-erbB2 proved a significant parameter for sensitive and specific detection of micrometastasis.

■ THE PLEIOTROPIC FUNCTION OF THE EGF AND c-erbB2 RECEPTOR PROTEINS

EGFR AND c-erbB2 IN ORGANOGENESIS, TISSUE REGENERATION AND REPAIR

All normal cells require mitogenic signals before an active proliferative state can be achieved. Distinct classes of signaling molecules, for instance soluble growth factors, extracellular matrix components, and cell-to-cell adhesion/interaction molecules, carry these signals to the cell. The erbB receptors on the cell membrane transduce growth stimulatory signals into the cell and trigger proliferation in physiological processes such as embryogenesis, organogenesis of nerves and the mammary gland, tissue regeneration and wound healing [90].

The human placenta is a rapidly growing organ that displays some similarities to invasive cancer. Immunohistochemistry has revealed that EGFR is intensively expressed in the villous cytotrophoblast in the first trimester. The c-erbB2 receptor is expressed in the first and third trimester along the apical membrane of the syncytiotrophoblast. Staining by the proliferation-associated marker Ki-67 has revealed proliferation in the EGFR-positive villous cytotrophoblast and

Cell count (x 1000)

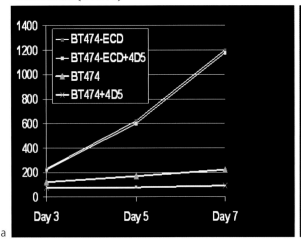

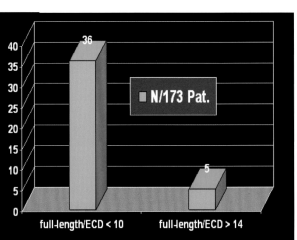

ratio (full-length/ECD)

Fig. 27.6a–b
27.6a Resistance of c-erbB2 overexpressing tumor cells to muMAb4D5 (analogous to Herceptin®) induced by c-erbB2 ECD overexpression [85].
27.6b Differential expression of alternatively spliced c-erbB2 mRNA (ECD) in peripheral blood stem cell collections (RT-PCR) [86, 87].

extravillous trophoblast, whereas most of the c-erbB2-positive cells were Ki-67 negative. These findings indicate a differential regulation of EGFR and c-erbB2 in the placenta with advancing pregnancy. Thus EGFR is more associated with proliferation and c-erbB2 with cellular differentiation. A complex regulation by hormones and growth factors can be postulated in which the erbB receptors are intimately involved [91].

Analogous to our growing knowledge of neuregulins (a large group of structurally related polypeptide factors), erbB receptor-mediated signaling pathways in normal somatic cell genesis, survival, proliferation and differentiation have been revealed. Independent efforts to identify factors responsible for stimulating c-erbB2 receptor phosphorylation have resulted in the discovery of three peptides: neu differentiation factor (ndf/heregulin), glial growth factor (ggf) and acetylcholine receptor inducing activity (aria). These are encoded by the same gene [92]. The collective term, neuregulins, indicates the importance of these factors in the nervous system. Many details of the rather diverse nrg-erbB signaling network have now been revealed, and its role in midgestation organogenesis as a key determinant in differentiation of several cell lineages is now assumed. The c-erbB3 and c-erbB4 proteins are direct nrg receptors, whereas EGFR and c-erbB2 function as co-receptors. The physiological function of the nrg-erbB signaling network comprises heart trabeculae formation, Schwann cell development, neuron migration in the brain, neuromuscular synapse signaling and also mammary gland lobuloalveolar morphogenesis. The underlying stromal mesenchymal cells are the main source of neuregulins in epithelial organogenesis.

The mammary gland is one of several organs in which major morphogenesis takes place after birth. During puberty, it involves branching and elongation, resulting in a ductal tree. A second budding phase during pregnancy generates the milk-producing lobuloalveolar structures. Analyses of organ cultures of the mouse mammary gland suggest that nrgs, whose expression peaks at pregnancy regulate the second morphogenic phase by stimulating lobuloalveolar budding and milk production. When cell pellets releasing nrgs were implanted within the mammary gland of prepubescent female mice, ductal branching and migration in the absence of exogenous steroid hormones could be induced [93]. Thus, nrgs appear to induce growth and inhibit differentiation of the primitive epithelial duct, but later in development these factors enhance mammary differentiation. The underlying signal diversification is based on a dynamic pattern of erbB receptor expression during cell fate determination, and morphogenic processes apparently dictate the nature of the cellular response. This could be substantiated by experimental data from mice. Tyrosine phosphorylation of EGFR and c-erbB2 could be detected in normal female mice but not in prepubertal mice. Furthermore, transgenic mice with impaired EGFR kinase activity, exhibited less mammary development than did wild-type mice [94].

HOMODIMER SIGNALING OF c-erbB2

The erbB cell surface receptors, which transduce growth-stimulatory signals into the cell interior, are themselves targets of deregulation during tumor pathogenesis. Dramatic examples of how the repertoire of erbB receptors is able to affect cell function are provided by several types of epithelial cancers. Overexpression of the c-erbB2 receptor in these tumors biases the formation of its differentially-acting heterodimers and induces proliferation at the expense of a differentiated phenotype.

Gross overexpression of c-erbB2 elicits ligand-independent phosphorylation and constitutive firing of the receptor. It has been shown in cellular model systems that tyrosine phosphorylation of the c-erbB2 receptors' autophosphorylation domain correlates well with its specific kinase activity and transforming potency [95]. The number of receptors expressed on the cell surface determines the level of tyrosine phosphorylation. Therefore, it could be concluded that a certain level of kinase activity is required for c-erbB2 to exert its transforming effect. Despite this data on c-erbB2 autophosphorylation and kinase activity, a particular threshold invariably correlated with the acquisition of the malignant phenotype is unknown in breast cancer. A first hint as to the method of acquisition may be provided by clinical trials on Herceptin® (the therapeutic anti-c-erbB2 antibody), in which patients benefited only when c-erbB2 was at least 3-fold overexpressed. In contrast, the rat homologue gene neu is oncogenically activated – as a result of autophosphorylation – due to a single point mutation (Val664Glu) in the region coding for the transmembrane domain of the receptor [96]. This point mutation of c-erbB2 has never been observed in human tumors. Autophosphorylation of the receptor in human tumors, and in consequence its oncogenic activation under conditions of overexpression, is related to the production of a putative ligand by an array of cell types or to a constitutive, unstimulated enzymatic activity. The latter possibility is supported by the finding that chronic activation of c-erbB2 is, at least in part, due to a strong upregulation of kinase activity exerted by its carboxy-terminal domain. The carboxy-terminal domain contains six tyrosine residues that can be phosphorylated by the kinase of the second c-erbB2 molecule in a homodimer. The major autophospho-

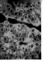

rylation site is the last tyrosine at position 1248. In vitro mutation of tyrosine 1248 to phenylalanine lowers tyrosine kinase activity and the transforming potential of the c-erbB2 receptor (see 'Heterodimer signaling of c-erbB2/EGF receptors' below). A strong mitotic signal pushing proliferation forward is mediated by the Grb2/Sos complex, which binds to the c-erbB2 autophosphorylation domain and increases the mitosis-activating protein kinase (MAPK) pathway. In particular, tyrosine phosphorylation of Shc results in a binding site for Grb2, a 24 kDa adapter protein that contains an SH2 domain between two SH3 domains. Grb2 associates with Sos via these SH3 domains. Sos is a 150 kDa guanyl nucleotide exchange factor for Ras, thus activating the MAPK pathway for example via RAS, RAF and MEK. Activated MAPKs migrate from the cytosol to the nucleus, where they phosphorylate a variety of proteins including the transcription factors Fos, Jun, and Myc. The activated proteins Jun and Fos form the active gene regulatory protein called activator protein-1 (AP-1), which turns on additional genes.

Although the participation of a ligand cannot be excluded at the present, it can be deduced from the published data that the level of c-erbB2 expression is critical in regulating the signaling ability of its constitutively active kinase. An imbalance in the equilibrium caused by overexpression above a critical threshold might, therefore, contribute to the progression of the cell along the malignant pathway.

Additionally to the activation of mitogenic pathways in breast cancer cells, c-erbB2 receptor signaling also inhibits apoptosis in taxol-treated breast cancer cells [97]. Taxol activates p34cdc2 kinase in MDA-MB-435 breast cancer cells, leading to cell cycle arrest at the G2/M phase and, subsequently, apoptosis. Overexpression of c-erbB2 receptor in MDA-MB-435 cells by transfection transcriptionally upregulates p21cip1, which associates with p34cdc2, inhibits taxol-mediated p34cdc2 activation, delays cell entrance into the G2/M phase, and thereby inhibits taxol-induced apoptosis.

The above-mentioned data indicates that c-erbB2 can increase cell growth either by activating mitosis-associated intracellular pathways or by inhibiting apoptosis pathways.

Additional experimental data have reaffirmed that c-erbB2 induces morphological changes in normal and cancer cells. An association of c-erbB2 with membrane glycoprotein complexes such as p60^{src}, p120^{abl} and microfilaments has been experimentally substantiated [98]. It can, therefore, be hypothesized that the formation of a signal transduction complex of c-erbB2 and the cytoskeleton at the signal transition from membrane to the cytoskeleton may represent a key event in cell shape changes.

HETERODIMER SIGNALING OF c-erbB2/EGF RECEPTORS

Overexpression of c-erbB2 leading to the dominant c-erbB2 receptor homodimer phenotype, as described above, is only present in about 15% of invasive cancers and 40–60% of DCIS. The transition of an in-situ carcinoma to the invasive phenotype can be attributed to the formation of distinct heterodimers of the erbB receptor family. This view is supported by the fact that the metastatic phenotype, which occurs regardless of clinical staging and histomorphology, mainly depends on the formation of c-erbB2/EGF receptor heterodimers. This phenotype escapes aggressive chemotherapy regimens and the new antibody-based c-erbB2 targeted therapies.

In breast cancer cell lines characterized by trans-endothelial invasiveness, constitutive coexpression of c-erbB2 and EGFR has been found [99–101]. These c-erbB2/EGF receptor heterodimers were found to be colocalized in areas of the cell undergoing extreme changes in shape. The c-erbB2 protein may therefore play a central role in the ability of breast cancer cells to invade extracellular matrices.

There are at least three major pathways of EGF/c-erbB2 heterodimer signaling mediating actin reorganization and reduction of adhesion [102]. The dominant pathway acts via direct binding of the protein phospholipase Cy1 (PLCy1 or phosphoinositide-specific PLC). Minor pathways recruit Grb2 and Sos to activate MAP kinases and are induced by the activation of PI3 kinase, which can also occur by heterodimerization of c-erbB2 with c-erbB3.

The ability of c-erbB2 to promote recycling of ligand-stimulated EGFR adds a further dimension to EGFR/c-erbB2 signaling [103].

Key events in the regulation of actin cytoskeleton activity are phosphoinositide (PI) synthesis and breakdown, the translocation and activation of actin binding proteins (ABPs) and changes in the cytoplasmic calcium concentration. Signaling of erbB receptors is connected to these events by the phosphoinositide-specific phospholipase Cy1 (PLCy1), which binds preferentially to the c-erbB2 receptor. Activation of PLCy1 is induced by ligand binding (for instance EGF) and phosphorylation of the c-erbB2/EGFR heterodimer. It is rapidly phosphorylated at three known sites – tyr771, tyr783 and tyr1254 – after binding. After its phosphorylation, PLCy1 dissociates from the receptor and translocates to the plasma membrane [104–107].

Catalytic breakdown of PIP2 by PLCy1 leads to the release of the actin-severing molecule gelsolin [108]. This process of gelsolin release was demonstrated in-situ in a specially designed immunofluorescence transendothelial-extracellular matrix invasion model.

In this model the invasive tumor cells are plated out on top of a monolayer of human umbilical vein endothelial cells (HUVEC), which are grown on a porous PET membrane (8 μm pores) coated with extracellular matrix. Gelsolin was shown to be released from the plasma membrane in response to c-erbB2 transphosphorylation. In SK-BR-3 cells, c-erbB2 and gelsolin were shown to be colocalized in areas where the cells were crawling out of the 8 μm pore of a PET membrane, in other words undergoing extreme changes in shape. F-actin was organized in a cross-weave opposite the 8 μm pore, indicating the formation of lamellipodia as the cell settled on the underside of the membrane. PLCγ1 also induces a reduction in cell adhesion and a local increase in lamellipodia extension rate. These observations indicate a role for PLCγ1 in cellular motility.

The exact role of all ABPs, like gelsolin, and other factors involved in actin polymerization is not yet fully understood and cannot be summarized directly due to the different types of cells used to model the effect of various proteins and signaling cascades. However, it is clear that erbB receptor tyrosine kinases play an important role in regulating the organization of the actin cytoskeleton. This effect is particularly interesting with respect to the migratory/invasive ability of certain tumor cells containing c-erbB2/EGF heterodimers.

CONCLUDING REMARKS: KEY STEPS IN BREAST CANCER ONCOGENESIS INDUCED BY EGFR AND THE c-erbB2 RECEPTOR

The above-mentioned experimental and clinical data provide evidence that, in the majority of cases, the molecular steps in breast cancer development and progression are dependent on erbB receptor signaling.

Allelic imbalances in the EGFR gene occur in morphologically normal breast tissue prior to cancerous change. These are extremely likely to be an early step in the pathway towards an invasive and metastatic breast cancer phenotype. Furthermore, the discovery of polymorphic sequences in intron 1 of the EGFR gene, which determine basal gene transcription (see 'Modulation of EGFR gene transcription' above), and the detection of allelic imbalances suggest that erbB receptor genes may be associated with a hereditary risk of breast cancer. Random genomic hits preferentially induce mutations and overexpression of EGFR and c-erbB2. Frequent overexpression of the c-erbB2 receptor represents a further carcinogenic step in poorly-differentiated DCIS. In parallel to EGFR allelic imbalances, amplification and overexpression of c-erbB2 is maintained in metastasis. In consequence, co-expression of c-erbB2 and EGFR is indica-

tive of invasive breast cancer, with enhanced cell migration and increased survival of cancer cells in peripheral blood and distant organs, leading to cancer metastasis.

The elucidation of the distinct molecular functions of these receptors will therefore greatly help in developing new therapies to improve prevention, monitoring and treatment of breast cancer. These therapies include the already published approaches targeting the receptors by antibodies or antibody constructs with toxins and liposomes. In addition, downregulation of receptor proteins can be achieved by intracellular antibody fragments, viral repressors or anti-sense oligonucleotides. In the future, these strategies will be supported by approaches targeting signals downstream from the receptors at various levels of the mitogenic and motogenic pathways, and signals involved in the maintenance of cellular homeostasis.

REFERENCES
1. Hesketh R. The Oncogene Handbook. London: Academic Press Ltd.; 1994.
2. Hanahan D, Weinberg RA. The hallmarks of cancer. Cell 2000;100: 57–70.
3. Slamon DJ, Clark GM, Wong SG, et al. Human breast cancer: correlation of relapse and survival with amplification of the HER-2/neu oncogene. Science 1987; 235: 177–82.
4. Gullick WJ, Berger MS, Bennett PL, Rothbard JB, Waterfield MD. Expression of the c-erbB2 protein in normal and transformed cells. Int J Cancer 1987; 40: 246–54.
5. Slamon DJ, Godolphin W, Jones LA, et al. Studies of the HER-2/neu proto-oncogene in human breast and ovarian cancer. Science 1989; 244: 707–12.
6. Allred DC, O'Connell P, Fuqua SAW, Kent Osborne C. Immunohistochemical studies of early breast cancer evolution. Breast Cancer Res Treat 1994; 32: 13–8.
7. Ignatoski KM, Lapointe AJ, Radany EH, Ethier SP. erbB2 overexpression in human mammary epithelial cells confers growth factor independence. Endocrinology 1999; 140: 3615–22.
8. Bargmann CI, Hung MC, Weinberg RA. The neu oncogene encodes an epidermal growth factor receptor-related protein. Nature 1986; 319: 226–30.
9. Kraus MH, Issing W, Miki T, Popescu NC, Aaronson SA. Isolation and characterization of ERBB3, a third member of the ERBB/epidermal growth factor receptor family: evidence for overexpression in a subset of human mammary tumors. Proc Natl Acad Sci U S A 1989; 86: 9193–7.
10. Plowman GD, Culouscou JM, Whitney GS, et al. Ligand-specific activation of HER4/p180erbB4, a fourth member of the epidermal growth factor receptor family. Proc Natl Acad Sci U S A 1993; 90: 1746–50.
11. Feldner JC, Brandt BH. Cancer cell motility – on the road from c-erbB2 receptor steered signaling to actin reorganization. Exp Cell Res 2002; 272: 93–108.

12. Krupp MN, Connolly DT, Lane MD. Synthesis, turnover, and down-regulation of epidermal growth factor receptors in human A431 epidermoid carcinoma cells and skin fibroblasts. J Biol Chem 1982; 257: 11489–96.

13. Carpenter G. Employment of the epidermal growth factor receptor in growth factor-independent signaling pathways. J Cell Biol 1999; 146: 697–702.

14. Alroy I, Yarden Y. The ErbB signaling network in embryogenesis and oncogenesis: signal diversification through combinatorial ligand-receptor interactions. FEBS Lett 1997;410: 83–6.

15. Alroy I, Yarden Y. The ErbB signaling network in embryogenesis and oncogenesis: signal diversification through combinatorial ligand-receptor interactions. FEBS Lett 1997; 410: 83–6.

16. Alroy I, Yarden Y. The ErbB signaling network in embryogenesis and oncogenesis: signal diversification through combinatorial ligand-receptor interactions. FEBS Lett 1997;410: 83–6.

17. Graus-Porta D, Beerli RR, Daly JM, Hynes NE. erbB2, the preferred heterodimerization partner of all ErbB receptors, is a mediator of lateral signaling. EMBO J 1997; 16: 1647–55.

18. Lenferink AE, Pinkas-Kramarski R, van de Poll ML, et al. Differential endocytic routing of homo- and hetero-dimeric ErbB tyrosine kinases confers signaling superiority to receptor heterodimers. EMBO J 1998; 17: 3385–97.

19. Klapper LN, Glathe S, Vaisman N, et al. The erbB2/HER2 oncoprotein of human carcinomas may function solely as a shared coreceptor for multiple stroma-derived growth factors. Proc Natl Acad Sci U S A 1999; 96: 4995–5000.

20. Feldner JC, Brandt BH. Cancer cell motility – on the road from c-erbB2 receptor steered signaling to actin reorganization. Exp Cell Res 2002; 272: 93–108.

21. Brandt BH, Roetger A, Dittmar T, et al. c-erbB2/EGFR as dominant heterodimerization partners determine a motogenic phenotype in human breast cancer cells. FASEB J 1999; 13: 1939–49.

22. Fisher B. Biological and clinical considerations regarding the use of surgery and chemotherapy in the treatment of primary breast cancer. Cancer 1977; 40: 574–87.

23. Klijn JG, Look MP, Portengen H, et al. The prognostic value of epidermal growth factor receptor (EGF-R) in primary breast cancer: results of a 10 year follow-up study. Breast Cancer Res Treat 1994; 29: 73–83.

24. Gasparini G, Boracchi P, Bevilacqua P, et al. A multi-parametric study on the prognostic value of epidermal growth factor receptor in operable breast carcinoma. Breast Cancer Res Treat 1994; 29: 59–71.

25. Sainsbury JR, Farndon JR, Needham GK, Malcolm AJ, Harris AL. Epidermal-growth-factor receptor status as predictor of early recurrence of and death from breast cancer. Lancet 1987; 1: 1398–402.

26. van de Vijver MJ, Peterse JL, Mooi WJ, et al. Neu-protein overexpression in breast cancer. Association with comedo-type ductal carcinoma in-situ and limited prognostic value in stage II breast cancer. N Engl J Med 1988; 319: 1239–45.

27. Slamon DJ, Clark GM, Wong SG, et al. Human breast cancer: correlation of relapse and survival with amplification of the HER-2/neu oncogene. Science 1987; 235: 177–82.

28. Ravdin PM, Chamness GC. The c-erbB2 proto-oncogene as a prognostic and predictive marker in breast cancer: a paradigm for the development of other macromolecular markers – a review. Gene 1995; 159: 19–27.

29. Gusterson BA, Gelber RD, Goldhirsch A, et al. Prognostic importance of c-erbB2 expression in breast cancer. International (Ludwig) Breast Cancer Study Group. J Clin Oncol 1992;10: 1049–56.

30. Muss HB, Thor AD, Berry DA, et al. c-erbB2 expression and response to adjuvant therapy in women with node-positive early breast cancer. N Engl J Med 1994; 330: 1260–6.

31. Brandt B, Vogt U, Schlotter CM, et al. Prognostic relevance of aberrations in the erbB oncogenes from breast, ovarian, oral and lung cancers: double-differential poly-merase chain reaction (ddPCR) for clinical diagnosis. Gene 1995; 159: 35–42.

32. Press MF, Bernstein L, Thomas PA, et al. HER-2/neu gene amplification characterized by fluorescence in-situ hybridization: poor prognosis in node-negative breast carcinomas. J Clin Oncol 1997; 15: 2894–904.

33. Brandt B, Roetger A, Heidl S, et al. Isolation of blood-borne epithelium-derived c-erbB2 oncoprotein-positive clustered cells from the peripheral blood of breast cancer patients. Int J Cancer 1998; 76: 824–8.

34. Holzman D. HER-2/neu gene bumped into the limelight. J Natl Cancer Inst 1996; 88: 147–8.

35. Baselga J. Clinical trials of Herceptin(trastuzumab). Eur J Cancer 2001; 37 Suppl 1: S18 – S24.

36. Niehans GA, Singleton TP, Dykoski D, Kiang DT. Stability of HER-2/neu expression over time and at multiple metastatic sites. J Natl Cancer Inst 1993; 85: 1230–5.

37. Baselga J. Clinical trials of Herceptin(trastuzumab). Eur J Cancer 2001; 37 Suppl 1: S18 – S24.

38. Bange J, Zwick E, Ullrich A. Molecular targets for breast cancer therapy and prevention. Nat Med 2001; 7: 548–52.

39. Baselga J. New therapeutic agents targeting the epidermal growth factor receptor. J Clin Oncol 2000; 18: 54S – 9S.

40. Hortobagyi GN. Developments in chemotherapy of breast cancer. Cancer 2000; 88: 3073–9.

41. Dancey JE, Freidlin B. Targeting epidermal growth factor receptor—are we missing the mark? Lancet 2003; 362: 62–4.

42. Yu D, Hamada J, Zhang H, Nicolson GL, Hung MC. Mechanisms of c-erbB2/neu oncogene-induced metas-tasis and repression of metastatic properties by adenovirus 5 E1A gene products. Oncogene 1992; 7: 2263–70.

43. Hung MC, Lau YK. Basic science of HER-2/neu: a review. Semin Oncol 1999; 26: 51–9.

44. Noonberg SB, Benz CC. Tyrosine kinase inhibitors targeted to the epidermal growth factor receptor subfamily: role as anticancer agents. Drugs 2000; 59: 753–67.

45. Harbeck N, Ross JS, Yurdseven S, et al. HER-2/neu gene amplification by fluorescence in-situ hybridization allows risk-group assessment in node-negative breast cancer. Int J Oncol 1999; 14: 663–71.

46. Roche PC, Ingle JN. Increased HER2 with U.S. Food and Drug Administration-approved antibody. J Clin Oncol 1999; 17: 434.

47. Maia DM. Immunohistochemical assays for HER2 overexpression. J Clin Oncol 1999; 17: 1650.

48. Bankfalvi A, Simon R, Brandt B, et al. Comparative methodological analysis of erbB2/HER-2 gene dosage, chromosomal copy number and protein overexpression in breast carcinoma tissues for diagnostic use. Histopathol 2000; 37: 411–9.

49. Bankfalvi A, Simon R, Brandt B, et al. Comparative methodological analysis of erbB2/HER-2 gene dosage, chromosomal copy number and protein overexpression in breast carcinoma tissues for diagnostic use. Histopathol 2000; 37: 411–9.

50. Dancey JE, Freidlin B. Targeting epidermal growth factor receptor – are we missing the mark? Lancet 2003; 362: 62–4.

51. Tidow N, Boecker A, Schmidt H, et al. Distinct amplification of an untranslated regulatory sequence in the EGFR gene contributes to early steps in breast cancer development. Cancer Res 2003; 63: 1172–8.

52. Stark GR, Wahl GM. Gene amplification. Annu Rev Biochem 1984; 53: 447–91.

53. Brandt B, Vogt U, Schlotter CM, et al. Prognostic relevance of aberrations in the erbB oncogenes from breast, ovarian, oral and lung cancers: double-differential polymerase chain reaction (ddPCR) for clinical diagnosis. Gene 1995; 159: 35–42.

54. Ro J, North SM, Gallick GE, et al. Amplified and overexpressed epidermal growth factor receptor gene in uncultured primary human breast carcinoma. Cancer Res 1988; 48: 161–4.

55. Brandt B, Vogt U, Schlotter CM, et al. Prognostic relevance of aberrations in the erbB oncogenes from breast, ovarian, oral and lung cancers: double-differential polymerase chain reaction (ddPCR) for clinical diagnosis. Gene 1995; 159: 35–42.

56. Berns EM, Klijn JG, van Putten WL, et al. c-myc amplification is a better prognostic factor than HER2/neu amplification in primary breast cancer. Cancer Res 1992; 52: 1107–13.

57. Brandt B, Vogt U, Schlotter CM, et al. Prognostic relevance of aberrations in the erbB oncogenes from breast, ovarian, oral and lung cancers: double-differential polymerase chain reaction (ddPCR) for clinical diagnosis. Gene 1995; 159: 35–42.

58. Brandt B, Vogt U, Schlotter CM, et al. Prognostic relevance of aberrations in the erbB oncogenes from breast, ovarian, oral and lung cancers: double-differential polymerase chain reaction (ddPCR) for clinical diagnosis. Gene 1995; 159: 35–42.

59. Brandt B, Vogt U, Schlotter CM, et al. Prognostic relevance of aberrations in the erbB oncogenes from breast, ovarian, oral and lung cancers: double-differential polymerase chain reaction (ddPCR) for clinical diagnosis. Gene 1995; 159: 35–42.

60. Brandt BH, Beckmann A, Gebhardt F, et al. Translational research studies of erbB oncogenes: selection strategies for breast cancer treatment. Cancer Lett 1997; 118: 143–51.

61. Brandt BH, Beckmann A, Gebhardt F, et al. Translational research studies of erbB oncogenes: selection strategies for breast cancer treatment. Cancer Lett 1997; 118: 143–51.

62. Ullrich A, Coussens L, Hayflick JS, et al. Human epidermal growth factor receptor cDNA sequence and aberrant expression of the amplified gene in A431 epidermoid carcinoma cells. Nature 1984; 309: 418–25.

63. Reiter JL, Threadgill DW, Eley GD, et al. Comparative genomic sequence analysis and isolation of human and mouse alternative EGFR transcripts encoding truncated receptor isoforms. Genomics 2001; 71: 1–20.

64. Simmen FA, Schulz TZ, Headon DR, et al. Translation in Xenopus oocytes of messenger RNA from A431 cells for human epidermal growth factor receptor proteins. DNA 1984; 3: 393–9.

65. Ilekis JV, Stark BC, Scoccia B. Possible role of variant RNA transcripts in the regulation of epidermal growth factor receptor expression in human placenta. Mol Reprod Dev 1995; 41: 149–56.

66. Clark AJ, Ishii S, Richert N, Merlino GT, Pastan I. Epidermal growth factor regulates the expression of its own receptor. Proc Natl Acad Sci U S A 1985; 82: 8374–8.

67. Deb SP, Munoz RM, Brown DR, Subler MA, Deb S. Wild-type human p53 activates the human epidermal growth factor receptor promoter. Oncogene 1994; 9: 1341–9.

68. Xu YH, Richert N, Ito S, Merlino GT, Pastan I. Characterization of epidermal growth factor receptor gene expression in malignant and normal human cell lines. Proc Natl Acad Sci U S A 1984; 81: 7308–12.

69. Ishii S, Xu YH, Stratton RH, et al. Characterization and sequence of the promoter region of the human epidermal growth factor receptor gene. Proc Natl Acad Sci U S A 1985; 82: 4920–4.

70. Maekawa T, Imamoto F, Merlino GT, Pastan I, Ishii S. Cooperative function of two separate enhancers of the human epidermal growth factor receptor proto-oncogene. J Biol Chem 1989; 264: 5488–94.

71. Gebhardt F, Zanker KS, Brandt B. Modulation of epidermal growth factor receptor gene transcription by a polymorphic dinucleotide repeat in intron 1. J Biol Chem 1999; 274: 13176–80.

72. Chi DD, Hing AV, Helms C, et al. Two chromosome 7 dinucleotide repeat polymorphisms at gene loci epidermal growth factor receptor (EGFR) and pro alpha 2 (I) collagen (COL1A2). Hum Mol Genet 1992; 1: 135.

73. Tidow N, Boecker A, Schmidt H, et al. Distinct amplification of an untranslated regulatory sequence in the EGFR gene contributes to early steps in breast cancer development. Cancer Res 2003; 63: 1172–8.

74. Gebhardt F, Zanker KS, Brandt B. Modulation of epidermal growth factor receptor gene transcription by a polymorphic dinucleotide repeat in intron 1. J Biol Chem 1999; 274: 13176–80.

75. Buerger H, Gebhardt F, Schmidt H, et al. Length and loss of heterozygosity of an intron 1 polymorphic sequence of EGFR is related to cytogenetic alterations and epithelial growth factor receptor expression. Cancer Res 2000; 60: 854–7.

76. Buerger H, Gebhardt F, Schmidt H, et al. Length and loss of heterozygosity of an intron 1 polymorphic sequence of EGFR is related to cytogenetic alterations and epithelial growth factor receptor expression. Cancer Res 2000; 60: 854–7.

77. Tidow N, Boecker A, Schmidt H, et al. Distinct amplification of an untranslated regulatory sequence in the EGFR gene contributes to early steps in breast cancer development. Cancer Res 2003; 63: 1172–8.

78. Tidow N, Boecker A, Schmidt H, et al. Distinct amplification of an untranslated regulatory sequence in the EGFR gene contributes to early steps in breast cancer development. Cancer Res 2003; 63: 1172–8.

79. Chen Y, Fischer WH, Gill GN. Regulation of the erbB2 promoter by RBPJkappa and NOTCH. J Biol Chem 1997; 272: 14110–4.

80. Bates NP, Hurst HC. An intron 1 enhancer element mediates oestrogen-induced suppression of ERBB2 expression. Oncogene 1997; 15: 473–81.

81. Chang CH, Scott GK, Kuo WL, et al. ESX: a structurally unique Ets overexpressed early during human breast tumorigenesis. Oncogene 1997; 14: 1617–22.

82. Taverna D, Antoniotti S, Maggiora P, et al. erbB2 expression in estrogen-receptor-positive breast-tumor cells is regulated by growth-modulatory reagents. Int J Cancer 1994; 56: 522–8.

83. Scott GK, Robles R, Park JW, et al. A truncated intracellular HER2/neu receptor produced by alternative RNA processing affects growth of human carcinoma cells. Mol Cell Biol 1993; 13: 2247–57.

84. Scott GK, Robles R, Park JW, et al. A truncated intracellular HER2/neu receptor produced by alternative RNA processing affects growth of human carcinoma cells. Mol Cell Biol 1993; 13: 2247–57.

85. Scott GK, Robles R, Park JW, et al. A truncated intracellular HER2/neu receptor produced by alternative RNA processing affects growth of human carcinoma cells. Mol Cell Biol 1993; 13: 2247–57.

86. Gebhardt F, Zanker KS, Brandt B. Modulation of epidermal growth factor receptor gene transcription by a polymorphic dinucleotide repeat in intron 1. J Biol Chem 1999; 274: 13176–80.

87. Park JW, Gebhardt F, Damon LE, Wolf J, Benz CC. Detection of breast cancer micrometastasis in bone marrow and peripheral blood stem cell collections. Proc Amer Soc Clin Oncology 1999; 37.

88. Gebhardt F, Zanker KS, Brandt B. Differential expression of alternatively spliced c-erbB2 mRNA in primary tumors, lymph node metastases, and bone marrow micrometastases from breast cancer patients. Biochem Biophys Res Commun 1998; 247: 319–23.

89. Gebhardt F, Zanker KS, Brandt B. Differential expression of alternatively spliced c-erbB2 mRNA in primary tumors, lymph node metastases, and bone marrow micrometastases from breast cancer patients. Biochem Biophys Res Commun 1998; 247: 319–23.

90. Hanahan D, Weinberg RA. The hallmarks of cancer. Cell 2000; 100: 57–70.

91. Muhlhauser J, Crescimanno C, Kaufmann P, et al. Differentiation and proliferation patterns in human trophoblast revealed by c-erbB2 oncogene product and EGF-R. J Histochem Cytochem 1993; 41: 165–73.

92. Burden S, Yarden Y. Neuregulins and their receptors: a versatile signaling module in organogenesis and oncogenesis. Neuron 1997; 18: 847–55.

93. Krane IM, Leder P. NDF/heregulin induces persistence of terminal end buds and adenocarcinomas in the mammary glands of transgenic mice. Oncogene 1996; 12: 1781–8.

94. Sebastian J, Richards RG, Walker MP, et al. Activation and function of the epidermal growth factor receptor and erbB2 during mammary gland morphogenesis. Cell Growth Differ 1998;9: 777–85.

95. Di Marco E, Pierce JH, Knicley CL, Di Fiore PP. Transformation of NIH 3T3 cells by overexpression of the normal coding sequence of the rat neu gene. Mol Cell Biol 1990; 10: 3247–52.

96. Hung MC, Lau YK. Basic science of HER-2/neu: a review. Semin Oncol 1999; 26: 51–9.

97. Yu D, Jing T, Liu B, et al. Overexpression of ErbB2 blocks Taxol-induced apoptosis by upregulation of p21Cip1, which inhibits p34Cdc2 kinase. Mol Cell 1998; 2: 581–91.

98. Carraway CA, Carvajal ME, Carraway KL. Association of the Ras to mitogen-activated protein kinase signal transduction pathway with microfilaments. Evidence for a p185(neu)-containing cell surface signal transduction particle linking the mitogenic pathway to a membrane-microfilament association site. J Biol Chem 1999; 274: 25659–67.

99. Roetger A, Merschjann A, Dittmar T, et al. Selection of potentially metastatic subpopulations expressing c-erbB2 from breast cancer tissue by use of an extravasation model. Am J Pathol 1998; 153: 1797–806.

100. Brandt BH, Roetger A, Dittmar T, et al. c-erbB2/EGFR as dominant heterodimerization partners determine a motogenic phenotype in human breast cancer cells. FASEB J 1999; 13: 1939–49.

101. Dittmar T, Husemann A, Schewe Y, et al. Induction of cancer cell migration by epidermal growth factor is initiated by specific phosphorylation of tyrosine 1248 of c-erbB2 receptor via EGFR. FASEB J 2002; 16: 1823–5.

102. Feldner JC, Brandt BH. Cancer cell motility – on the road from c-erbB2 receptor steered signaling to actin reorganization. Exp Cell Res 2002; 272: 93–108.

103. Lenferink AE, Pinkas-Kramarski R, van de Poll ML, et al. Differential endocytic routing of homo- and hetero-dimeric ErbB tyrosine kinases confers signaling superiority to receptor heterodimers. EMBO J 1998; 17: 3385–97.

104. Chen P, Xie H, Sekar MC, Gupta K, Wells A. Epidermal growth factor receptor-mediated cell motility: phospholipase C activity is required, but mitogen-activated protein kinase activity is not sufficient for induced cell movement. J Cell Biol 1994; 127: 847–57.

105. Chen P, Murphy-Ullrich JE, Wells A. A role for gelsolin in actuating epidermal growth factor receptor-mediated cell motility. J Cell Biol 1996; 134: 689–98.

106. Schewe Y, Dittmar T, Brandt BH, Zanker KS. The phospholipase Cy (PLCy) plays a key role in the migration of her-2/neu positive breast cancer cells. Proc Amer Assoc Cancer Res 2001; 42: 921.

107. Dittmar T, Husemann A, Schewe Y, et al. Induction of cancer cell migration by epidermal growth factor is initiated by specific phosphorylation of tyrosine 1248 of c-erbB2 receptor via EGFR. FASEB J 2002; 16: 1823–5.

108. Brandt BH, Roetger A, Dittmar T, et al. c-erbB2/EGFR as dominant heterodimerization partners determine a motogenic phenotype in human breast cancer cells. FASEB J 1999; 13: 1939–49.

INDEX